Cesarean Delivery

Cesarean Delivery
A Comprehensive Illustrated Practical Guide

Edited by

Gian Carlo Di Renzo, MD, PhD
Founder and Director of the Permanent International and European
School in Perinatal, Neonatal and Reproductive Medicine (PREIS)
and Professor and Chairman, Department of Obstetrics and Gynecology
and Director, Centre for Perinatal and Reproductive Medicine
Santa Maria della Misericordia University Hospital
Perugia, Italy

Antonio Malvasi, MD
Professor, Department of Obstetrics and Gynecology
Santa Maria Hospital
GVM Care & Research
Bari, Italy
and Adjunct Professor, International Translational Medicine
and Biomodelling Research Group
Department of Applied Mathematics
Moscow Institute of Physics and Technology (State University)
Moscow Region, Russia

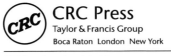

CRC Press
Taylor & Francis Group
Boca Raton London New York

CRC Press is an imprint of the
Taylor & Francis Group, an **informa** business

CRC Press
Taylor & Francis Group
6000 Broken Sound Parkway NW, Suite 300
Boca Raton, FL 33487-2742

© 2017 by Taylor & Francis Group, LLC
CRC Press is an imprint of Taylor & Francis Group, an Informa business

No claim to original U.S. Government works

Printed on acid-free paper
Version Date: 20160912

International Standard Book Number-13: 978-1-4822-2633-1 (Hardback)

This book contains information obtained from authentic and highly regarded sources. While all reasonable efforts have been made to publish reliable data and information, neither the author[s] nor the publisher can accept any legal responsibility or liability for any errors or omissions that may be made. The publishers wish to make clear that any views or opinions expressed in this book by individual editors, authors or contributors are personal to them and do not necessarily reflect the views/opinions of the publishers. The information or guidance contained in this book is intended for use by medical, scientific or health-care professionals and is provided strictly as a supplement to the medical or other professional's own judgement, their knowledge of the patient's medical history, relevant manufacturer's instructions and the appropriate best practice guidelines. Because of the rapid advances in medical science, any information or advice on dosages, procedures or diagnoses should be independently verified. The reader is strongly urged to consult the relevant national drug formulary and the drug companies' and device or material manufacturers' printed instructions, and their websites, before administering or utilizing any of the drugs, devices or materials mentioned in this book. This book does not indicate whether a particular treatment is appropriate or suitable for a particular individual. Ultimately it is the sole responsibility of the medical professional to make his or her own professional judgements, so as to advise and treat patients appropriately. The authors and publishers have also attempted to trace the copyright holders of all material reproduced in this publication and apologize to copyright holders if permission to publish in this form has not been obtained. If any copyright material has not been acknowledged please write and let us know so we may rectify in any future reprint.

Except as permitted under U.S. Copyright Law, no part of this book may be reprinted, reproduced, transmitted, or utilized in any form by any electronic, mechanical, or other means, now known or hereafter invented, including photocopying, microfilming, and recording, or in any information storage or retrieval system, without written permission from the publishers.

For permission to photocopy or use material electronically from this work, please access www.copyright.com (http://www.copyright.com/) or contact the Copyright Clearance Center, Inc. (CCC), 222 Rosewood Drive, Danvers, MA 01923, 978-750-8400. CCC is a not-for-profit organization that provides licenses and registration for a variety of users. For organizations that have been granted a photocopy license by the CCC, a separate system of payment has been arranged.

Trademark Notice: Product or corporate names may be trademarks or registered trademarks, and are used only for identification and explanation without intent to infringe.

Visit the Taylor & Francis Web site at
http://www.taylorandfrancis.com

and the CRC Press Web site at
http://www.crcpress.com

Printed and bound in the United States of America by Publishers Graphics, LLC on sustainably sourced paper.

We express our sincere thanks to our professional teachers, many of whom watching us from Heaven, because they taught us the art of medicine, surgery and clinical practice, constantly pushing us to further scientific research. And, even more, we thank God for giving us the ability to illustrate the moments of clinical and surgical professional life from forty years of practice with our patients.

Gian Carlo Di Renzo
Antonio Malvasi

Acknowledgments

We are particularly thankful to our friend Prof. Michael Stark who has developed the concept of minimal surgery for cesarean delivery, making the procedure safer than before. He has also inspired us to produce this book through the continuing interaction within NESA (New European Surgery Academy), of which he is the Founder and President.

The editors are also grateful to Antonio Dell'Aquila, who teamed up with them in creating the marvelous illustrations for this book.

Gian Carlo Di Renzo
Antonio Malvasi

Contents

Contributors ix

1 Epidemiologic trends internationally: Maternal and perinatal morbidity and mortality 1
Ana Pilar Betrán and Mario Merialdi

2 Laparotomies and cesarean delivery 11
Gian Carlo Di Renzo, Shilpa Nambiar Balakrishnan, and Antonio Malvasi

3 Hysterotomies during cesarean delivery 39
Antonio Malvasi, Shilpa Nambiar Balakrishnan, and Gian Carlo Di Renzo

4 Fetal extraction during cesarean delivery 57
Gian Carlo Di Renzo, Antonio Malvasi, and Andrea Tinelli
    Cephalic extraction 57
    Breech presentation 76
    Fetal extraction with instruments 98
    Anomalous presentation 112

5 Placental removal and uterine exteriorization techniques 123
Antonio Malvasi and Gian Carlo Di Renzo

6 Suture of uterine incisions 145
Antonio Malvasi and Gian Carlo Di Renzo

7 Optimal cesarean delivery of the twenty-first century 161
Michael Stark

8 Fibroids and myomectomy in cesarean delivery 173
Andrea Tinelli and Antonio Malvasi

9 Management of placenta previa and/or accreta 189
Graziano Clerici and Laura Di Fabrizio

10 The proactive use of balloons for management of postpartum hemorrhage in cesarean delivery 199
Yakov Zhukovskiy

11 Exceptional situations after cesarean delivery and postpartum hemorrhage 207
José M Palacios-Jaraquemada

12 Dystocia and intrapartum ultrasound in cesarean delivery 215
Gian Carlo Di Renzo, Chiara Antonelli, Irene Giardina, and Antonio Malvasi

13 Dystocia and cesarean delivery: New perspectives in the management of labor and the prevention of cesarean delivery 225
Antonio Malvasi, Gian Carlo Di Renzo, and Eleonora Brillo

14 Shoulder dystocia and cesarean delivery 237
Enrico Ferrazzi

15 Multiple pregnancy and cesarean birth 257
Gian Carlo Di Renzo, Giulia Babucci, and Antonio Malvasi

16 Cesarean delivery for the preterm neonate 277
Gabriele D'Amato, Savino Mastropasqua, and Elena Pacella

17 The neonate from cesarean delivery 297
Ola Didrik Saugstad

18 General anesthesia for cesarean delivery: Indications and complications 307
Krzysztof Kuczkowski, Yayoi Ohashi, and Tiberiu Ezri

19 Local anesthesia for cesarean delivery: Epidural, spinal, and combined spinal–epidural anesthesia 323
Krzysztof Kuczkowski, Toshiyuki Okutomi, and Rie Kato

20 Characteristics of the postcesarean delivery uterine scar 341
Antonio Malvasi and Gian Carlo Di Renzo

21 Vaginal birth after cesarean delivery 355
Antonio Malvasi, Gian Carlo Di Renzo, and Laura Di Fabrizio

22 Forensic aspects of cesarean delivery 365
Antonio Malvasi and Gian Carlo Di Renzo

Index 393

Contributors

Chiara Antonelli
Department of Obstetrics and Gynecology
Centre for Perinatal and Reproductive Medicine
Santa Maria della Misericordia University Hospital
University of Perugia
Perugia, Italy

Giulia Babucci
Department of Obstetrics and Gynecology
Centre for Perinatal and Reproductive Medicine
Santa Maria della Misericordia University Hospital
University of Perugia
Perugia, Italy

Shilpa Nambiar Balakrishnan
Consultant Obstetrician and Gynaecologist
Prince Court Medical Centre
Kuala Lumpur, Malaysia

Ana Pilar Betrán
Department of Reproductive Health
and Research
World Health Organization
Geneva, Switzerland

Eleonora Brillo
Department of Obstetrics and Gynecology
Centre for Perinatal and Reproductive Medicine
Santa Maria della Misericordia University Hospital
University of Perugia
Perugia, Italy

Graziano Clerici
Department of Obstetrics and Gynecology
Santa Maria della Misericordia University Hospital
Perugia, Italy

Gabriele D'Amato
Neonatal Intensive Care Unit, UTIN
Di Venere Hospital
Bari, Italy

Laura Di Fabrizio
Department of Obstetrics and Gynecology
Centre for Perinatal and Reproductive Medicine
Santa Maria della Misericordia University Hospital
Perugia, Italy

Gian Carlo Di Renzo
Department of Obstetrics and Gynecology
Centre for Perinatal and Reproductive Medicine
Santa Maria della Misericordia University Hospital
Perugia, Italy

Tiberiu Ezri
Department of Anesthesia
Tel Aviv University
Halochamim, Israel

Enrico Ferrazzi
Department of Woman, Mother and Neonate
Buzzi Children's Hospital
University of Milan
Milan, Italy

Irene Giardina
Department of Obstetrics and Gynecology
Centre for Perinatal and Reproductive Medicine
Santa Maria della Misericordia University Hospital
Perugia, Italy

Rie Kato
Division of Anesthesiology and Reanimatology for Paturients/Fetuses/Infants
Research and Development Center for New Medical Frontiers
Kitasato University School of Medicine
and
Division of Obstetric Anesthesia
Center for Perinatal Medicine
Kitasato University Hospital
Kitasato, Japan

Krzysztof Kuczkowski
Texas Tech University Health Sciences Center
Paul L. Foster School of Medicine
El Paso, Texas

Antonio Malvasi
Department of Obstetrics and Gynecology
Santa Maria Hospital
GVM Care & Research
Bari, Italy

and

International Translational Medicine and Biomodelling
Research Group
Department of Applied Mathematics
Moscow Institute of Physics and Technology
(State University)
Moscow, Russia

Savino Mastropasqua
Paediatrics and Neonatology Unit, UTIN
La Madonnina Clinical Hospital
Bari, Italy

Mario Merialdi
Maternal and Newborn Health
Global Health BD
Franklin Lakes, New Jersey

Yayoi Ohashi
Department of Anaesthesia and Pain Medicine
Royal Perth Hospital
Perth, Australia

Toshiyuki Okutomi
Division of Obstetric Anesthesia
Center for Perinatal Care
Child Health and Development
Kitasato University Hospital
Kitasato, Japan

Elena Pacella
Department of Sense Organs
Sapienza University of Rome
Rome, Italy

José M Palacios-Jaraquemada
Department of Gynaecology and Obstetrics
CEMIC University Hospital
University of Buenos Aires
Buenos Aires, Argentina

Ola Didrik Saugstad
Department of Pediatric Research
Oslo University Hospital
University of Oslo
Oslo, Norway

Michael Stark
The New European Surgical Academy
The ENSAN Hospitals Group
Berlin, Germany

Andrea Tinelli
Department of Obstetrics and Gynaecology
Vito Fazzi Hospital
Lecce, Italy

and

Department of Applied Mathematics
Moscow Institute of Physics and Technology
State University
Moscow, Russia

Yakov Zhukovskiy
Gynamed Ltd.
Moscow, Russia

Epidemiologic trends internationally
Maternal and perinatal morbidity and mortality

ANA PILAR BETRÁN and MARIO MERIALDI

INTRODUCTION

A cesarean delivery can be a life-saving surgical procedure for both mother and baby when complications arise during pregnancy or delivery. The unprecedented, dramatic, and medically unjustified increase in its use over recent decades has transformed this surgery into one of the most controversial topics in modern obstetric practice [1,2].

In 1985, a panel of experts was set up to review and issue recommendations for the appropriate technology for birth at a meeting organized by the World Health Organization (WHO) in Fortaleza, Brazil [3]. These experts concluded that "there is no justification for any region to have a cesarean delivery rate higher than 10%–15%." This reference was based on the scarce evidence available then and the fact that some of the countries with the lowest perinatal mortality rates had, at that time, cesareans section rates lower than 10%. Despite this recommendation and the lack of evidence that increased rates improve maternal and perinatal outcomes, and some studies showing that higher rates could be linked to negative maternal and perinatal outcome [4–6], cesarean delivery rates continue to rise, particularly in high- and middle-income countries, with no sign of curbing the trend [7–10]. Additional concerns and controversies around this include inequities observed in the use of the procedure, not only between countries but also within countries [11–13], the cost that unnecessary cesarean deliveries impose on financially deficient health systems [10], and the multifactorial web of factors underlying this phenomenon, which is not fully understood.

In 2009, WHO published a handbook for monitoring emergency obstetric care [14]. For the first time since 1985, it was acknowledged that "although WHO has recommended since 1985 that the rate of caesarean deliveries not exceed 10%–15% there is no empirical evidence for an optimum percentage or range of percentages, despite the growing body of research that shows a negative effect of high rates," and advised that "very low and very high rates of cesarean delivery can be dangerous. Pending further research, users of the handbook might want to continue to use a range of 5%–15% or set their own standards."

EPIDEMIOLOGICAL DATA AND TRENDS WORLDWIDE

The first accounts of the increase of cesarean delivery rates date back to 1976, with the compilation of data from the 1940s to the 1970s in hospitals in the United States [15,16]. In the early 1980s, Placek and colleagues reported a national rise in cesareans in the United States, from 4.5% in 1965 to 10.4% in 1975 and 16.5% in 1980 [17], showing that this increase was not restricted to particular hospitals. A number of later studies presented and compared cesarean delivery rates in a small number of industrialized countries where data were available, along with their indications, starting in the 1980s [18,19]. One of the first global attempts to systematically compile national-level estimates of cesarean delivery worldwide was published in 2007 to map practices on the mode of delivery, and reported data for 126 countries, which represented nearly 90% of all live births globally [7].

Table 1.1, from that 2007 study, shows the global, regional, and subregional cesarean delivery rates according to WHO geographical regional divisions at that time. Globally, 15% of the deliveries were by cesarean delivery at the time of these estimates. At national level, rates were highest in Latin and North America, where almost 30% and 25% of the deliveries were by cesarean, respectively. The lowest rates were in Africa, where the proportion of cesarean deliveries was 3.5%. These averages, however, mask wide variations between subregions and countries. For instance, the rate of cesarean delivery in Southern Africa (14.5%) contrasts sharply with the rates seen in Middle, Western, and Eastern Africa (1.8%, 1.9%, and 2.3%, respectively). Likewise, the variation within Asia is striking. Although the average rate of cesarean deliveries in the region is 15.9%, very low rates in South-Central (5.8%) and South-Eastern Asia (6.8%) contrast sharply with the very high rate seen in Eastern Asia (40.5%) which is mainly driven by cesarean deliveries in China.

Latin America has classically been the region with the highest cesarean delivery rates in the world, with Brazil leading this rise, followed closely by Chile and Mexico. In 2010, over 50% of all Brazilians were delivered by cesarean delivery, a 20% increase in just 4 years since 2006 [20], and over 80% of all deliveries are by cesarean delivery in the private sector.

Figure 1.1a and b shows the cesarean delivery rates of the countries included in the 2007 analysis and which countries fall within the 10%–15% range. The design of the upper panel in log scale allows one to better visualize the countries in the lower spectrum of cesarean rates. Again, African countries are clearly pictured in this area; Chad, Ethiopia, Madagascar, and Niger present the lowest rates, all below 1%. It is worth mentioning that only two African countries present rates above 10%, namely, Egypt and South Africa. In contrast, Figure 1.1b (in natural scale) enhances the visualization of those countries with higher cesarean delivery use. Brazil, China, Italy, and

Table 1.1 Cesarean delivery rates by region and subregion and coverage of the estimates

Region/subregion[a]	Births by cesarean delivery (%)	Range, minimum to maximum (%)	Coverage of estimates[b] (%)
World total	15.0	0.4–40.5	89 (74)[c]
More developed regions	21.1	6.2–36.0	90
Less-developed countries	14.3	0.4–40.5	89 (72)[c]
Least-developed countries	2.0	0.4–6.0	74
Africa	**3.5**	**0.4–15.4**	**83**
Eastern Africa	2.3	0.6–7.4	93
Middle Africa	1.8	0.4–6.0	26
Northern Africa	7.6	3.5–11.4	84
Southern Africa	14.5	6.9–15.4	93
Western Africa	1.9	0.6–6.0	95
Asia	**15.9**	**1.0–40.5**	**89 (65)[c]**
Eastern Asia	40.5	27.4–40.5	90 (0.31)[c]
South-Central Asia	5.8	1.0–10.8	93
South-Eastern Asia	6.8	1.0–17.4	83
Western Asia	11.7	1.5–23.3	75
Europe	**19.0**	**6.2–36.0**	**99**
Eastern Europe	15.2	6.2–24.7	100
Northern Europe	20.1	14.9–23.3	100
Southern Europe	24.0	8.0–36.0	97
Western Europe	20.2	13.5–24.3	100
Latin America and the Caribbean	**29.2**	**1.7–39.1**	**92**
Caribbean	18.1	1.7–31.3	78
Central America	31.0	7.9–39.1	98
South America	29.3	12.9–36.7	90
Northern America	**24.3**	**22.5–24.4**	**100**
Oceania	**14.9**	**4.7–21.9**	**92**
Australia/New Zealand	21.6	20.4–21.9	100
Melanesia	4.9	4.7–7.1	87
Micronesia	na[d]	na	0
Polynesia	na	na	0

[a] Countries categorized according to the UN classification. Countries with a population of less than 140,000 in 2000 are not included.
[b] Refers to the proportion of live births for which nationally representative data were available.
[c] Figures within parentheses represent coverage excluding data from China.
[d] na = data not available.

Mexico all had cesarean rates higher than 35% at the time of that study.

Other estimates have been published by WHO in the 2014 World Health Statistics [21]. All regional estimates show an increase in the use of cesarean delivery except for Africa where the average rate is still 4%. In the Americas and Europe, present rates of cesarean deliveries are 36% and 24%, respectively.

CONSEQUENCES OF GLOBAL INEQUALITIES

One of the negative consequences of the unprecedented cesarean delivery rate increase is the diversion of human and financial resources from other equally, if not more, important health interventions [22]. Alternately, it is argued that the indiscriminate reduction of cesarean deliveries could have a negative effect on maternal and perinatal outcomes, and could be seen as a disrespect of women's autonomy and preferences [23].

As presented above, there is a wide variation in cesarean delivery use between and within countries [24–27]. This use follows the health-care inequity pattern of the world: underuse in low-income settings, and adequate or even unnecessary use in middle- and high-income settings [7,8,13,28]. In 2012, Gibbons et al. analyzed the resource-use implications of such inequality. The authors showed that 0.8–3.2 million additional cesarean deliveries are needed every year in low-income countries, where 60% of the world's births occur, and in middle- and

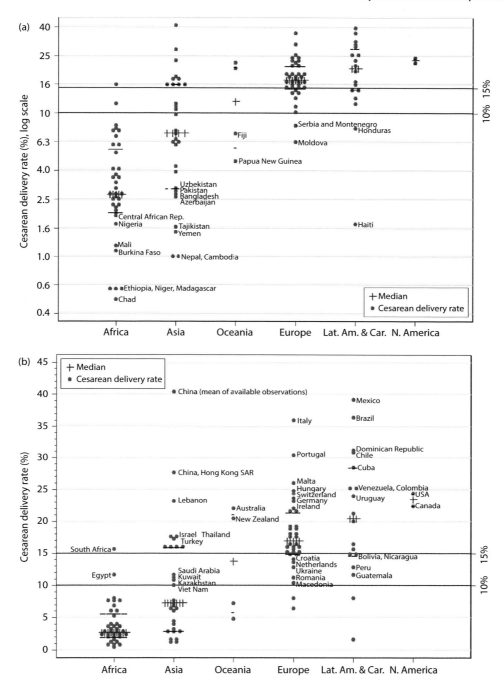

Figure 1.1 (a, b) Dot-plots of cesarean delivery rate by region, showing median and interquartile range; log scale (upper) and natural units (lower). Selected regional outliers identified with text labels.

high-income countries, where 37.5% of the births occur, there is a yearly excess of 4.0–6.2 million cesarean deliveries [11]. Based on these data, the reduction of cesarean delivery rates to 15% would lead to a $2.32 billon savings, while $432 million would be necessary to attain a 10% rate where needed. However, within countries, the extent to which the overuse of cesarean delivery among certain segments of the population affects the health-care system and the delivery of the intervention to those most in need is unknown [29].

CESAREAN DELIVERY AND MATERNAL AND PERINATAL OUTCOMES

Undoubtedly a cesarean delivery can resolve life-threatening situations for both the mother and the baby. However, in normal, uncomplicated deliveries, there is controversy about the harm that can potentially be inflicted with this surgery, as some studies have shown increased maternal mortality and morbidity [30]. The consequences of overusing cesarean delivery are unclear, and the question "what is the association between cesarean delivery and maternal and perinatal outcomes when the cesarean delivery may not be considered medically necessary?" is pending. The answer to this question is not a straightforward process for different reasons. It involves the consideration of multiple short- and long-term outcomes, for both mother and baby, some of which may be competing. Randomized controlled trials where pregnant women are randomly assigned to vaginal delivery or cesarean delivery have yet to be designed in an ethical, feasible, and useful manner. This has been a source of controversy and a reason for creativity for many years [31–33]. A survey involving all consultant obstetricians and heads of midwifery in the United Kingdom reported that only a minority would support a randomized trial of planned cesarean delivery compared with planned vaginal delivery [31]. In noninterventional studies, such as observational designs, comparing women by their eventual route of delivery is not appropriate. Although complications are more frequent in women who had a cesarean delivery compared with those who had a vaginal delivery, it is difficult to assess to what extent the cesarean delivery was the cause or the consequence of the negative outcome. Methodologically, it is a challenge to isolate the morbidity specifically caused by the route of delivery.

At the ecological level, several studies have been published presenting the association between cesarean delivery rates and maternal and newborn outcomes [7–9,34,35]. These types of study compare groups rather than individuals, and for this reason, the results are often difficult to interpret epidemiologically [36]. A valid conclusion at population level should not be taken as valid at the individual level, and associations at population level should not be extrapolated at the individual level to avoid the ecological fallacy. Cross-sectional comparisons of cesarean delivery rates versus maternal, infant, and neonatal mortality indicators at country level have been published using different statistical techniques. Overall, authors have found that in settings with high maternal and neonatal mortality rates, which usually also show low or very low use of cesarean delivery, there is an inverse and statistically significant association between the rate of cesarean delivery and mortality—that is, as cesarean delivery rates increase, mortality decreases. However, in countries with lower levels of maternal and newborn mortality, which tend to be the countries with higher cesarean delivery rates, this association is not found [8,35], and some authors have hypothesized a positive correlation showing that higher cesarean delivery rates are associated with higher maternal, newborn, and infant mortality [7]. One ecological study used nationally representative longitudinal data from 19 countries with low maternal mortality rates to explore what is the optimal rate for medically necessary cesarean deliveries [34]. Data from the last three decades for countries in Northern and Western Europe, North America, Australia, New Zealand, and Japan adjusted for human development index (HDI) and gross domestic product (GDP) confirmed the sharp increase in cesarean delivery rate in these countries and showed that once cesarean deliveries reach 10%–15%, further increases in this rate had no impact on maternal, neonatal, and infant mortality at population level. However, before reaching these levels, maternal, neonatal, and infant mortality decreased substantially as cesarean delivery rates increased. Besides the longitudinal nature of this study, a critical part of its design was that it only included countries with reliable statistics where women can receive a cesarean delivery whenever needed, thus reducing the confounding effect of socioeconomic and health system factors that are often at the root of the low cesarean delivery levels in high-mortality countries.

In search of constructive steps and keeping in mind all the aforementioned limitations, WHO designed the Global Survey on Maternal and Perinatal Health to assess the risks and benefits associated with cesarean delivery compared with vaginal delivery. This was a multicountry, facility-based cross-sectional study that took place in 2004–2005 in Africa and Latin America and in 2007–2008 in Asia. The WHO Global Survey included data for 290,610 births in 24 countries [37]. Individual-level analysis in the Latin American countries showed that cesarean delivery independently reduced the overall risk in breech presentations and risk of intrapartum fetal death in cephalic presentations, but increased the risk of severe maternal and neonatal morbidity and mortality in cephalic presentations [5]. Analysis at facility level showed that rates of cesarean delivery were positively associated with postpartum antibiotic treatment and severe maternal mortality and morbidity, fetal mortality rates, as well as higher number of babies admitted to the intensive care unit for 7 days or longer [6]. Figures 1.2 through 1.4 show the adjusted association between rate of cesarean delivery and maternal morbidity and mortality index and postnatal treatment with antibiotics (Figure 1.2), the adjusted association between rate of cesarean delivery and intrapartum death and neonatal mortality (Figure 1.3), and the adjusted association between rate of cesarean delivery and neonatal admission to intensive care for 7 days or more and preterm delivery (Figure 1.4). Although these analyses are not free of bias and limitations, the large sample size and the extensive statistical adjustment for many confounding factors and the consistent and strong trend reported support the validity of the results.

In the Asian Global Survey data (109,101 deliveries in 122 recruiting facilities in nine countries) all deliveries were carefully classified into spontaneous, operative vaginal delivery, antepartum cesarean delivery without indications, antepartum cesarean delivery with indications, intrapartum cesarean delivery without indications, and intrapartum cesarean delivery with indications [4]. Compared with vaginal delivery, the adjusted risk of maternal mortality and morbidity index (any of the following: maternal mortality, admission to intensive care unit, blood transfusion, hysterectomy, or internal iliac artery ligation) was increased for operative vaginal delivery (odds ratio [OR] 2.1, 95% confidence interval [CI] 1.7–2.6) and all types of cesarean delivery (antepartum without indication OR 2.7, CI 1.4–5.5; antepartum with indication

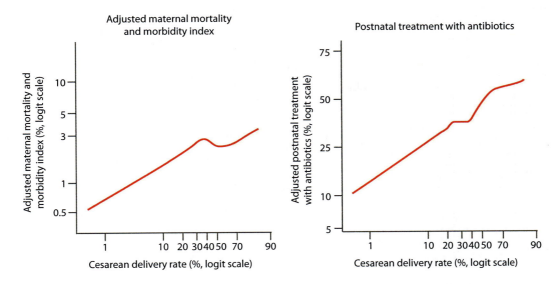

Figure 1.2 Association between rate of cesarean delivery and maternal morbidity and mortality index and postnatal treatment with antibiotics. Rates of outcomes adjusted by proportions of primiparous women, previous cesarean delivery, gestational hypertension or preeclampsia or eclampsia during current pregnancy, referral from other institution for pregnancy complications or delivery, breech or other noncephalic fetal presentation, and epidural during labor, along with complexity index for institution and type of institution in multiple linear regression analysis. Curves based on LOWESS smoothing applied to scatterplot of logit of rates of cesarean delivery versus logit of adjusted probability of each outcome.

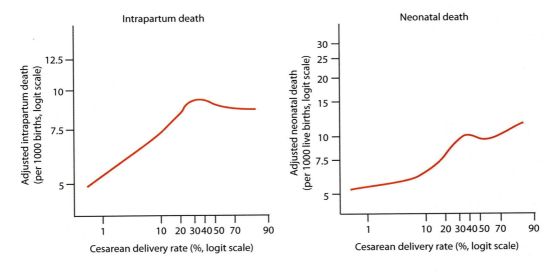

Figure 1.3 Association between rate of cesarean delivery and intrapartum death (per 1000 births) and neonatal mortality (per 1000 live births). Mortality rates adjusted by proportions of primiparous women, previous cesarean delivery, gestational hypertension or preeclampsia or eclampsia during current pregnancy, referral from other institution for pregnancy complications or delivery, breech or other noncephalic fetal presentation, and epidural during labor, along with complexity index for institution and type of institution in multiple linear regression analysis.

OR 10.6, CI 9.3–12.0; intrapartum without indication OR 14.2, CI 9.8–20.7; intrapartum with indication OR 14.5, CI 13.2–16.0). Based on these findings, the authors concluded that "to improve maternal and perinatal outcomes, cesarean delivery should be done only when there is a medical indication" [4, pp. 494–495].

Although the WHO Global Survey was conducted in middle- and low-income countries and was facility based, studies in high-income countries at population level offer similar results. In a population-based study in California in 2005–2007 with over 1.5 million live singleton births, compared with vaginal delivery, primary cesarean, repeat cesarean, and vaginal birth after cesarean (VBAC) had higher rates of severe morbidity [38]. However, in this same study, women delivered vaginally had higher rates of pelvic floor morbidity (defined as *International Classification of Diseases, Ninth Revision* (ICD-9) codes for episiotomy, third- and fourth-degree laceration, vulvar

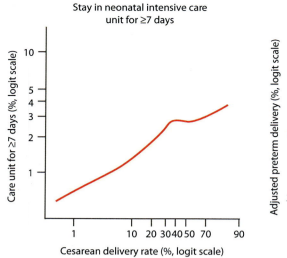
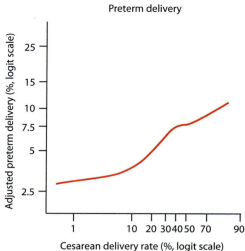

Figure 1.4 Association between rate of cesarean delivery and neonatal admission to intensive care for 7 days or more and preterm delivery. Rates of outcomes adjusted by proportions of primiparous women, previous cesarean delivery, gestational hypertension or preeclampsia or eclampsia during current pregnancy, referral from other institution for pregnancy complications or delivery, breech or other noncephalic fetal presentation, and epidural during labor, along with complexity index for institution and type of institution in multiple linear regression analysis.

or perianal hematoma, or other trauma or indication of third or fourth laceration on the birth certificate) than those delivered by cesarean.

A prospective nationwide population-based cohort study in the Netherlands attempted to evaluate the risk of severe acute maternal morbidity related to mode of delivery [39]. Severe acute maternal morbidity including intensive care unit admission, uterine rupture, eclampsia, and major obstetric hemorrhage was analyzed over a 2-year period (2004–2006) in more than 350,000 deliveries registered in the country. The investigators found a significantly higher risk of severe acute maternal morbidity in women who had an elective cesarean delivery compared to those who attempted a vaginal delivery (6.4 per 1000 versus 3.9 per 1000, respectively; OR 1.7, 95% CI 1.4–2.0).

Several studies have analyzed temporal trends in peripartum hysterectomy. In Italy, a 15-year study over 1.2 million women reported an increase over time from 0.57 to 0.88 per 1000 deliveries in 1996 and 2010, respectively [40]. Authors noted that women who underwent cesarean delivery had a fivefold increase in their risk of hysterectomy than those who had a vaginal delivery (OR 5.66, 95% CI 4.91–6.54). A similar large study in the United States between 1997 and 2005 concluded that mode of delivery as well as prior obstetric history are major risk factors for peripartum hysterectomy. Compared to women having a vaginal birth, those delivered by primary cesarean delivery had twice the risk of having a hysterectomy (OR 2.20, CI 1.80–26.69) while in those having a repeat section the risk was four times higher (OR 4.51, CI 3.76–5.40) [41]. Other population-based analysis in Italy, China, and the Netherlands arrived at similar results [39,42,43].

FACTORS CONTRIBUTING TO TRENDS OF CESAREAN DELIVERY

Despite worldwide concern, controversies, and investigations, the determinants of rising cesarean delivery rates remain unclear and warrant urgent, focused, and country-specific attention. Causes for this trend are multifactorial and involve complex interactions between maternal and pregnancy characteristics, such as increasing maternal age, obesity, and excessive gestational weight gain and multiple pregnancies [44–47], as well as administrative, economic, social, and clinical factors including differences in thresholds for intervention at institutional and practitioner levels and fear of litigation [48,49]. Maternal request is cited as being one of the key factors driving the cesarean delivery increase [48,50–54]. However, contrary to this popular belief, a systematic review of the literature reports that only 16% of over 17,000 women across a range of countries prefer cesarean delivery [55]. Factors associated with cesarean delivery preference include younger age, nulliparity, lower instruction, and a previous delivery by cesarean [55–57].

Higher cesarean delivery preference may in part be explained by the increasing perceived safety of cesarean delivery, especially in countries with a high cesarean delivery rate. Although the relative risks for complications of cesarean delivery are still several times higher than in a vaginal delivery [4,58–60], the absolute risks for maternal or perinatal morbidity and mortality are very small, and may contribute to the sense of the safety of this surgery and to the rising rates of cesarean delivery, especially in developed countries. The media also contributes to the portrayal of cesarean delivery as a simple and low-risk procedure. For instance, most articles published in popular Brazilian and Spanish women's magazines over the last 20 years do not use optimal sources of information and fail to report important perinatal and long-term maternal risks of cesarean delivery, such as iatrogenic prematurity and increased risk for placenta previa/accreta in future pregnancies [61,62].

MONITORING CESAREAN DELIVERY RATES AT LOCAL LEVEL

The proportion of deliveries by cesarean delivery at country level is a useful indicator, and as such, its use is promoted and recommended by international agencies to monitor emergency obstetric care, access, and quality [14,63]. This indicator provides information that can be used for guiding policy and programs as well as planning for the necessary resources. In addition, the information is relatively easier to obtain compared with other maternal health indicators, as women can be expected to remember more dependably the type of delivery than, for example, if the care provider at birth was formally skilled, the number of antenatal care visits they attended, or the antenatal test performed [64]. Also, the reliability of the information obtained through demographic and health surveys (mainly in developing countries) has been assessed to be of sufficient precision at the national level [65]. However, there are limitations, and the data presented above needs to be interpreted with caution. Monitoring, reporting, and analyzing national rates can mask important within-country variation; not only the well-identified urban versus rural differences but also variation within hospitals and districts [12,13,66,67]. Potentially appropriate levels of cesarean delivery rates of about 15% do not indicate that those women who need a cesarean delivery are getting it, which should be the goal of health providers, instead of achieving a specific percentage or rate at the country level. Moreover, the population rate of cesarean deliveries does not assess the quality of the intervention, the appropriateness of the technique, the adequate capacity of the facility, or the adequate capacity and training of the health-care providers.

Monitoring cesarean delivery rates at subnational level (e.g., hospital-level) is essential to understand trends and associated factors. Despite this critical need, the lack of a standardized, internationally accepted classification system to monitor and compare rates in a replicable and action-oriented manner has precluded advances in this direction. Classifications based on indications for cesarean delivery have been the most frequently used [68]. The rationale for this is that in order to understand whether the cesarean delivery is necessary or not, we need to know why it was performed in the first place. Theoretically, these types of classifications are easy to implement because the "causes" of the cesarean are routinely reported in the medical records, but the drawbacks for international comparison are multiple. Indicators are neither mutually exclusive nor totally inclusive, unless an extensive list of indications is provided. Moreover, the definitions of some of the most common conditions leading to cesarean (e.g., dystocia, fetal distress) are poorly described or unclear, thus hindering reproducibility by different clinicians. Last, the utility of this classification to change clinical practice is questionable because many of the indications cannot be prospectively identified.

A systematic review of available classification systems conducted by WHO and published in 2011 found and evaluated 27 different classifications. This review concluded that "women-based classification in general, and Robson's classification, in particular, would be in the best position to fulfil current international and local needs and that efforts to develop an internationally applicable cesarean delivery classification would be most appropriately placed in building upon this classification" [68, p. 1]. The system proposed by Robson in 2001 classifies women into 10 groups based on their obstetric characteristics (parity, previous cesarean delivery, gestational age, onset of labor, fetal presentation, and number of fetuses) without needing the indication for cesarean delivery [69]. The system can be applied prospectively, and its categories are totally inclusive and mutually exclusive so that every woman who is admitted for delivery can be immediately classified based on these few basic characteristics that are usually routinely collected by obstetric care providers worldwide (see Table 1.2).

Table 1.2 Description of the Robson 10-group classification system for cesarean delivery

Group	Women included
1	Nulliparous with single cephalic pregnancy, ≥37 weeks' gestation in spontaneous labor
2	Nulliparous with single cephalic pregnancy, ≥37 weeks' gestation who either had labor induced or were delivered by cesarean delivery before labor
3	Multiparous without a previous uterine scar, with single cephalic pregnancy, ≥37 weeks' gestation in spontaneous labor
4	Multiparous without a previous uterine scar, with single cephalic pregnancy, ≥37 weeks' gestation who either had labor induced or were delivered by cesarean delivery before labor
5	All multiparous with at least one previous uterine scar, with single cephalic pregnancy, ≥37 weeks' gestation
6	All nulliparous women with a single breech pregnancy
7	All multiparous women with a single breech pregnancy including women with previous uterine scars
8	All women with multiple pregnancies including women with previous uterine scars
9	All women with a single pregnancy with a transverse or oblique lie, including women with previous uterine scars
10	All women with a single cephalic pregnancy <37 weeks' gestation, including women with previous scars

A systematic review assessed the use of the Robson classification worldwide and the experiences by the users as well as the adaptations, modifications, and recommendations suggested [70]. Despite the lack of official endorsement by any international organizations or institution or formal guidelines, the use of the Robson classification is increasing rapidly and spontaneously. Users find it simple, robust, clear, flexible, easy to implement, and clinically relevant. As the variables necessary to construct this classification are readily available even in developing countries, this system can be potentially used at all levels, i.e., national, regional, and hospital levels. All these are clear advantages in the current international scenario with a highly prioritized need for standardization of the collection and analysis of cesarean delivery data. This is an essential step to assess what is the most appropriate range of cesarean delivery rates to obtain the best maternal and perinatal outcomes, regardless of the level of the health system and of the country.

REFERENCES

1. Editorial: What is the right number of caesarean sections? *Lancet* 1997;349:815–6.
2. Caesarean delivery—The first cut isn't the deepest. *Lancet* 2010;375(9719):956.
3. World Health Organization (WHO). Appropriate technology for birth. *Lancet* 1985;2(8452):436–7.
4. Lumbiganon P, Laopaiboon M, Gulmezoglu AM et al. Method of delivery and pregnancy outcomes in Asia: The WHO global survey on maternal and perinatal health 2007–2008. *Lancet* 2010;375:490–9.
5. Villar J, Carroli G, Zavaleta N et al. Maternal and neonatal individual risks and benefits associated with caesarean delivery: Multicentre prospective study. *BMJ* 2007;335(7628):1025.
6. Villar J, Valladares E, Wojdyla D et al. Cesarean delivery rates and pregnancy outcomes: The 2005 WHO global survey on maternal and perinatal health in Latin America. *Lancet* 2006;367(9525):1819–29.
7. Betran AP, Merialdi M, Lauer JA et al. Rates of caesarean delivery: Analysis of global, regional and national estimates. *Paediatr Perinat Epidemiol* 2007;21:98–113.
8. Althabe F, Sosa C, Belizan JM, Gibbons L, Jacquerioz F, Bergel E. Cesarean delivery rates and maternal and neonatal mortality in low-, medium-, and high-income countries: An ecological study. *Birth* 2006;33(4):270–7.
9. Belizan JM, Althabe F, Barros FC, Alexander S. Rates and implications of caesarean deliverys in Latin America: An ecological study. *BMJ* 1999;319:1397–402.
10. Gibbons L, Belizan JM, Lauer J, Betran AP, Merialdi M, Althabe F. The global numbers and costs of additionally needed and unnecessary caesarean deliverys performed per year: Overuse as a barrier to universal coverage. *World Health Report*. Geneva, Switzerland: World Health Organization; 2010.
11. Gibbons L, Belizan JM, Lauer JA, Betran AP, Merialdi M, Althabe F. Inequities in the use of cesarean delivery deliveries in the world. *Am J Obstet Gynecol* 2012;206(4):331, e1–19.
12. Cavallaro FL, Cresswell JA, Franca GV, Victora CG, Barros AJ, Ronsmans C. Trends in cesarean delivery by country and wealth quintile: Cross-sectional surveys in southern Asia and sub-Saharan Africa. *Bull World Health Organ* 2013;91(12):914–22D.
13. Ronsmans C, Holtz S, Stanton C. Socioeconomic differentials in caesarean rates in developing countries: A retrospective analysis. *Lancet* 2006;368(9546):1516–23.
14. World Health Organization, United Nations Population Fund (UNFPA), UNICEF, and Mailman School of Public Health, Averting Maternal Death and Disability (AMDD). *Monitoring Emergency Obstetric Care: A Handbook*. Geneva, Switzerland: World Health Organization; 2009.
15. Hibbard LT. Changing trends in cesarean delivery. *Am J Obstet Gynecol* 1976;125(6):798–804.
16. Jones OH. Cesarean delivery in present-day obstetrics. Presidential address. *Am J Obstet Gynecol* 1976;126(5):521–30.
17. Placek PJ, Taffel S, Moien M. Cesarean section delivery rates: United States, 1981. *Am J Public Health* 1983;73(8):861–2.
18. Notzon FC, Cnattingius S, Bergsjo P et al. Cesarean section delivery in the 1980s: International comparison by indication. *Am J Obstet Gynecol* 1994;170(2):495–504.
19. Notzon FC, Placek PJ, Taffel SM. Comparisons of national cesarean-section rates. *N Engl J Med*. 1987;316(7):386–9.
20. Saúde Md. Pesquisa Nacional de Demografía e Saúde da Criança e da Mulher. *Sistema de Informações de Nascidos Vivos—SINASC*. 2011. http://svs.aids.gov.br/cgiae/sinasc/
21. World Health Organization (WHO). *World Health Statistics 2014*. Geneva, Switzerland: WHO; 2014.
22. Wagner M. Fish can't see water: The need to humanize birth. *Int J Gynaecol Obstet* 2001;75(Suppl 1):S25–37.
23. Sachs BP, Castro MA. The risk of lowering cesarean-delivery rate. *New Engl J Med* 1999;340:54–57.
24. European Perinatal Health Report. Health and Care of Pregnant Women and Babies in Europe. 2010. http://www.europeristat.com/images/doc/EPHR2010_w_disclaimer.pdf
25. Hanley GE, Janssen PA, Greyson D. Regional variation in the cesarean delivery and assisted vaginal delivery rates. *Obstet Gynecol* 2010;115(6):1201–8.
26. Clark SL, Belfort MA, Hankins GD, Meyers JA, Houser FM. Variation in the rates of operative delivery in the United States. *Am J Obstet Gynecol* 2007;196(6):526 e1–5.
27. Victorian Government Department of Health (DoH). *Victorian Maternity Services Performance Indicators. Complete Set for 2008–9*. Victoria, Australia: Victorian Government DoH; 2010.
28. Althabe F, Belizan JM. Caesarean delivery: The paradox. *Lancet* 2006;368(9546):1472–3.

29. Stanton C, Ronsmans C, Baltimore Group on C. Recommendations for routine reporting on indications for cesarean delivery in developing countries. *Birth* 2008;35(3):204–11.
30. Clark SL, Belfort MA, Dildy GA, Herbst MA, Meyers JA, Hankins GD. Maternal death in the 21st century: Causes, prevention, and relationship to cesarean delivery. *Am J Obstet Gynecol* 2008;199(1):36 e1–5; discussion 91–2 e7–11.
31. Lavender T, Kingdon C, Hart A, Gyte G, Gabbay M, Neilson JP. Could a randomised trial answer the controversy relating to elective caesarean delivery? National survey of consultant obstetricians and heads of midwifery. *BMJ* 2005;331(7515):490–1.
32. Ecker JL. Once a pregnancy, always a cesarean? Rationale and feasibility of a randomized controlled trial. *Am J Obstet Gynecol* 2004;190(2):314–8.
33. Feldman GB, Freiman JA. Prophylactic cesarean delivery at term? *N Engl J Med* 1985;312(19):1264–7.
34. Ye J, Betran AP, Vela MG, Souza JP, Zhang J. Searching for the optimal rate of medically necessary cesarean delivery. *Birth* 2014;41(3):237–44.
35. Zizza A, Tinelli A, Malvasi A et al. Cesarean delivery in the world: A new ecological approach. *J Prev Med Hyg* 2011;52(4):161–73.
36. Rothman KJ, Greenland S. *Modern Epidemiology*. Philadelphia, PA: Lippincott-Raven; 1998.
37. Shah A, Faundes A, Machoki M et al. Methodological considerations in implementing the WHO Global Survey for Monitoring Maternal and Perinatal Health. *Bull World Health Organ* 2008;86(2):126–31.
38. Lyndon A, Lee HC, Gilbert WM, Gould JB, Lee KA. Maternal morbidity during childbirth hospitalization in California. *J Matern Fetal Neonatal Med* 2012;25(12):2529–35.
39. van Dillen J, Zwart JJ, Schutte J, Bloemenkamp KW, van Roosmalen J. Severe acute maternal morbidity and mode of delivery in the Netherlands. *Acta Obstet Gynecol Scand* 2010;89(11):1460–5.
40. Parazzini F, Ricci E, Cipriani S et al. Temporal trends and determinants of peripartum hysterectomy in Lombardy, Northern Italy, 1996–2010. *Arch Gynecol Obstet* 2013;287(2):223–8.
41. Spiliopoulos M, Kareti A, Jain NJ, Kruse LK, Hanlon A, Dandolu V. Risk of peripartum hysterectomy by mode of delivery and prior obstetric history: Data from a population-based study. *Arch Gynecol Obstet* 2011;283(6):1261–8.
42. Stivanello E, Knight M, Dallolio L, Frammartino B, Rizzo N, Fantini MP. Peripartum hysterectomy and cesarean delivery: A population-based study. *Acta Obstet Gynecol Scand* 2010;89(3):321–7.
43. Wei Q, Zhang W, Chen M, Zhang L, He G, Liu X. Peripartum hysterectomy in 38 hospitals in China: A population-based study. *Arch Gynecol Obstet* 2014;289(3):549–53.
44. Weiss JL, Malone FD, Emig D et al. Obesity, obstetric complications and cesarean delivery rate—A population-based screening study. *Am J Obstet Gynecol* 2004;190(4):1091–7.
45. Kiel DW, Dodson EA, Artal R, Boehmer TK, Leet TL. Gestational weight gain and pregnancy outcomes in obese women: How much is enough? *Obstet Gynecol* 2007;110(4):752–8.
46. Fitzsimmons BP, Bebbington MW, Fluker MR. Perinatal and neonatal outcomes in multiple gestations: Assisted reproduction versus spontaneous conception. *Am J Obstet Gynecol* 1998;179(5):1162–7.
47. Bragg F, Cromwell DA, Edozien LC et al. Variation in rates of cesarean delivery among English NHS trusts after accounting for maternal and clinical risk: Cross sectional study. *BMJ* 2010;341:c5065.
48. Cohain JS. Documented causes of unneCesareans. *Midwifery Today Int Midwife* 2009(92):18–9, 63.
49. Sakala C, Yang YT, Corry MP. Maternity care and liability: Pressing problems, substantive solutions. *Womens Health Issues* 2013;23(1):e7–13.
50. Graham WJ, Hundley V, McCheyne AL, Hall MH, Gurney E, Milne J. An investigation of women's involvement in the decision to deliver by caesarean delivery. *Br J Obstet Gynaecol* 1999;106(3):213–20.
51. Jackson NV, Irvine LM. The influence of maternal request on the elective cesarean delivery rate. *J Obstet Gynaecol* 1998;18(2):115–9.
52. Mould TA, Chong S, Spencer JA, Gallivan S. Women's involvement with the decision preceding their cesarean delivery and their degree of satisfaction. *Br J Obstet Gynaecol* 1996;103(11):1074–7.
53. Usha Kiran TS, Jayawickrama NS. Who is responsible for the rising cesarean delivery rate? *J Obstet Gynaecol* 2002;22(4):363–5.
54. Wilkinson C, McIlwaine G, Boulton-Jones C, Cole S. Is a rising cesarean delivery rate inevitable? *Br J Obstet Gynaecol* 1998;105(1):45–52.
55. Mazzoni A, Althabe F, Liu NH et al. Women's preference for caesarean delivery: A systematic review and meta-analysis of observational studies. *BJOG* 2011;118(4):391–9.
56. Karlstrom A, Nystedt A, Johansson M, Hildingsson I. Behind the myth—Few women prefer cesarean delivery in the absence of medical or obstetrical factors. *Midwifery* 2011;27(5):620–7.
57. Torloni MR, Betran AP, Montilla P et al. Do Italian women prefer cesarean delivery? Results from a survey on mode of delivery preferences. *BMC Pregnancy Childbirth* 2013;13:78.
58. American College of Obstetricians and Gynecologists (ACOG). ACOG Committee Opinion No. 394, December 2007. Cesarean delivery on maternal request. *Obstet Gynecol* 2007;110(6):2.
59. Deneux-Tharaux C, Carmona E, Bouvier-Colle MH, Breart G. Postpartum maternal mortality and cesarean delivery. *Obstet Gynecol* 2006;108(3 Pt 1):541–8.
60. Marshall NE, Fu R, Guise JM. Impact of multiple cesarean deliveries on maternal morbidity: A systematic review. *Am J Obstet Gynecol* 2011;205(3):262 e1–8.

61. Torloni M, Campos Mansilla B, Merialdi M, Betran A. What do popular Spanish women's magazines say about caesarean delivery? A 21-year survey. *BJOG* 2014;121(5):548–55.
62. Torloni MR, Daher S, Betran AP et al. Portrayal of cesarean delivery in Brazilian women's magazines: 20 year review. *BMJ* 2011;342:d276.
63. Bailey PE, Paxton A. Program note. Using UN process indicators to assess needs in emergency obstetric services. *Int J Gynaecol Obstet* 2002;76:299–305.
64. Tomeo CA, Rich-Edwards JW, Michels KB et al. Reproducibility and validity of maternal recall of pregnancy-related events. *Epidemiology* 1999;10(6):774–7.
65. Stanton CK, Dubourg D, De Brouwere V, Pujades M, Ronsmans C. Reliability of data on caesarean deliverys in developing countries. *Bull World Health Organ* 2005;83(6):449–55.
66. Stanton C, Ronsmans C. Caesarean birth as a component of surgical services in low- and middle-income countries. *Bull World Health Organ* 2008;86(12):A.
67. Feng XL, Wang Y, An L, Ronsmans C. Cesarean delivery in the People's Republic of China: Current perspectives. *Int J Women's Health* 2014;6:59–74.
68. Torloni MR, Betran AP, Souza JP et al. Classifications for cesarean delivery: A systematic review. *PLoS One* 2011;6(1):e14566.
69. Robson MS. Classification of caesarean deliverys. *Fetal Matern Med Rev* 2001;12(1):23–39.
70. Betran AP, Vindevoghel N, Souza JP, Gulmezoglu AM, Torloni MR. A systematic review of the Robson classification for caesarean delivery: What works, doesn't work and how to improve it. *PLoS One* 2014;9(6):e97769.

Laparotomies and cesarean delivery

GIAN CARLO DI RENZO, SHILPA NAMBIAR BALAKRISHNAN, and ANTONIO MALVASI

INTRODUCTION

The ability to extract the fetus by laparotomy was a significant step in moving away from traditional obstetrics and towards modern maternal–fetal medicine. Caesarean delivery can currently be considered as the operation women the world over are most likely to undergo.

OPENING THE ABDOMINAL WALL

Different surgical techniques for carrying out cesarean deliveries have been described, and consequently, several types of incisions are used to access the abdominal cavity. Regardless of the type of access, the surgical technique must comply with certain basic requirements. It must adequately expose the uterus, allow the fetus to be easily accessed and extracted, reduce the risk of postsurgical complications, and allow for an aesthetically pleasing result. The urgency of the operation, the patient's body mass index (BMI), previous abdominal operations, and the experience of the surgeon are other factors that play a role in determining the type of surgery.

There are two types of cutaneous incisions: transverse (Pfannenstiel, Maylard, Cherney, Joel-Cohen) and longitudinal (median or paramedian). Most cesarean deliveries are carried out with a transverse incision of the skin and the muscle fascia using a technique introduced by Pfannenstiel in 1900 [1].

As a surgical technique, the traditional Pfannenstiel incision involves the transverse cutting of the skin (Figure 2.1a) and subcutaneous tissue (Figure 2.1b) along the suprasymphyseal fold of the abdomen, the Bumm pelvic line, along a straight or slightly curved cut approximately 15-cm long. The transverse cutaneous incisions in the Pfannenstiel laparotomy are obviously performed in the same area, but along different lines close to the area. The type of incision performed is a function of different factors, such as the patient's health, weight, size of the gravidic abdomen, and the preference and experience of the surgeon.

Generally, all Pfannenstiel transverse incisions during cesarean delivery are carried out in the Malgaigne triangle area. This region has the approximate shape of an isosceles triangle that points down to the pubic symphysis and with its base at the top: along the top it is defined by the Bumm pelvic fold and on the sides and bottom by the two groin-femoral folds. Whichever way the incisions are carried out, closer to the base or to the apex of the Malgaigne triangle, they have a slight upward concavity and are parallel to the elastic fibers of the dermis and therefore respect this area's superficial layer anatomy.

After performing hemostasis of the main blood vessels, which may be required, the front tissue sheath of the rectus muscles is exposed and cut transversely the same length as the cutaneous incision (Figures 2.2a, b, and c). The sheath is then separated from the muscle layer: while the fascia is kept taut, the aponeurosis edges are detached laterally to the median raphe, which is then cut (Figures 2.3a and b). The separation is completed by detaching with fingers or with the help of a wad of gauze on forceps. This maneuver likely results in some bleeding due to damage to the fascia perforator vessels (Figures 2.4a, b, and c).

The rectus muscles are separated along the median line up to the base of the pyramidal muscles which are sectioned sagitally in the point of union, without detaching them from the ipsilateral rectus muscle. The transversalis fascia and the peritoneum are cut vertically, being careful to avoid the bladder. In fact when the bladder is empty, the bottom is approximately at the level of the upper margin of the pubic symphysis. Locating the space of Retzius, especially during a repeated cesarean delivery, prevents damage to the dome of the bladder. This virtual space is located in front of the external side of the parietal peritoneum. It is above the bladder and characterised by lax cellular tissue which can be easily detached by finger fracture. It also keeps the dome of the bladder away from the laparotomy (Figure 2.5).

In addition to aesthetic reasons, the transverse incision has numerous advantages that vary depending on the direction and location of the opening of the abdomen. It is the incision that best adapts to the various abdominal wall structures and therefore is able to facilitate the mending of damaged tissues. The skin is cut parallel to the elastic and collagen fibers of the dermis. Retraction of the cutaneous margins will be minimized, and they will be able to fit together more easily. The rectus muscle sheath is also cut along the direction of the fibers. It is therefore more of a separation than a delivery of the fibers. These surgical maneuvers can be carried out because the Pfannenstiel laparotomy is performed below the arched line in a place where the rectus muscle fascia is replaced by a thin layer constituted by the transversalis fascia (Figure 2.6).

Anatomical and functional damage is considerably less than that resulting from longitudinal sections and can be repaired without compromising resistance of the fascia, which is in fact the most important structure in terms of postoperative dehiscence. This complication occurs much less frequently than in vertical incisions.

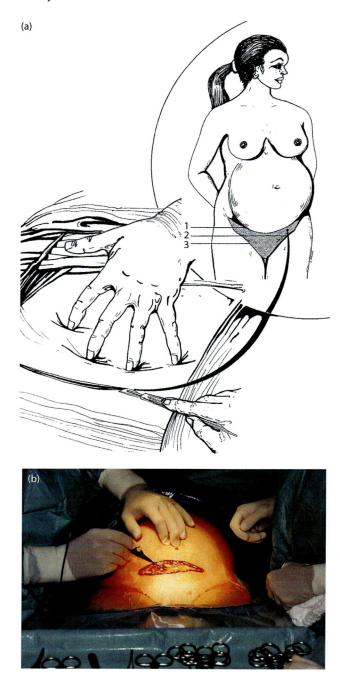

Figure 2.1 (a) Skin incision in the Pfannenstiel laparotomy. (This incision is performed parallel to the elastic and collagen fiber of the derma of the cutis.) Inset: the Malgaigne triangle described by three lines: (1) pubic line, (2) inguinal–femoral left line, and (3) inguinal–femoral right line. (b) Skin incision in the Pfannenstiel laparotomy of the subcutaneous tissue with electric scalpel at cesarean delivery. (Modified from Malvasi A, Di Renzo GC. *Semeiotica Ostetrica*, Rome, Italy: CIC Edizioni Internazionali; 2012.)

In fact the fascia opening is parallel to the tension lines of the wide abdomen muscles (Figures 2.7a and b), so contractions do not stretch the suture, as in the sagittal sections, but are instead lateral and therefore in the same direction as the cut. In fact, in longitudinal incisions the frequency of laparotomy wound dehiscence is eight times greater [2].

It is uncertain whether this surgical approach is also beneficial in terms of immediate postoperative complications: Wall and colleagues have observed in the vertical incision, in 239 obese patients, a greater incidence of parietal complications, as opposed to the transverse incision [3]. Houston and colleagues, in a retrospective study, again in obese patients, did not observe any difference [4]. However, the postoperative course is improved, as the transverse incisions are frequently less painful. Because the wound is remote from the diaphragm, the localized pain is not worsened by breathing. Moreover, use of the oblique muscles

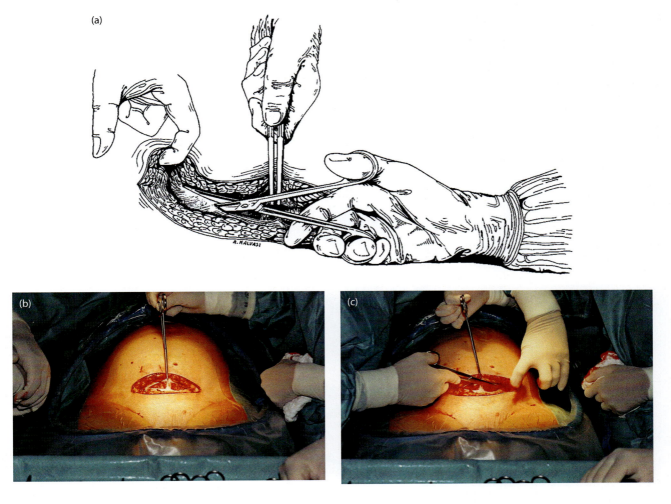

Figure 2.2 (a) Section of the anterior right rectus fascia and anterior right fascia of oblique muscle, with curved Mayo scissor during Pfannenstiel laparotomy. (b) Extension of the incision of the fascia at right of the patient at the oblique muscle, with curved Mayo scissors during Pfannenstiel laparotomy. (c) Extension of the incision of the fascia at the left of the abdomen.

of the abdomen does not cause the wound margins to separate and therefore does not cause pain. Postoperative ileus is less frequent and/or less serious. This can likely be attributed to the fact that, because the operating field is at the center of the abdominal incision, the "trauma" of the intestinal loops is not as great as that during the vertical incision. Cutaneous adhesion is more rapid and solid, in part due to the lesser frequency of septic complications [3]. Consequently, the surgical scar will be straighter and less visible. With regard to the disadvantages of the transverse incision, some authors have noted that, especially in obese patients, exposure of the uterus is not optimal. The limited visibility can be improved by making adequate use of the cutaneous incision and separating, vertically and laterally, the rectus muscles from their sheath.

The difficulties in extracting the fetus in the Pfannenstiel incision, when the length of the cutaneous delivery is at least 15 cm, are in fact minimal and statistically comparable to the Mackenrodt–Maylard technique [5]. A study by Finan and colleagues has shown that the fetus extraction time is not related to the type of incision but is instead related to its length: an Allis clamp placed between the retractor handles indicates the correct length of the incision (15 cm), whether transverse or longitudinal [6].

The opening of the abdomen is not as rapid with a traditional transverse incision as with a longitudinal incision and may cause increased blood loss. This, however, remains limited as it involves the larger branches of the external pudendal and superficial inferior epigastric arteries. For this reason some authors believe it should be contraindicated in case of coagulopathy or preeclampsia. A clinical trial, however, has brought to light how, in terms of infections and/or hematomas, in patients affected by the hemolysis, elevated liver enzymes, and low platelet count (HELLP) syndrome the frequency of complications of the laparotomy wound is not influenced by the type of cutaneous incision [7]. Past studies have not shown a significant statistical difference between the two types of incisions in terms of the need for blood transfusions, the variations of hemoglobin, and incidence of fever [8].

The transverse incision according to Mackenrodt–Maylard can be used in the event a wider opening becomes

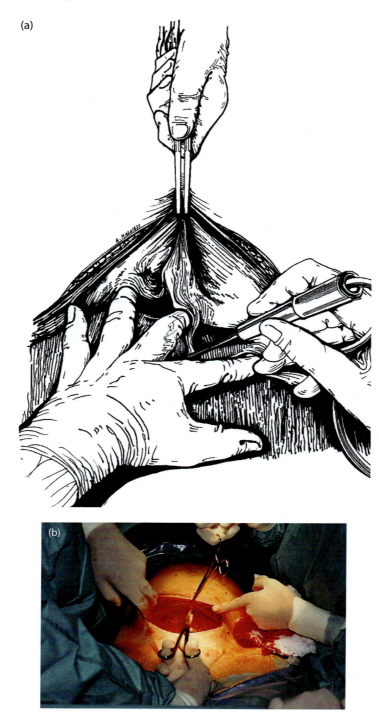

Figure 2.3 (a) Detachment of the alba-line with the electric scalpel while the assistant produces traction of the upper sectioned fascia. (b) Incision of the alba-line of the muscles by Mayo scissors.

necessary [9,10]. The Mackenrodt–Maylard laparotomy, described in 1901–1907, involves the incision of the skin and of the subcutaneous tissue from one anterior superior iliac spine to the other, following a slight upward concavity. After the fascia is cut transversely, the rectus muscles are separated, for a short length, along the median line and are then isolated below the muscle venter up to the lateral margin of the muscles. This level shows the underlying lower epigastric vessels which some authors would rather tie and deliver to reduce blood loss. This, however, is not essential. The rectus muscles are then cut transversely with scissors or electric scalpel, starting from the medial margin. The upper stump is secured to the above aponeurotic fascia. This prevents an excessive retraction of the severed muscle venters which would make it difficult to bring them closer together during suturing. After thorough hemostasis of the severed muscle, the transversalis fascia and peritoneum are opened transversely (Figures 2.8a and b).

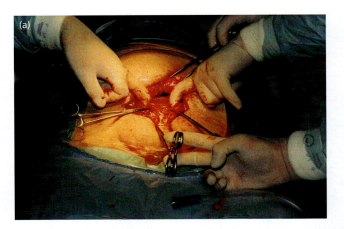
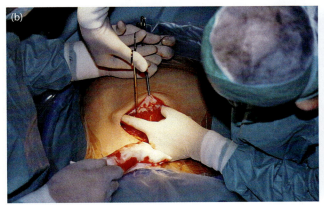
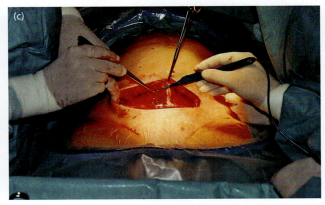

Figure 2.4 (a) Digital stretching by the surgeon and the assistant of the muscles and parietal plane exposition. (b) Incision of the fascia over the skin and subcutaneous line incision, to facilitate extraction of the fetus. (c) Hemostasis with electric scalpel of the abdominal vessels.

A variant of the Mackenrodt–Maylard technique was described by Cherney in 1941 [11]. The Cherney laparotomy involves the resectioning of the rectus muscles at the pubic insertion: after the fascia is cut transversely, the lower layer is detached up to the pubis. Once the muscular plane is displayed, the pyramidal muscles are separated from the rectus muscles up to the base and the quadrilateral tendons of the latter are cut at the pubic insertion located between the iliac spines and the symphysis (Figure 2.9).

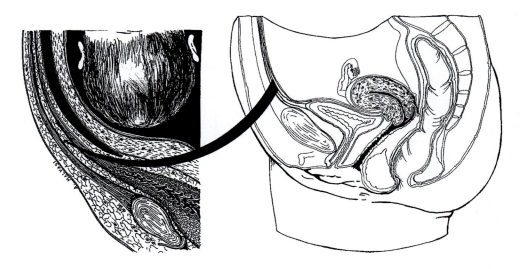

Figure 2.5 Sagittal section of the female pregnant pelvis (left) and nonpregnant pelvis (right). The curved black line indicates the abdominal fascia. (Modified from Malvasi A, Di Renzo GC. *Semeiotica Ostetrica*, Rome, Italy: CIC Edizioni Internazionali; 2012.)

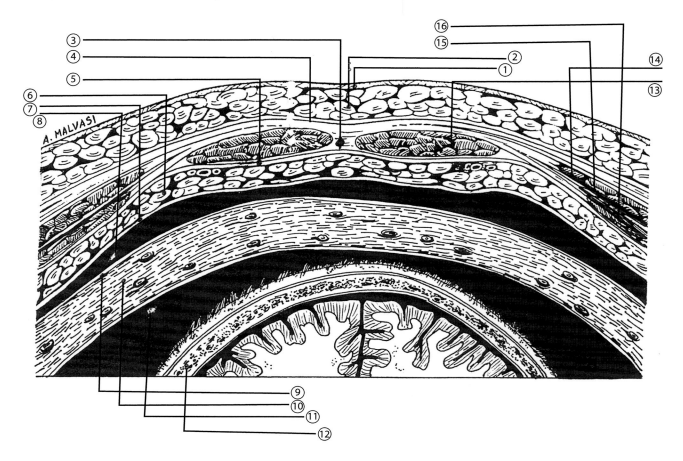

Figure 2.6 Frontal anatomic section of abdominal wall, under the arcuate line and the pregnant uterus at pregnancy term. Laparotomies for cesarean delivery are performed under the arcuate line. 1 = skin; 2 = subcutaneous tissue of anterior subumbilical abdominal wall; 3 = abdominal fascia of rectus abdominis muscles (linea alba); 4 = anterior abdominis fascia, of right rectus muscle; 5 = fascia transversalis; 6 = subperitoneal tissue; 7 = anterior parietal peritoneum; 8 = peritoneal cavity; 9 = visceral uterine peritoneum; 10 = anterior uterine wall (lower uterine segment, at pregnancy term); 11 = amniotic cavity; 12 = fetal head (right parietal fetal skull, of the fetus in cephalic presentation); 13 = left rectus muscle; 14 = left external oblique muscle; 15 = transverse muscle; 16 = left internal oblique muscle.

Low incisions in women who have already been subjected to previous pelvic surgery may result in intraoperative problems due to scar reaction (Figure 2.10).

The Mackenrodt–Maylard procedure allows an adequate exposure of the uterus, although doubts regarding the transverse delivery of the rectus muscles have limited its use. In fact this type of incision may result in extensive muscular damage and in unexpected lesions of the underlying vessels [12].

Ayers and Morley, instead, have not noticed differences in terms of surgical morbidity [5] between the Pfannenstiel technique and the sectioning of rectus muscles (Figure 2.10). These authors therefore believe that the Mackenrodt–Maylard technique is safe and should be highly recommended whenever there are situations involving a particular risk (e.g., macrosomia, twins) These require wide surgical exposure in order for the cesarean delivery to be nontraumatic.

Giacalone and colleagues have also shown, in a randomized study, that in terms of postoperative pain and perisurgical complications, the Maylard technique does not present statistical differences compared to the Pfannenstiel incision [13]. The clinical and objective evaluation of the strength of the abdominal wall, performed after the operation, has also evidenced similar results.

An alternative to the traditional abdomen opening according to Pfannenstiel, is the Joel-Cohen transverse incision [14]. The main idea behind this procedure is to respect the anatomy of the abdominal wall as much as possible with the use of the "stretching" technique. This method is based on two basic concepts:

- Perform a minimum incision in order to reduce surgical duration and improve healing.
- Morbidity is not affected by the position of the incision but by dieresis and unnecessary suturing of tissues.

New procedures have also been described, such as the one proposed by the Misgav Ladach General Hospital in Jerusalem [15,16]. This surgical technique, known in Italy as the "Caesarean delivery according to Stark," has adopted the Joel-Cohen transverse incision.

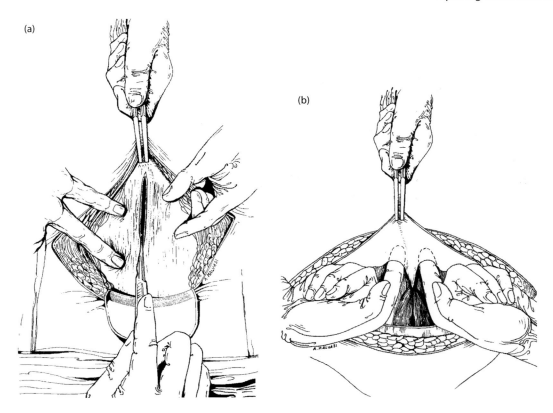

Figure 2.7 (a) Longitudinal incision of the fascia in a transverse laparotomy with scalpel during cesarean delivery. (b) Detachment of the fascia by the surgeon with two fingers, before the longitudinal incision.

The Joel-Cohen laparotomy is a surgical technique in which a straight cutaneous incision is performed approximately 3 cm below the level of the anterior superior iliac spines, approximately 2–3 cm above the point of the Pfannenstiel incision (Figure 2.11). After the cutaneous incision the subcutaneous tissues are cut centrally, for 2–3 cm, in an area in which there are no significant vessels (Figure 2.12). This incision can also be performed in case of previous surgical interventions, without excision of the laparotomy scar. Once the fascia is exposed, use fingers to widen the subcutaneous tissue in order to expose an area of at least 4–5 cm, thereby protecting the lateral epigastric vessels (Figure 2.13). The fascia is cut centrally for 2–3 cm, open scissors are inserted beneath the subcutaneous tissue, and the incision is extended, on both sides, a few centimeters beyond the cutaneous incision so that the fascia opening is larger than the cutaneous opening (Figure 2.14). Use index fingers to detach the fascia cranially and caudally to provide more room for the next maneuver (Figure 2.15).

The rectus muscles are widened by laterally stretching them until at least 10–12 cm of peritoneum are exposed. In this maneuver, the surgeon and assistant both insert their index and middle fingers under the muscles and simultaneously widen the subcutaneous tissue with a bilateral manual pull until there is a sufficient opening (Figure 2.16). If greater strength is required to perform this maneuver, as occurs for obese women or for repeated operations, the index and middle fingers of the other hand, of both surgeon and assistant, can be placed over the first hand (Figure 2.17). It is not recommended to place fingers from both hands next to each other as that increases the odds of vessels being damaged, with resulting hematomas.

The parietal peritoneum can be opened by finger fracture and then by stretching the opening, preferably in the transverse direction (to avoid damage to the bladder during the pull), or carefully in the cephalocaudal direction, until the lower uterine segment is adequately exposed (Figure 2.18). This type of abdominal opening has many advantages:

- Rapid extraction of the fetus [17]
- Shorter total duration of the intervention [18–22]
- Extremely limited blood loss [19,20,23]
- Reduction in postoperative pain [19,21]
- Rapid mobilization and recovery of the intestinal transit of the patient [22]
- Reduction in postoperative morbidity [15,16,18]
- Less suture material used [22,23]
- Shorter period of hospitalization [16,22]

As Stark explains, the rationale for using the Joel-Cohen laparotomy, and in particular the stretching of the abdominal wall tissues, is that many anatomical structures include vessels and nerve fibres that have a certain degree of elasticity. This stretching method opens tissues without causing lesions and, after the lateral traction, the still-intact blood vessels can frequently be seen running

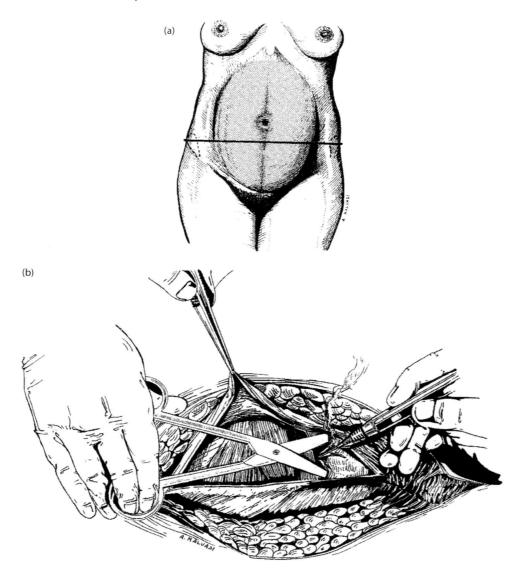

Figure 2.8 (a) Incision line of the Mackenrodt–Maylard laparotomy. (b) Mackenrodt–Maylard laparotomy: the left rectus muscle transverse section with electric scalpel. ([a] Modified from Malvasi A, Di Renzo GC. *Semeiotica Ostetrica*, Rome, Italy: CIC Edizioni Internazionali; 2012.)

from one wall of the laparotomy breach to the other. The blood vessels and nerve fibres are attached like musical instrument strings and can be easily moved from their seat without bleeding and with minimal tissue damage.

Even though there is wide consensus on this type of technique, some authors stress that the Pfannenstiel technique should not be considered outdated. Franchi and colleagues in a randomized study have not noticed significant statistical differences in the duration of the intervention, in intra- and postoperative complications, and in neonatal neurological development between the Pfannenstiel and Joel-Cohen techniques [17]. The authors conclude that even though the fetus can be extracted more quickly in the Joel-Cohen technique, there are no advantages for the mother or fetus, and that therefore one technique cannot be preferred over the other. In the Joel-Cohen technique the incision is higher and less aesthetic than in the traditional technique. This problem, however, has also been studied by Stark who modified the technique and lowered the cutaneous incision line.

The longitudinal incision has traditionally been used to carry out a cesarean delivery [24]. From a surgical point of view, in the longitudinal incision the abdomen is cut from the pubic symphysis to the navel for a length of at least 15 cm (Figures 2.19a, b, and c). If necessary, a wider opening can be achieved by extending the incision and moving around and to the left of the navel (Figure 2.20). In a similar manner, subcutaneous tissue is sectioned with a scalpel blade or with an electric scalpel to limit and control bleeding (Figures 2.21a and b). The incision is extended to the aponeurosis, while checking the terminal branches of the external pudendal and superior epigastric arteries for any bleeding. Once the fascia along the linea alba is exposed, a short central segment is cut (Figure 2.22). After the fascia

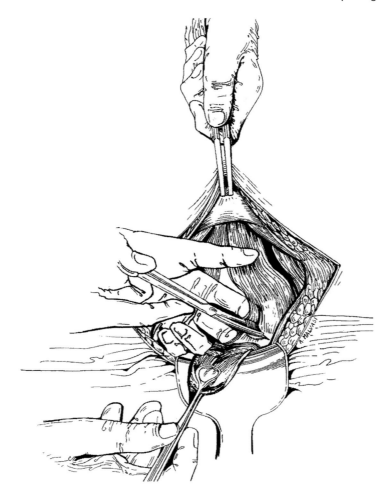

Figure 2.9 The Cherneyn laparotomy: the rectus muscles were sectioned at the pubic bone insertion. This laparotomy is performed at cesarean delivery in case of placenta accreta and/or increta.

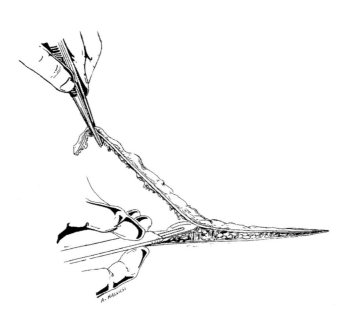

Figure 2.10 Hypertrophic skin removal with scissor during repeat cesarean delivery.

is separated from the rectus muscles, thus creating a "tunnel," it is divided vertically for a length equal to the cutaneous incision.

The rectus muscles must be separated by blunt dissection, for example, with closed scissors and then, to complete, with the index fingers. If the separation takes place exactly along the connecting line, there will not be any blood loss (Figure 2.23). Widening the muscle venters exposes the transversalis fascia, the deep layer of the transverse muscle that covers the preperitoneal fat. After carefully dividing it, expose and then cut the peritoneum.

The urachus that runs along the external side of the peritoneum from the navel to the bladder indicates the median line to be followed during the incision (Figure 2.24). This type of access to the abdominal cavity is applied vertically to the various layers of the abdomen and provides wide exposure of the operating area. The incision is quick, simple, and results in less blood loss than in the transverse incision due to the smaller number of vessels in this area (Figure 2.25). It has the advantage that it can be extended should it become necessary during the intervention. For this reason it is occasionally preferred in obese or weak patients, or in an emergency. This type of access

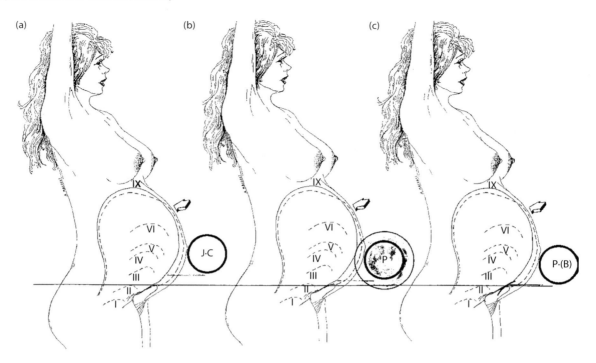

Figure 2.11 Laparotomies of (a) Joel-Cohen, (b) Pfannenstiel, and (c) lower Pfannenstiel. (Modified from Malvasi A, Di Renzo GC. *Semeiotica Ostetrica*, Rome, Italy: CIC Edizioni Internazionali; 2012.)

is also preferred when the cesarean delivery is carried out with local anesthesia [25]. This incision however is at high risk of postoperative dehiscence and incisional hernia [2] due to the limited strength of the aponeurosis along the median line, and to the stress on the wound that originates from the contraction of abdominal muscles and from the intra-abdominal pressure increase that inevitably follows a laparotomy.

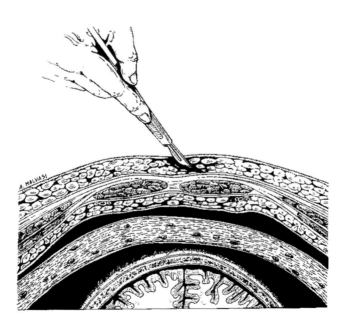

Figure 2.12 Joel-Cohen laparotomy at cesarean section: skin incision and fat fissure incision at central laparotomy area.

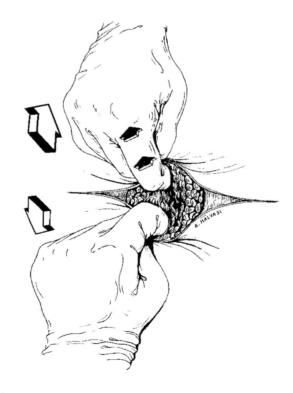

Figure 2.13 Stretching of subcutaneous tissue in the incision area with fingers index up and down.

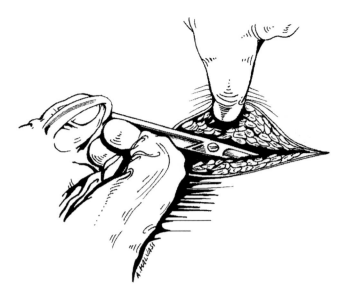

Figure 2.14 Section of the anterior fascia layer with Mayo scissors.

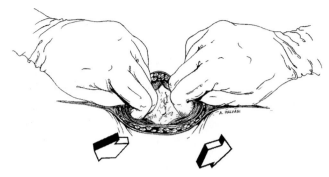

Figure 2.16 Stretching of abdominal muscles at cesarean delivery.

The linea alba is formed by the fusion of the terminal aponeurotic fibers originating from the external oblique, internal oblique, and transverse muscles on both sides of the abdomen. It is therefore the thinnest and weakest part of the fascia. The sagittal delivery of this structure would result in greater anatomical damage. Even a thorough reconstruction may be inadequate and create conditions that might favor, or even cause, dehiscence of the wound.

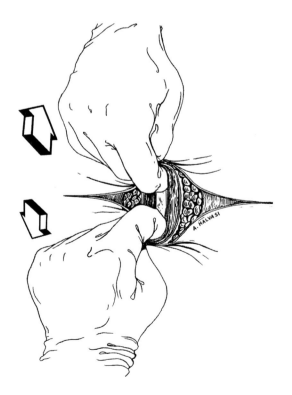

Figure 2.15 Caudocranial stretching of the fascia to make the next maneuver easier.

Inadequate vascularization along the median line does not help in achieving a quick and effective consolidation of the edges. The aesthetic result of the vertical incision is certainly not as satisfying as that of the transverse incision.

The paramedian incision is performed laterally to the median line, usually on the right. The anterior sheath of the rectus muscle is divided and isolated up to the connecting medial margin with the contralateral muscle. However, this type of incision is not widely used as it greatly alters the innervation and vascularization of the medial segment of the corresponding rectus muscle. This incision is certainly more solid than the median one [26]; however, the aesthetic result of the scar is not satisfactory. Other transverse laparotomies are used during a cesarean delivery.

The general principle behind these other laparotomies and/or their variants is to perform a low cutaneous incision, to move the subcutaneous fatty tissue upward, and to deliver the fascia as high as possible, in order to have sufficient access to the operating field.

The Kustner laparotomy, described in 1896, consists of a transverse incision that involves only the skin and a vertical incision of the underlying layers. [27]. The cutaneous incision is performed in the suprasymphyseal area. The subcutaneous tissue is detached and mobilized cranially. The fascia is cut longitudinally along the linea alba in order to separate the rectus muscles along the median line. The parietal peritoneum is cut in a similar longitudinal manner (Figure 2.26).

This incision is preferred for aesthetic reasons, but it is not surgically advantageous as the operating field has a limited view compared to the Pfannenstiel laparotomy [28]. The low Pfannenstiel laparotomy (Nichols DH):

> …in patients in which it is essential that the incision be as concealed as possible the surgeon can perform a "low Pfannenstiel," during which the incision is carried out a finger width below the pubic hair. The abdominal wall and the subcutaneous tissue are separated in the cranial direction from the rectus fascia which can be cut transversely as in the classic Pfannenstiel… [29].

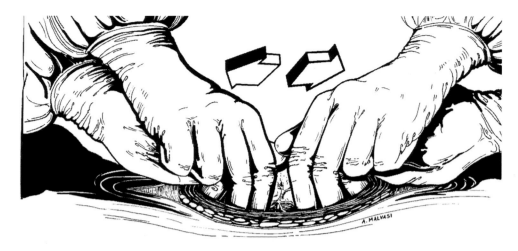

Figure 2.17 Bimanual stretching with the handsoverlapped, by surgeon and assistant, during laparotomy.

An important phase of the modified laparotomy is the preparation of the fascia, as accurately described by F. Novak:

> …detach the fascia from the rectus by blunt disdelivery until there are four deep pockets; pull the Allis clamps upwards two by two, first the upper ones then the lower ones, and then cut the linea alba connective tissue, longitudinally, respectively, at the top as close to the navel as possible, and at the bottom at the symphysis. The pyramidal muscles are not to be detached from the fascia… [30].

The *modified Joel-Cohen* laparotomy that we perform has the following surgical phases:

1. Transverse cutaneous incision 12–15 cm long: performed 99 times on the Bumm suprapubic skinfold, 32 times one finger width below the pubic hair line (a "low" Pfannenstiel).

Lower incisions were performed only after a thorough preoperative ultrasound examination.

The purpose of separating the incision location in three groups, while using in each case the "stretching" technique, was to verify the increasing difficulty of the abdominal opening compared to Joel-Cohen.

- The subcutaneous tissue is cut with an upward beveled incision, along the median line transversely for 3 cm (Figure 2.27). At the same time the operator, with the

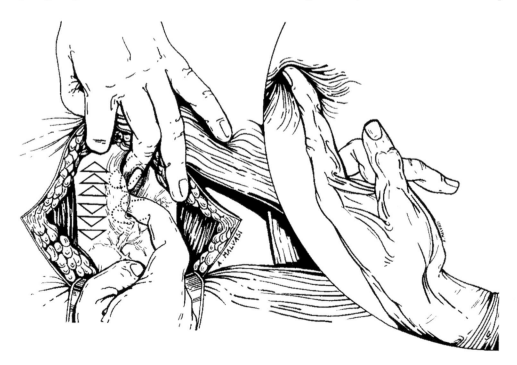

Figure 2.18 Parietal peritoneum opened with fingers transversely and longitudinally to avoid bladder couple injuries. (Modified from Malvasi A et al., *J Matern Fetal Neonatal Med* 2007.)

Opening the abdominal wall 23

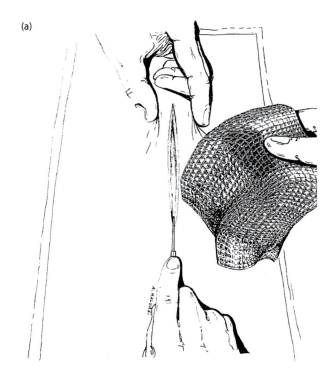

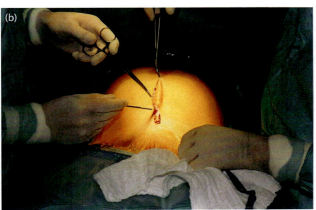

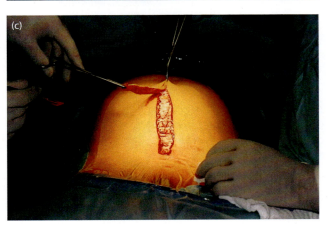

Figure 2.19 (a) Longitudinal skin incision at longitudinal laparotomy during cesarean delivery, extended 15 cm from pubic symphysis. (b) Incision of skin scar in longitudinal laparotomy during repeat cesarean delivery. (c) Excision and removal of the skin scar longitudinally during repeat cesarean delivery.

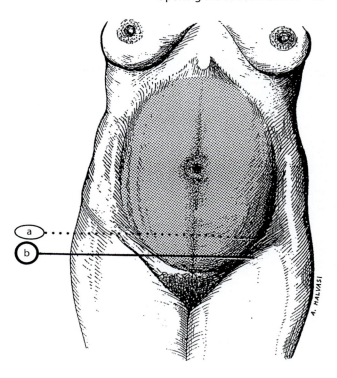

Figure 2.20 Up-extension of longitudinal laparotomy with excision left around umbilicus: (a) incision of Joel-Cohen; (b) Pfannenstiel incision

index finger of the other hand, performs a finger fracture of the subcutaneous tissue in an upward median direction for 3 cm (Figure 2.28) until exposing the fascia (Figure 2.29). Then, while the assistant lifts upward and in the cranial direction the upper edge of the incision, the operator cuts the fascia with the scalpel along the median line (Figure 2.30) for 3 cm (for 5–6 cm for thick subcutaneous tissue).

It is important to note that due to the beveled opening of the subcutaneous tissue, the fascia incision is well above the level of the cutaneous incision.

- After reopening the edges of the fascia with two Kocher forceps, perform an endoscopic incision with straight Mayo scissors (Figure 2.31) (if curved, the tips should point up along the direction of the fascia fibers). However, the cut must be extended for 4 cm beyond the cutaneous incision so that the opening of the fascia layer is larger than the cutaneous one (the *reverse cone incision*).
- Observe the median raphe of the pyramidal muscles (the lower the fascia incision, the farther one is from the fibrous apex of the pyramidal muscles). After inspecting and digitally isolating this fibrous union (Figure 2.32), one or two Mayo scissor snips are enough to cut through (Figure 2.33) and then "tunnel" up with the index finger until reaching the medial edges of the rectus muscles.
- The surgeon then performs a slight "stretching" in the caudal cranial direction, pulling slightly more in the cranial direction and performing a blunt detachment of the pyramidal muscles (Figure 2.34).

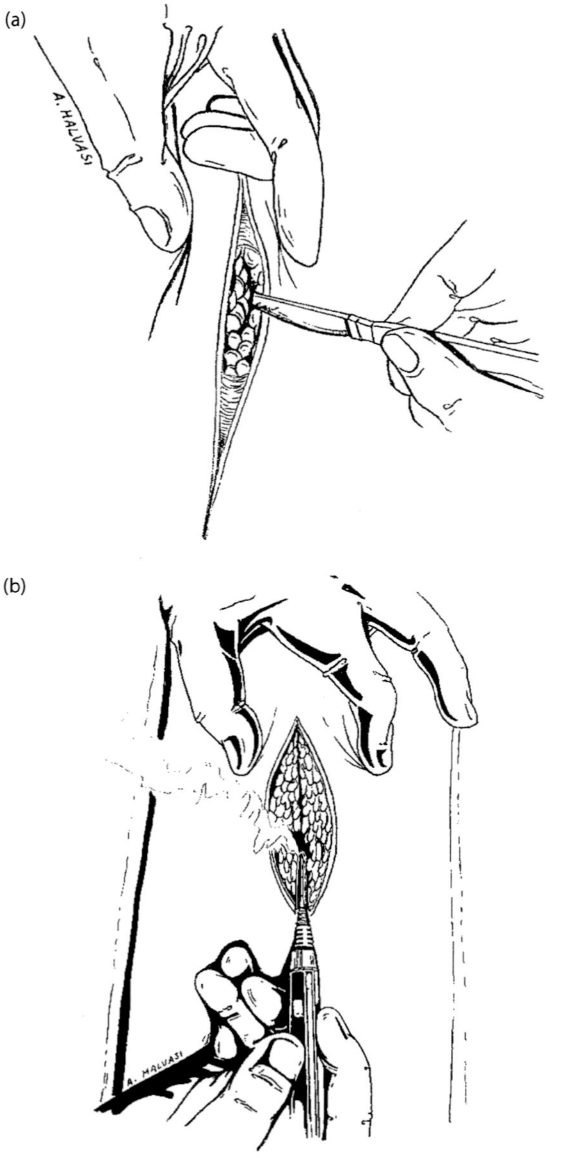

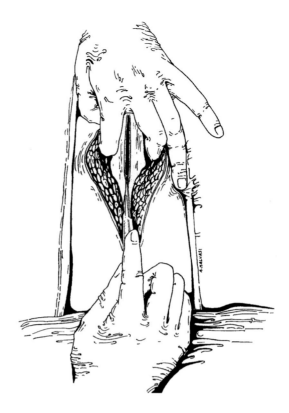

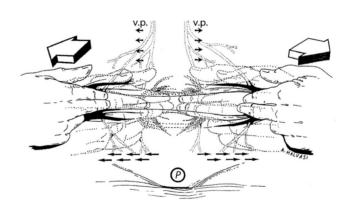

Figure 2.21 (a) Longitudinal laparotomy: section of the skin and subcutaneously with scissors. (b) Longitudinal laparotomy at cesarean delivery and hemostasis with electric scalpel.

Figure 2.22 Longitudinal laparotomy and alba-line of the fascia incision with scalpel.

Figure 2.23 Gentle stretching of rectus muscles, to epigastric vessels, avoiding the injuries in longitudinal laparotomy. (Modified from Malvasi A et al. Rome, Italy: CIC Edizioni Internazionali; 1998.)

- Although disapproved by Stark [14,18,30], this maneuver does not actually modify the vascular anatomy of the abdominal wall because of the lower incision and the small pulling force.
- This is followed by the combined midlateral "cross stretching" performed by surgeon and assistant, as described by Joel-Cohen (Figure 2.35). The combined vertical and horizontal stretching has given it the "cross stretching" name.
- After "stretching" the surgeon checks the wideness of the breach and opens the peritoneum by finger fracture (Figure 2.36).
- Once the fetal extraction, placental removal, uterine externalization, and cleaning of the cavity are completed, suture only the fascia and skin.

The Joel-Cohen laparotomy, applied by Stark to the cesarean delivery following the Misgav Ladach method, has had two main comparisons over the years: the Pfannenstiel laparotomy and the unavoidable modifications in surgical techniques, by several authors, brought about by the aesthetic and functional requirements which vary in relation to the social context of the pregnant woman and gynecologist. Moreover, studies described in literature frequently compare the traditional cesarean

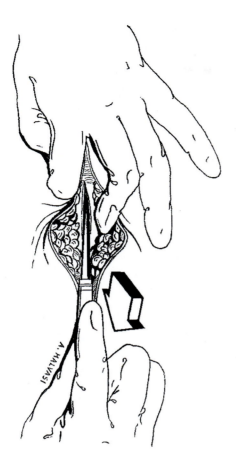

Figure 2.24 Incision with scalpel of the parietal peritoneum scarred in repeat cesarean delivery.

delivery with the Misgav Ladach method, thereby including the Pfannenstiel and Joel-Cohen laparotomies. Thus the study is subject to a—at times—high number of variables, in comparison to which the differences due to laparotomies do not appear as significant in terms of intraoperative and postoperative course.

Given the extensive use of both the Joel-Cohen laparotomy and its modifications, it seems appropriate to summarize the current situation by looking at the literature (Table 2.1). Ansaloni et al. [39] have in fact observed a shorter surgery duration and fewer infections (6.2% in the first versus 20% in the second with $p = 0.01$) in the Misgav Ladach technique compared to the traditional technique. Moreira et al. [40] have observed that the time between cutaneous incision and fetal extraction is significantly shorter for Misgav Ladach (5 minutes and 26 seconds versus 6 minutes and 20 seconds). They have also conducted a cost–benefit analysis in the maternity and gynecological clinic in Dakar (Senegal), which showed a 15 Euro reduction in costs in the Misgav Ladach technique compared to the traditional technique. The Misgav Ladach technique was introduced in Italy in 1996 [41]. The same-year results from an Italian multicentric study on 1356 operations showed, among other results, that the Joel-Cohen laparotomy was superior in terms of surgical duration and fetal extraction [42].

The Misgav Ladach method, in fact, contains two innovative principles: the Joel-Cohen laparotomy and the nonclosure of the peritoneum, both of which have also been assessed and described by other authors. Lorentzen et al. [43] maintain that the peritoneum closure in laparotomies

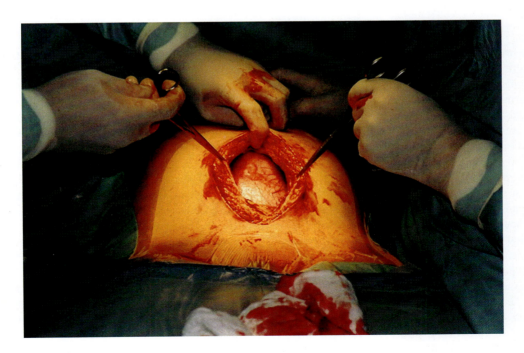

Figure 2.25 The longitudinal laparotomy permits optimal exposure of the uterus uterine wall in case of urgent cesarean delivery.

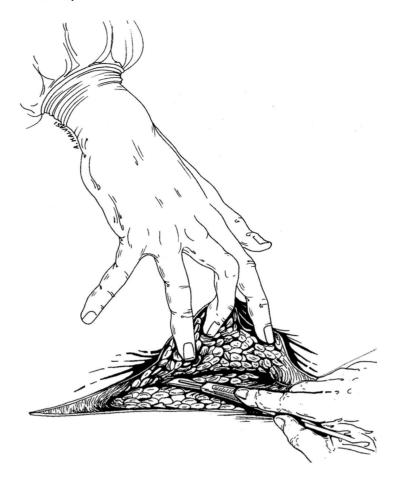

Figure 2.26 Kustner laparotomy: transverse incision of the skin in the suprasymphyseal zone, dissection of the subcutaneous tissue and cranial incision band longitudinally along the central line, separating the rectus muscle in the midline; longitudinally incised similarly the parietal peritoneum.

is based more on common practice than on scientific evidence. Holmgren et al. [44] have confirmed the importance of the Joel-Cohen laparotomy in the Misgav Ladach method in terms of surgical duration, blood loss, fetal extraction, and postoperative morbidity. Lazarov et al. [45] have assessed the advantages of not suturing the peritoneum and visceral parietal in 170 gynecological laparotomies and 45 cesarean sections.

Darj and Nordstrom [19] have demonstrated that the Misgav Ladach surgical phases are shorter than the traditional method (12.5 minutes versus 26 minutes). This reduction is especially true in the Joel-Cohen laparotomy, so much so that the authors liken it to the "Pfannenstiel method." Popiela et al. [46] state that the Misgav Ladach technique compared to the Pfannenstiel cesarean delivery (traditional cesarean section) shows a reduction in surgical duration, hospitalization, and postoperative morbidity. Zienkowicz et al. [47] have noted that the opening of the abdominal wall with the Joel-Cohen laparotomy causes less trauma and therefore has a shorter convalescence. Gaucherand et al. [48] report a statistically significant lower incidence of abdominal wall hematomas in the Joel-Cohen laparotomy compared to other transverse laparotomies during a cesarean delivery.

In Italy, Grignaffini et al. [49] and Corosu et al. [50] modified the Misgav Ladach method (Stark method) by performing a Pfannenstiel laparotomy instead of a Joel-Cohen, whereas Messalli et al. [51] have shown the superiority of the Stark method to the traditional one.

Li et al. [52] carried out further technical modifications to the Misgav Ladach, consisting of a 2–3 cm transverse incision of the fascia, an incision of the uterine segment directly on the visceral peritoneum, double-layer suturing of the uterine breach, and continuous suture of the skin.

Fatusic et al. [53] report a lower incidence of abdominal wall infections in Misgav Ladach versus the traditional method (4.54% versus 9% with $p < 0.05$). Instead Studzinski [54] does not report differences in the two methods in terms of wall infections. Redlich and Koppe [55] have, similarly, not observed in the two laparotomies significant differences in the formation of hematomas. Gaucherand et al. [48], on the contrary, have seen a reduction in parietal blood pools in the Joel-Cohen laparotomy, as have Heidenreich and Borgmann [56].

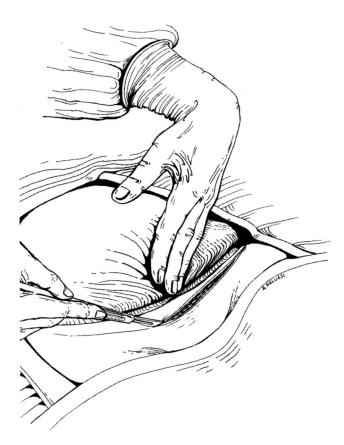

Figure 2.27 Joel-Cohen modified laparotomy: the subcutaneous tissue incised with a scalpel on the median line for 3 cm transversely upward. (Modified from Malvasi A et al. Rome, Italy: CIC Edizioni Internazionali; 1998.)

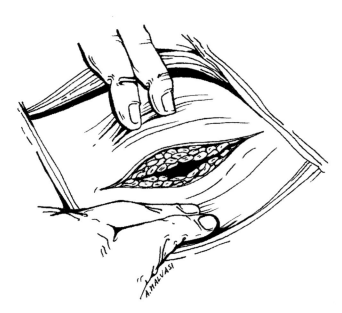

Figure 2.28 Joel-Cohen modified laparotomy: the first operator uses the index finger of one hand to simultaneously detach the subcutaneous tissue and with the other fingers, 7–8 cm upward. (Modified from Di Renzo GC. *Trattato di Ostetricia e Ginecologia*, Rome, Italy: Verduci Editore; 2009.)

A study on the preferred surgical techniques of English gynecologists carried out by Tully et al. [57] has shown that the Pfannenstiel laparotomy is normally preferred in cesarean sections, though Joel-Cohen laparotomies are carried out in emergency cases. Olezczuk et al. [58] note the superiority of the Joel-Cohen laparotomy over Pfannenstiel even in cesarean sections with twins. Following its description [14], the Joel-Cohen laparotomy has also been adopted in gynecology and has undergone modifications [59].

CLOSURE OF THE ABDOMINAL WALL

Traditionally the abdominal wall closure is performed by layers.

- The suture of the peritoneum, along with that of the transversalis fascia, starts from the upper margin (Figure 2.37).
- A continuous suture is usually employed (e.g., Vicryl 2.0 or 3.0).
- The suture line on the internal surface of the peritoneum must remain as smooth as possible. This prevents adherence to the omentum and to the intestinal loops.
- The suture must therefore be carried out so that the two internal sides of the serosa are brought together due to eversion of the peritoneal margins.
- The rectus muscles are brought together with a suture that brings the edges into contact. The suture is not as that might damage fibers and cause postoperative hematomas.
- In the Mackenrodt-Maylard technique the muscle venters obviously need to be sutured. If hemostasis of the muscular fascia is insufficient subfascial drainage may be required [60].
- The aponeurotic fascia is then closed with a continuous suture (Figure 2.37).
- Some authors prefer separate stitches when there is a risk of wound dehiscence.
- The subcutaneous tissue and skin are then sutured. The skin can be closed with different techniques: detached nonabsorbable stitches, absorbable or nonabsorbable intradermal sutures (Figure 2.38), metal staples, or biological glue.
- The method and type of opening during a cesarean delivery have been the source of controversy as has been the closure of the abdominal wall.
- One of the most debated issues is the closure of the peritoneum.

In the 1970s Ellis and colleagues had an unfavorable opinion on peritonization [61]. According to these authors, the peritoneum must not be sutured, because it closes spontaneously and reforms rapidly thus avoiding any adhesion.

Experimental studies conducted on animals have in fact shown that suturing the peritoneum increases tissue ischemia, necrosis, inflammation, and foreign-body reaction to suturing materials. In fact Elkins and colleagues [62] have examined histological samples at 4, 8, 12, 24, and 48

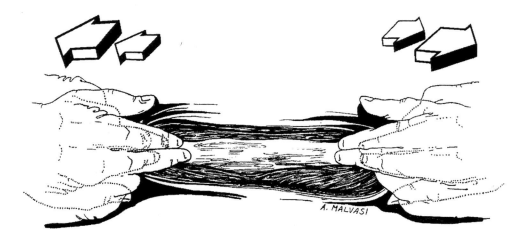

Figure 2.29 Joel-Cohen modified laparotomy: lateral stretching of the subcutaneous to highlight the fascia. (Modified from Malvasi A et al. Rome, Italy: CIC Edizioni Internazionali; 1998.)

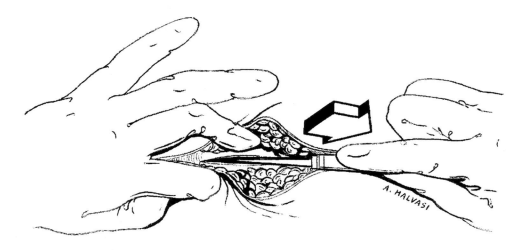

Figure 2.30 Joel-Cohen modified laparotomy: while the assistant raises the upper edge of the incision, the operator with the scalpel cuts the fascia in the midline for 3 cm (if the subcutaneous is fat also for 5–6 cm).

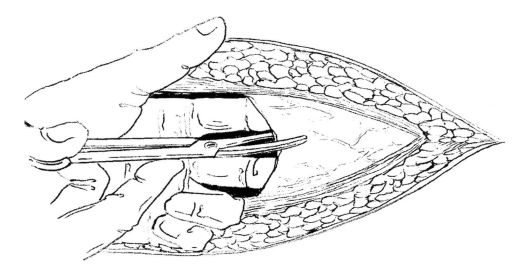

Figure 2.31 Joel-Cohen modified laparotomy: the edge of the fascia is incised with Mayo scissors, with the finger guide that separates them from the muscular tissue.

Closure of the abdominal wall 29

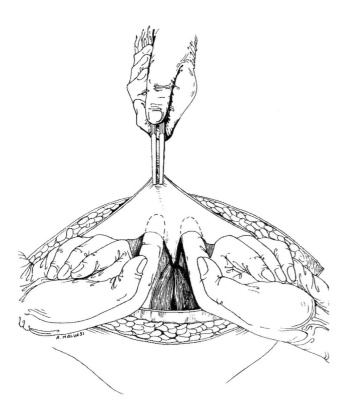

Figure 2.32 Joel-Cohen modified laparotomy: digital insolation of the fibrous bridge median to the rectus muscles.

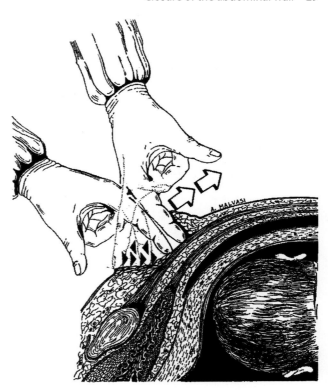

Figure 2.34 Joel-Cohen modified laparotomy: stretching of the muscle in caudal–cranial direction; by pulling cranially it dissects bluntly up the pyramidal muscles.

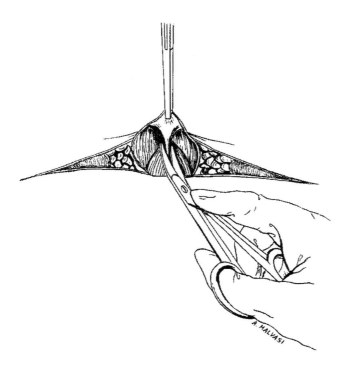

Figure 2.33 Joel-Cohen modified laparotomy: resection with scissors of the fibrous bridge.

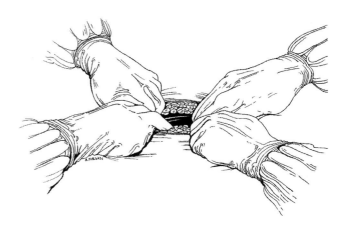

Figure 2.35 Joel-Cohen modified laparotomy: medial-lateral combined stretching between the operator and the assistant, as indicated by Joel-Cohen, the combination of vertical and horizontal stretching is called "cross stretching."

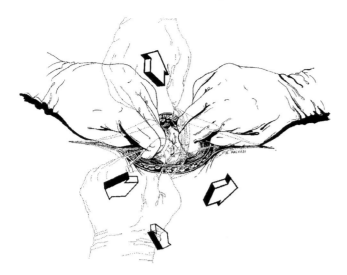

Figure 2.36 Joel-Cohen modified laparotomy: "cross stretching" combined with the opening of the peritoneum by finger fracture.

hours and at 5, 7, and 14 days following peritoneal damage on rabbits. The authors comment:

> ….no superficial fibrin was visible approximately 24 hours after the intervention and other reactions gradually diminished over time, except in the electrocauterisation areas in which the reactions continued during the three weeks of the study. The peritoneal excision area without suturing showed a decrease in necrotic tissue within 24 hours, and within 48 hours the tissue that was first damaged showed fibroblasts and consistent mesothelial integrity, that is, peritonization….

These factors may slow the recovery process and are important precursors to adhesion; peritoneal margins instead repair quickly without suture, with a low risk of infections and with adhesion less likely. Various studies in literature are therefore against the closure of the peritoneum [63,64]. The cesarean delivery according to Stark does not involve the closure of the visceral and parietal peritoneum. Studies performed by this author show a significant reduction in postoperative adhesion compared to the traditional technique [65]. Also shown is a reduction in postoperative morbidity: 7% in the Joel-Cohen technique versus 19.8% in the Pfannenstiel procedure [18]).

There is no general agreement in literature on the outcome of peritonization.

Chanrachakul and colleagues, in a randomized study on 60 patients who underwent a cesarean delivery with longitudinal incision, have not seen any difference in postoperative pain between a sutured and nonsutured peritoneum [66]. These authors have also not observed variations in terms of surgical duration, incidence of postoperative complications, recovery of intestinal transit, and length of hospital stay.

Pietrantoni and colleagues have also not observed differences between sutured and nonsutured peritoneum in a prospective study on 248 cesarean sections according to Pfannenstiel. Only surgical durations were significantly reduced (48.1 + 1.2 minutes for the open group versus 53.2 + −1.4 minutes for the closed group $p < 0.05$).

This study did not show any difference in terms of immediate or long-term postoperative complications, endometritis, and recovery of intestinal transit and length

Table 2.1 Several of the transverse laparotomies less frequently used during a cesarean delivery, in addition to the ones described previously.

Author	Surgical procedure	Year
Novak [29]	Transverse incision on the upper edge of the pubic symphysis	1973
	Subcutaneous incision with upper detachment of 4 cm and opening of the fascia at the same level (or as high as possible)	
Stark [15]	Transverse skin incision	1994
	2-cm incision	
	Along the median line of the subcutaneous tissue	
	Endoscopic transverse delivery of the fascia	
	Stretching of the subcutaneous tissue and muscles	
Turner-Warwick [31]	V-shaped incision	1974
	Transverse incision of skin and cutaneous tissue in Pfannenstiel position	
	Fascia cut with a V-shaped incision with apex pointing down	
	Rectus muscles and peritoneum sectioned longitudinally	
Pandolfo, Malinas, and colleagues [32]	Skin incision with low concavity and subsequent opening of layers, as in Pfannenstiel	1977
Mouchel [33]	Transverse incision of all layers, including the rectus muscles immediately above the pyramidal muscles	1981
Racinet and Favier [34]	"Inverted cone" incision: fascia opened laterally 3 cm beyond the cutaneous incision	1984
Chow [35]		1983
Ferrari [36]	Lower Joel-Cohen cutaneous incision	1996
Malvasi and colleagues [37,38]	Cross stretching (Figure 2.36)	1997

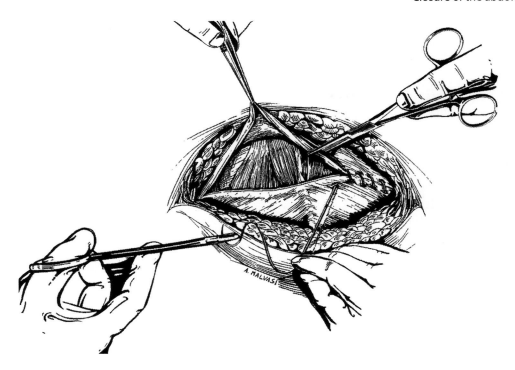

Figure 2.37 Suture in the transverse laparotomy for closing the abdominal wall: suture of the fascia.

of hospital stay. There was, however, an increase in the exposure to anesthetics and in costs, to the point that authors advise to leave the parietal peritoneum open.

Pietrantoni and colleagues [67] estimate that the cost of a single suture of the parietal peritoneum (36-in 3.0 polyglactin) is $14.30—15.1% of the total cost of a cesarean delivery, thereby saving approximately $100,286 a year in sutures, surgical durations, and anesthesia.

Cochrane Library has also published a review on this subject [68]. Nine clinical trials were examined, for a total of 1811 patients who underwent a cesarean delivery during which the visceral and/or parietal peritoneum was either

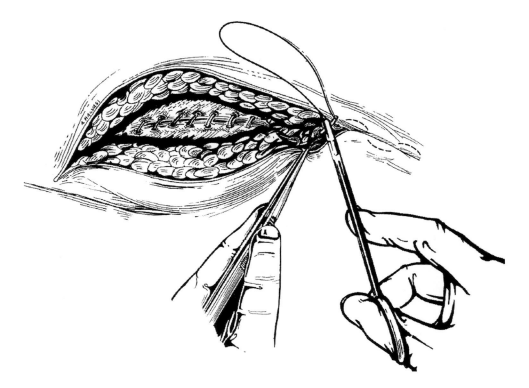

Figure 2.38 Skin and the subcutaneous tissue intradermal suture.

sutured or not sutured. The purpose of the review was to highlight differences in intra- and postoperative outcomes, both immediate and long term. In terms of results, it should be noted that

- Surgical duration decreased when neither or one of the two layers were sutured: the nonclosure of both layers shortened the intervention by 7.33 minutes.
- The incidence of febrile complications and the period of hospitalization were significantly reduced when either both layers were not closed or only the visceral peritoneum was closed.
- The trend regarding the need for analgesia and the incidence of parietal infections points to the nonclosure as being preferable.
- Data pertaining to endometritis are highly variable.

No other statistical difference has been noticed. The long-term follow-up analyzed in a single clinical trial did not show significant variations. The reviewers came to the conclusion that

- The short-term outcome of patients improves if the peritoneum is not closed.

- Long-term studies are limited, though results obtained from other procedures support the need to not suture the peritoneum.
- Currently there is no evidence that supports the time and costs needed for a peritoneum closure.

Although laparotomies are becoming less frequent, when they are carried out—as opposed to the parietal peritoneum which can be done with a continuous suture (Figure 2.39)—the interrupted suture of the fascia is preferred (Figure 2.40) as there is a greater tendency toward dehiscence.

With regard to the abdominal rectus muscles, Michael Stark holds that the muscular venters must not be sutured. A study conducted by the same author has highlighted how, in this procedure, a simplification of the intervention and a reduction in surgical duration does not result in an increase in morbidity and in postsurgical pain [65]. In the technique according to Stark the intervention is completed by suturing the subcutaneous tissue and skin with three Donati stitches; four Allis clamps are applied on the skin edges and are removed after 5–7 minutes (Figure 2.41).

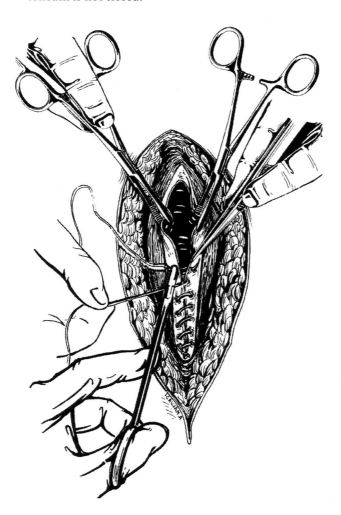

Figure 2.39 Continued suture of the visceral peritoneum in the longitudinal laparotomy.

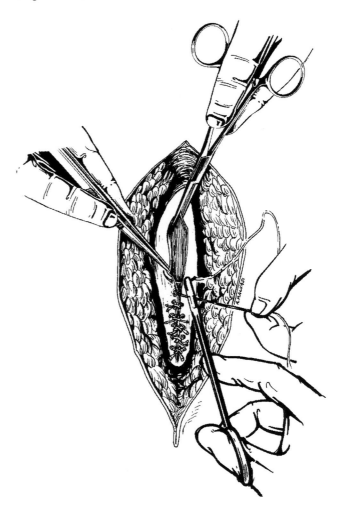

Figure 2.40 Apposition of the abdominal muscles in the course of the longitudinal laparotomy.

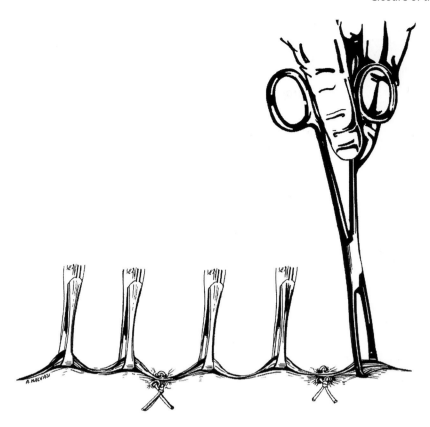

Figure 2.41 In cesarean delivery using the Stark technique, the intervention ends by suturing the subcutaneous tissue and skin with three Donati points; four Allis clamps are then applied on the skin edges, which are subsequently removed after 5–7 minutes.

The usefulness of subcutaneous tissue closure has been reassessed. Studies conducted on animals, in fact, had led to the belief that closure of the Camper fascia with the addition of extraneous materials might predispose the wound to infections and facilitate postsurgical dehiscence. However, literature has not confirmed this experimental data: there are no clinical studies on humans that have substantiated this hypothesis [69].

Not closing the Camper fascia instead might result in an increased risk of seroma and hematomas, as well as facilitate superficial wound dehiscence. From this point of view, pregnancies, due to the vascularization and edema of tissues, are at particular risk. Moreover, pathologies such as preeclampsia may increase the deposit of extracellular fluids and predispose the patient to a hemorrhagic diathesis.

A randomized clinical trial was carried out on 438 patients in whom the nonclosure of subcutaneous tissue was compared to synthesis by means of continuous suture with absorbable suture material. Closure of the fascia Camper proved to be better as it is associated with a lower incidence of wound dehiscence [70].

Similar studies have been conducted on obese patients, well known to be at risk of dehiscence of the laparotomy scar [71]. Results have shown how, even in this instance, closure of the subcutaneous tissue reduces the incidence of wound dehiscence, seroma formation, and infections.

Cochrane Library reviewers have also contributed their opinion on this matter [72]. Seven trials were analyzed, in which 2056 patients underwent a cesarean section. The intent of the review was to highlight differences in postsurgical outcomes, both short and long term, in relation to

- Different techniques used for the stitching of the muscle layer
- Closure or nonclosure of the Camper fascia
- Different surgical techniques and materials employed in the suturing of the Camper fascia

The results show that

- The risk of hematoma and seroma is reduced with the closure of the Camper fascia.
- The overall risk of parietal complications (hematomas, seromas, infections, dehiscence) is also reduced with the suturing of the subcutaneous adipose tissue.
- There was no difference in the incidence of parietal infections.
- There are no long-term data available.
- There are no studies available regarding different techniques or suture material used for the closure of the muscle layer or Camper fascia.

The reviewers therefore came to the conclusion that the closure of the Camper fascia reduces parietal complications. Given what we currently know, it can be stated that the closure of the subcutaneous tissue, even though surgical durations are somewhat lengthened, should be recommended as it has significant advantages, especially in obese patients. It is, however, difficult, in light of how few studies are found in literature, to pass judgment on skin suturing methods.

A Cochrane Library review studied the effects of techniques and suturing materials used for cutaneous synthesis and the time needed to complete these techniques [73]. A single randomized study was selected by the authors: the closure of the skin with staples was compared to intradermal suture with absorbable material [74]. Although surgical durations were shorter in the first method, the intradermal suture reduced the postsurgical pain and had better aesthetic results.

Due to the limited information currently available, the best method for skin closure after a cesarean delivery cannot be conclusively determined.

The Cochrane Library has published a review on the topic of parietal drain [75]. The purpose of the study was to determine the effects of parietal drain and to compare the different types of drain. Seven studies were chosen in which 1993 patients underwent a cesarean delivery. These were the results:

- The use of drainages did not determine any differences in the risk of infection, febrile morbidity, and endometritis.
- There is some evidence that indicates that when drainage is not used, the cesarean delivery is shortened by 5 minutes and that there might be a slight decrease in blood loss.

The reviewers therefore concluded that

- There is no evidence that the regular use of parietal drainage is beneficial to patients who undergo a cesarean delivery.
- In light of the limited number of selected studies, it cannot be determined whether drainage is useful when hemostasis is deemed insufficient.
- There is no data on which type of drainage is best.

CONCLUSIONS

Every surgical procedure is composed of hundreds of movements, every gesture has a purpose, meaning and history. It is important to examine each phase of every intervention in order to determine its necessity and effectiveness in relation to its purpose… [15].

With these words spoken at the World Congress of Obstetrics and Gynaecology in 1994, Michael Stark introduced a new type of cesarean delivery, which soon became known as the "cesarean delivery according to Stark."

This technique, based on the stretching philosophy, has undeniable advantages, but also disadvantages, which must be carefully assessed during the surgical choice. In this regard, it must be stressed how the limited visibility of the pelvis may be a reason to choose traditional techniques, especially in an emergency situation or when wide exposure of the operating field is needed, such as for anomalies in the fetus, twin pregnancy, or fetal macrosomia.

The aesthetic outcome should not be underestimated, as the Joel-Cohen incision is higher on the abdominal wall compared to the Pfannenstiel incision. The Michael Stark technique, in which a lower cutaneous incision is performed, is currently being used to overcome this problem.

The advantages of the cesarean delivery according to Stark, mainly due to rapid execution and to better results in terms of maternal morbidity, suggest that this technique may become more common in the future.

The ideal laparotomy is chosen by the surgeon to achieve an optimal incision, easy fetal extraction and rapid suture of the uterus.

Currently transverse laparotomies are commonly used during cesarean deliveries, even in repeated ones [76]. Longitudinal laparotomies are reserved for repeated laparotomies or for special cases, as in the presence of myomas or pathological placentation, or for combined interventions, as later hernias and laparocele ventral hernias are more frequent [77].

Until 20 years ago the preferred transverse laparotomy, among those who practised cesarean deliveries, was the Pfannenstiel [78]. This method has been modified in an attempt to lower the transverse incision and therefore achieve a more aesthetic result. At times, the Pfannenstiel overlaps with the Kustner laparotomy, which is more widely used in gynecological interventions. The low incision of the skin results in a greater upward detachment of the muscle fascia layer. In the Pfannenstiel laparotomy this inevitably involves perforator vessels, branches of the superficial epigastric artery, which may cause hemostasis and resulting complications.

In obese patients and in the presence of associated uterine pathologies, for example myomas, the Cherney or Maylard incision can occasionally be performed, with transverse delivery of the abdominal wall muscles [77,79]. However, the Joel-Cohen laparotomy has become more common. This laparotomy consists of a central incision of the subcutaneous tissue along a front and upper transiliac line, which falls below the arched line—that is, in the area in which the rear fascia of the rectus muscles is particularly thin [80].

Performing a central incision at this level makes it possible to perform a mid-lateral separation of the tissues of the abdominal wall without the need for excessive incisions, as is the case for the Pfannenstiel laparotomy [81]. The stretching of tissues also results in the mid-lateral separation of the vascular branches of the superficial epigastric arteries, which usually remain intact up to the end of the laparotomy. An incision at this level also allows for hysterotomy and fetal extraction without the use of retractors, along with suture and uterine externalization. Furthermore, a common practice is to not suture the parietal peritoneum or muscles and, generally, to fit together skin and subcutaneous tissue with two or three stitches [81–88].

An always more frequent problem, especially in industrialized countries, is the cesarean delivery in obese and diabetic patients, and their outcome. In these cases it is preferable to perform a fascia suture with separate stitches to avoid dehiscence and postsurgical laparocele ventral hernias. Another problem in these patients is the healing of the fatty subcutaneous tissue, for which some believe it is useful to add surgical drains in the subcutaneous tissue. Some authors believe that in these patients it is unnecessary to perform a multilayer stitch of the subcutaneous tissue, rather it is sufficient to fit together the edges of the Cooper fascia, especially evident in obese patients, without significant hematomas, adiponecrosis, or dehiscence. Skin suturing did not show any difference among the various techniques, including conventional sutures and staples [89].

REFERENCES

1. Pfannenstiel J. Ueber die vorteile des suprasymhysaeren fascien-querschnitt fuer die gynaecologishe koliotomien, zugleich ein beitrag zu der indikationsstellung der operationswege. *Samml. Klin, Vort. (Nevefolge) Gynaek.* No. 68–98 (*Klin. Vort. N.F.* No. 268, Gynaek. No. 1900; 97).
2. Mowat J, Bonnar J. Abdominal wound dehiscence after Caesarean delivery. *Br Med J* 1971;2:256–7.
3. Wall PD, Deucy EE, Glantz JC, Pressman EK. Vertical skin incisions and wound complications in the obese parturient. *Obstet Gynecol* 2003;102:952–6.
4. Houston MC, Raynor BD. Postoperative morbidity obese parturient woman: Supraumbilical and low transverse abdominal approaches. *Am J Gynecol* 2000;182:1033–5.
5. Ayers JW, Morley GW. Surgical incision for caesarean section. *Obstet Gynecol* 1987;70:706–8.
6. Finan MA, Mastrogiannis DS, Spellacy WN. The Allis test for easy caesarean delivery. *Am J Obstet Gynecol* 1991;164:772–5.
7. Briggs R, Chari RS, Mercer B, Sibai B. Postoperative incision complications after caesarean delivery in patients with antepartum syndrome of haemolysis, elevated liver enzymes, and low platelets (HELLP): Does delayed primary closure make a difference? *Am J Obstet Gynecol* 1996;175:893.
8. Haeri AD. Comparison of transverse and vertical skin incisions for caesarean section. *S Afr Med J* 1976;52:3.
9. Mackenrodt A. Die radikaloperation des gebarmutterscheidenkerebes mit. Ausraumung des Bekens. *Verh Dtsch Gynakol* IX:139, 1901. In: A cura di: Hg Robert. *Noveau Traité de technique chirurgicale. L'incision trasversale avec deliverydes droits.* Tome XIV Gynecologie. 3° Edit. Paris, France: Masson; 197757–8.
10. Maylard AE. Direction of abdominal incision. *Br Med J* 1907;2:895.
11. Cerney LS. A modified transverse incision for low abdominal operation. *Surg Gynecol Obstet* 1940;72:92.
12. O'Grady JP, Veronikis DK, Chervenak FA, McCullough LB, Kanaan CM, Tilson JL. Caesarean delivery. In: O'Grady JP, Gimovsky ML eds. *Operative Obstetrics.* Baltimore, MD: Williams and Wilkins; 1995: 239–87.
13. Giacalone PL, Daures JP, Vignal J, Herisson C, Hedon B, Laffargue F. Pfannenstiel versus Maylard incision for caesarean delivery: A randomized controlled trial. *Obstet Gynecol* 2002;99:745–50.
14. Joel-Cohen S. *Abdominal and Vaginal Hysterectomy. New Technique Based on Time and Motion Studies.* London, UK: W. Heineman, Medical Books; 1972:170.
15. Stark M. Technique of Caesarean section: The Misgav Ladach method. In: Popkin DR, Peddle LJ. eds. *Women's Health Today: Perspectives on Current Research and Clinical Practice. Proceedings of the XIV F.I.G.O. World Congress of Gynecology and Obstetrics,* Montreal, September 1994. New York, NY: Parthenon; 1994:81–85.
16. Stark M, Chavkin Y, Kupfersztain C, Guedj P, Finkel AR. Evaluation of combinations of procedures in cesarean section. *Int J Gynecol* 1995;48:273–6.
17. Franchi M, Ghezzi F, Raio L, Di Naro E, Miglierina M, Agosti M, Bolis P. Joel-Cohen or Pfannenstiel incision at cesarean delivery: Does it make a difference? *Acta Obstet Gynecol Scand* 2002;81:1040–6.
18. Stark M, Finkel AR. Comparison between the Joel-Cohen and Pfannenstiel incisions in caesarean section. *Eur J Obstet Gynecol Reprod Biol* 1994;53:121–2.
19. Darj E, Nordstrom ML. The Misgav Ladach method for caesarean delivery compared to the Pfannenstiel method. *Acta Obstet Gynecol Scand* 1999;78:37–41.
20. Wallin G, Fall O. Modified Joel-Cohen technique for caesarean delivery. *Br J Obstet Gynaecol* 1999; 106:221–6.
21. Mathai M, Ambersheth S, George A. Comparison of two transverse abdominal incisions for caesarean delivery. *Int J Gynaecol Obstet* 2002;78:47–9.
22. Ferrari AG, Frigerio LG, Candotti G, Buscaglia M, Petrone M, Taglioretti A, Calori G. Can Joel-Cohen incision and single layer reconstruction reduce caesarean delivery morbidity? *Int J Gynaecol Obstet* 2001;72:135–43.
23. Bjorklund K, Kimaro M, Urassa E, Lindmark G. Introduction of the Misgav Ladach caesarean delivery at an African tertiary centre: A randomised controlled trial. *Br J Obstet Gynaecol* 2000;107:209–16.
24. Myerscough PR. Caesarean section: Sterilization: Hysterectomy. In: Myerscough PR, ed. *Munro Kerr's Operative Obstetrics,* 10th ed. London, UK: Balliere Tindall; 1982:295–319.
25. World Health Organization (WHO)/United Nations Population Fund (UNFPA)/UNICEF/World Bank. *Managing Complications in Pregnancy and Childbirth: A Guide for Midwives and Doctors.* Geneva, Switzerland: WHO; 2000.
26. Kendall SW, Brennan TG, Guillou PJ. Suture length to wound length ratio and the integrity of midline and lateral paramedian incisions. *Br J Surg* 1991;78:705–7.
27. Kustner O. Der suprasymphysare kreuzschnitt, eine methode der coeliotomie bei wenig umfanglichen affektioen der weiblichen bekenorgane. *Monatsschr*

Geburtsh Gynakol 1896;4:197. In: A cura di: I. Vandelli C. A. Bruno, *Chirurgia Ginecologica ed Ostetrica. Semeiotica e Tecnica Operatoria.* Vol. II, Cap.: 7. Ediz. Roma: CIC; 1983:335–40.

28. Nichols DH. Incisioni. In: A cura di: DH. Nichols, *Chirurgia Ginecologica ed Ostetrica.* (Ediz. Ital. A. Ferrari); Roma: CIC, Ediz. Internaz.; 1995:156.
29. Novak F. Pfannenstiel bassa. (Tecniche operatorie laparotomiche). In: *Tecniche Chirurgiche Ginecologiche.*, Padova: Piccin Nuova Libraria S.p.a; 1998:212–4.
30. Stark M, Joel-Cohen S. Evaluation of alternative procedure for caesarean delivery. *XIII World Congress of Gynecology and Obstetrics; Int J Gynecol Obstet* 1991; Abstract 1701.
31. Turner-Warwick R. The functional anatomy of the urethra. In: Droller MJ, ed. *The Surgical Management of Urologic Disease.* St. Louis, MO: Mosby-Year Book; 1992.
32. Malinas J, Payan R, Malinas Y. 94 observations d'incision sous-pubienne selon S.M. Pandolfo. *Rev. Fr. Gynéc. Obstét.* 1977;72 (11):413–5.
33. Mouchel J. Incision transversale transrectale en pratique gynécologique et obstétricale. 673 observations. *Nouv Press Med* 1981;10(6):413–5.
34. Racinet C, Favier M. Technique. *La césarienne: Indications, techniques, complications.* Chapter 5. Paris, France: Masson Edit; 1984:55–63.
35. Chow KK. Passaggi operativi in dettaglio. Eseguire un'apertura addominale. Evoluzione dell'incisione cutanea. In: *Il taglio cesareo: Sicurezza, costo e benefici.* Roma, Italy: CIC Ediz Ital; 1996:12–13, 14–33, 148–162.
36. Ferrari A, Frigerio L, Origoni M, Candotti G, Mariani A, Petrone M. Modified Stark procedure for caesarean section. *Pelvic Surg* 1996;5:239–44.
37. Malvasi A, Traina V, Baldini D, Caringella G, Totaro P. The modified Joel-Cohen laparotomy in caesarean delivery by Stark. In: Pachì A. ed. *Medicina Fetale '97,* Rome, Italy: CIC Edit Intern; 1997:325–35.
38. Malvasi A, Totaro P, Casiero I, Traina V. Repeat caesarean section: Joel-Cohen or Pfannenstiel laparotomy? *IInd International Congress on Controversies in Obstetrics and Gynecology.* Rome, Italy: CIC Edit Intern; 1999:145–9.
39. Ansaloni L, Brundisini R, Morino G, Kiura A. Prospective, randomized, comparative study of Misgav Ladach versus traditional caesarean delivery at Nazareth Hospital, Kenya. *World J Surg* 2001;25:1164–72.
40. Moreira P, Moreau Jc, Faye Me, Ka S, Kane Gueye Sm, Faye Eo, Dieng T, Diadhaiou F. Comparison of caesarean techniques: Classic versus Misgav Ladach caesarean. *J Gynecol Obstet Biol Reprod* 2002;31:572–6.
41. Stark M. The Misgav Ladach method for caesarean section. *Atti del LXXII Congr SIGO, XXXVII Congr AOGOI, IV Congr.* S.R.L. Firenze: AGUI; Scientific Press Edit; 1996:177–81.
42. Gigliotti B, Bennici S, Capotorto A et al. Taglio cesareo rapido secondo Stark. Risultati di un gruppo di studio italiano su 1356 interventi. *Atti del LXXII Congr SIGO, XXXVII Congr AOGOI, IV Congr.* S.R.L. Firenze: AGUI; Scientific Press Edit; 1996: 1059–63.
43. Lorentzen U, Philipsen JP, Langhoff-Roos J, Hornnes PJ. Surgical technique in caesarean section. Evidence or tradition? *Ugeskr Laeger* 1998;20:2517–20.
44. Holmgren G, Sjoholm L, Stark M. The Misgav Ladach method for caesarean delivery: Method description. *Acta Obstet Gynecol Scand* 1999;78:615–21.
45. Lazarov L, Mangurova S, Koleva I, Tsankova V, Naidenova S, Lazarova G. Gynecological interventions and caesarean delivery without suturing of the peritoneum (visceral and parietal). *Akush Ginekol* 1999;38:20–22.
46. Popiela A, Panszczyk M, Korzeniewski J, Baranowski W. Comparative clinical analysis of caesarean delivery technique by Misgav Ladach method and Pfannenstiel method. *Ginecol Pol* 2000;71:255–7.
47. Zienkowicz Z, Suchocki S, Sleboda H, Bojarski M. Caesarean delivery by the Misgav Ladach with the abdominal opening surgery by Joel-Cohen method. *Ginekol Pol* 2000;7:284–7.
48. Gaucherand P, Bessai K, Sergeant P, Rudigoz RC. Towards simplified caesarean section. *J Gynecol Obstet Biol Reprod* 2001;30:348–52.
49. Grignaffini A, Bazzani F, Rinaldi M, Azzoni D, Vadora E. Innovations of the Stark method for caesarean section. Comparison of techniques. *Minerva Ginecol* 1999;51:475–82.
50. Corosu R, Roma B, Marziali M, Di Roberto R. Modifications to the technique of caesarean delivery after Stark. *Minerva Ginecol* 1998;50:391–5.
51. Messalli Em, Cobellis L, Pizerno G. Caesarean delivery according to Stark. *Minerva Ginecol* 2001;53:367–71.
52. Li M, Zou L, Zhu J. Study on modification of the Misgav Ladach method for caesarean section. *J Tongij Med Univ* 2001;21:75–77.
53. Fatusic Z, Kuriak A, Jasarevic E, Hafner T. The Misgav Ladach method: A step forward in operative technique in obstetrics. *J Perinat Med* 2003;31:395–8.
54. Studzinski Z. The Misgav Ladach method for caesarean delivery compared to the Pfannenstiel technique. *Ginekol Pol* 2002;73:672–6.
55. Redlich A, Koppe I. The "gentle caesarean section"— An alternative to the classical way of sectio. A prospective comparison between the classical technique and the method of Misgav Ladach. *Zentralbl Gynakol* 2001;123:638–43.
56. Heidenreich W, Borgmann U. Results of the Misgav Ladach caesarean section. *Zentralbl Gynakol* 2001;123:634–7.
57. Tully L, Gates S, Brocklehust P, Mckenzie-Mcharg K, Ayers S. Surgical techniques used during cesarean delivery operations: Results of a national survey of practice in the UK. *Eur J Obstet Gynecol Reprod Biol* 2002;102:120–6.

58. Oleszczuk J, Leszczynska-Gorzelak B, Michalach B, Pietras G. Delivery of twins by cesarean delivery with the Misgav Ladach method. *Ginekol Pol* 2000;71:1417–21.
59. Katsulov A, Nedialkov K, Koleva ZH et al. The Joel-Cohen (Misgav Ladach) method—A new surgical technique for cesarean delivery and gynaecological laparotomy. *Akush Ginekol* 2000;29(1):10–13.
60. Loong RLC, Rogers MS, Chang AMZ. A controlled trial on wound drainage in caesarean section. *Aust NZJ Obstet Gynecol* 1988;28:266.
61. Ellis H, Heddle R. Does the peritoneum need to be closed at laparotomy? *Br J Surg* 1977;64:733–6.
62. Elkins TE, Stovall TG. A histologic evaluation of peritoneal injury and repair: Implications for adhesion formation. *Obstet Gynecol* 1987;70:225–8.
63. Irion O, Luzuy F, Bèguin F. Nonclosure of the visceral and parietal peritoneum at cesarean section: A randomised controlled trial. *Br J Obstet Gynaecol* 1996;103:690–4.
64. Nagele F, Karas H, Spitzer D. Closure or nonclosure of the visceral peritoneum at cesarean delivery. *Am J Obstet Gynecol* 1996;174:1366–70.
65. Stark M. Adhesion-free cesarean section. *World J Surg* 1992;17:419.
66. Chanrachakul B, Hamontri S, Herabutya Y. A randomized comparison of postcesarean pain between closure and nonclosure of peritoneum. *Eur J Obstet Gynecol Reprod Biol* 2002;101:31–35.
67. Pietrantoni M, Parsons MT, O'Brien WF, Collins E, Knuppel RA, Spellacy WN. Peritoneal closure or nonclosure at cesarean. *Obstet Gynecol* 1991; 77:293–6.
68. Bamigboye AA, Hofmeyr GJ. Closure versus nonclosure of the peritoneum at caesarean section. *Cochrane Database Syst Rev*. 2003;(4):CD000163.
69. Hussain SA. Closure of subcutaneous fat: A prospective randomized trial. *Br J Surg* 1990;77:107.
70. Del Valle GO, Combs P, Qualls C, Curet LB. Does closure of Camper fascia reduce the incidence of post-cesarean superficial wound disruption? *Obstet Gynecol* 1992;80:1013–6.
71. Naumann RW, Hauth JC, Owen J. Subcutaneous tissue approximation in relation to wound disruption after cesarean delivery in obese women. *Obstet Gynecol* 1995;85:412–6.
72. Anderson ER, Gates S. Techniques and materials for closure of the abdominal wall in caesarean section. *Cochrane Database Syst Rev* 2004 October 18;(4):CD004663.
73. Alderdice F, McKenna D, Dornan J. Techniques and materials for skin closure in caesarean delivery (Cochrane review). In: *The Cochrane Library*. Chichester, UK; John Wiley & Sons, Ltd.; Issue 4, 2004.
74. Frishman GN, Schwartz T, Hogan JW. Closure of Pfannenstiel skin incisions. Staples vs. subcuticular suture. *J Reprod Med* 1997;42:627–30.
75. Gates S, Anderson E. Wound drainage for caesarean section. *Cochrane Database Syst Rev* 2005;(1):CD004549.
76. Hofmeyr GJ, Mathai M, Shah A, Novikova N. Techniques for caesarean section. *Cochrane Database Syst Rev* 2008;(1):CD004662.
77. Dodd JM, Anderson ER, Gates S. Surgical techniques for uterine incision and uterine closure at the time of caesarean section. *Cochrane Database Syst Rev* 2008(3):CD004732.
78. Loos MJ, Scheltinga MR, Mulders LG, Roumen RM. The Pfannenstiel incision as a source of chronic pain. *Obstet Gynecol* 2008;111(4):839–46.
79. Nabhan AF. Long-term outcomes of two different surgical techniques for cesarean. *Int J Gynaecol Obstet* 2008100(1):69–75. Epub 2007 October 1.
80. Stark M, Hoyme UB, Stubert B, Kieback D, di Renzo GC. Post-cesarean adhesions—Are they a unique entity? *J Matern Fetal Neonatal Med* 2008; 21(8):513–6.
81. Mathai M, Hofmeyr GJ, Mathai NE. Abdominal surgical incisions for caesarean section. *Cochrane Database Syst Rev* 2007;(1):CD004453.
82. Malvasi A, Tinelli A, Serio G, Tinelli R, Casciaro S, Cavallotti C. Comparison between the use of the Joel-Cohen incision and its modification during Stark's cesarean section. *J Matern Fetal Neonatal Med* 200720(10):757–61.
83. Hofmeyr JG, Novikova N, Mathai M, Shah A. Technique for caesarean section. *Am J Obstet Gynecol* 2009;201(5):431–44.
84. Hudić I, Bujold E, Fatušić Z, Skokić F, Latifagić A, Kapidžić M, Fatušić J. The Misgav-Ladach method of cesarean section: A step forward in operative technique in obstetrics. *Arch Gynecol Obstet* 2012; 286(5):1141–6.
85. Naki MM, Api O, Celik H, Kars B, Yaşar E, Unal O. Comparative study of Misgav-Ladach and Pfannenstiel-Kerr cesarean techniques: A randomized controlled trial. *J Matern Fetal Neonatal Med* 2011;24(2):239–44.
86. Gedikbasi A, Akyol A, Ulker V, Yildirim D, Arslan O, Karaman E, Ceylan Y. Cesarean techniques in cases with one previous cesarean delivery: Comparison of modified Misgav-Ladach and Pfannenstiel-Kerr. *Arch Gynecol Obstet* 2011;283(4):711–6.
87. CORONIS Collaborative Group, Abalos E, Addo V, Brocklehurst P et al. Caesarean delivery surgical techniques (CORONIS): A fractional, factorial, unmasked, randomised controlled trial. *Lancet* 2013;382(9888):234–48.
88. Le Dû R, Bernardini M, Agostini A, Mazouni C, Shojai R, Blanc B, Gamerre M, Bretelle F. Comparative evaluation of the Joel-Cohen cesarean delivery versus the transrectal incision. *J Gynecol Obstet Biol Reprod (Paris)* 2007;36(5):447–50. Epub 2007 February 28.
89. Mackeen AD, Berghella V, Larsen ML. Techniques and materials for skin closure in caesarean section. *Cochrane Database Syst Rev* 2012;11:CD003577. doi:10.1002/14651858.CD003577

FURTHER READING

Belci D, Kos M, Zoricić D, Kuharić L, Slivar A, Begić-Razem E, Grdinić I. Comparative study of the "Misgav Ladach" and traditional Pfannenstiel surgical techniques for cesarean section. *Minerva Ginecol* 2007;59(3):231–40.

Caesarean section: New ideas. *NU News in Health Care Developing Countries*. I.C.H. University Hospital, Uppsala, Sweden, 3/1995 (9):35.

Dahlke JD, Mendez-Figueroa H, Rouse DJ, Berghella V, Baxter JK, Chauhan SP. Evidence based surgery for cesarean delivery: An updated systematic review. *Am J Obstet Gynecol* 2013 March 1. doi:10.1016/j.ajog.2013.02.043.

Galli P, Malvasi A, Di Renzo GC. Metodologia clinica propedeutica alla chirurgia ostetrico-ginecologica convenzionale. In: Di Renzo GC (ed.), *Trattato di Ginecologia ed Ostetricia*, Roma: Verduci Edit. Cap.175; 2133–74. 2009.

Ho Imgren G, Sjoholm L. The Misgav Ladach method of caesarean section: Evolved by Michael Stark in Jerusalem. *Trop Doctor* 1996;26:1–7.

Kulas T, Habek D, Karsa M, Bobić-Vuković M. Modified Misgav Ladach method for cesarean section: Clinical experience. *Gynecol Obstet Invest* 2008;65(4):222–6.

Makoha FW, Fathuddien MA, Felimban HM. Choice of abdominal incision and risk of trauma to the urinary bladder and bowel in multiple caesarean sections. *Eur J Obstet Gynecol Reprod Biol* 2006;125(1):50–3.

Mathai M, Hofmeyr GJ. Abdominal surgical incisions for caesarean section. *Cochrane Database Syst Rev* 2007;(1):CD004453.

Racă AM, Rack R, Cărbunaru O, Munteanu M, Râcă N. Subcutaneous fat tissue drainage in obese pregnant women after caesarean delivery. *Rev Med Chir Soc Med Nat Iasi* 2011;115(2):434–7.

Tixier H, Thouvenot S, Coulange L, Peyronel C, Filipuzzi L, Sagot P, Douvier S. Cesarean delivery in morbidly obese women: Supra o subumbilical transverse incision? *Acta Obstet Gynecol Scand* 2009;88(9):1049–52.

Toledo J, Giron JJ, Dominguez A, Kunnakerry J, Alterkawi A. Laparotomies in gynecology using the Joel-Cohen technique. *Rev Med Univ Navarra* 1981;25:29–32.

Hysterotomies during cesarean delivery

ANTONIO MALVASI, SHILPA NAMBIAR BALAKRISHNAN,
and GIAN CARLO DI RENZO

> …In case of a difficult birth the sides of the woman are cut and from the opening the fetus is extracted…
>
> (Maimonides, 1135–1204)

HISTORICAL NOTES AND EVOLUTION

In the collective imagination, the uterine delivery coincides with the cesarean delivery or abdominal birth. At the beginning of the eighteenth century, fear of infections led doctors to develop techniques that would prevent or at least limit contact between the uterine incision and the peritoneal cavity. One of the solutions was the extraperitoneal cesarean delivery.

This method was used for the first time by Ritgen in 1821, unsuccessfully, as the patient died. Skene was the first to successfully complete this intervention in New York, in 1876. And in 1907 in Cologne, Frank performed 13 interventions that were successful, as the mothers survived. Frank's technique was later improved upon, with excellent results, by Latzko and Sellheim.

In the 1930s, Americans Waters and Norton further perfected that which would become the most used extraperitoneal technique.

The advent of modern chemo-antibiotic therapies has, nowadays, basically eliminated this surgical approach.

Most surgeons, initially, performed a longitudinal (vertical) laparotomy to open the uterine cavity (Figure 3.1) [1].

This approach avoided a dangerous lateral disdelivery and allowed a sufficiently wide opening for safe extraction of the fetus. Among the disadvantages was potentially severe bleeding, the possibility of the incision extending down toward the bladder and vagina, and an increased risk of uterine rupture in later pregnancies.

In 1871 Vincenzo Balocchi described the longitudinal hysterotomy technique in the following manner: "…The uterus is to be cut, layer after layer, until the surface of the egg is reached; then with the left index finger reach between the egg and the internal surface of the uterus and with a rimmed knife cut this viscus, high and low, the same length as the external wound. Once this is done and while the assistants make sure to secure the walls of the venter above it, immediately rupture the membranes and extract the fetus."[2]

The author describes in detail how to cut the abdominal and uterine walls while carefully avoiding the spread of amniotic liquid into the abdominal cavity, as it was thought to cause puerperal infections.

In particular, he describes the opening of the uterus up to the membranes, cut last, the uterine incision of the front side of the uterus (not the fundus) to improve wound healing. Above all he describes bringing the abdominal wall into contact with the uterine wall to avoid the spread of amniotic liquid into the abdominal cavity (Figure 3.2).

The longitudinal hysterotomy was certainly a further step forward in the cesarean delivery technique, especially compared to the Porro method. As Gall wrote, "As powerful and ingenious as Porro's contribution was to the development of the surgical technique, utero-ovarian amputation was not the ideal method—as Schroerer correctly defined it—as it was a transition between the traditional Caesarean delivery and one that belonged to a distant future" [3].

In 1882 Kehrer envisaged the possibility of a low transverse incision at the level of the internal cervical orifice. He believed that a hysterotomy performed at this level would improve morbidity due to the anteflexion tendency of the uterus.

Kehrer thus described the low transverse incision on the lower uterine segment, which is still today accurate: "The low transverse incision of the uterus also allows for a smaller cut of the abdominal wall compared to the traditional method, which required a longer incision, as the uterine body had to be cut higher. Benefits of a small incision are evident: intestinal loops do not occupy the operating zone and the peritoneum is less exposed and, consequently, less subject to cooling and mechanical irritation" [4].

After a lengthy debate between Sanger and Kehrer, Sanger was able to publish the innovative hysterotomic technique in 1881 before Kehrer [5].

The Kehrer incision did not become as popular as the Fritsch incision, in which a transverse hysterotomy was performed on the uterine fundus; the subsequent development of this technique constituted a fundamental improvement in modern cesarean delivery techniques.

In 1926 Kerr popularized the transverse incision on the lower uterine segment, as opposed to the higher traditional incision [6].

Kerr primarily introduced this method with the aim of decreasing uterine ruptures in subsequent pregnancies, but he was also convinced that compared to the low vertical incision, there was a reduction in blood loss, breach infection, and bladder lacerations.

Many surgeons had previously proposed this technique at the end of the eighteenth and beginning of the nineteenth centuries, but only after Kerr's publication did the method gain in popularity and become widely used up to the present day [1].

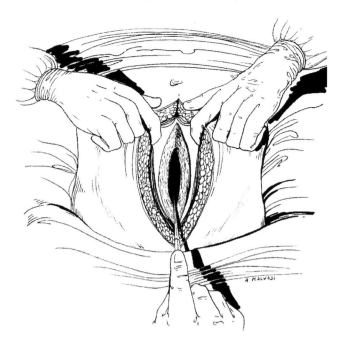

Figure 3.1 Traditional vertical incision of the uterus at full-term pregnancy.

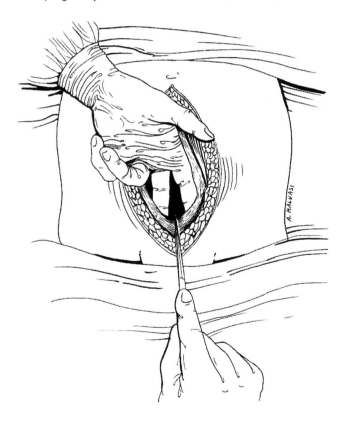

Figure 3.2 Longitudinal incision of the anterior wall along its entire surface which reaches the membranes. The membranes used to be cut only after the abdominal wall was set against the uterine wall to avoid amniotic fluid from "contaminating" the abdominal cavity, as it was erroneously believed at the time that this would result in an infection of the peritoneum.

Current hysterotomic techniques

The first phase of any hysterotomy is the exposure of the uterine viscus that will be cut.

The lateral walls can be widened with lateral valves, an orthostatic retractor, or simply, with a suprapubic valve.

In the past when cesarean deliveries were performed under general anesthesia, the surgeon could use the Trendelenburg position to keep the intestinal loops from the operating field. Conversely, with the current use of regional anesthesia techniques, the Trendelenburg position is not used during a cesarean delivery, because it is the second operator that, if necessary, keeps the intestinal loops from the surgical field.

Miyabe and Sato have shown that, during a cesarean delivery, the Trendelenburg position, compared to the traditional supine decubitus, is likewise not effective against sudden cases of arterial hypotension linked to spinal anesthesia [7].

Conversely, Setayesh et al. have shown that in elective cesarean deliveries the Trendelenburg position increases the onset and spreading to the spine of "single-shot" epidural anesthesia [8].

Once the operating field is adequately exposed it is best to not apply protective abdominal pads, as they are not deemed necessary and there is a risk of them not being removed.

In this regard, Stark, in describing the Misgav Ladach method, has repeatedly demonstrated that the use of laparotomy pads is not only useless but is also potentially harmful for at least two reasons: the possibility of leaving them in the abdomen, and their "abrasive" effect on the peritoneal surface, which predisposes to postsurgical intraperitoneal adherences [9]. In fact, in Stark's review of the literature, he cites Down's studies on the foreign-body effect of laparotomy pads [10,11] while he also refers to Larsen's studies on the antibacterial properties of amniotic fluid [12,13].

Harrigill et al., with regard to the presence of amniotic fluid in the abdominal cavity during a cesarean delivery, have shown that in cesarean deliveries after 37 weeks, irrigating with 500–1000 mL of normal saline versus nonirrigation does not statistically affect maternal morbidity [14].

In certain cases, however, laparotomy gauze can be used after it is dampened with saline solution and, in particular, after securing it to the operating field to prevent it from being left in the abdomen. If pads, however, are placed in the abdomen, two are more than sufficient and can be placed laterally, starting from the exclusion of the right paracolic gutter, continuing above the hysterotomy and ending with the left paracolic gutter [15].

However, the application of laparotomy gauze in the abdomen has not yet been codified in the technical description of cesarean delivery and remains an individual choice (Figure 3.3). Any uterine rotation must be detected and corrected to avoid an asymmetrical incision of the wall, so that the prevesical visceral serosa can be cut and downwardly detached to better expose the lower uterine segment.

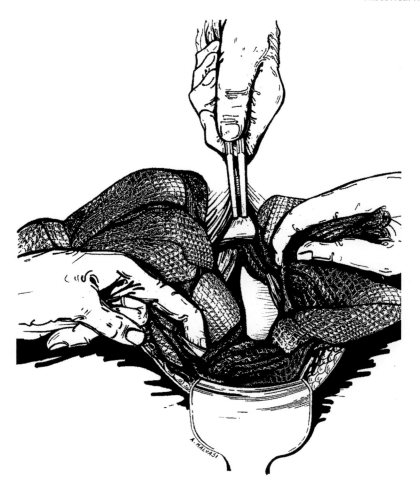

Figure 3.3 Two laparotomy gauzes are applied in the paracolic–uterine gutters; one is applied before the incision of the vesicouterine plica followed by another applied before the incision of the uterine wall.

The incision of the vesicouterine fold must take into account the anatomical characteristics of the lower uterine segment. In fact, differences can be observed in fold detachment in elective cesarean deliveries compared to emergency cesarean deliveries.

In the first elective cesarean delivery, the lower uterine segment has not completed the anatomical modification of its anterior uterine portion. As a result, the "detachable" area of the vesicouterine fold is smaller and in a low position so that consequently the surgical detachment is difficult and, if performed close to the adherence area to the uterus of the visceral peritoneum, may frequently cause bleeding from the lower uterine segment or from the prevesical vessels.

In these cases, to avoid loose cellular tissue infiltration from the fold, it is preferable to carry out hemostasis with a Moynihan clamp by placing a free thread around the vascular mouth (Figure 3.4).

In a cesarean delivery with advanced cervical expansion and pregnant woman in labor, the vesicouterine fold is clearly visible and can be easily detached from the lower uterine segment by blunt disdelivery with Mayo scissors and/or by finger fracture (Figures 3.5 through 3.7). In case of cesarean delivery, once the expansion is complete, the fold is edematous and is accompanied by transudate in the vesicouterine space, which, before the incision, is drained with a laparotomy pad or aspirator.

In this case the fold is positioned above the uterus, next to the dome of the bladder and in a high position due to the extension of the anterior wall of the uterine segment and the subsequent expansion and leveling of the cervix. For this reason the parietal peritoneum must be cut in a higher position to avoid accidental lesions to the bladder.

Before performing the hysterotomy make sure that the vesical catheter is well positioned and that the urinary bladder has been emptied so that dangerous complications are avoided. In case of obstructed labor with Bandl's ring, the fold may be in a higher position, so the incision must be placed correctly to avoid infamous vesical lesions [16].

In this regard Racinet and Favier wrote: "Keep in mind the vesical risk, especially when the intervention is carried out during labour: locating the urachus is rather useful: when one is on the urachus one cannot be on the bladder.... The incision must be carried out decisively, without hesitation. It involves various layers, since the

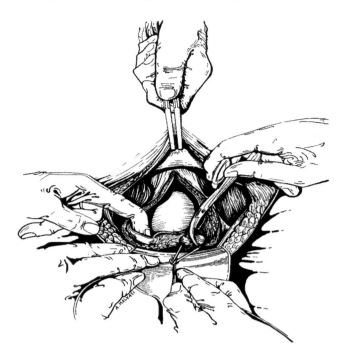

Figure 3.4 Forcipressure and ligation of a prevesical vessel during the opening of the peritoneal peritoneum at the level of the prevesical space (Retzius space).

serosa is located in different layers due to the gravidic edema. A hesitant incision will meet these successive layers" [15].

During a repeated cesarean delivery the vesicouterine fold is usually tightly adherent to the anterior side of the lower uterine segment. Frequently they constitute a single entity: Phipps et al. have reported 42 vesical lesions on thousands of cesarean deliveries (incidence 0.28%), even though the only significant risk factor seems to be the previous cesarean delivery (67% versus 32%, $p < 0.01$) [17].

In case of severe intraperitoneal adhesion, some authors believe that the extraperitoneal cesarean delivery technique may be useful. This is however limited to the surgeon's degree of familiarity with the technique [18], because it requires that the bladder be isolated and downwardly detached outside of the peritoneal cavity.

Ezechi et al. [19] have observed that there is less bleeding from the transverse incision when uterine externalization is achieved after the fetal extraction. In case of iterative cesarean delivery, the detachment layer between the uterine segment wall and the dome of the bladder (normally tightly adherent to each other) must be located and the bladder pushed downward, staying away from both prevesical and newly formed vessels.

Generally, during detachment of the fold, a part of the anterior side of the lower uterine segment is slightly exposed, sufficiently enough for the subsequent hysterorrhaphy with hemostasis.

In fact in the case of anomalous bleeding, which requires more free space, it is preferable to push the fold down away

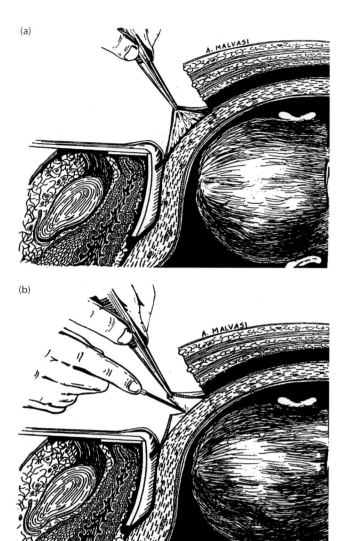

Figure 3.5 The vesicouterine plica is held by forceps, lifted (sagittal section in [a]), and cut with a scalpel blade (sagittal section in [b]).

from the dome of the bladder to facilitate hemostasis without the risk of accidentally including part of the dome of the bladder in the uterine suture (Figure 3.8).

When performing a cesarean delivery, some surgeons, instead, do not consider it practical to cut only the peritoneal fold, or to leave it open, but consider it useful to suture both the uterine muscle and the peritoneal serosa in a single layer (*mass closuring* technique).

In light of the above, the vesicouterine fold can be isolated and detached in several ways. However, each of the described methods, while taking into account variables tied to tradition, training, and preference of the surgeon, are logical and surgically valid, as long as the detachment area between uterus and bladder is located.

For these reasons the vesicouterine fold can be lifted with surgical clamps in different points, in order to locate the most detachable area of the uterus (Figure 3.9).

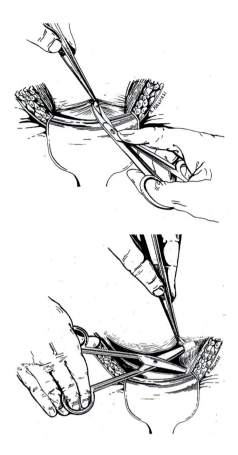

Figure 3.6 Vesicouterine plica held by forceps, (a) incision with Mayo scissors, and (b) leftward extension of the visceral peritoneal incision.

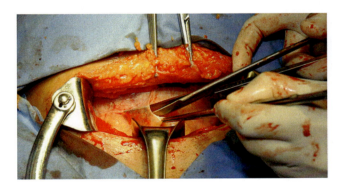

Figure 3.7 The vesicouterine plica is detached through blunt dissection by widening the outer, noncutting edge of Mayo scissors.

The fold can then be cut with a scalpel (Figure 3.10) being careful to point the scalpel blade upward, or it can be clamped and cut with Mayo scissors (Figure 3.5).

Some obstetricians, especially during an emergency, prefer to cut the visceral peritoneum together with the lower uterine segment without performing preliminary surgery (Figure 3.11).

After incision of the visceral peritoneum a finger fracture detachment of the vesicouterine fold can be performed

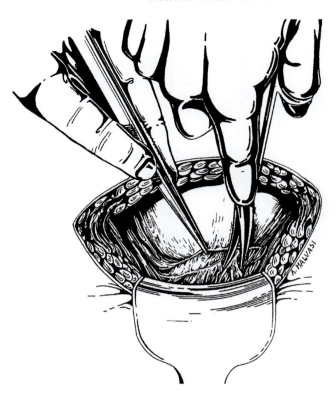

Figure 3.8 The vesicouterine plica adheres to the lower uterine segment, due to a previous cesarean delivery, and is detached with Mayo scissors.

in the mid-lateral direction (Figure 3.12). If detachment by finger fracture of the vesicouterine fold is difficult to carry out, laparotomy gauze or a swab on a clamp can be used (Figures 3.13 and 3.14).

Generally, the vesicouterine fold is compressed by the lower abdominal valve so as to have more room in the uterine incision area. This is especially true if the uterine incision is performed in the lower part of the anterior wall of the lower uterine segment (Figure 3.15).

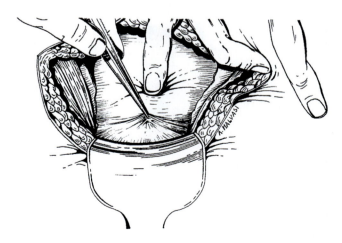

Figure 3.9 Forceps are used on the vesicouterine plica to locate the best detachment area.

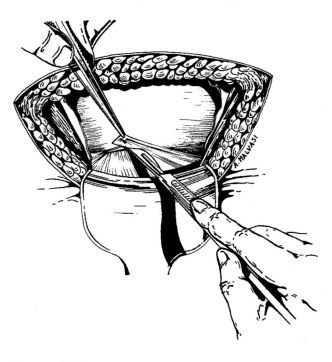

Figure 3.10 The vesicouterine plica is held by forceps and is cut with a scalpel blade.

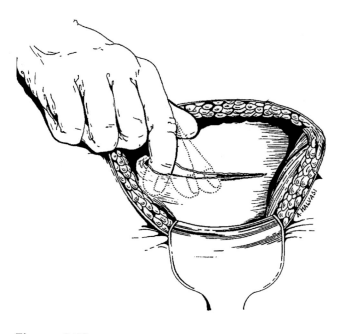

Figure 3.12 Digital detachment of the vesicouterine plica from the external side of the lower uterine segment.

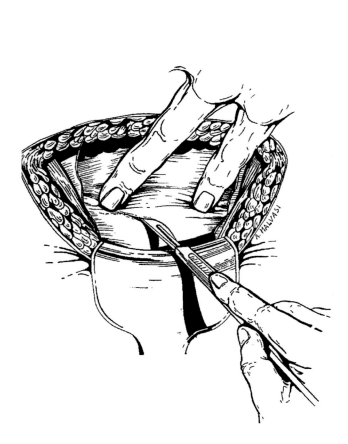

Figure 3.11 Direct incision with a scalpel blade of the visceral peritoneum and of the lower uterine segment without detaching the plica.

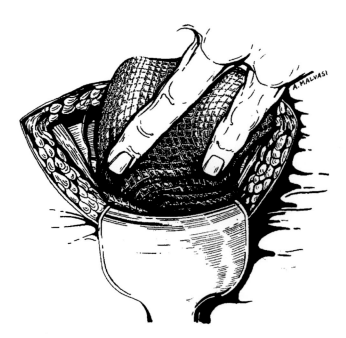

Figure 3.13 Downward detachment of the vesicouterine plica with the help of a laparotomy pad.

The placenta must first be located by ultrasound scanning before starting the intervention in order to, if possible, avoid encountering it during the hysterotomy [20,21], as previously described (Figure 3.16) by Denhez et al. [20] and Boehm et al. [21].

Once the anterior part of the placenta of the lower uterine segment is located, even when not previa, to prevent accidental iatrogenic fetal lesions safety surgical maneuvers must be performed to reduce bleeding from the

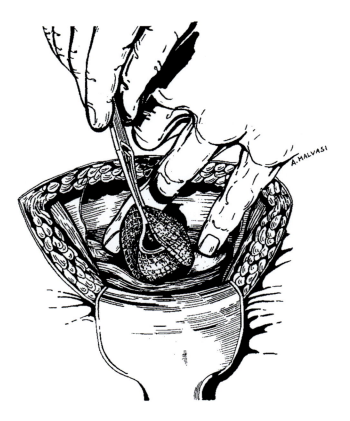

Figure 3.14 Downward detachment of the vesicouterine plica that adheres to the lower uterine segment, using a swab mounted on ring forceps.

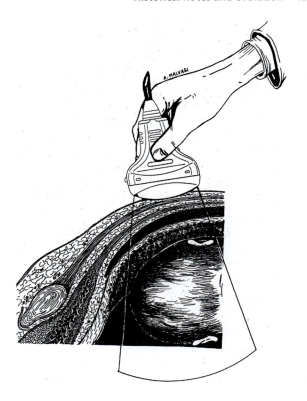

Figure 3.16 A transabdominal convex ultrasound probe is used to locate the placenta in relation to the lower uterine segment before the cesarean delivery is performed.

incision, which is already highly vascularized by the placental bed.

These techniques, though operator dependent, require some common surgical measures.

Some prefer a central incision on the lower uterine segment without marking a preventive line. This is true especially for varix that, if cut and bleeding, "hide" and make it difficult to continue the hysterotomy.

During the incision any bleeding from the placental bed can be controlled by the surgeon or second operator with laparotomy gauze pressed on the hemorrhagic vessels, or by draining blood with an aspirator placed on the edges of the incision (Figure 3.17).

In both cases this avoids an incision being carried out blindly, especially when the lower uterine segment is somewhat thick, as in elective cesarean deliveries.

The hysterotomy continues progressively until reaching the last thin layer of myometrium before the membranes: at this point, after reducing blood loss from the breach it is recommended to penetrate the uterine cavity strongly with the index finger, thus completing the hysterotomy by blunt disdelivery in a bloodless manner to avoid fetal lesions (Figure 3.18).

In studying accidental fetal lesions that occur during cesarean deliveries, Okaro and Anya report a 0.55% frequency and link these to the surgical technique employed during the hysterotomy [22].

Other safety maneuvers that can be performed during a hysterotomy include the blunt use of the opposite end of the scalpel so that during a hysterotomy the membranes can be identified (Figure 3.19). However, if it is difficult to widen the uterine breach with fingers, the index and middle fingers of the left hand (if the operator is right-handed) can be placed under the uterine wall to cut and the incision can be extended with Mayo scissors (Figure 3.20).

Before a hysterotomy it is, however, always important to control the fetal position by touch.

The type of incision depends on numerous factors such as position and size of the fetus, location of the placenta,

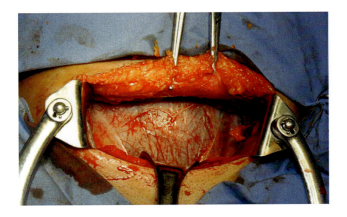

Figure 3.15 Exposure of the lower uterine segment.

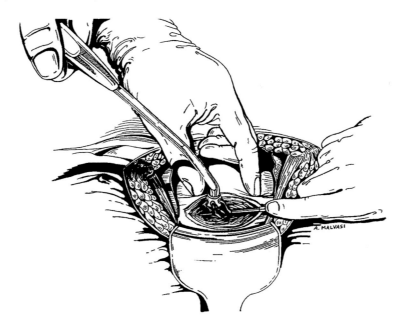

Figure 3.17 Central incision of the uterine breach: the second operator uses the aspirator to drain any excess blood while the first surgeon performs the incision.

presence of fibrous tumors, and development of the lower uterine segment.

In light of the above, an important consideration is the wideness (width) of the hysterotomy so that the fetus can be extracted without trauma.

Iffy and Pantages describe two cases in New Jersey of Erb's palsy that occurred during a cesarean delivery: one occurred after the manual repositioning of the head after the forceps and ventouse failed, the other occurred during an elective cesarean delivery with numerous adherences

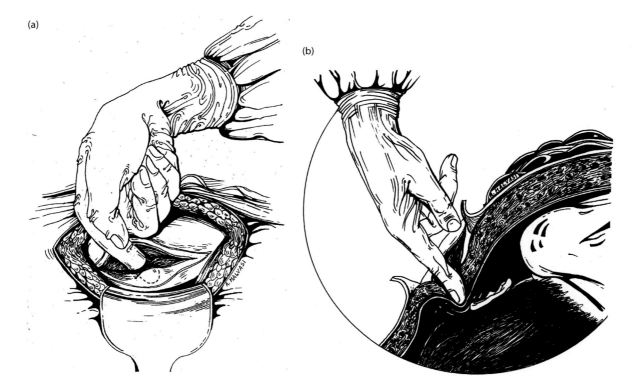

Figure 3.18 (a and b) Opening of the uterine breach: the index finger penetrates to the last layer of the myometrium and reaches the amniochorial membranes.

Historical notes and evolution 47

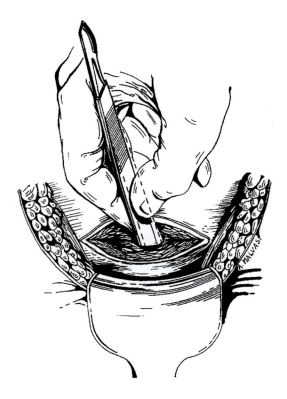

Figure 3.19 The tail end of the scalpel is used to open the uterine breach along its last layer and next to the amniochorial membranes.

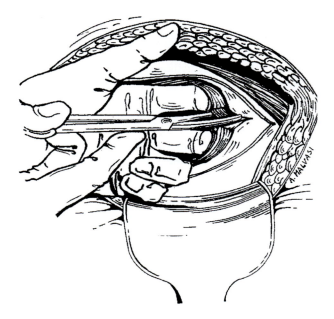

Figure 3.20 If, after the central incision is completed, the surgeon deems the lower uterine segment to be too thick for it to be opened digitally, he will laterally extend the incision using Mayo scissors and will protect the presenting part with the index and middle fingers of the other hand inserted below the incision area.

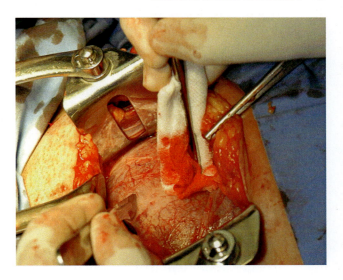

Figure 3.21 Initial phase of the transverse incision of the lower uterine segment and detachment of the visceral peritoneum from the segment itself.

and small uterine breach [23]. Dessolle et al. have shown that the emergency cesarean delivery is the main cause of accidental fetal lesions [24].

With regard to the type of hysterotomy, the Kerr incision with transverse incision on the lower uterine segment is currently the most common (Figure 3.21) [3].

The Kerr hysterotomy technique has numerous advantages due to the features of the anatomical region in which the incision is performed: greater elasticity of the myometrium, lower blood circulation, lower thickness, and muscle fibers that run parallel to the incision.

This type of hysterotomy provides undeniable advantages, such as simplicity of the suture, less blood loss, less adherence, and improved wound healing.

The Kerr hysterotomy variants used in obstetrics are the following: arcuate incision with lower convexity and oblique diagonal incision of the lower segment (Figure 3.22).

The reason alternative techniques are used is to obtain incisions that are parallel to the prevalent direction of the muscle venters so that the fibers are not cut but are instead separated.

The greatest drawback of the street transverse incision is the risk of lateral extension with damage to the uterine vessels that results in severe hemorrhage. This does not happen with the arcuate incision.

When the transverse incision must be extended, a "J" or upside-down "T" can be carried out with a scalpel (Figure 3.23).

Complications observed by these surgeons, resulting from the incision extension technique, are shown in Table 3.1.

Boyle and Gabbe study

As for the lesser-used vertical incision technique, there is the low vertical incision (according to De Lee) (Figure 3.24) and the traditional vertical incision (according to Sanger).

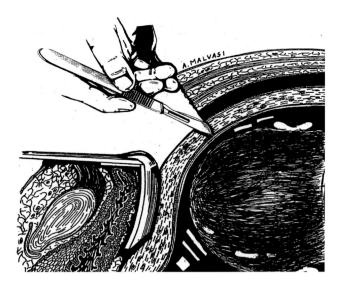

Figure 3.22 Incision of the uterus with exposed lower convexity and sagittal section.

The low vertical incision is performed in the lower part of the uterine segment, but if necessary it can be extended to the uterine fundus.

A hysterotomy can be performed in the traditional vertical incision by cutting the anterior uterine wall up

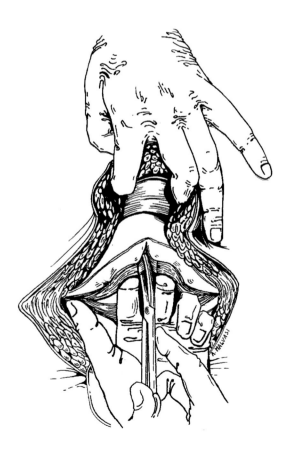

Figure 3.23 Upward widening of the "T" incision of the uterine breach.

Table 3.1 Complications related to the low transverse incision extension technique identified in the 1996 Boyle and Gabbe study

Complication	Number of cases
Insufficiently developed uterine segment	12
Fetus head blocked in mid pelvis	6
Shoulder dystocia	3
Fetal anomalies	2
Placenta praevia	1
Uterine dextrorotation	1
Head entrapment in breech presentation	9
Breech presentation with insufficiently developed uterine segment	6
Shoulder presentation	5
Vertex and arm composite presentation	3
Second twin shoulder presentation	2
Shoulder presentation, premature rupture of membranes (PROM), oligohydramnios	2
Transverse/transverse twin	1
Vertex-foot composite presentation second twin	1
Breech second twin	1
Breech presentation with arm at incision level	1
Total	56

to the fundus. This technique is rarely used because, as previously mentioned, it presents a higher risk of maternal morbidity and of uterine rupture in later pregnancies compared to the low vertical incision and the low transverse incision.

The difference between the low vertical hysterotomy, limited to the noncontractile part of the myometrium, and the extended hysterotomy in the higher and contractile part of the myometrium (longitudinal hysterotomy) cannot be determined with an objective analysis, but only subjectively by the surgeon.

The biggest downside of the low vertical incision is that it can extend to the fundus (becoming a traditional vertical incision) or down to the bladder, cervix, and vagina.

In 1998 Halperin reported a 6% rate of dehiscence in 70 pregnancies after a traditional cesarean delivery and no dehiscence in 70 pregnancies following the transverse incision of the uterus [25]. Patterson published a retrospective study in 2003 on over 19,000 cesarean deliveries (Figure 3.26), 98.5% of which were performed with low transverse incision, 1.1% with traditional technique, and 0.4% with an upside-down "T" uterine incision: maternal morbidity (puerperal infections, blood transfusions, hysterectomies, and transfer to intensive care) was significantly higher in the "traditional" and "T" incisions compared to the low transverse incision (Figure 3.25) [26].

Greene et al. [27], due to the greater morbidity and mortality in the vertical incision and its variants, have

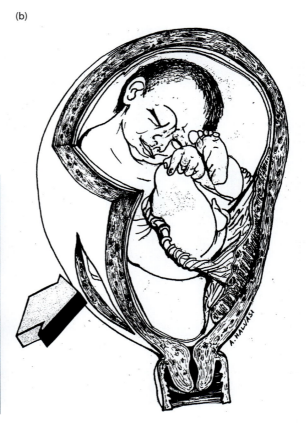

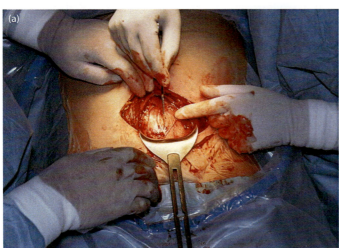

Figure 3.24 Low vertical incision: (a) intraoperative photograph and (b) schematic diagram in relation to the fetus.

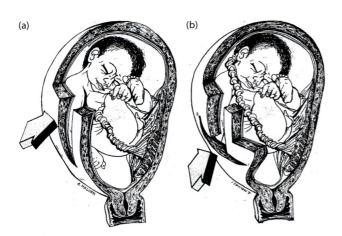

Figure 3.25 (a) High (complete) longitudinal incision and (b) upside-down T incision. The arrows indicate the uterine incisions in cesarean section.

underscored the need to properly inform patients who undergo this type of cesarean delivery in order to avoid later medical and legal disputes.

Due to the greater percentage of hysterectomies and intensive care treatment in the traditional technique, provided there is sufficient lower uterine segment, it is recommended, even in very premature births, to transversely cut the uterus and, if necessary, to extend the T incision.

The currently accepted prerequisites for carrying out a traditional vertical incision are as follows:

- Insufficiently developed lower uterine segment for cases in which extended intrauterine manipulation is required (e.g., pre-term breech presentation, shoulder presentation)
- Pathology of the lower uterine segment, which precludes the transverse incision (e.g., a voluminous myoma)
- Strongly adherent bladder
- Certain anomalous fetal presentations, such as posterior dorsum shoulder presentation

The literature also contains unusual incisions such as the "J" incision (Figure 3.27) as well as incisions of the back part of the uterus [28] or on the fundus (as described by Shukunami et al.), which prevent bleeding from placenta previa [29].

With regard to the type of incision of the uterine part, the hysterotomy is typically performed with a scalpel.

Various techniques are used to minimize damage to the fetus during incision of the myometrium even though none of these have been proven conclusively.

Generally, a hysterotomy is performed with a scalpel by progressively narrowing the myometrium in a limited central area and stretching it upward with gauze or a wad. This maneuver, commonly used in most operating rooms, progressively reveals the layers, minimizes bleeding, increases

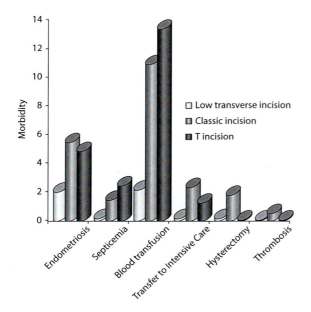

Figure 3.26 Percentage of maternal morbidity in the Patterson study.

exposure, and facilitates the separation of uterine tissue from the membranes and skin of the fetus (Figure 3.28). It has been suggested that the use of a blunt scalpel and serrated blade limits the risk of harm to the fetus, though this does not seem especially necessary (Figure 3.29) [8].

Another technique is applying Allis clamps to the lower and upper edges of the myometrial incision, lifting them, and therefore simplifying the hysterotomy.

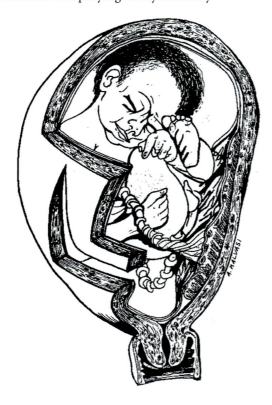

Figure 3.27 "J" incision.

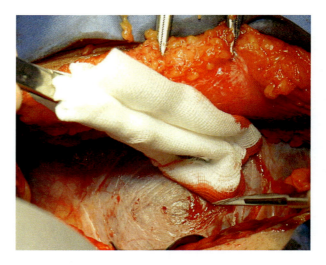

Figure 3.28 Gauze on a clamp stretches the first layers of the myometrium which are cut in the upper part; this reduces bleeding and facilitates the incision of the deeper layers.

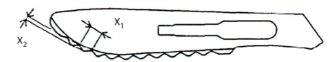

Figure 3.29 Blunt blade scalpel proposed by Ishii in 1999.

Sometimes the barrier is so thin that it can be dissected by simply pressing the end of the scalpel handle, used as a blunt blade, or by pressing blunt scissors against it. The scissors once inside the cavity can be opened by the operator to widen the myometrial fibers and extend the hysterotomy incision (Figure 3.30).

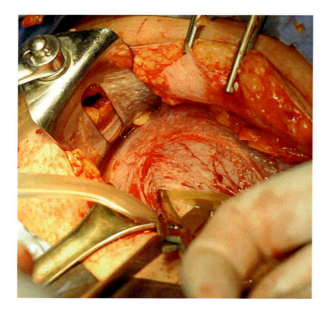

Figure 3.30 Blunt scissors are opened in order to widen the breach and drain the amniotic fluid.

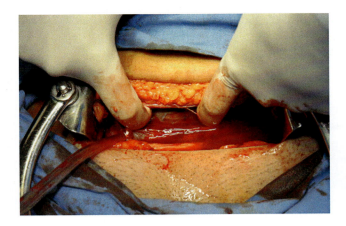

Figure 3.31 Blunt widening of the breach with digital traction.

The maneuver with blunt scissors that opens the innermost layer of the myometrium is a delicate technique that requires surgical experience as it may result in iatrogenic fetal damage.

Once inside the uterine cavity the incision can be extended by myometrial delivery with the use of blunt scissors or by digitally pulling the edges upward and laterally (Figure 3.31).

In case of a thin uterine segment, the bilateral digital pull (Figure 3.32) can be carried out with the index fingers of both of the surgeon's hands. In the presence instead of a thicker segment, as in an elective cesarean delivery, it can be carried out with the index and middle fingers of both hands (Figure 3.34) [30].

When the incision on the segment is carried out in an unusually high position and the segment is not especially thin, after performing latero-lateral digital traction, some obstetricians perform a careful caudal cranial pull to widen the hysterotomy breach (Figure 3.33) [31].

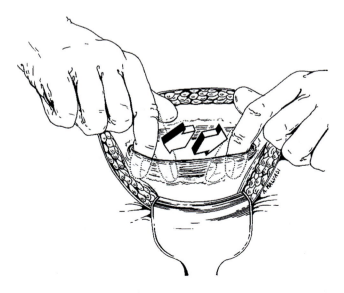

Figure 3.32 Latero-lateral digital widening of the uterine breach in the cesarean delivery hysterotomy.

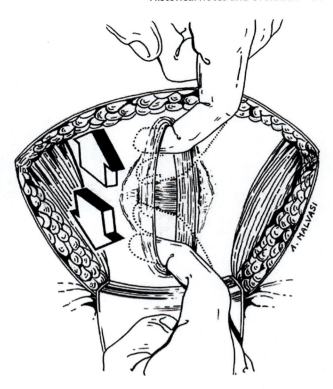

Figure 3.33 Latero-lateral digital widening of the uterine breach with a careful caudal cranial pull.

In 2002 Magann showed, in a randomized prospective study on over 900 patients who underwent a cesarean delivery, that the blunt extension of the breach, compared to an incision performed with scissors, is associated with a significant reduction in bleeding, transfusions, and involuntary extension of the breach (Figure 3.35 and Table 3.2) [30].

However, these data were not reflected in a study conducted by Rodriguez in 1994, which did not show any difference between the two methods [31].

Hameed et al., instead, have shown that the extension of the uterine breach with sharp instruments is more precise and has wide margins of safety [32]. Furthermore, literature describes the extension of the uterine incision with the Auto Suture poly-CS automatic stapler: the instrument is placed between the membranes and the uterine walls after performing a small hysterotomy; the stapler then creates two rows of absorbable stitches on the uterine walls, and the hysterotomy is done between the two stitches in order to minimize blood loss [33].

However, a randomized clinical study as well as a study by Cochrane have not shown any significant benefit to this method that instead increases costs and fetus extraction time [34].

When the uterine segment is cut and widened, especially during dystocic labor, the face or ear of the fetus can be seen. Consequently, all safety maneuvers must be put into effect to avoid iatrogenic lesions, especially after rupture of the membranes (Figure 3.36).

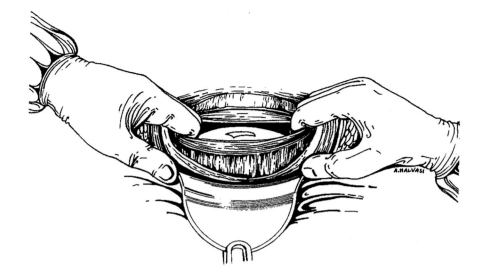

Figure 3.34 Latero-lateral extension of the uterine breach using the index and middle fingers of both hands.

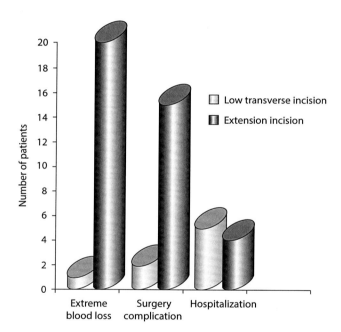

Figure 3.35 Number of patients with complications and average hospitalization period resulting from the incision extension technique versus a control group.

Table 3.2 The Magann study shows an increase in blood loss and in complications when the scissor cut is used to widen the uterine breach

Complication	Scissor cut (in 470 patients)	Blunt cut (in 475 patients)
Average blood loss (mL)	886	843
Transfusions (number of patients)	9	2
Extension of uterine scar		
1–3 cm	57	20
>3 cm	69	24
Wide ligament lacerations (number of patients)	16	7
Cervical lacerations (number of patients)	15	8
Postpartum endometritis (number of patients)	66	51

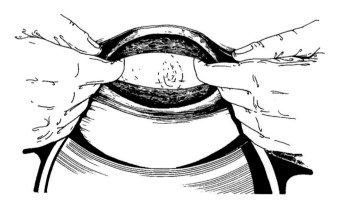

Figure 3.36 Digital opening of the uterine breach in which the fetus right cheek and ear can be seen underneath the chorionic membranes.

The last surgical phase that completes the uterine incision, before proceeding with the fetal extraction, is the opening of the amniochorial membranes (Figure 3.37). As mentioned, this phase requires special attention to prevent iatrogenic damage to the fetus. Various techniques can be used to cut the amniotic sac: a careful incision can be performed with a surgical clamp, which is safer for the underlying fetal parts, or it can be carefully opened with a scalpel (Figure 3.38). Some obstetricians, instead, prefer to use fingers to open the amniotic sac in front of the uterine breach (Figure 3.39) so that it can be opened with as little

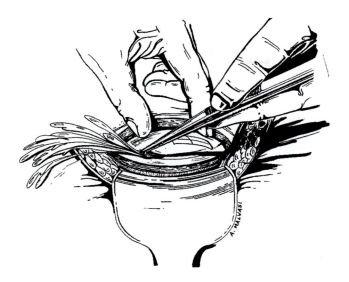

Figure 3.37 Opening of the amniotic sac with surgical forceps.

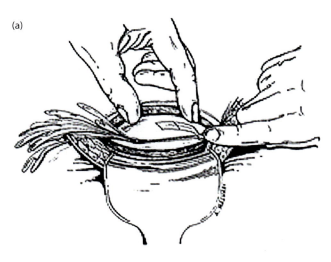

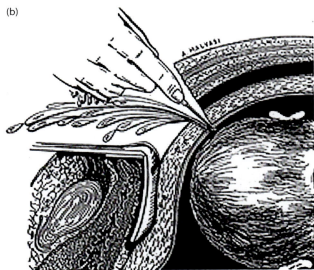

Figure 3.38 Incision of amniochorial membranes with a scalpel: (a) frontal section and (b) sagittal section.

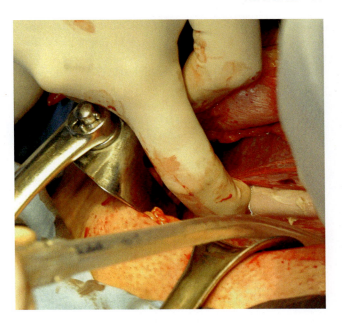

Figure 3.39 Opening of amniochorial membranes with fingers and draining of the amniotic fluid with disposable aspirator.

trauma as possible. The membranes, however, are difficult to grasp, especially when they adhere to the presented part.

CONCLUSIONS

The literature describes different types of hysterotomy incisions during a cesarean delivery; the longitudinal incision has been replaced by the commonly used transverse incision of the lower uterine segment [35]. The transverse incision is performed with sharp instruments along its entire extension. The central incision is then followed by a blunt extension [36]. Some authors maintain that there is no difference between the two methods [37]. In this regard, several related methods are described in the literature [38], even though the authors favor the blunt incision [39–41].

A point that is being currently debated is the direct hysterotomy incision of the visceral peritoneum, as opposed to after the detachment of the uterine vesical fold [41–47].

Another substantial problem is the hysterotomy with whole versus ruptured membranes. If ruptured, a series of safety maneuvers are required to avoid iatrogenic fetal lesions [48].

Hysterotomies have special surgical characteristics in preterm cesarean deliveries [26,30,49].

The literature describes special types of uterine incisions for anomalous situations (e.g., placenta previa, myoma previa, adherences, etc.) [50–55].

REFERENCES

1. Galbert HA, Bey M. History and development of cesarean operation. *Obstet Gynecol Clin North Am* 1988;15:591–605.
2. Balocchi V. *Ostetricia per gli studenti di medicina e chirurgia*. IV Edizione. Milano, Italy: Ernesto Oliva Editore; 1871:820–2.

3. Gall P. *Il Taglio Cesareo Addominale. Studio Clinico-Storico.* Bologna, Italy: Sez. IV. L. Cappelli Editore; 1922:53–59.
4. Kehrer FA. Uber ein modifiziertes Verfahren beim Kaiserschnitt. *Arch Gynekol Bd* 1882;19:117.
5. Sanger M. Zur Reabilitierung des klassischen Kaiserschnittes etc. *Arch F Gyn* 1882;19:370.
6. Kerr JMM. The technique of cesarean delivery, with special reference to the lower uterine segment incision. *Am J Obstet Gynecol* 1926;12:729–34.
7. Miyabe M, Sato S. The effect of head-down tilt position on arterial blood pressure after spinal anesthesia for caesarean delivery. *Reg Anesth* 1997;22:239–42.
8. Setayesh AR, Kholdebarin AR, Moghadam MS, Setayesh HR. The Trendelenburg position increases the spread and accelerates the onset of epidural anesthesia for Caesarean delivery. *Can J Anesth* 2001;48:890–3.
9. Stark M. Technique of Caesarean delivery: The Misgav Ladach method. In: Popkin DR, Peddle LJ, eds. *Women's Health Today: Perspectives on Current Research and Clinical Practice. Proceedings of the XIV F.I.G.O. World Congress of Gynecology and Obstetrics.* New York, NY: Parthenon; 1994:81–85.
10. Down RH, Whitehead R, Watts JM. Do surgical packs cause peritoneal adhesions? *Aust NZ J Surg* 1979;49:379–82.
11. Down RH, Whitehead R, Watts JM. Why do surgical packs cause peritoneal adhesions? *Aust NZ J Surg* 1980;50:83–85.
12. Larsen B, Davis B, Charles D. Critical assessment of antibacterial properties of human amniotic fluid. *Gynecol Obstet Invest* 1984;18:100–4.
13. Larsen B, Galask RP. Host resistance to intraamniotic infection. *Obstet Gynecol Surv* 1975;30:675–91.
14. Harrigill KM, Miller HS, Haynes DE. The effect of intraabdominal irrigation at cesarean delivery on maternal morbidity: A randomized trial. *Obstet Gynecol* 2003;101:80–85.
15. Favier M, Racinet C. *La Cèsarienne: Indications, techniques, complications.* Chapter 5. Paris: Masson; 1984:63–65.
16. Chhabra S, Gandhi D, Jaiswal M. Obstructed labour: A preventable entity. *J Obstet Gynecol* 2000;20:151–3.
17. Phipps MG, Watabe B, Clemons JL, Weitzen S, Myers DL. Risk factors for bladder injury during caesarean delivery. *Obstet Gynecol* 2005;105:156–60.
18. Zabransky F, Grossmannova H. Extraperitoneal cesarean delivery—An alternative or routine? *Ceska Gynecol* 2001;66:187–9.
19. Ezechi OC, Kalu BK, Njokanma FO, Nwokoro CA, Okeke GC. Uterine incision closure at cesarean delivery: A randomized comparative study of intraperitoneal closure and closure after temporary exteriorisation. *West Afr J Med* 2005;24:41–43.
20. Denhez M, Bouton JM, Engelman P, Dupray DM. Placental localisation: Screening and prognosis. *J Gynecol Obstet Biol Reprod* 1981;10:335–47.
21. Boehm FH, Fleischer AC, Barrett JM. Sonographic placental localization in the determination of the site of uterine incision for placenta previa. *J Ultrasound Med* 1982;1:311–4.
22. Okaro JM, Anya SE. Accidental incision of the fetus at caesarean delivery. *Niger J Med* 2004;13:56–58.
23. Iffy L, Pantages P. Erb's palsy after delivery by Caesarean section. (A medico-legal key to a vexing problem). *Med Law* 2005;24:655–61.
24. Dessole S, Cosmi E, Balata A, Uras L, Caserta D, Capobianco G, Ambrosini G. Accidental fetal lacerations during caesarean delivery: Experience in an Italian level III university hospital. *Am J Obstet Gynecol* 2004;191:1673–7.
25. Halperin ME, Moore DC, Hannah WJ. Classical versus low-segment transverse incision for preterm caesarean delivery: Maternal complications and outcome of subsequent pregnancies. *Br J Obstet Gynecol* 1998;95:990–6.
26. Patterson LS, O'Connell CM, Baskett TF. Maternal and perinatal morbidity associated with classic and inverted T cesarean incisions. *Obstet Gynecol* 2002;100:633.
27. Greene RA, Fizpatrick C, Turner MJ. What are the maternal implications of a classical caesarean delivery? *J Obst Gynecol* 1988;18:345–7.
28. Picone O, Fubini A, Doumerc S, Frydman R. Caesarean delivery by posterior due to torsion of the pregnant uterus. *Obstet Gynecol* 2006;107:533–5.
29. Sukunami K, Hattori K, Nishijima K, Kotsuji F. Transverse fundal uterine incision in a patient with placenta increta. *J Matern Fetal Neonatal Med* 2004;16:355–6.
30. Magann EF, Chauhan SP, Bufkin L et al. Intraoperative haemorrhage by blunt versus sharp expansion of the uterine incision at caesarean delivery: A randomised clinical trial. *BJOG* 2002;109:448.
31. Rodriguez AI, Porter KB, O'Brien WF. Blunt versus sharp expansion of the uterine incision in low-segment transverse cesarean delivery. *Am J Obstet Gynecol* 1994;171:1022.
32. Hameed N, Ali MA. Maternal blood loss by expansion of uterine incision at caesarean delivery—A comparison between sharp and blunt techniques. *J Ayub Med Coll Abbottabad* 2004;16:47–50.
33. Wilkinson C, Enkin MW. Absorbable staples for uterine incision at caesarean section. *Cochrane Database Syst Rev.* 2000;(2):CD000005.
34. Dodd JM, Anderson ER, Gates S. Surgical techniques for uterine incision and uterine closure at the time of caesarean delivery. *Cochrane Database Syst Rev* 2008;(3):CD004732.
35. Greene RA, Fitzpatrick C, Turner MJ. What are the maternal implications of a classical caesarean delivery? *J Obstet Gynaecol* 1998;18(4):345–7.
36. Abalos E, Addo V, Sharma JB, Matthews J, Oyieke J, Masood SN, El Sheikh MA. The CORONIS Trial. International study of caesarean delivery surgical

techniques: A randomised fractional, factorial trial. *BMC Pregnancy Childbirth* 2007;7:24.
37. Hidar S, Jerbi M, Hafsa A, Slama A, Bibi M, Khaïri H. The effect of uterine incision expansion at caesarean delivery on perioperative haemorrhage: A prospective randomised clinical trial. *Rev Med Liege* 2007;62(4):235–8.
38. Cromi A, Ghezzi F, Di Naro E, Siesto G, Loverro G, Bolis P. Blunt expansion of the low transverse uterine incision at cesarean delivery: A randomized comparison of 2 techniques. *Am J Obstet Gynecol* 2008;199(3):292.e1–6.
39. Hameed N, Ali MA. Maternal blood loss by expansion of uterine incision at caesarean delivery—A comparison between sharp and blunt techniques. *J Ayub Med Coll Abbottabad* 2004;16(3):47–50.
40. Chicaud B, Roux C, Rudigoz RC, Huissoud C. Blunt or sharp expansion of cesarean delivery: A comparative study. *Gynecol Obstet Biol Reprod (Paris)*. 2013;42(4):366–71.
41. Xu LL, Chau AM, Zuschmann A. Blunt vs. sharp uterine expansion at lower segment cesarean delivery delivery: A systematic review with meta-analysis. *Am J Obstet Gynecol* 2013;208(1):62.e1–8. doi:10.1016/j.ajog.2012.10.886
42. Hohlagschwandtner M, Ruecklinger E, Husslein P, Joura EA. Is the formation of bladder flap at caesarean necessary? A randomized trial. *Obstet Gynecol* 2001;98:1089–92.
43. Berghella V, Baxter JK, Chauhan SP. Evidence-based surgery for cesarean delivery. *Am J Obstet Gynecol* 2005;193(5):1607–17.
44. Mahajan NN. Justifying formation of bladder flap at cesarean delivery? *Arch Gynecol Obstet* 2009;279(6):853–5.
45. Malvasi A, Tinelli A, Gustapane S, Mazzone E, Cavallotti C, Stark M, Bettocchi S. Surgical technique to avoid bladder flap formation during cesarean delivery. *G Chir* 2011;32(11–12):498–503.
46. Tuuli MG, Odibo AO, Fogertey P, Roehl K, Stamilio D, Macones GA. Utility of the bladder flap at cesarean delivery: A randomized controlled trial. *Obstet Gynecol* 2012;119(4):815–21.
47. Walsh CA. Evidence-based cesarean technique. *Curr Opin Obstet Gynecol* 2010;22(2):110–5.
48. Alexander JM, Leveno KJ, Hauth J et al. Fetal injury associated with cesarean delivery. *Obstet Gynecol* 2006;108(4):885–90.
49. Rochelson B, Pagano M, Conetta L, Goldman B, Vohra N, Frey M, Day C. Previous preterm cesarean delivery: Identification of a new risk factor for uterine rupture in VBAC candidates. *J Matern Fetal Neonatal Med* 2005;18(5):339–42.
50. Picone O, Fubini A, Doumerc S, Frydman R. Caesarean delivery by posterior hysterotomy due to torsion of the pregnant uterus. *Obstet Gynecol* 2006;107(2 Pt 2):533–5.
51. Nishijima K, Shukunami K, Arikura S, Kotsuji F. An operative technique for conservative management of placenta accreta. *Obstet Gynecol* 2005;105(5 Pt 2):1201–3.
52. Shukunami K, Hattori K, Nishijima K, Kotsuji F. Transverse fundal uterine incision in a patient with placenta increta. *J Matern Fetal Neonatal Med* 2004;16(6):355–6.
53. Ward CR. Avoiding an incision through the anterior previa at cesarean delivery. *Obstet Gynecol* 2003;102(3):552–4.
54. Sparic R, Lazovic B. Inevitable cesarean myomectomy following delivery through posterior hysterotomy in a case of uterine torsion. *Med Arh* 2013;67(1):75–76.
55. Kotsuji F, Nishijima K, Kurokawa T, Yoshida Y, Sekiya T, Banzai M, Minakami H, Udagawa Y. Transverse uterine fundal incision for placenta praevia with accreta, involving the entire anterior uterine wall: A case series. *BJOG* 2013;120(9):1144–9.

FURTHER READING

Boyle JG, Gabbe SG. T and J vertical extensions in low tranverse caesarean births. *Obstet Gynecol* 1996;87:238–43.

Field CS. Surgical techniques for cesarean delivery. *Obstet Gynecol Clin North Am* 1988;15:657–72.

Ishii S, Endo M. Blunt-edged, notched scalpel for caesarean incision. *Obstet Gynecol* 1999;94:469.

Villeneuve MG, Khalife S, Marcoux SA, Blanchet P. Surgical staples in Caesarean delivery: A randomized controlled trial. *Am J Obstet Gynecol* 1990;163:1646.

Fetal extraction during cesarean delivery

GIAN CARLO DI RENZO, ANTONIO MALVASI, and ANDREA TINELLI

Cephalic extraction

.... when the obstetrician ruptures the membranes the assistant who is responsible for distancing the margins of the wound must keep the abdominal walls in close contact with the uterine walls. This is immediately followed by the extraction of the fetus in which the first presenting part is grabbed…

(P. Cazeaux, 1845)

INTRODUCTION

The incision of the lower uterine segment, the improvement of extraction methods, the development of anesthesiological and neonatal resuscitation techniques, antibiotics, and hemoderivatives have in the twentieth century consolidated the cesarean delivery and reduced its complications [1–4].

Fetal extraction during cesarean delivery has been seen in myths, legends, and religions of various cultures as completely distinct from vaginal delivery.

In historical iconographic representations, fetal extraction has been loaded with religious and mythological meanings, such as the birth of gods and demigods, or the birth of the "Antichrist." These, in fact, were extracted from the maternal "womb" instead of being born the "natural" way, and for this reason the extraction had to have been performed by those—divinities or people of the cloth—capable of performing this act, instead of by common people.

In modern times, now that certain ideas tied to the "abdominal birth" are part of the past, it is generally thought that abdominal delivery of the fetus is a safe act and therefore without any particular risk.

In reality some authors observe that that is not the case, as both maternal and fetal lesions are possible even during fetal extraction from cesarean delivery.

Prerequisites for a proper fetal extraction during cesarean delivery, whether elective or emergency, are an adequate exposure of the operating field and a good position on the operating bed in relation to operator needs. It is essential for fetal extraction that the surgeon is well positioned in relation to the pregnant woman lying on the operating table: right-handed surgeons must be to the right of the patient, and left-handed surgeons must be to the left.

By positioning himself or herself on the right side of the patient, the operator will be able to properly perform the maneuvers, and in particular be able to properly position the hand and provide a "lever effect" on the presenting part (Figure 4.1).

An adequate laparotomy in relation to the case that required a cesarean delivery is needed to achieve a good fetal extraction.

In addition, it must be noted that most cesarean deliveries currently are performed with the pregnant mother under spinal, epidural, or combined spinal epidural (CSE) anesthesia, and therefore with a conscious patient who is following the birth of the child and is aware of the surgical maneuvers [1–4].

FETAL EXTRACTION

Essentially extraction must deal with three types of presentations [5,6]:

- Cephalic
- Breech
- Transverse (shoulder)

The extraction may at times be instrumental—that is, assisted by obstetric instruments such as forceps and vacuum extractor. As a general rule the anesthesiologist may need to resort, in case of difficulties, to pharmacological relaxation of the uterus.

FETAL EXTRACTION IN CEPHALIC PRESENTATION
Introduction

Once the incision of the uterine breach is carried out and the capacity is checked to be adequate, the operator must insert his fingers in the uterine cavity and place them between the wall and the fetal head: the fingers are placed under the presenting part and provide an outward lever effect.

The assistant removes the suprapubic valve, when used, so that all the space available in the pubic area can be utilized.

The operator provides three subsequent movements to the cephalic pole:

- Raising the presenting part to the level of the uterine incision—that is, in the direction of the uterine body (Figure 4.2)
- Positioning in the occipital-pubic direction (Figure 4.3)
- Progressing toward the surface—that is, toward the uterine breach (Figure 4.4)

To facilitate the extraction of the fetal head the operator must position his hands in relation to the presentation.

Position of the fetal head

Figures 4.5 through 4.11 depict the various positions of the fetal head during cesarean extraction and the

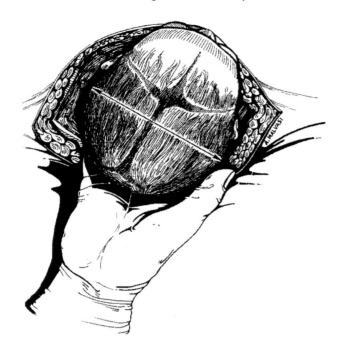

Figure 4.1 Positioning of the right hand of the operator on the presenting part to provide the "lever effect" (on the head) and to facilitate the disengagement and, therefore, the fetal extraction, with sacral rotation of the occiput.

corresponding position of the fetal head in vaginal delivery. The rationale is that the fetal head can have various positions in both the elective cesarean delivery and in dystocic labor. However, to facilitate the extraction the operator should verify the position of the fetal head, and the extraction should then take this position into account, as during vaginal delivery.

Extracting the head along its axis will facilitate the subsequent extraction of the shoulders, as the biparietal diameter is parallel to the bisacromial diameter. This serves to avoid excessive or anomalous rotation that could harm the fetus or cause uterine tears.

Position of the operator's hand

During fetal extraction, the operator when right handed will use his or her right hand and will stand to the right of the patient. On the contrary, if the operator is left handed he or she will use his or her left hand (Figure 4.12).

The operator's hand must enter the breach and insert itself under the fetal head with fingers spread (Figure 4.13).

In the next surgical phase the surgeon's hand must function as an inclined plane on which the fetal head slides, from bottom to top, under the "vis a tergo" of the assistant or of the operator (Figure 4.14).

Therefore, the main phases that characterize the posture of the surgeon's hand are inserting and positioning the hand in the uterus and holding and lifting the fetal head (Figure 4.15).

To facilitate extraction of the head, the assistant normally exerts a small amount of pressure on the uterine fundus. Less frequently, in case of a relatively easy extraction, the operator can assist the progress of the extraction by placing his or her left hand on the anterior uterine wall (Figure 4.16).

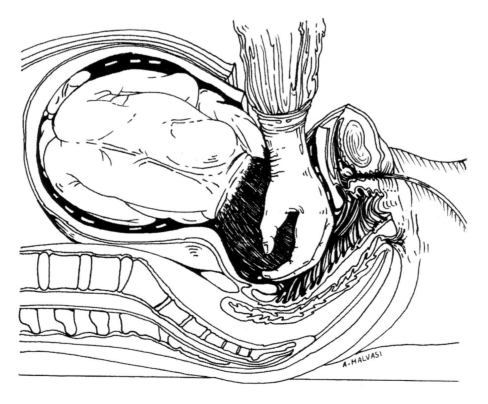

Figure 4.2 Raising of the presenting part (cephalic) to the level of the uterine incision to facilitate fetal extraction.

Fetal extraction in cephalic presentation 59

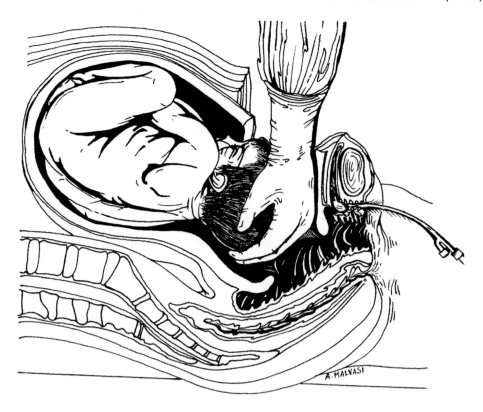

Figure 4.3 Positioning of the operator's hand in the occipital–pubic direction on the presenting part to have a better hold on the fetal head.

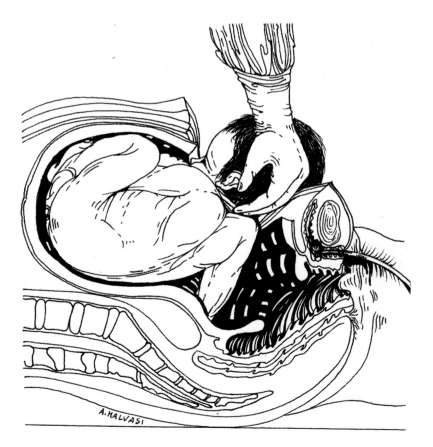

Figure 4.4 Progression, guided by the surgeon, of the presenting part toward the uterine breach.

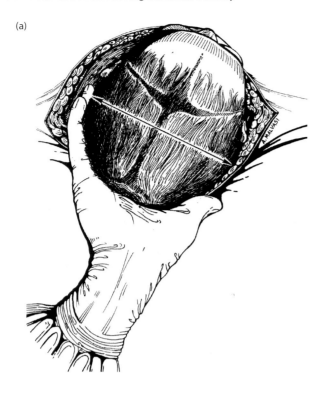

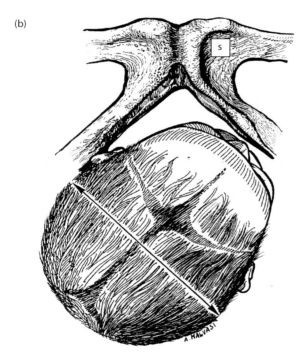

Figure 4.5 (a) Extraction from the uterine breach on incision of the fetal head in right occiput posterior position; (b) corresponding fetal head in vaginal delivery (S = pubic symphysis, front view).

The assistant simultaneously assists the operator by exerting a gradual and constant pressure on the uterine fundus in the craniocaudal direction, to help the head pass through the hysterotomy breach. This pressure must be applied only when the presenting part is firmly engaged in the uterine incision.

The externalized head slides on the palm of the hand supporting it

With regard to the fundal pressure applied by the assistant on the fetal head, it should be noted that the more the pressure required by the surgeon increases, the more the rules for adequate extraction have not been observed, a typical case being a narrow laparotomy breach.

Correct extraction of the head, in case of anomalies of the fetal head position, may require additional maneuvers, which however avoid maternal and fetal damage.

In case of normally flexed head the surgeon must gradually and delicately reduce the flexion before extracting it (Figure 4.17).

The fetus in face presentation has a longitudinal lie. The presentation is cephalic, but the presenting part is the face and the attitude is of complete extension.

The chin is the presenting part and the presenting diameter is the submento bregmatic diameter (ca. 9.5 cm). The incidence of face presentation is under 1%, the majority if which are secondary as the head extends during labor and frequently upon entry at the pelvis.

Approximately 70% of face presentations are in the anterior–transverse position, and 30% are in the posterior–transverse position. Diagnosis is performed with traditional obstetric maneuvers but can also be assisted by intrapartum ultrasound.

In case of face presentation it is mandatory to perform a cesarean delivery. In fact the different types of face presentation and the maneuvers to modify this presentation, including the application of forceps, appear nowadays to be outdated (Figure 4.18).

In frontal presentation the fetus has a longitudinal lie, and presentation is cephalic, but the presenting part is the forehead and the attitude is of partial extension (circa 50%). This contrasts with face presentation in which the extension is complete.

The forehead is the presenting part, and the presenting diameter is the mentovertical diameter (circa 13.5 cm), which is the longest anterior–posterior diameter of the fetal head. The incidence of face presentation is under 1%. Primitive forehead presentations are rare; however, these presentations frequently develop during labor.

Because the frontal presentation is a partial extension of the head, frequently it is transitory. In fact the head can subsequently flex, thereby transforming to occipital presentation, or it can instead completely extend into a face presentation. Therefore, for frontal presentation, the presentation diagnosis and the subsequent evolution in occipital or face presentation is especially important. In the first case especially for pluriparous women, vaginal delivery is a possibility. In case of face presentation and therefore of a stop in the

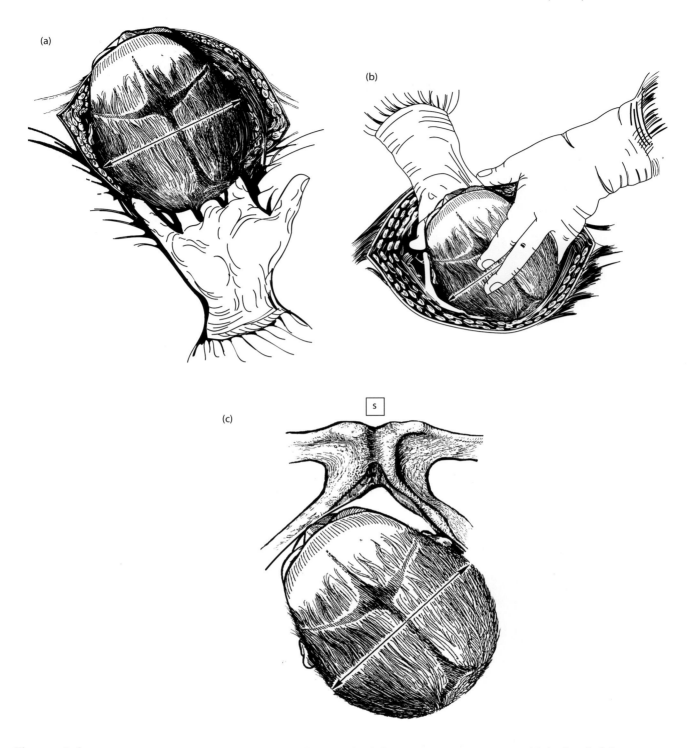

Figure 4.6 Extraction from the uterine breach of the fetal head in left occiput posterior position; (a) the hand of the operator facilitates the extraction of the head from this position; (b) the operator extracts the fetal head from the breach along with the shoulders; (c) corresponding fetal head in vaginal delivery (S = symphysis).

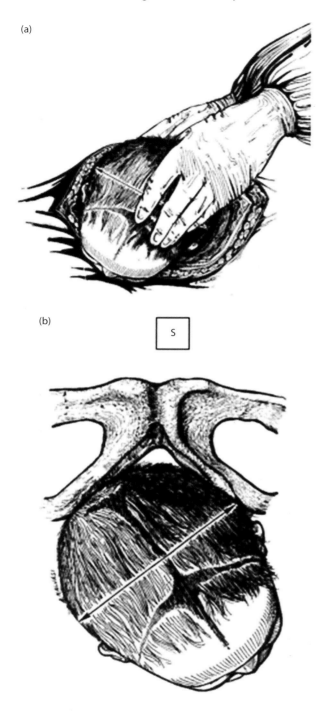

Figure 4.7 (a) Extraction from the uterine breach of the fetal head in right occiput anterior position; (b) corresponding fetal head in vaginal delivery (S = symphysis).

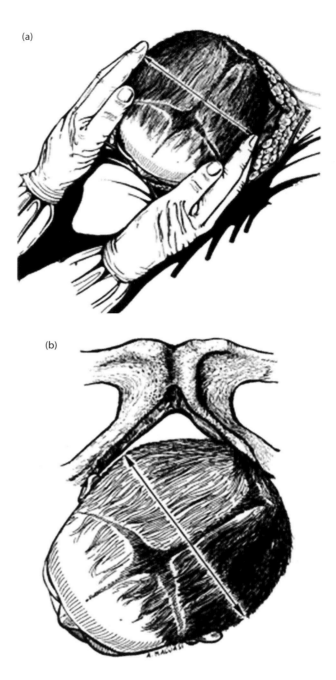

Figure 4.8 (a) Extraction from the uterine breach of the fetal head in left occiput anterior position; (b) corresponding fetal head in vaginal delivery (S = symphysis).

progression of the presenting part, and with the possibility of fetal distress, a cesarean delivery is mandatory.

In case of bregma presentation, the fetus has a longitudinal lie and the cranium is slightly deflected, halfway between extension and flexion. The occiput and the forehead are at the same level in the pelvis, and for this reason the bregma presentation is also called the "intermediate vertex presentation." The leading part is the vertex; the presenting part is the bregma. The presenting diameter is the occipital frontal diameter measuring 11 cm, and because it is longer than the suboccipitobregmatic diameter, it is less favorable. For this reason the bregma presentation has a slower progression and a higher incidence of the presenting part stopping in the birth canal.

The prognosis of vaginal delivery therefore is generally positive, except in those infrequent cases in which the bregmatic presentation transforms into a frontal or face presentation, which requires operative delivery, in particular with cesarean delivery.

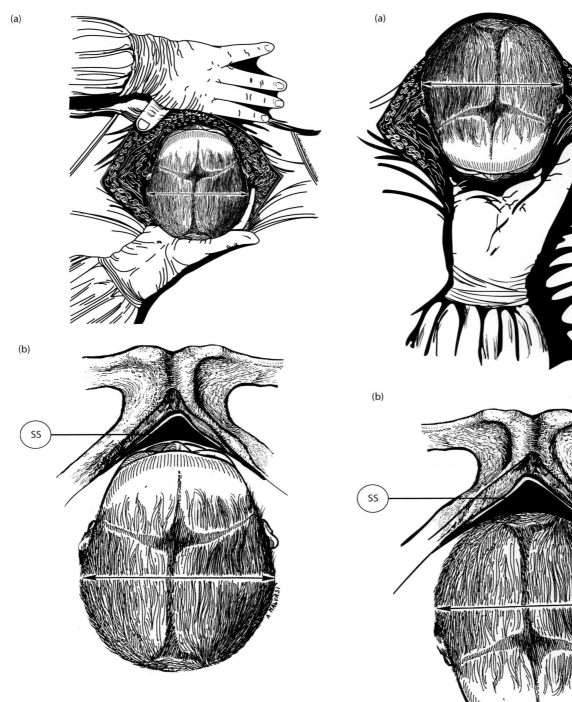

Figure 4.9 (a) Extraction from the uterine incision of the fetal head in median or longitudinal occiput posterior position; (b) corresponding fetal head in vaginal delivery (SS = subsymphyseal area). The extraction can be facilitated by the application of pressure by the first operator on the upper part of the uterine incision. This maneuver, however, does not encounter the obstacles that the pubic symphysis encounters from behind and below a rigid structure such as the pubic symphysis, as occurs in vaginal delivery.

Figure 4.10 (a) Extraction from the uterine incision on breach of the fetal head in occiput median anterior position; (b) corresponding fetal head in vaginal delivery (bottom right) (SS = subsymphyseal area).

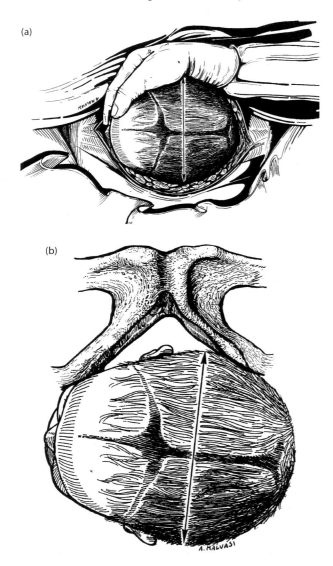

Figure 4.11 (a) Extraction from the uterine breach of the fetal head in left occiput transverse position; (b) corresponding fetal head in vaginal delivery.

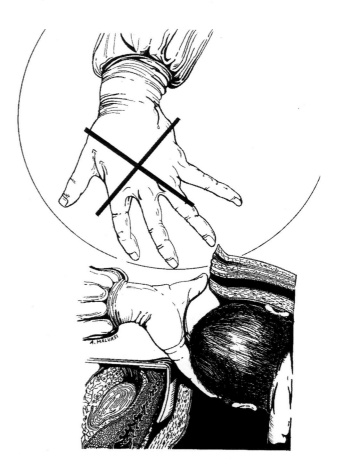

Figure 4.12 Extraction from the uterine breach of the fetal head with the left hand, with left-handed operator placed to the left of the patient and not vice versa (image at top).

Obviously frontal and face presentations, and especially bregma presentations, may be complicated by asynclitism or by the association of an upper limb, which increases the diameter (already unfavorable) in relation to the pelvic diameter, thereby presenting complicating factors that require operative delivery.

The bregma attitude at times may be further complicated by the hooking of the jaw on the symphysis or on the promontory, which stops the descent and halts the progression of the head inside the birth canal.

In case of hyperextended head, the operator must prevent further extension by inserting his or her flattened hand in the uterine cavity and letting the head slip up and out (Figure 4.18).

In case of occiput posterior position, the hand of the operator is inserted "cup-like" in the uterine cavity, reaches the fetal occiput, lifts the head, and brings it up and out (Figure 4.19).

In case of association with an upper limb, the operator must, before the extraction, move up the limb placed in front of the head to prevent the volumes of both fetal parts from blocking the extraction, as well as tearing the uterine breach (Figure 4.20).

Among the most common anomalies of fetal head position are anterior and posterior asynclitism: the operator must therefore align the fetal head (especially in posterior presentations) and then perform the extraction. The direction of the fetal head (up and back) would otherwise complicate the extraction process (Figures 4.21 and 4.22).

In terms of the height of the presenting part, there are two distinct situations:

- *Head deeply engaged*: This condition occurs in those situations in which the mother is moved from the labor and/or delivery room to the operating room during advanced labor, for reasons of fetal distress or, more frequently, dystocia.

  The situation in which the head is engaged and the uterine incision is at the level of the fetal neck or shoulder is the most difficult in terms of extraction. In such a situation the operator must grab the fetal vertex and bring it up, moving it along the axis of the uterus in

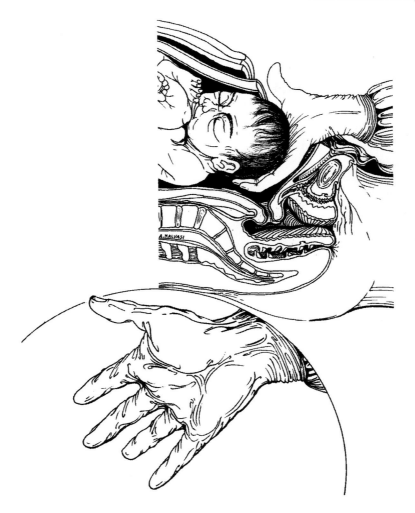

Figure 4.13 Posture of the operator's hand ready for the extraction of the fetal head.

the caudocranial direction, while avoiding lever movements on the symphysis.

At times engagement of the head is such that it is difficult to insert the hand in the virtual space between the fetal head and the posterior side of the pubic symphysis (Figure 4.23). In fact it is necessary to be very careful when inserting a hand deep into the birth canal to reach the fetal vertex, in order to reduce the likelihood of transverse and longitudinal tears on the lower uterine segment, already thin due to the advanced and dystocic labor. If this maneuver is ineffective, further vaginal pushing maneuvers are required: the assistant must insert a hand into the vagina and push the head back in the cranial direction (Figure 4.24).

The next phase requires a strong push from the bottom (vaginally) by the assistant. With this maneuver, the operator can reach the fetal vertex and perform the extraction (Figure 4.25). This maneuver takes place in case of a "failed" application of forceps or ventouse and in which the head is located at the mid strait and is wedged between mid strait and inferior strait, or due to strong Kristeller maneuvers carried out for vaginal delivery.

It should be noted that this particular condition is the result of an erroneous evaluation of the progression of labor and of the presenting part and of an erroneous prediction of vaginal delivery which could lead to medicolegal consequences. The risks can be reduced through the use of intrapartum ultrasound. In fact this method can diagnose dystocia even before digital evaluation, resulting in the indication of a cesarean delivery.

An extreme and infrequent external maneuver is the Zavanelli maneuver that is performed with the fetal head outside the rima vulvae. This maneuver is performed with Type II shoulder dystocia—that is, when the fetus is "expelled." In other words the fetus is beyond the rima vulvae (*turtle sign*), but the fetal shoulders remain above the superior strait—that is the anterior shoulder is under the pubic symphysis and the posterior shoulder is above the promontory. Should these dramatic circumstances occur, perform a wide abdominal parietal incision and try to perform a rapid vertex or breech extraction of the fetus, while the assistant tries to move the head to the pelvic cavity to free it from the suffocating vulvovaginal grip.

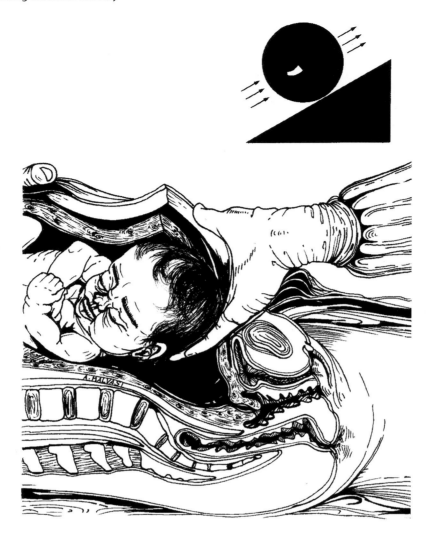

Figure 4.14 The surgeon's hand, assisted by the push on the uterine fundus, is like an inclined plane on which slides the fetal head.

Complex and prolonged maneuvers almost inevitably result in strain to the nearby bladder involved in the fetal extraction maneuvers. Therefore, the presence of blood in the vesical catheter or in the urinary bladder should not worry the surgeon. If anything the vesical catheter must be kept beyond the standard postsurgical time to allow the bladder to spontaneously resume function. In fact the pressure of the fetal head and the extraction maneuvers frequently result in bladder retention during the postpartum or early puerperium period.

The consequences of the Zavanelli maneuvers on the fetus can instead be much more serious. Some authors in fact describe fetal column fractures at the cervical level in the attempt to reposition the fetal head in the birth canal, with the death of the fetus [7]. In addition, other authors, in trying to reduce the danger of the Zavanelli maneuver, have proposed a repositioning of the head (even partial) in the vaginal canal in the (successful) attempt to rotate the shoulders with the McRoberts or Wood maneuver, in order to extract the fetus from the laparotomy breach [8]. However, an important aspect remains, and that is that, currently, the Zavanelli maneuver (and its modifications) is an extreme obstetric maneuver, and the possibility of associated fetal damage must be contemplated [9,10].

The Zavanelli maneuver, however, is the last obstetric opportunity to resolve in a relatively short amount of time a compromised situation. Gherman et al. underscore the importance of recognizing shoulder dystocia and proceeding with appropriate maneuvers before resorting to the Zavanelli maneuver [11].

- *Head too high*: If the cephalic vertex is too high and can be pushed back, it will be difficult to hold onto and fetal extraction will be easier if performed with version and breech extraction. With high fetal head, as occurs during an elective cesarean delivery, the assistant should exert pressure on the uterine fundus to bring the fetal head closer to the hand of the operator and to move it toward the hysterotomy breach.
  - *High head and narrow uterine breach*: When the uterine breach is at the limit between the body and the lower uterine segment, the thickness of the

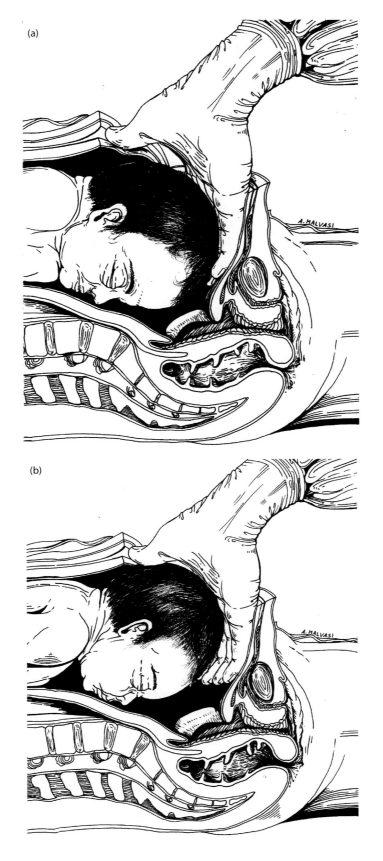

Figure 4.15 (a) Insertion and positioning of the hand in the uterus; (b) holding and lifting the fetal head.

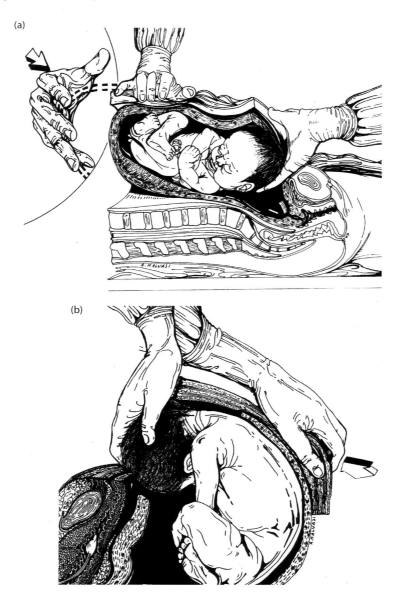

Figure 4.16 (a) The assistant normally exerts a small amount of pressure on the uterine fundus. (b) Less frequently, in case of a relatively easy extraction, the operator with his or her left hand can assist the progress of the extraction. The arrows indicate the hand direction of this maneuver.

myometrium, the presence of adherences in case of previous cesarean deliveries, the presence of obstacles such as myomaprevium, inadequate position of the fetal head, and other circumstances may require a strong push on the fetal fundus, as during a Kristeller maneuver that can be performed even though normally it is prohibited. However, in order to extract a difficult fetal head, it is essential that the head rotate around the axis that brings the occiput next to the operator's hand that functions as a lever on which slides the fetal head that then disengages from the "abdominal birth canal."

- *Fetal extraction with the left hand*: This must be performed only by left-handed operators. Right-handed operators would find the extraction maneuver to be difficult and ineffective.

In case of *fetal macrosomia*, some authors recommend moving the cephalic extremity toward a face presentation in relation to the uterine breach: the index and middle fingers of the operator are inserted in the oral cavity of the fetus—being careful to place them at the base of the tongue and not on the palate to avoid traumatic lesions—and rotate the fetus until the mouth is visible [12] (Figures 4.26 through 4.29), by rotating along the median line (Figure 4.30).

After the fetal head has emerged the same amount of attention must be paid to the extraction of the shoulders, which is carried out in a similar manner to vaginal extraction. The operator with his hands symmetrically holds the fetal head at the level of the fetal cheeks (Figure 4.31). As during vaginal delivery, the posterior and anterior shoulders emerge after performing tilting movements

Fetal extraction in cephalic presentation 69

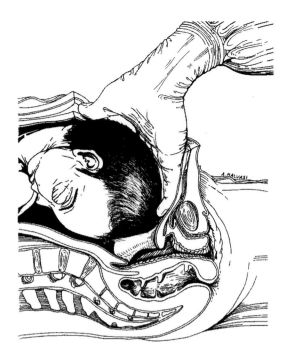

Figure 4.17 Posterior flexion of the head, which the operator must align before the extraction.

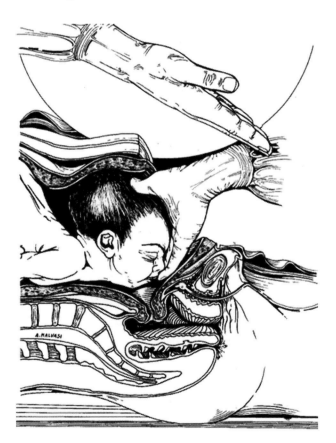

Figure 4.18 Head with mentum posterior position in face presentation. The head hyperextended in occiput anterior position and pushed by the fundal pressure applied by the assistant slides on the hand of the surgeon (above) preventing any further flexion.

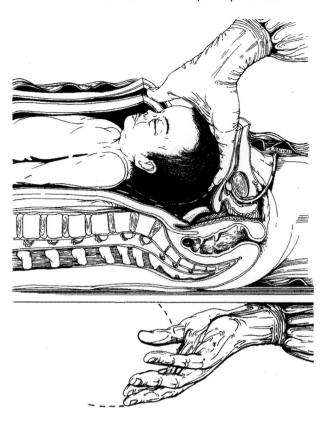

Figure 4.19 Occiput posterior position and extraction of the fetal head with "cup-like" position of the surgeon hand (below).

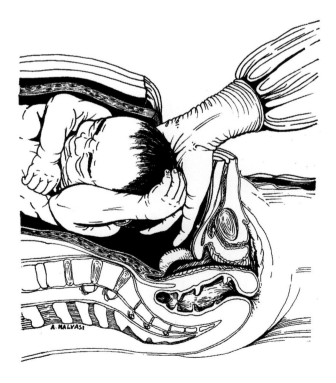

Figure 4.20 Fetal extraction with association of the upper left limb, which must be pushed up and back to facilitate extraction of the head.

70 Fetal extraction during cesarean delivery

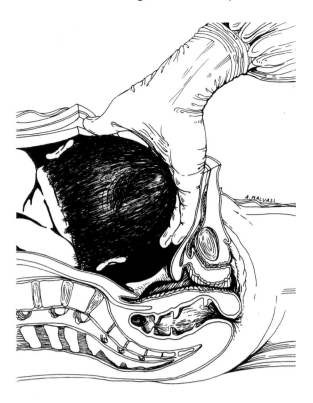

Figure 4.21 Extraction of the fetal head in anterior asynclitism: the operator's hand pushes the fetal head up before disengagement, as extraction of the cephalic extremity is unlikely to occur in the asynclitic position, of full cervical dilatation.

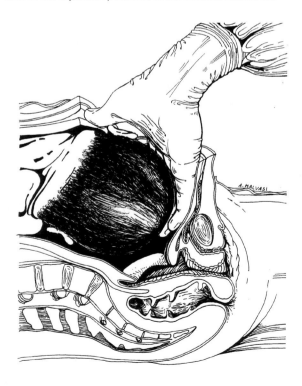

Figure 4.22 Extraction of the presenting part in posterior asynclitism: the hand of the operator must penetrate deeply into the birth canal in order to carry out the extraction, in advanced second-labor stage.

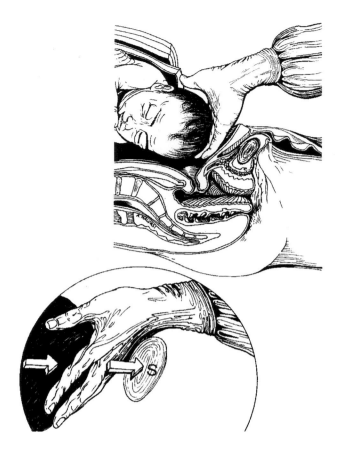

Figure 4.23 Extraction of the fetal head engaged in the pelvic cavity. The hand must be inserted in the virtual space between the fetal head and the posterior side of the pubic symphysis (bottom image, S = symphysis)

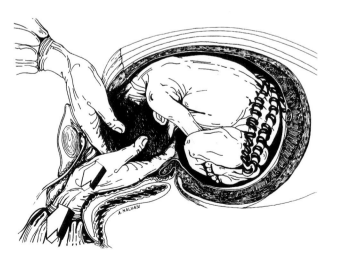

Figure 4.24 Fetal head deeply engaged in the pelvic cavity extraction: with hand inserted in the vagina the assistant pushes the fetal head so that the operator can insert his or her hand in the uterine breach and position it under the fetal head.

Fetal extraction in cephalic presentation 71

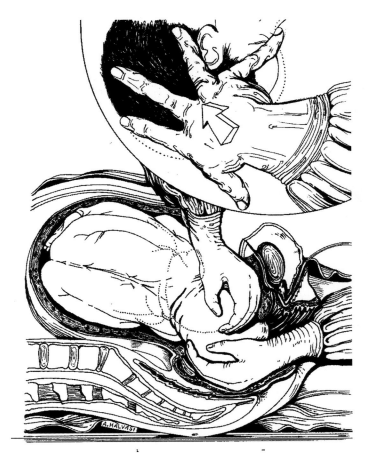

Figure 4.25 The next phase requires a strong push from the vagina on the fetal head by the assistant, while the operator extracts the fetal head by lifting it up and out.

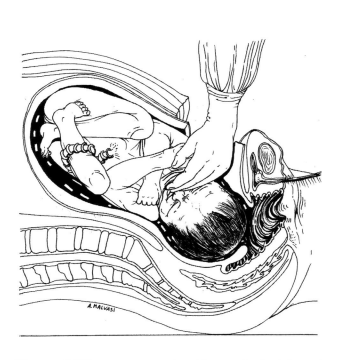

Figure 4.26 The operator's hand locates the fetal rima oris before appropriately inserting the fingers in the buccal cavity.

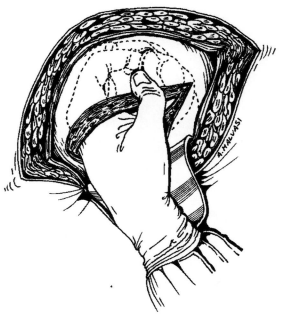

Figure 4.27 The operator's hand, once the index finger locates the fetal lips through the uterine breach, applies the index finger, or index finger together with the middle finger, directed toward the fetal palate in order to perform the extraction maneuver.

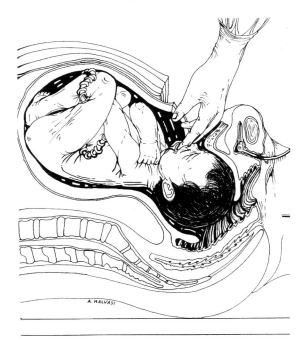

Figure 4.28 The operator, once the index and middle fingers have been inserted in the buccal cavity of the fetus, rotates the fetal head.

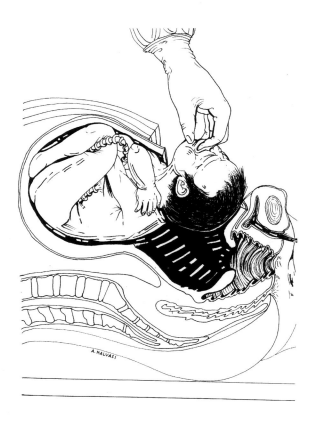

Figure 4.30 Once the fetal head has been hooked with fingers inserted in the buccal cavity, the obstetrician exerts a slight traction in an external and upward direction, thereby extracting the fetal head.

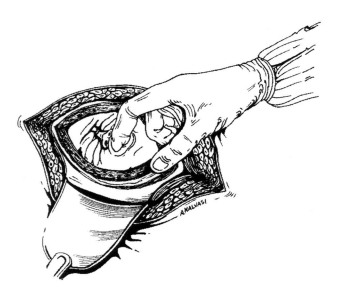

Figure 4.29 When the fetal head appears in the hysterotomy opening, the surgeon can move the fetal head along the median line by inserting his index finger in the buccal cavity.

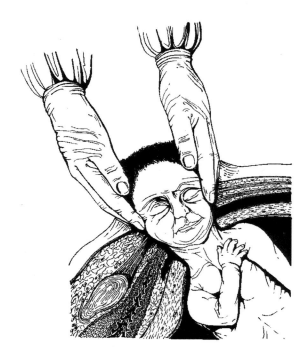

Figure 4.31 The surgeon uses his hands to perform an anchoring maneuver of the fetal cheeks in order to extract the head. He must feel which of the two fetal shoulders can be more easily extracted (sagittal section at top).

(Figure 4.32). The shoulders must emerge, as during vaginal extraction, by positioning the bisacromial diameter transversely, along the main axis of the hysterotomy and laparotomy. If the shoulder extraction is perpendicular to the laparotomy and hysterotomy incisions, the operator

Fetal extraction in cephalic presentation

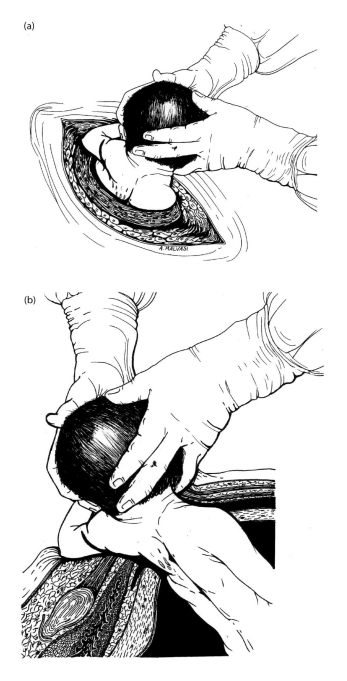

Figure 4.32 (a and b) Tilting movements help the shoulders emerge (the left shoulder is here shown emerging first). (Modified from Malvasi A, Di Renzo GC. *Semeiotica Ostetrica*, Rome, Italy: CIC Edizioni Internazionali; 2012.)

may pull excessively on the brachial plexus. The resulting damages performed during cesarean delivery are described in the literature.

It is therefore recommended to accompany the extraction of the shoulders with additional maneuvers in which the uterine breach is widened and extended in the inferior–superior direction (Figure 4.33). Should these maneuvers also prove to be insufficient, one can opt, as a last resort, for version and breech extraction of the fetus [13,14].

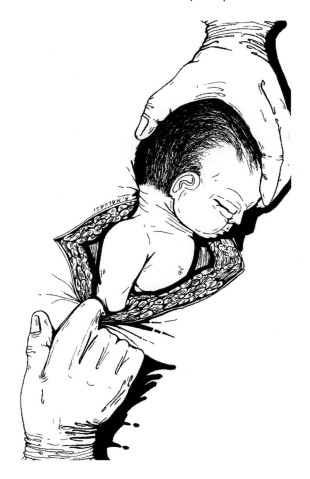

Figure 4.33 Tilting movements to help the shoulders emerge, in this case, before extraction.

Some operators perform extraction with the help of laparotomy retractors. This seldom-used practice can, however, during the extraction cause fetal damage against the rigid parts of the instrument. For this reason soft retractors have been designed and used, such as the Pelosi retractor [15,16] that, according to the author, is useful in assisting fetal extraction (Figure 4.34).

Risks of fetal extraction

Fetal damages in the manual extraction during cesarean delivery are rare (2%) and include [17–23]

- Damage to the brachial plexus
- Long bone fractures
- Tendinous lesions
- Penetration of the epistropheus in brain structures

Fetal damage tied to instrumental extraction is comparable to the damage that occurs vaginally:

- Cephalohematomas
- Scalp abrasion
- Cephalic phlegmons
- Parietal fracture
- Intracranial hemorrhage

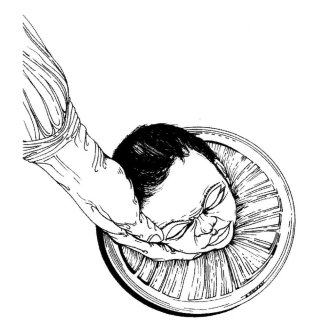

Figure 4.34 Soft Pelosi retractor for fetal extraction during cesarean delivery.

Conclusions

Extraction in cephalic presentation during cesarean delivery is the most common. The cephalic extraction phases are the following: lifting of the fetus to the level of the uterine incision, that is in the direction of the uterine body, positioning in the occipital–pubic direction, and progressing toward the surface of the uterine breach [24,25]. The goal of these steps is to not damage the fetus and to not cause maternal damage or bleeding. Cephalic extraction must take into account the position of the fetal head and shoulders and try to bring the biparietal diameter parallel to the bisacromial diameter.

Special cases, such as fetal head that is deflected, hyperflexed, or with sacral rotation of the occiput require additional measures and maneuvers [26–28].

Special attention must be paid in case of engaged head, which, in extreme cases, requires the combined action of the assistant who pushes the fetal head back and of the first operator who extracts the head from the breach, while trying to minimize damage [28,29]. An alternative is version and subsequent breech extraction [30].

Instead, if the head can be pushed back, head rotation maneuvers may be required. These maneuvers bring the head closer to the breach to facilitate its extraction [31].

Shoulder extraction must also follow the pattern of shoulder extraction during vaginal delivery, by extracting the anterior and posterior shoulder along the main axis of the hysterotomy and laparotomy.

The occiput posterior position should be diagnosed before incision of the uterine breach and before extraction [32–38] in order to prevent damage to the fetus [39–45].

REFERENCES

1. Drife J. The start of life: A history of obstetrics. *Postgrad Med J* 2002;78:311–5.
2. Lévy J. Chirurgie obstétricale. Nouveau traité de technique chirurgicale. Tomo XIV, *Gynecologie*. II edition. Paris: Masson; 1973:chapitre XL, 770–84.
3. Martella E, Quirino R. Operazioni ostetriche. *La clinica ostetrica e ginecologica, volume 1, Ostetricia*. Masson editore, II edizione; 1996:capitolo 21, 817–65.
4. Sevell JE. *Caesarean Delivery—A Brief History*. Bethesda, MD: National Library of Medicine; 1993.
5. Gagliardi L e Cerruti G. Taglio cesareo. Tecnica chirurgica. Volume XVI/2, Chirurgia ostetrica e ginecologica. UTET; 1986:1021–30.
6. Hema KR, Johanson R. Techniques for performing caesarean delivery. *Best Pract Res Clin Obstet Gynaecol* 2001;1:17–47.
7. Ross MG, Beall MH. Cervical neck dislocation associated with the Zavanelli maneuver. *Obstet Gynecol* 2006;108(3 Pt 2):737–8.
8. Zelig CM, Gherman RB. Modified Zavanelli maneuver for the alleviation of shoulder dystocia. *Obstet Gynecol* 2002;100(5 Pt 2):1112–4.
9. Kenaan J, Gonzalez-Quintero VH, Gilles J. The Zavanelli maneuver in two cases of shoulder dystocia. *J Matern Fetal Neonatal Med* 2003;13(2):135–8.
10. Vollebergh JH, van Dongen PW. The Zavanelli manoeuvre in shoulder dystocia: Case report and review of published cases. *Eur J Obstet Gynecol Reprod Biol* 2000;89(1):81–84.
11. Gherman RB, Chauhan S, Ouzounian JG, Lerner H, Gonik B, Goodwin TM. Shoulder dystocia: The unpreventable obstetric emergency with empiric management guidelines. *Am J Obstet Gynecol* 2006;195(3):657–72.
12. Cesarean delivery and postpartum hysterectomy. In: Cunningham FG, Gant NF, Leveno KJ, Gilstrap III LC, Hauth JC, Wenstrom KD, eds. *Williams Obstetrics*, 21st ed., Int ed; 2002, Chapter 23:537–63.
13. Warenski JC. A technique to facilitate delivery of the high-floating head at cesarean delivery. *Am J Obstet Gynecol* 198115;139(6):625–7.
14. Levy R, Chernomoretz T, Appelman Z, Levin D, Or Y, Hagay ZJ. Head pushing versus reverse breech extraction in cases of impacted fetal head during Cesarean delivery. *Eur J Obstet Gynecol Reprod Biol* 20051;121(1):24–6.
15. Pelosi MA 2nd, Pelosi MA 3rd. Pelosi minimally invasive technique of cesarean delivery. *Surg Technol Int* 2004;13:137–46.
16. Pelosi MA 3rd, Pelosi MA. A simplified method of cesarean delivery. *N J Med* 1998;95(3):37–45.
17. National Collaborating Centre for Woman's and Children's Health. *Cesarean Section. Clinical Guidelines*. London, UK: RCOG Press; April 2004.

18. Zuspan FP, Quilligan EJ. *Douglas-Stromme Operative Obstetrics*, 5th ed. Norwalk, CT: Appleton and Lange; 1988.
19. Fuller DA, Raphael JS. Extensor tendon lacerations in a preterm neonate. *J Hand Surg Am* 1999;24:628–32.
20. Towner D, Castro MA, Eby-Wilkens E, Gilbert WM. Effect of mode of delivery in nulliparous women on neonatal intracranial injury. *N Engl J Med* 1999;341:1709–14.
21. McFarland LV, Raskin M, Daling JR, Benedetti TJ. Erb/Duchenne's palsy: A consequence of fetal macrosomia and method of delivery. *Obstet Gynecol* 1986;68:784–8.
22. World Health Organization (WHO). *Cesarean Delivery. Managing Complications in Pregnancy and Childbirth*. Geneva, Switzerland: WHO; 2003:8. http://www.who.it.
23. Soutoul JH, Bertrand J, Pierre F. *Le gynécologue obstétricien face au juge*. Bruxelles, France: Institut Shering; 1989:222.
24. Landesman R, Graber EA. Abdomino-vaginal delivery: Modification of the cesarean delivery operation to facilitate delivery of the impacted head. *Am J Obstet Gynecol* 198415;148(6):707–10.
25. Khosla AH, Dahiya K, Sangwan K. Cesarean delivery in a wedged head. *Indian J Med Sci* 2003;57(5):187–91.
26. Iffy L, Apuzzio JJ, Cohen-Addad N, Zwolska-Demczuk B, Francis-Lane M, Olenczak J. Abdominal rescue after entrapment of the aftercoming head. *Am J Obstet Gynecol* 1986;154(3):623–4.
27. Pollard JK, Leaphart WL, Braun TE, Capeless EL. Hysterotomy to effect vaginal delivery with mentum anterior head entrapment. *Obstet Gynecol* 1996;87(5 Pt 2):822–3.
28. Blickstein I. Difficult delivery of the impacted fetal head during cesarean delivery: Intraoperative disengagement dystocia. *J Perinat Med* 2004;32(6): 465–9.
29. Chopra S, Bagga R, Keepanasseril A, Jain V, Kalra J, Suri V. Disengagement of deeply engaged fetal head during cesarean delivery in advanced labor conventional method versus reverse breech extraction. *Acta Obstet Gynecol Scand* 2009;88(10):1163–6.
30. Frass KA, Al Eryani A, Al-Harazi AH. Reverse breech extraction versus head pushing in cesarean delivery for obstructed labor. A comparative study in Yemen. *Saudi Med J* 2011;32(12):1261–6.
31. Goodlin RC. Anterior vaginotomy: Abdominal delivery without a uterine incision. *Obstet Gynecol* 1996;88(3):467–9.
32. Malvasi A, Tinelli A, Stark M. Intrapartum sonography sign for occiput posterior asynclitism diagnosis. *J Matern Fetal Neonatal Med* 2011;14.24(3):553–4.
33. Ghi T, Youssef A, Pilu G, Malvasi A, Ragusa A. Intrapartum sonographic imaging of fetal head asynclitism. *Ultrasound Obstet Gynecol* 2012;26.39(12): 238–40.
34. Malvasi A, Tinelli A, Brizzi A et al. Intrapartum sonography head transverse and asynclitic diagnosis with and without epidural analgesia initiated early during the first stage of labor. *Eur Rev Med Pharmacol Sci* 2011;15(5):518–23.
35. Barbera AF, Tinelli A, Pacella E, Malvasi A. Occiput posterior position and intrapartum sonography. In: Antonio Malvasi, ed. *Intrapartum Sonography for Labor Management*. New York, NY: Springer; 2012:61–72. Cap. 5.
36. Malvasi A, Tinelli A, Barbera A, Eggebø TM, Mynbaev OA, Bochicchio M, Pacella E, Di Renzo GC. Occiput posterior position diagnosis vaginal examination or intrapartum sonography? A clinical review [published online September 13, 2013]. *J Matern Fetal Neonatal Med* 2014;27(5):520–6.
37. Barbera AF, Tinelli A, Malvasi A. Asynclitism: Clinical and intrapartum diagnosis in labor. In: Malvasi A, ed. *Intrapartum Sonography for Labor Management*. New York, NY: Springer; 2012:73–86.
38. Malvasi A, Di Renzo G C., Tinelli A, Laterza F. *Ecografia Intrapartum ed il Parto*. 2012; Rome: G Laterza. Chapters 5 and 7.
39. Dessole S, Cosmi E, Balata A, Uras L, Caserta D, Capobianco G, Ambrosini G. Accidental fetal lacerations during cesarean delivery: Experience in an Italian level III university hospital. *Am J Obstet Gynecol* 2004;191(5):1673–7.
40. Okaro JM, Anya SE. Accidental incision of the fetus at caesarean delivery. *Niger J Med* 2004;13(1):56–8.
41. Urzaiz Rodríguez E. The tragedy of vertex delivery occipito-posterior position 1955. *Ginecol Obstet Mex* 2012;80(9):625–9.
42. Malvasi A, Tinelli A, Brizzi A, Guido M, Martino V, Casciaro S, Celleno D, Frigo MG, Stark M, Benhamou D. Intrapartum sonography for occipito posterior detection in early low dose combined spinal epidural analgesia by sufentanil and ropivacaine. *Eur Rev Med Pharmacol Sci* 2010;14(9):799–806.
43. Tinelli A, Gustatane S, Giacci F, Dell'Edera D, Malvasi A. Intrapartum sonography and clinical risk management. In: Malvasi A, ed. *Intrapartum Sonography for Labor Management*. New York, NY: Springer; 2012:133–48.
44. Malvasi A, Stark M, Ghi T, Farine D, Guido M, Tinelli A. Intrapartum sonography for fetal head asynclitism and trasverse position: Sonographic signs and comparison of diagnostic performance between transvaginal and digital examination. *J Matern Fetal Neonatal Med* 2012;25(5):508–12.
45. Malvasi A, Di Renzo GC. *Semeiotica Ostetrica*. Rome: CIC Ediz. Intern. Cap.12. Travaglio patologico; 2012:483–501.

FURTHER READING

Bofill JA, Lencki SG, Barhan S, Ezenagu LC. Instrumental delivery of the fetal head at the time of elective repeat caesarean: A randomized pilot study. *Am J Perinatol* 2000;17:265–9.

Hankins GD, Clark SM, Munn MB. Cesarean delivery on request at 39 weeks: Impact on shoulder dystocia, fetal trauma, neonatal encephalopathy, and intrauterine fetal demise. *Semin Perinatol* 2006;30(5):276–87.

Racinet C, Bouzid F. Tagli cesarei. Encycl Med Chir. Elsevier, Paris, Ginecologia—Ostetricia, 41900; 1994:21.

Breech presentation

> … extraction is performed by traction on the emerging parts of the fetus. Frequently stronger pulls are required and at times the child may be subjected to lesions during the extraction.
>
> (e. Bumm. *Trattato Completo di Ostetricia*, Vol II, 4th ed., 1924)

INTRODUCTION

Delivery with breech presentation, in its variant forms, is common and up to a few years ago was performed vaginally.

An analysis of the scientific literature shows that the incidence of breech presentation during gestation is reduced, generally, from about 20% around the 28th week to 3%–4% at full term, while taking into account that approximately 96.5% of children are born in cephalic presentation (0.1% face and 0.03% forehead), with 0.28% transverse presentation and 0.08% mixed presentation [1].

These statistics show that there is spontaneous intrauterine fetal version during the third trimester of pregnancy, though should breech presentation persist beyond the 37th week the probability of spontaneous version is almost nil.

Generally, contributing factors to the persistence of this anomalous presentation are prematurity, multiple pregnancy, fetal macrosomia with anomalous full-term presentation (fetal–pelvic disproportion with fetus in breech presentation after 37 weeks), polio (polyhydramnios), oligohydramnios, type of placental insertion (placenta praevia or paracornual fundus), fetal cranial malformations (hydrocephalus or anencephaly), uterine malformations, and large myomas [2].

The greater incidence of feto-neonatal morbidity and mortality in case of breech presentation can be attributed to traumas related to the delivery (asphyxiation or musculoskeletal lesions), to prematurity, and to congenital malformations [3]. The literature contains many cases of brachial plexus and sternocleidomastoid muscle strain, bone fractures (prevalently of the clavicle), and intracranial hemorrhage [4].

A breech presentation diagnosis improves prehension of the fetal breech and allows a better division of the extraction phases, thereby decreasing the risk of iatrogenic maternal–fetal lesions.

In recent years there has been a radical shift in terms of delivery methods in case of breech presentation. Breech delivery has in fact always been represented in clinical practice as a major problem in terms of maternal–fetal outcome.

From the beginning to less than 50 years ago, vaginal obstetrics was predominant in delivery rooms. In fact the significant risks associated with carrying out a cesarean delivery for breech delivery meant that the doctor needed a profound understanding of semiotics and considerable manual skills. With the advent of antibiotic therapy, and the progress in instrumental diagnostics and modern abdominopelvic surgery, traditional vaginal obstetrics has been definitively replaced by abdominal surgical obstetric options [5].

This trend has been further consolidated by modern legal medicine, which has been the decisive factor in the replacement of vaginal breech delivery with cesarean delivery [6]. Nowadays in fact, cesarean delivery is considered a means by which to reduce maternal and fetal–neonatal problems and is the most common way to carry out deliveries in many European countries and in North America, despite the well-known risks of maternal morbidity and mortality related to this surgical intervention [5,6].

Generally speaking, breech extraction through the abdomen follows the same rules as vaginal breech delivery. The same can be said for establishing the breech position in relation to pelvic diameters. It is clear that breech extraction performed with a cesarean delivery is not as difficult as vaginal delivery due to the shortness of the uterine breach and due to the fact that the fetus does not have to move through a rigid canal containing narrow passages, such as the pelvis [7].

BREECH PRESENTATION DIAGNOSIS

Breech presentation diagnosis can be determined clinically through external palpation maneuvers but is currently diagnosed mainly through ultrasound (Figure 4.35).

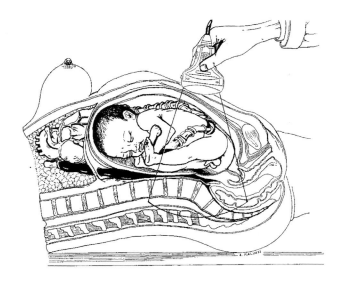

Figure 4.35 Breech presentation diagnosis (incomplete, buttocks variant) obtained with transabdominal ultrasound before a cesarean delivery.

Breech presentations can be divided into (Figures 4.36 and 4.37)

- *Complete*: Legs of the fetus flexed on the thighs, thighs flexed on the abdomen, crossed feet.
- *Incomplete*: When one of the elements of complete presentation is missing; these include the following variants: *buttocks* (thighs flexed on the abdomen and legs extended in front of the trunk); *knees* (thighs extended on the trunk and legs flexed on the thighs); *feet* (thighs and legs, both partially extended); *mixed*.

Depending on the type of presentation at the pelvic inlet there may be different presenting fetal parts:

- Buttocks and feet (complete breech presentation).
- Buttocks (incomplete breech presentation: buttocks variant).
- Knees (incomplete breech presentation: knees variant).
- Feet (incomplete breech presentation: feet variant).
- In case of mixed variant small parts, such as a foot and a knee, a buttock and a foot may be presented.
- Buttocks and feet (complete breech presentation).

The breech presentation diagnosis, with its complete, incomplete, and mixed variants, is more significant for vaginal delivery than for a cesarean delivery. However, because most breech deliveries in primigravidae are carried out, as has been mentioned, abdominally, in order to properly extract the fetus it is always recommended to determine the presentation before carrying out the cesarean delivery. This is especially important in cases of fetal macrosomia or, on the contrary, in cases of cesarean delivery on a preterm fetus, so that the appropriate maneuvers can be performed and iatrogenic fetal lesions, as well as medical and legal disputes, can be avoided.

BREECH EXTRACTION MANEUVERS

Even though breech extraction during a cesarean delivery is not as difficult as vaginal extraction, to avoid maternal-fetal lesions, the operator must perform the same extraction maneuvers during the breech extraction that are performed for vaginal extraction.

In fact the different characteristics of the uterine breach and of the type of laparotomy compared to the complexity of the birth canal facilitate these maneuvers. These, however, must be carried out properly in order to avoid tears in the uterine breach as well as fetal distortions and fractures.

In order to extract the fetus, and depending on the type of presentation, one of the following obstetric maneuvers are to be carried out.

Hooking the fetal inguinofemoral region

Once the uterine breach is open the first maneuver to perform for the buttocks-only variant is hooking the fetal inguinofemoral region.

First it is necessary to palpate with the index and middle finger the fetal breech, in order to locate the inguinofemoral plica of the fetus (Figure 4.38). The obstetrician must then insert his index finger in the inguinofemoral plica of the fetus (Figure 4.39). The operator then inserts the middle finger in the plica and firmly hooks the inguinofemoral area (Figure 4.40).

The hooking maneuver of the inguinofemoral plicae, therefore of the buttocks, must then proceed as in the vaginal delivery, according to the various presentations:

- Posterior transverse sacroiliac (Figure 4.41)
- Posterior right sacroiliac (Figure 4.42)
- Anterior transverse sacroiliac (Figure 4.43)
- Anterior left sacroiliac (Figure 4.44)
- Left longitudinal sacroiliac (Figure 4.45)
- Right longitudinal sacroiliac (Figure 4.46)

Breech presentation "buttocks-only" variant

In the complete buttocks variant hold the fetal pelvis with both hands: fingers should lay on the anterosuperior crista iliaca and the palms on the sacrum to minimize the risk of damage to the soft abdominal tissues of the fetus. This maneuver, actually, is performed in two steps. The first step is to locate the position of breach and to insert fingers along the inguinal fetal plicae. The second maneuver consists in hooking the breach and positioning the bitrochanteric diameter parallel to the transverse hysterotomic axis.

The operator continues the breech extraction maneuver, complete buttocks variant, by holding the breech with the index and middle fingers placed on the fetal anterior iliac spines. If possible the bitrochanteric transverse diameter is brought parallel to the uterine breach (transverse direction) to facilitate the extraction (see Figure 4.46).

Breech presentation "incomplete buttocks" variant

The images in the text describing the breech presentation, feet variant, complete or incomplete, are shown for instructional purposes. They show the breech and the feet for the various positions of the presenting part in relation to the uterine breach, as though from a vaginal point of view.

In reality, once the inferior uterine segment is cut only the feet can be seen while the breech can be seen subsequently once the lower limbs have been extracted.

In the first phase of the breech extraction, incomplete buttocks variant, the presenting fetal foot must be located. In order to do this the operator must insert his hand through the uterine breach and, by palpation, distinguish the fetal foot from the hand (Figure 4.47). The differential diagnosis of hand and foot will prevent the lowering of the upper limb instead of the lower limb, which would complicate breech extraction. If the hand is close to the lower limb the operator should push it back up so that it does not engage the uterine breach along with the lower limbs.

Locating the fetal foot generally facilitates the extraction of the contralateral limb, which is, however, carried out as the feet variant, when the operator has also lowered the lower contralateral limb and placed it parallel to the

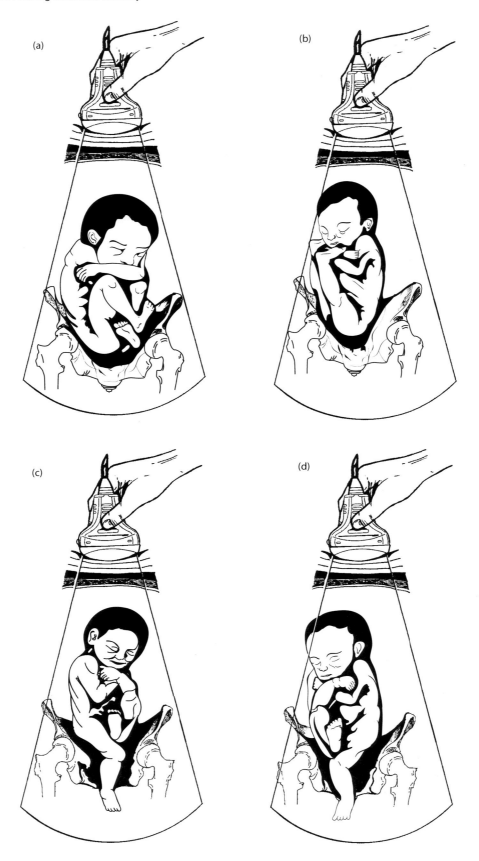

Figure 4.36 Breech presentation variant: (a) complete breech presentation; (b) incomplete breech presentation buttocks variant; (c) mixed incomplete breech presentation right foot and left buttock variant; (d) mixed incomplete breech presentation left foot and right buttock variant. (Modified from Malvasi A, Di Renzo GC. *Ecografia intraparto ed il parto*, Bari, Italy: Editori Laterza; 2012.)

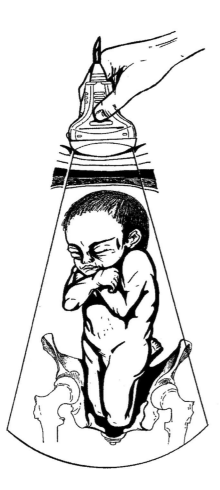

Figure 4.37 Breech presentation variant: incomplete breech presentation, knees variant. (Modified from Malvasi A, Di Renzo GC. *Ecografia intraparto ed il parto*, Bari, Italy: Editori Laterza; 2012.)

presenting limb (Figure 4.48: incomplete breech presentation, buttocks variant, anterior right sacroiliac; Figure 4.49: incomplete breech presentation, buttocks variant, anterior right sacroiliac).

In the breech presentation incomplete feet variant, at times, the foot is not visible, especially in longitudinal or oblique presentations. When extraction is difficult due to the feet not being readily available and/or visible, the operator must turn it into a feet variant breech presentation. Specifically, once the operator has inserted his hand through the uterine breach into the uterine cavity, he must feel the fetal feet and then hook them. At this point of the maneuver, the surgeon must use the index and middle fingers of his hand to hook the fetal ankle and move the feet toward the uterine breach (Figure 4.50).

As mentioned, the extraction, even during a cesarean delivery, must be carried out according to the obstetric rules codified in the Obstetric Semiotics of traditional vaginal extraction, which we describe later.

When both limbs (or only a single lower limb) are high, making it difficult for the surgeon to hook them, the obstetrician is forced to carry out the Pinard maneuver (Figure 4.51).

In this maneuver, in which the feet are moved toward the hysterotomy, two fingers are placed at the hollow of the fetal knee and the thigh and knee are pushed laterally in relation to the median line. By doing this the limb flexes and, normally, the foot moves toward the back of the operator's hand.

After the maneuver, wait for the buttocks to be expelled and then grab the feet and proceed with the (complete or incomplete) breech extraction, as previously described.

Fetal extraction, in case of breech presentation incomplete variant, can be problematic if pulling the foot, during

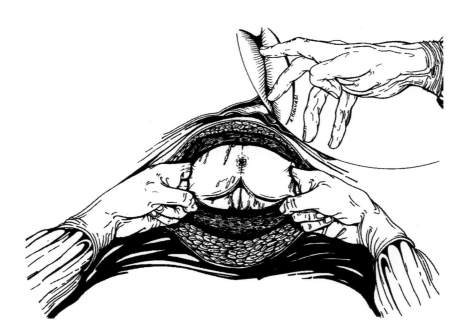

Figure 4.38 The operator with his right hand (image at top right) locates the right fetal inguinofemoral area (anterior sacroiliac presentation).

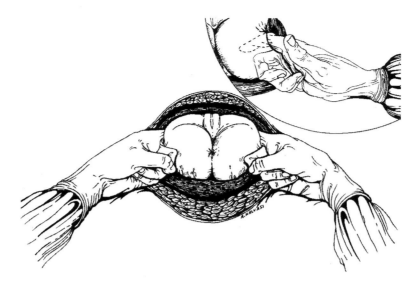

Figure 4.39 The operator inserts the index finger of the right hand (image at top right) into the right fetal inguinofemoral area (posterior sacroiliac presentation).

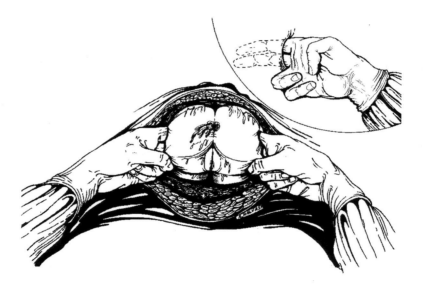

Figure 4.40 The operator then inserts the index finger next to the middle finger of the right hand (image at top right) in the right fetal inguinofemoral area (anterior sacroiliac presentation).

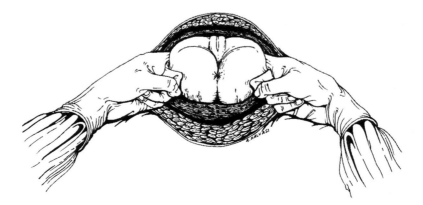

Figure 4.41 Fetal hooking maneuver (initial phase) in incomplete breech presentation, buttocks variant (posterior transverse sacroiliac): using the index fingers the operator hooks both sides of the fetal hips along the inguinal plicae.

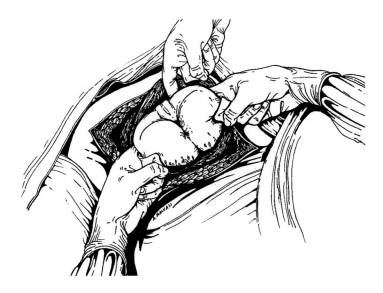

Figure 4.42 Fetal hooking maneuver (initial phase) in incomplete breech presentation, buttocks variant (posterior right sacroiliac): using the index fingers the operator hooks both sides of the fetal hips along the inguinal plicae.

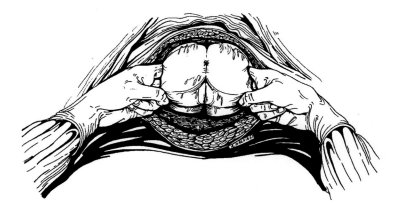

Figure 4.43 Fetal hooking maneuver (initial phase) in incomplete breech presentation, buttocks variant (anterior transverse sacroiliac fetal position): using the index and middle fingers the operator hooks both sides of the fetal hips along the inguinal plicae.

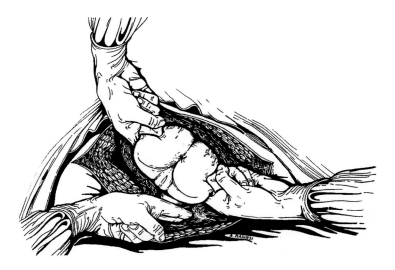

Figure 4.44 Fetal hooking maneuver (initial phase) in incomplete breech presentation, buttocks variant (anterior left sacroiliac): using the index fingers the operator hooks both sides of the fetal hips along the inguinal plicae.

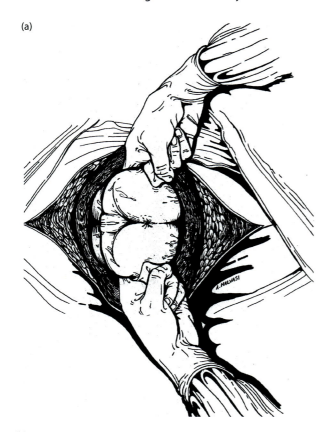

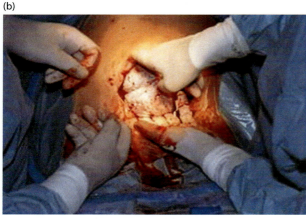

Figure 4.45 Left longitudinal sacroiliac position: in transverse positions of the complete buttocks variant, extraction is carried out by locating the fetal crista iliaca, followed by hooking (a) and extracting them. This can be done with the left hand of the operator, which is positioned in the suprapubic area and acts as a cleavage plane (b).

the extraction of the lower limb closer to the hysterotomy, results in the other lower limb being blocked. The surgeon must then make sure that the limb that has been pushed, or that has not descended, simultaneously follows the previously extracted lower limb. The extraction will otherwise be problematic or even impracticable without causing fetal damage, as the lower limb in the uterine cavity constitutes a sort of barrier (Figure 4.52).

In fact certain mixed maneuvers can be performed for a breech presentation incomplete variant, as though a normal breech extraction or a "big breech extraction" were to be performed.

The foot closer to the uterine breech can be lowered by pulling downward in order to disengage the anterior hip. This is followed by an upward pull that creates space between the posterior hip and the uterine wall so that the foot of the limb that did not descend can be held (Figure 4.53). Once the operator feels the foot, he or she must surround the ankle with his or her index and middle fingers and pull to lower the lower limb in the uterine cavity (Figure 4.54).

During these maneuvers, the fetus normally rotates in the direction of the major axis of the hysterotomy and laparotomy incision. This will also create more space for the following maneuvers.

Breech presentation "complete buttocks" variant

In the breech presentation complete buttocks variant, both feet are brought together immediately below the uterine breach. This presentation can have various positions in relation to the uterine breach, as during vaginal extraction (Figures 4.55 through 4.57).

In the breech presentation feet variant, the operator inserts his or her hand in the uterine cavity and locates the fetal feet. While the operator lifts the uterine breach with his or her left hand to increase the available space (maneuver that can be performed by the assistant), he or she uses his or her right hand to grab the feet and extract them from the breach. In extracting the legs the bitrochanteric diameter positions itself along the major axis of the uterine breach (Figure 4.58).

The surgeon must then place his or her hands symmetrically on the lower limbs of the fetus. The thumbs are pointing in the medial direction and are applied on the posterior side of the thighs up to the gluteal sulcus. The remaining fingers firmly hold the fetal inguinofemoral area (Figure 4.59). Properly positioning the hands on the gluteus will prevent accidental iatrogenic damage to the lower limbs of the fetus, such as the fracture of one of the femurs.

In case of neglected labor due to breech presentation with advanced or complete expansion and with a fetus that cannot be delivered vaginally (e.g., macrosomic fetus) the modified Piper maneuver can be performed.

The progression of the trunk with posteriors dorsum can be problematic as it results in an abnormal delivery mechanism of the shoulder and head. Therefore, the rotation maneuvers, which will be described below, can be difficult or impossible to perform. Therefore, the Piper method is used in breech delivery in case of posterior sacral rotation in advanced labor with feet presentation (Figures 4.60 and 4.61).

The fetus is pushed upward, so that the feet are at the height of the uterine breach; therefore, once the lower limbs are held, rotation is achieved by pulling and rotating the legs (Figure 4.62).

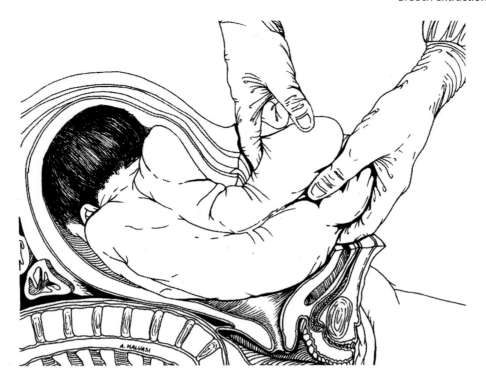

Figure 4.46 Fetal hooking maneuver in incomplete breech presentation, buttocks variant (subsequent phase): to complete the extraction, hold the fetal pelvis with both hands; the index and middle fingers should lay on the anterosuperior crista iliaca and the thumbs on the sacrum to minimize the risk of damage to the soft abdominal tissues of the fetus. However, if possible, the bitrochanteric diameter should be brought parallel to the major diameter of the hysterotomy and of the laparotomy incision. This will facilitate the extraction of the breech and the fetal trunk (right longitudinal sacroiliac presentation).

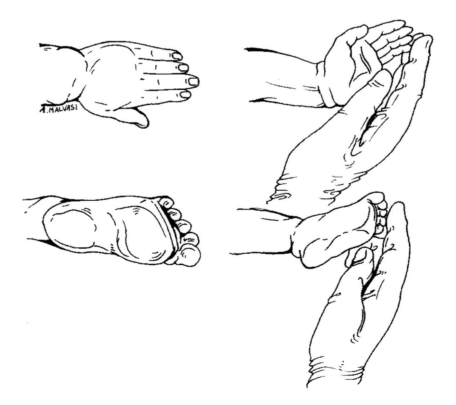

Figure 4.47 Maneuvers for locating the fetal hand and foot: the operator can distinguish the hand, which has long and more flexible fingers, from the foot, which is not as flexible and has short toes.

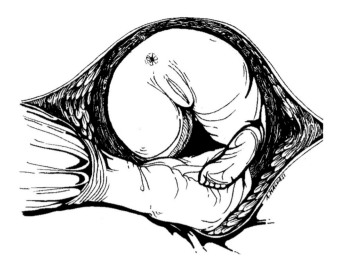

Figure 4.48 Fetal hooking maneuver (initial phase) in incomplete breech presentation, buttocks variant (anterior right sacroiliac): the operator hooks the right fetal foot.

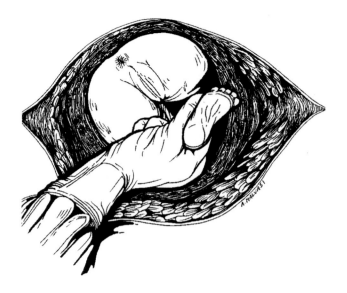

Figure 4.49 Fetal hooking maneuver (initial phase) in incomplete breech presentation, buttocks variant (anterior right sacroiliac): the operator hooks the left foot (posterior), which is the easiest fetal part to hold.

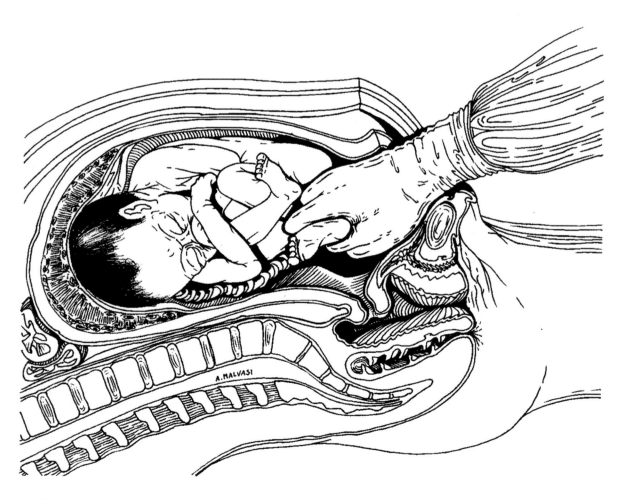

Figure 4.50 Complete breech extraction maneuver feet variant: the surgeon with the index and middle fingers of his right hand must hook the fetal ankle and holding one foot (or preferably both) move the feet toward the uterine breach.

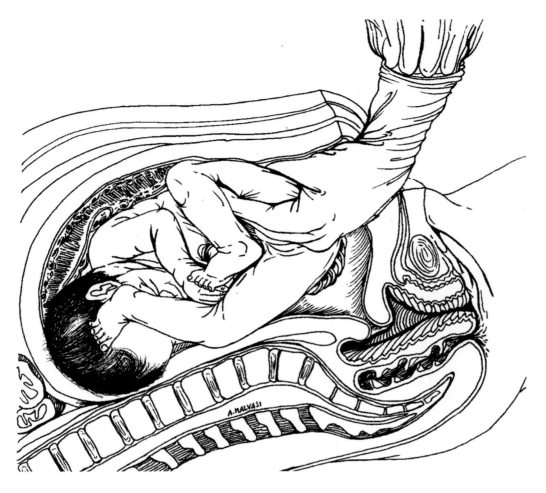

Figure 4.51 In the Pinard maneuver, which is performed to move the fetal feet toward the hysterotomy, two fingers are placed at the hollow of the fetal knee, and the thigh and knee are pushed laterally in relation the median lime. In so doing the limb flexes and, normally, the foot moves toward the back of the operator's hand.

Extraction of the fetus from the uterine breach

Once the glutei are extracted perform the following maneuvers to extract the trunk:

- Delicately pull the fetus until its bisacromial diameter—positioned in an anterior–posterior direction—reaches the uterine breach (Figures 4.63 through 4.65).
- To extract the shoulders—first the anterior and the posterior (Figure 4.66)—gently slide the curved finger from the subaxillary region to the subhumeroulnar region and extract the upper limb once the shoulder has emerged; move the fingers along the fetal neck and anchor them on both sides of the shoulders and pull in an upward direction (Figure 4.67).
- Delicately pull the funicle to create a loop to avoid it stretching, so that the umbilical cord can be "freed" and the funicle loops can be extracted to prevent them (to the extent possible) from being compressed by the fetal body against the uterine breach. This would reduce the supply of blood flow which, if the following maneuvers take longer than expected, must be avoided (Figure 4.68).

The most widely used maneuver to extract the head is the Mauriceau–Smellie–Veit maneuver: after rotating the face in the posterior direction, the operator from the left side of the patient places the first and third fingers of his or her left hand on the cheekbones of the fetus (Figure 4.69) and inserts the index finger in the mouth. With this finger the operator exerts a slight downward pressure on the jaw and flexes the head toward the fetal thorax (Figure 4.70). With his or her right hand the operator lowers the fetal body on the mother's abdomen, while the assistant exerts pressure on the uterine fundus to facilitate the descent of the fetal head (Figure 4.71).

In the Wigand–Martin variant, the operator exerts suprapubic pressure with his or her contralateral hand in the direction of the fetal head to facilitate its spontaneous descent (Figure 4.72).

Extraction of the fetal head, even in breech extraction during a cesarean delivery, is a critical phase and must be carried out in a short amount of time and with a proper sequence of maneuvers. In fact when the shoulders emerge from the uterine breach the breach itself becomes a sort of muscular ring (with a certain degree of rigidity) around the

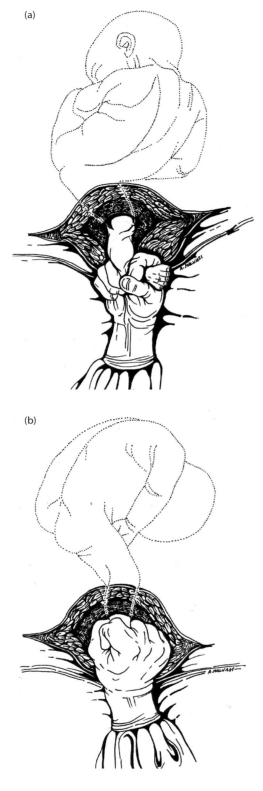

Figure 4.52 Breech extraction incomplete buttocks variant posterior right sacroiliac position in which the lower left limb has not descended and has not followed the lower left limb held by the operator (a). The operator must lower the lower limb that has been pushed or that has not descended (b). The extraction will otherwise be problematic or even impracticable without causing fetal damage.

neck of the fetus. The fetus with the help of the operator must "slip out" from this ring. The Mauriceau maneuver has the advantage of allowing the operator to modulate both the pulling maneuvers on the jaw and the pulling and lifting maneuvers on the fetal neck. However, the assistant must be told when and where to perform the pushing maneuver.

The Wignard maneuver has the advantage of allowing the extraction of the fetal head without the help of the assistant. However, what is lacking are the directional forces on the neck of the fetus and, if necessary, a stronger push.

The Wignard maneuver, if necessary, can become a modified Mauriceau maneuver: in fact, in the Wignard maneuver, the hand of the operator that is pressing on the suprapubic area can move to the fetal neck in order to upwardly move the head as in the Mauriceau maneuver.

During the fetal extraction, when carried out properly and even more so when not carried out properly (Figure 4.73), one or both of the limbs can be blocked. Should that occur, one must proceed according to traditional semiotics and lower the blocked limb.

In the example shown, the right upper fetal limb is blocked with a top-down movement—that is, a descent block. Initially, the right upper limb had risen alongside the head; the forearm then dropped behind the occiput toward the upper part of the fetal dorsum.

The upper limb or limbs can also be blocked with a bottom-up movement, also known as an ascent block.

Initially, the upper limb was lowered along the side of the fetus; the forearm then moved behind the dorsum and was forced to move in an upward direction (Figure 4.74).

This second type of block can be more difficult to resolve and requires greater attention because the upper limb is hyperextended up and toward the back.

Generally, when the upper limbs are blocked the arms are in front of the face. The maneuver to lower the arms consists of the following: a thumb is placed in the axillary cavity and the index and middle fingers, parallel to the fetal arm, held it against the fetal head. The goal is to have two leverage points: the first being the scapulohumeral articulation that is rotated and the second being the elbow articulation that is flexed.

In the ascent block—that is, when the upper limb is pushed back against the fetal occiput—the fundamental phase of the maneuver is, initially, the rotation of the elbow articulation, so that the arm from posterior moves to anterior position, followed by the lever movement, with fulcrum in the scapulohumeral articulation, to lower the arm.

Version through external maneuvers with fetus in breech presentation

The trend in modern obstetrics is not to deliver a breech presentation vaginally, but rather to reduce the incidence of cesarean deliveries in primigravidae with breech presentation, through version in case of a single fetus in breech presentation.

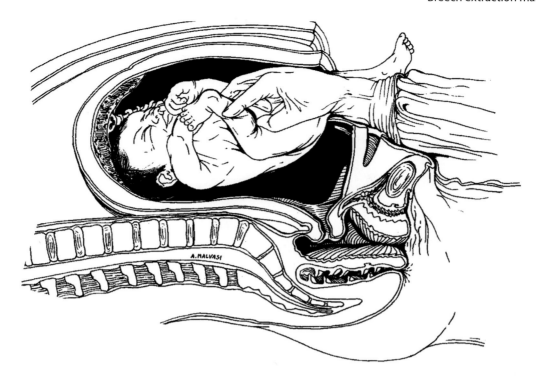

Figure 4.53 Touching and holding the blocked foot in the breech extraction incomplete variant. The foot close to the uterine breech can be lowered by pulling downward in order to disengage the anterior hip. This is followed by an upward pull that creates space between the posterior hip and the uterine wall so that the holding maneuver can be performed on the foot of the limb that did not descend.

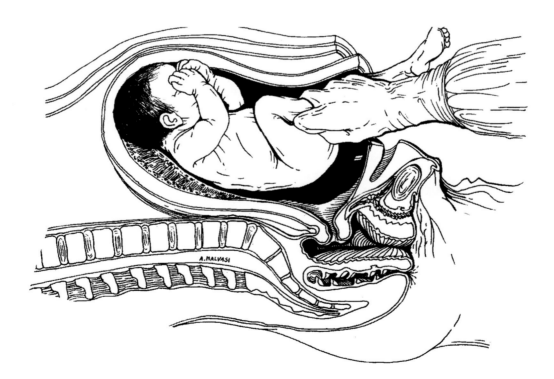

Figure 4.54 Maneuver for lowering the lower limb (subsequent phase): the operator feels the foot and then must surround the ankle with his or her index and middle fingers and pull to lower the lower limb in the uterine cavity. During these maneuvers the fetus normally rotates (in the figure the fetus moves to the posterior transverse sacroiliac position) in the direction of the major axis of the hysterotomy and laparotomy incision. This will also create more space for the following maneuvers.

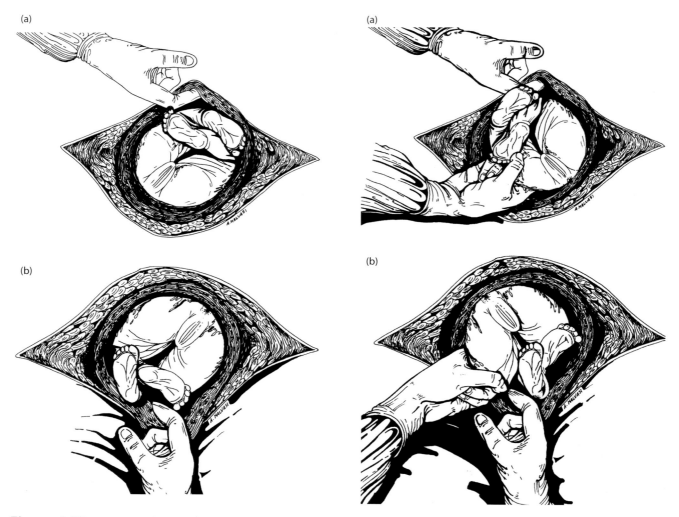

Figure 4.55 Complete presentation feet variant after incision of the lower uterine segment: (a) posterior right sacroiliac variant and (b) anterior left sacroiliac variant.

Figure 4.56 Complete presentation feet variant, (a) left posterior sacroiliac; (b) right anterior sacroiliac variant.

Some studies have shown that external cephalic version (ECV) is effective in reducing the incidence of breech presentations in full-term pregnant women and therefore of Cesarean deliveries performed for this purpose.

The American College of Obstetricians and Gynecologists (ACOG) in 2001 [7] and the Royal College of Obstetricians and Gynaecologists (RCOG) in 2006 [1] have included ECV among the standard procedures in the management of full-term breech presentations, thereby allowing the maneuver to be provided to all pregnant women with breech presentation, in normal full-term pregnancies.

The version of the fetus from breech to cephalic position, in order to restore the best presentation for vaginal delivery, is a technique that has been applied for years [8–11] and is also contained in the latest Royal College guidelines from December 2006 [1] (level of evidence I A). In fact, in many Anglo-Saxon birth centers, ECV is routinely provided upon request. According to clinico-epidemiological studies [12–16], ECV, in the cases examined, reduces the incidence of breech delivery to under 1% with a concurrent reduction in the number of cesarean deliveries (especially true when the intervention is systematically performed for this presentation) [17].

As mentioned, ECV is a method that has been known for a very long time. In Italy, however, modern obstetrics has limited its use and few apply it for fear of complications and medicolegal repercussions. The essential conditions needed for this maneuver are the following: placenta preferably at the fundal level or inserted at the back, a normal amount of amniotic fluid, intact amniochorial membranes, a reassuring fetal cardiogram, no contractile activity of the patient's uterine muscles, the fetus must be actively moving in an ultrasound examination, with the dorsum in a lateral position [1,7,15,16]. The mother obviously must not have excessive abdominal subcutaneous panniculus adiposus [1,7].

The contraindications of ECV can be classified as maternal, fetal or adnexal, or conversely, absolute or relative. Absolute maternal contraindications are the following:

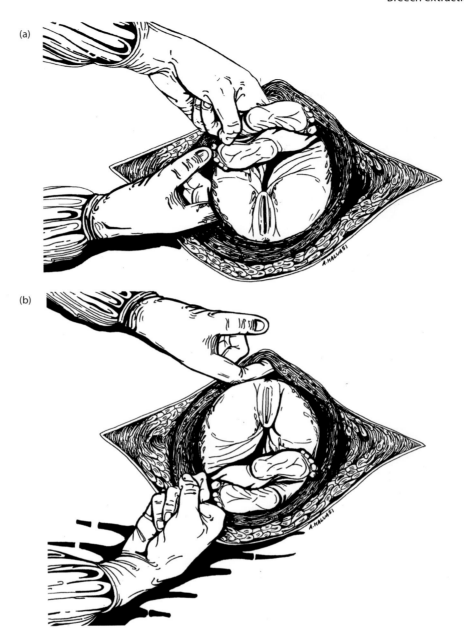

Figure 4.57 Complete presentation feet variant, (a) posterior transverse sacroiliac; (b) anterior transverse sacroiliac.

indications for an elective cesarean delivery, birth canal anomalies, previous nontransverse hysterotomy, and lack of informed consent of the pregnant mother. Relative maternal contraindications are gestational age under 36 weeks, maternal pathologies (such as hypertension, diabetes, gestosis, hyperthyroidism, etc.), previous hysterotomy or metrorrhagias during pregnancy, and uterine malformations.

Absolute fetal contraindications instead are the following: twin pregnancy or serious fetal anomalies (hydrocephalus, anencephaly, heart disease, etc.) and nonreassuring fetal cardiogram before the ECV procedure. The relative contraindications are the following: delay in intrauterine growth or estimated fetal weight over 4000 grams and incomplete breech variant.

Absolute contraindications of fetal adnexa are the following: abnormal placental insertion (placenta praevia), significant oligohydramnios (under 50), or premature rupture of the membranes. Relative contraindications include placenta with anterior insertion [1,7,15,16].

Before beginning any maneuver, the obstetrician must make sure that the fetus is in good health with ultrasound and cardiotocography (CTG) exams, to be repeated after the ECV at predetermined intervals of 3 or 6 hours.

To perform this method the pregnant woman must have an empty bladder, be lying supine with slightly flexed legs, and have signed an informed consent. Some obstetricians prefer the woman to be in a slight Trendelenburg position, and others prefer the lateral decubitus position. In any case it is best that the pelvis be slightly raised (to facilitate

90 Fetal extraction during cesarean delivery

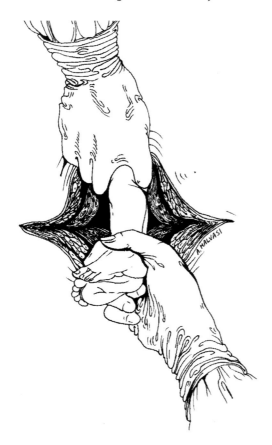

Figure 4.58 The operator inserts his or her hand in the uterine cavity and locates the fetal feet. While the operator lifts the uterine breach with his or her left hand to increase the available space, the right hand is used to grab the feet and extract them from the breach, thus extracting the legs.

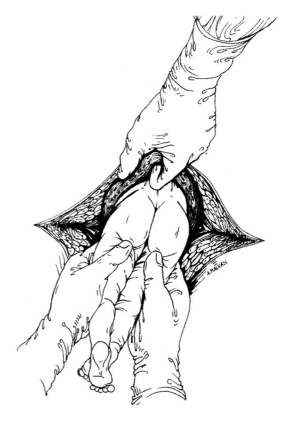

Figure 4.59 The surgeon applies his or her hands on the lower limbs of the fetus. The thumbs are pointing in the medial direction and are applied on the posterior side of the thighs up to the gluteal sulcus. The remaining fingers firmly hold the fetal inguinofemoral area.

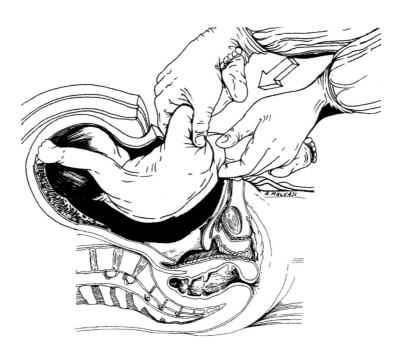

Figure 4.60 First phase of the Piper maneuver: the fetus is pushed upward.

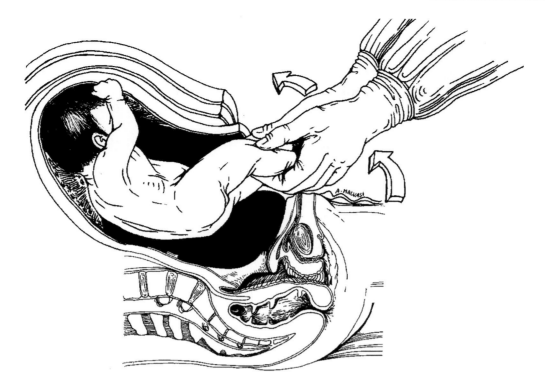

Figure 4.61 Second phase of the Piper maneuver: the fetus is pushed upward with breech rotation.

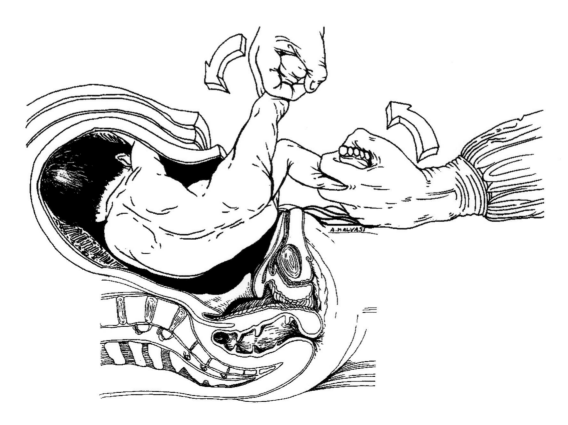

Figure 4.62 Third phase of the Piper maneuver: rotation is achieved by pulling the front leg.

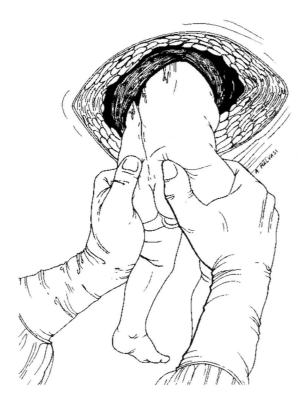

Figure 4.63 In this maneuver, the fetus is delicately pulled until its bisacromial diameter is positioned in a latero-lateral direction, along the major axis of the uterine breach.

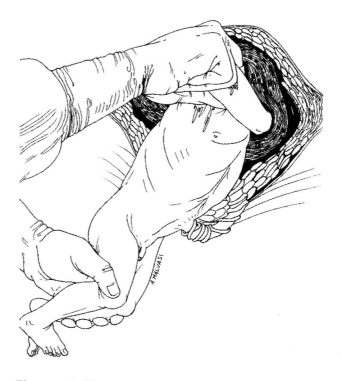

Figure 4.65 Disengagement maneuver of the anterior shoulder.

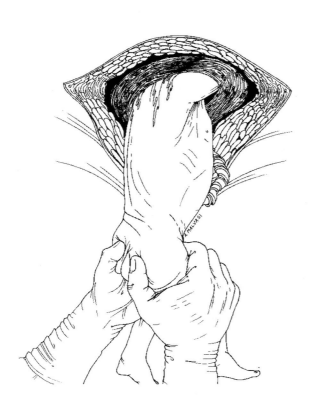

Figure 4.64 By pulling the fetus downward, the shoulders will engage and the axillary cavity and anterior arm will emerge.

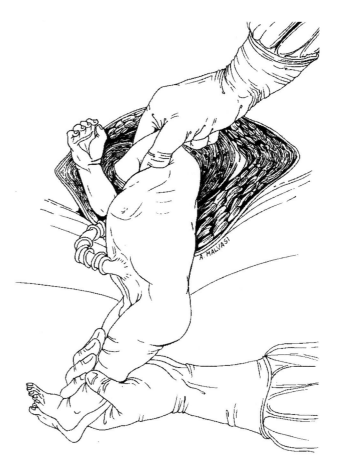

Figure 4.66 Disengagement maneuver of the posterior shoulder after the fetal body has been rotated by 90°.

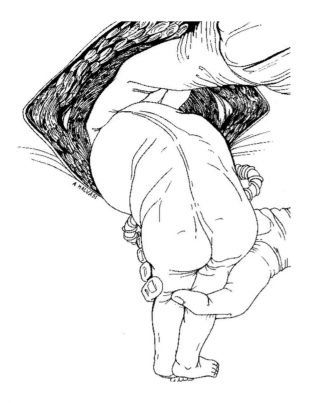

Figure 4.67 Anchoring maneuver of the fetal shoulders in which the fingers of the surgeon applied on both sides of the fetal shoulders pull in a forward and upward direction.

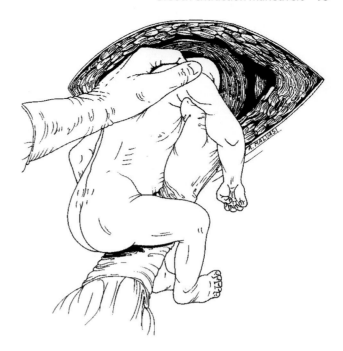

Figure 4.69 First phase of the Mauriceau maneuver: the surgeon, with his or her right hand, locates the buccal cavity of the fetus and inserts his or her index and middle fingers.

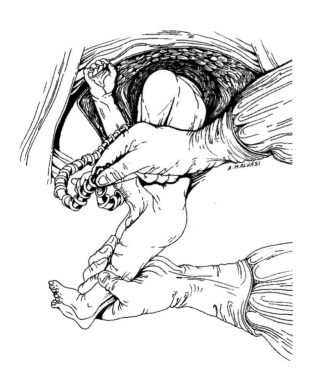

Figure 4.68 After disengagement of both shoulders, and before disengaging the head, the umbilical cord must be "freed" so that the funicle loops can be extracted to prevent them (to the extent possible) from being compressed by the fetal body against the uterine breach.

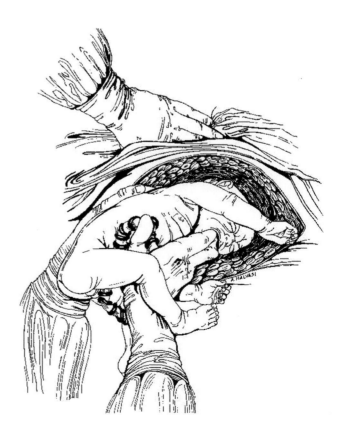

Figure 4.70 Second phase of the Mauriceau maneuver: the surgeon simultaneously pulls up with his or her left hand on the neck, while the right hand placed in the fetal mouth disengages the head from the uterine breach.

94 Fetal extraction during cesarean delivery

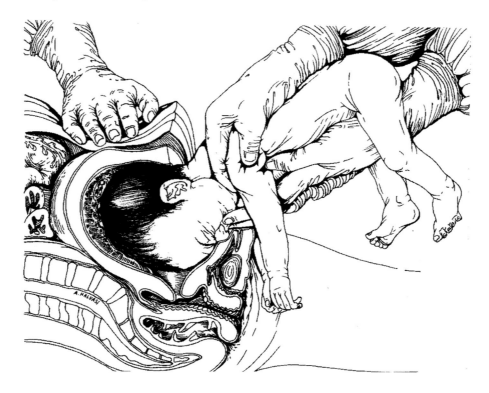

Figure 4.71 Mauriceau maneuver: the operator inserts the index and middle finger of the left hand in the mouth of the fetus and exerts some pressure on the jaw, while with the right hand he or she pulls on the neck and lifts the fetus high (left-handed operator). The assistant maintains a constant suprapubic pressure to facilitate the maneuvers of the operator.

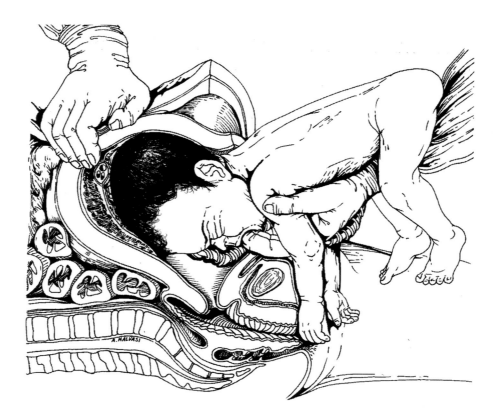

Figure 4.72 Wignard maneuver: the operator carefully pulls the jaw with the index and middle finger of the left hand placed in the fetal mouth, and with the right hand on the suprapubic area gradually pushes the head.

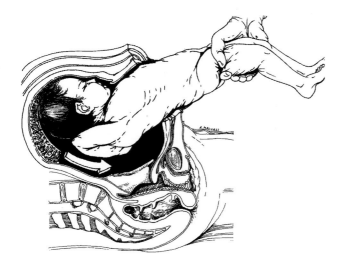

Figure 4.73 The right upper fetal limb is blocked with a top-down movement—that is, a descent block. Initially, the right upper limb had risen alongside the head; the forearm then dropped behind the occiput toward the upper part of the fetal dorsum. By touching the axillary cavity one can feel that it is wide and nearly flat.

the disengagement of the breech) and that the pregnant woman be infused with a tocolytic drug (to maximize relaxation of the uterine muscles) [17,18].

The obstetrician places his or her nearly flat hands on the two fetal poles and applies a constant pressure in the attempt to turn the fetus with an anterior (craniocaudal) or posterior (caudocranial) movement. The rotation of the fetus is easier in the direction that accentuates the flexion of the trunk, in the direction in which the fetus "sees," which is also the shortest distance for cephalic

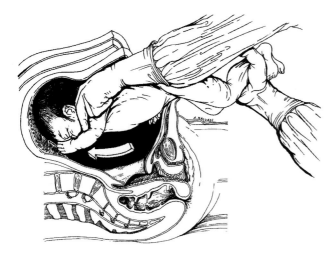

Figure 4.74 The left upper limb is blocked with a bottom-up movement—that is, an ascent block. Initially, the upper limb was lowered along the side of the fetus; the forearm then moved behind the dorsum and was forced to move in an upward direction. By touching the axillary cavity one can feel that it is narrow and deep, which differentiates this from the ascent block.

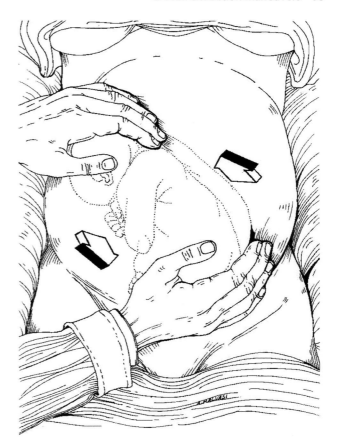

Figure 4.75 External cephalic version of fetus in breech presentation with left anterior fetal dorsum.

presentation (Figures 4.75 and 4.76). Some obstetricians prefer to exert pressure only on the fetal dorsum or only on one fetal pole (breech or cephalic extremity).

During the entire rotation of the fetus, it is necessary to check the fetal heart rate with CTG and for any vaginal blood loss (due to detachment of the placenta, a rare but possible event). For this reason the rotation should be performed in completely safe conditions, with a team ready to intervene should a cesarean delivery become necessary [19]. In most cases ECVs are carried out normally and do not cause discomfort for the woman: should this not happen the maneuvers must be immediately suspended, and if necessary, regional anaesthesia must be applied.

After the maneuver, it is recommended to use tocolytics, such as nifedipine, terbutaline, or atosiban, to relax the uterus [17–19].

Risks and complications in the use of ECV include placental trauma, which can cause a partial or complete detachment of the placenta from the insertion site: this occurs in 1% to 4.5% of cases and apparently is due to excessive force applied during the ECV maneuver [20,21]. The force that is applied during the ECV determines an increase in pressure in the intervillous space, which results in the rupture of vessels and the formation of retroplacental hematoma. It is therefore recommended to never exert too much force during the version [22].

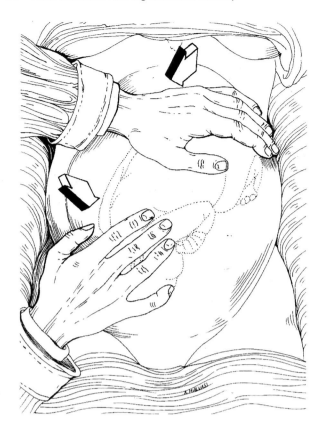

Figure 4.76 The fetus after the version maneuver has turned in the anterior direction (craniocaudal) with dorsum to the right and breech at top left.

Another risk associated with ECV is the wrapping of the funicles around the fetal neck, as confirmed by studies. Furthermore, version reduces the greater frequency of funicle complications associated with breech delivery, in which the incidence of prolapsed funicle is 3–20 times that of cephalic delivery [1,7,20].

ECV rarely causes rupture of the amniotic sac, though there is an increase in changes to fetal heart rate recorded with a cardiotocograph after an ECV. It has been established that version maneuvers modify the heart rate in 20%–40% of cases. These changes, however, are transitory and disappear 15 minutes after the maneuvers end [23].

Last, the frequency of hemorrhage or fetal–maternal transfusion is between 2% and 30%: it has been demonstrated that ECV can cause a transfusion between fetus and mother. For this reason at the end of the procedure anti-D immunoglobulins are administered to women with Rh-negative blood type.

The percentage of positive outcome of the maneuver, when correctly performed, is around 70%–90% [1,7,24].

It is apparent that ECV is simpler in earlier stages, but it is also true that by intervening before the 32nd–34th week many fetuses, which would have spontaneously turned in the uterus, would be subjected to this maneuver. The scientific literature reports that once version occurs at the 37th week or later, very few fetuses return to the breech presentation [25].

Conclusions

Normally fetuses in breech presentation spontaneously turn to other presentations up to the 37th week [26]. After this date the fetus is unlikely to change the initial presentation [27]. In some countries, physicians resort to external cephalic version, assisted by tocolytic betamimetics [28].

In modern obstetrics, breech presentation, in most cases, leads to delivery by cesarean delivery [28,29]. Due to medical and legal risks tied to vaginal birth complications [30], most obstetricians prefer abdominal delivery to assisted vaginal delivery [31–33].

Generally, cesarean delivery of a breech presentation can be planned after the 38th week of gestation and outside of labor [34,35]. However, some reviews and trials have evaluated the possibility of providing vaginal birth to patients who are strongly motivated, without pathologies in the anamnesis, with maternal and fetal well-being, and not at risk of the complications inherent with this maneuver. These studies have concluded that there is no difference for these selected patients in the maternal–fetal outcome [1,7,36–39].

Maneuvers for delivery of the fetus in breech presentation, during a cesarean delivery, are the same as those during assisted vaginal delivery. Similarly, external cephalic version maneuvers are basically the same as those that were performed in the past [8–11] to avoid fetal damage [40]. External cephalic version is an obstetric intervention that is still used in some countries, and it reduces the incidence of cesarean deliveries. It favors the rotation of the fetus from breech to cephalic present and is without particular risks. It is recommended for those cases in which the patient requests it [1,7,12–16].

REFERENCES

1. Royal College of Obstetricians and Gynaecologists (RCOG). *The Management of Breech Presentation.* Guideline No. 20b; December 2006.
2. Ghosh MK. Breech presentation: Evolution of management. *J Reprod Med* 2005;50:108–16.
3. Doyle NM, Riggs JW, Ramin SM, Sosa MA, Gilstrap LC 3rd. Outcomes of term vaginal breech delivery. *Am J Perinatol* 2005;22:325–8.
4. Cheng M, Hannah M. Breech delivery at term: A critical review of the literature. *Obstet Gynecol* 1993;82:605–18.
5. Hannah ME, Hannah WJ, Hewson SA, Hodnett ED, Saigal S, Willan AR. Planned caesarean delivery versus planned vaginal birth for breech presentation at term: A randomised multicentre trial. Term Breech Trial Collaborative Group. *Lancet* 2000;356(9239):1375–83.
6. International Federation of Gynecology and Obstetrics. Recommendations of the FIGO Committee on Perinatal Health on guidelines for the management of breech delivery. *Eur J Obstet Gynecol Reprod Biol* 1995; 58:89–92.

7. Committee on Obstetric Practice. ACOG committee opinion. Mode of term singleton breech delivery. Number 265, December 2001. American College of Obstetricians and Gynecologists. *Int J Gynaecol Obstet* 2002;77(1):65–66.
8. Friedlander D. External cephalic version in the management of breech presentation. A report on 706 patients treated by this method. *Am J Obstet Gynecol* 1966;95(7):906–13.
9. Berg D, Kunze U. Critical remarks on external cephalic version under tocolysis. Report on a case of antepartum fetal death. *J Perinat Med* 1977;5(1):32–38.
10. Van Dorsten JP, Schifrin BS, Wallace RL. Randomized control trial of external cephalic version with tocolysis in late pregnancy. *Am J Obstet Gynecol* 1981;141(4):417–24.
11. Morrison JC, Myatt RE, Martin JN Jr, Meeks GR, Martin RW, Bucovaz ET, Wiser WL. External cephalic version of the breech presentation under tocolysis. *Am J Obstet Gynecol* 1986;154(4):900–3.
12. Grootscholten K, Kok M, Oei SG, Mol BW, van der Post JA. External cephalic version-related risks: A meta-analysis. *Obstet Gynecol* 2008;112(5):1143–51.
13. Hutton EK, Saunders CA, Tu M, Stoll K, Berkowitz J; Early External Cephalic Version Trial Collaborators Group. Factors associated with a successful external cephalic version in the early ECV trial. *J Obstet Gynaecol Can* 2008;30(1):23–28.
14. Doyle NM, Riggs JW, Ramin SM, Sosa MA, Gilstrap LC 3rd. Outcomes of term vaginal breech delivery. *Am J Perinatol* 2005;22:325–8.
15. International Federation of Gynecology and Obstetrics. Recommendations of the FIGO Committee on Perinatal Health on guidelines for the management of breech delivery. *Eur J Obstet Gynecol Reprod Biol* 1995;58:89–92.
16. Hutton EK, Hofmeyr GJ. External cephalic version for breech presentation before term. *Cochrane Database Syst Rev* 2006;(1):CD000084.
17. Kok M, Bais JM, van Lith JM, Papatsonis DM, Kleiverda G, Hanny D, Doornbos JP, Mol BW, van der Post JA. Nifedipine as a uterine relaxant for external cephalic version: A randomized controlled trial. *Obstet Gynecol.* 2008;112(2 Pt 1):271–6.
18. Collaris R, Tan PC. Oral nifepidine versus subcutaneous terbutaline tocolysis for external cephalic version: A double-blind randomised trial. *BJOG.* 2009;116(1):74–80.
19. Abenhaim HA, Varin J, Boucher M. External cephalic version among women with a previous cesarean delivery: Report on 36 cases and review of the literature. *J Perinat Med* 2009;37(2):156–60.
20. Sela HY, Fiegenberg T, Ben-Meir A, Elchalal U, Ezra Y. Safety and efficacy of external cephalic version for women with a previous cesarean delivery. *Eur J Obstet Gynecol Reprod Biol* 2009;142(2):111–4.
21. Boucher M, Marquette GP, Varin J, Champagne J, Bujold E. Fetomaternal hemorrhage during external cephalic version. *Obstet Gynecol* 2008;112(1):79–84.
22. Khoo CL, Bollapragada S, Mackenzie F. Massive fetomaternal hemorrhage following failed external cephalic version: Case report. *J Perinat Med* 2006;34(3):250–1.
23. Salani R, Theiler RN, Lindsay M. Uterine torsion and fetal bradycardia associated with external cephalic version. *Obstet Gynecol* 2006;108(3 Pt 2):820–2.
24. Higgins M, Turner MJ. How useful is external cephalic version in clinical practice? *J Obstet Gynaecol* 2006;26(8):744–5.
25. Ben-Meir A, Elram T, Tsafrir A, Elchalal U, Ezra Y. The incidence of spontaneous version after failed external cephalic version. *Am J Obstet Gynecol* 2007;196(2):157.
26. Westgren M, Edvall H, Nordström L, Svalenius E, Ranstam J. Spontaneous cephalic version of breech presentation in the last trimester. *Br J Obstet Gynaecol* 1985;92(1):19–22.
27. Fonseca L, Monga M. Spontaneous version following preterm premature rupture of membranes. *Am J Perinatol* 2006;23(4):201–3.
28. Cluver C, Hofmeyr GJ, Gyte GM, Sinclair M. Interventions for helping to turn term breech babies to head first presentation when using external cephalic version. *Cochrane Database Syst Rev* 2012;1:CD000184.
29. Palencia R, Gafni A, Hannah ME et al.; Term Breech Trial Collaborative Group. The costs of planned cesarean versus planned vaginal birth in the Term Breech Trial. *CMAJ* 2006;174(8):1109–13.
30. Hofmeyr GJ, Hannah ME. Planned caesarean delivery for term breech delivery. *Cochrane Database Syst Rev* 2003;(3):CD000166.
31. Nassar N, Roberts CL, Barratt A, Bell JC, Olive EC, Peat B. Systematic review of adverse outcomes of external cephalic version and persisting breech presentation at term. *Paediatr Perinat Epidemiol* 2006;20(2):163–71.
32. Golfier F, Vaudoyer F, Ecochard R, Champion F, Audra P, Raudrant D. Planned vaginal delivery versus elective caesarean delivery in singleton term breech presentation: A study of 1116 cases. *Eur J Obstet Gynecol Reprod Biol* 2001;98(2):186–92.
33. Su M, Hannah WJ, Willan A, Ross S, Hannah ME; Term Breech Trial Collaborative Group. Planned caesarean delivery decreases the risk of adverse perinatal outcome due to both labour and delivery complications in the Term Breech Trial. *BJOG* 2004;111(10):1065–74.
34. Liu S, Liston RM, Joseph KS, Heaman M, Sauve R, Kramer MS; Maternal Health Study Group of the Canadian Perinatal Surveillance System. Maternal mortality and severe morbidity associated with low-risk planned cesarean delivery versus planned vaginal delivery at term. *CMAJ* 2007;176(4):455–60.

35. Lau TK, Lo KW, Rogers M. Pregnancy outcome after successful external cephalic version for breech presentation at term. *Am J Obstet Gynecol* 1997;176(1 Pt 1):218–23.
36. Kumari AS, Grundsell H. Mode of delivery for breech presentation in grandmultiparous women. *Int J Gynaecol Obstet* 2004;85(3):234–9.
37. Phipps H, Roberts CL, Nassar N, Raynes-Greenow CH, Peat B, Hutton EK. The management of breech pregnancies in Australia and New Zealand. *Aust N Z J Obstet Gynaecol* 2003;43(4):294–7.
38. Molkenboer JF, Reijners EP, Nijhuis JG, Roumen FJ. Moderate neonatal morbidity after vaginal term breech delivery. *J Matern Fetal Neonatal Med* 2004;16(6):357–61.
39. Gilbert WM, Hicks SM, Boe NM, Danielsen B. Vaginal versus cesarean delivery for breech presentation in California: A population-based study. *Obstet Gynecol* 2003;102(5 Pt 1):911–7.
40. Capobianco G, Virdis G, Lisai P, Cherchi C, Biasetti O, Dessole F, Meloni GB. Caesarean delivery and right femur fracture: A rare but possible complication for breech presentation. *Case Rep Obstet Gynecol* 2013;2013:613709. doi:10.1155/2013/613709.

FURTHER READING

Doumouchtsis SK, Arulkumaran S. Are all brachial plexus injuries caused by shoulder dystocia? *Obstet Gynecol Surv* 2009 Sep;64(9):615–23.

Goffinet F, Carayol M, Foidart JM et al. PREMODA Study Group. Is planned vaginal delivery for breech presentation at term still an option? Results of an observational prospective survey in France and Belgium. *Am J Obstet Gynecol* 2006;194:1002–11.

Fetal extraction with instruments

> …any obstetrician that extracts a fetus from the uterine breach must remember this. If a caesarean delivery is performed to protect the brain of the baby from the trauma which would occur vaginally, or for obstetric reasons, special attention must be paid when removing the body and the head. Any trauma that occurs during a Caesarean delivery cannot be justified."
>
> (R. Durfee, in *Gynecologic and Obstetric Surgery*. DH Nichols, 1993)

EXTRACTION WITH INSTRUMENTS

When all extraction attempts do not succeed, instruments such as forceps and ventouse (vacuum extractor) must be used. An extraction with instruments is always preferable to a widening of the hysterotomy breach as the pedunculi of the uterine arteries can be damaged [1].

Besides those specific cases during a cesarean delivery in which the fetal head needs to be extracted with instruments, some operators prefer to disengage the head from the uterine breach using a ventouse. The phases and methods, however, are those of the vaginal delivery.

Some operators use single-use vacuum extractors. These offer certain advantages as they are smaller and can be better handled than traditional vacuum extractors. In addition, subjective pressure can be applied on the scalp, and when necessary, the device can be deactivated manually.

In using forceps during a cesarean delivery, greater attention must be paid to application time and traction methods. The latter, however, have phases that are comparable to those of vaginal delivery. The use of forceps or vacuum extractor should be considered only when manual maneuvers fail [2–4].

There are certain conditions that may lead to its use:

- Cephalic presentation:
  - The fetal head is too high, meaning it cannot be firmly held and maneuvered—even with fundal pressure.
  - The head is deeply engaged in the superior strait and cannot be easily pushed out.
- Breech presentation: hyperflexion of the fetal head.

Using forceps

Short forceps with crossed branches and sliding mechanism (Pajot or Smellie) or with divergent branches (Suzor) can be used.

As an alternative, a single forceps branch may be used as a lever, with the pubic symphysis functioning as a fulcrum. Some authors [5] do not recommend it as it might widen the hysterotomy breach and have fetal repercussions (cephalohematomas).

There are two different types of cephalic presentation, depending on whether the fetal occiput is anterior or posterior.

Application of forceps during a cesarean delivery

The figures in the text refer to the application of forceps during a cephalic presentation:

- Slide the left branch of the forceps along the palm side of the technician's left hand (Figures 4.77 and 4.78).
- Move the branch forward along the cheek of the fetus (Figure 4.79).
- Insert the right branch using the same technique (Figure 4.80).
- Cross the two branches (Figure 4.81): the branches should have an upward concavity in case of anterior occiput and downward concavity in case of posterior occiput.
- Quickly and delicately extract the head of the fetus (Figure 4.82) by pulling on the crossed branches of the forceps directed upwards while the contralateral hand lowers the edges of the uterine breach so that the head can more easily disengage from it.
- The next phase may require the use of a single branch that functions as a lever between breach and head, allowing the head to emerge (Figure 4.83).

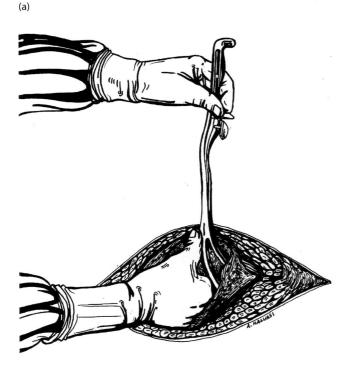

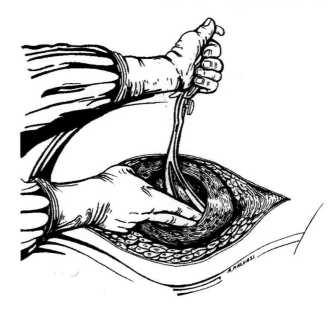

Figure 4.78 Deep positioning, from top to bottom, of the left branch.

- In the event of cephalic presentation, in which it is difficult to manually extract the head, forceps are used by applying the branches directly and symmetrically on the head of the fetus. This maneuver is made easier by the better visibility of the presented part through the uterine breach and the easier palpation of the scalp sutures compared to vaginal delivery, even in the event of posterior occiput presentation (Figures 4.84 and 4.85).
- A single branch of the forceps may be used when extraction of the head from the uterine breach proves to be especially difficult. The branch is placed between the head of the fetus and the Doyen autostatic valve to increase leverage. If necessary, the operator or assistant can apply external pressure on the uterine fundus, which allows the presented parts to slide on the forceps branch that functions as a lever (Figure 4.86).

In case of breech presentation use Piper forceps or, better yet, Piper forceps modified according to Laufe. The modified forceps have divergent branches that are shorter and easier to handle than the conventional version [6].

The method for applying forceps to the head is similar to the one used in vaginal delivery:

- The assistant is tasked with lifting the fetal body so that the head and uterine breach are visible.
- As when applying this method to the vaginal delivery, insert the left branch along one side of the fetal face, in which the palm side of the technician's hand is used as a guide.
- Perform the same procedure with the right branch.
- Once the forceps are applied, flexion of the head is achieved by delicately lifting the legs and lowering the fetal head toward them.
- The extraction is completed by pulling externally and lifting the gripped part.

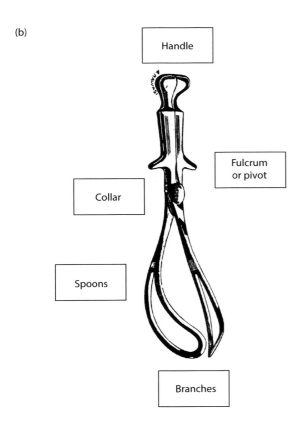

Figure 4.77 The left branch is inserted and guided by the operator's right hand (a); illustration of the Naegele forceps and its various parts, with an upward and forward curvature of the branches and of the apex of the branches compared to other types of forceps (b).

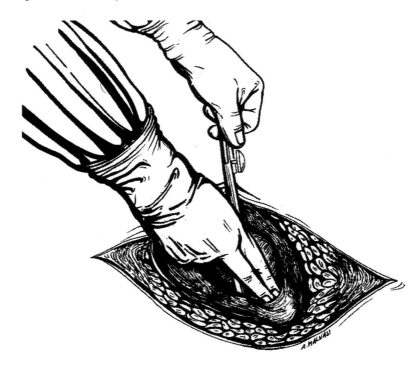

Figure 4.79 The operator positions the left branch of the forceps, slides it around the fetal cheek, and lowers the branch handle.

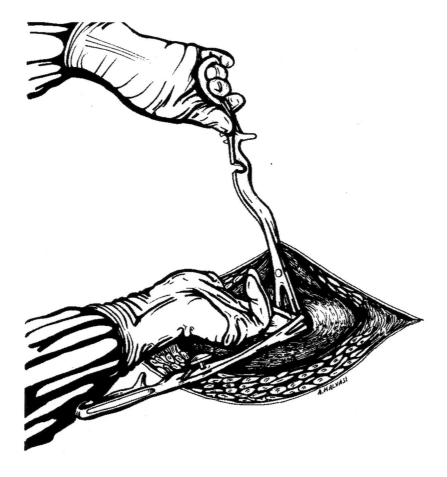

Figure 4.80 The operator inserts the right branch of the forceps.

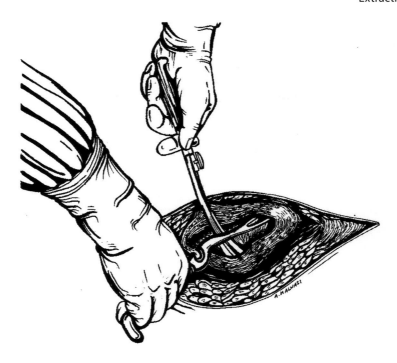

Figure 4.81 The operator maneuvers the forceps branches.

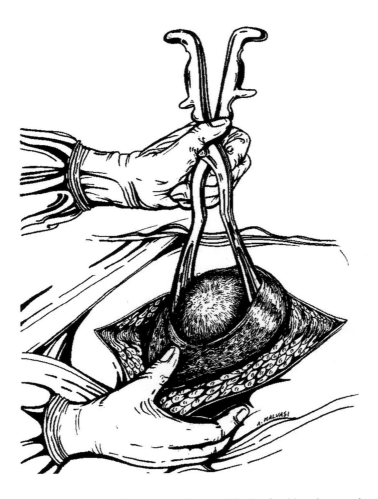

Figure 4.82 The operator performs the extraction: as the left hand lifts the fetal head upward to facilitate the extraction, the right hand lowers the lower edge of the uterine breach.

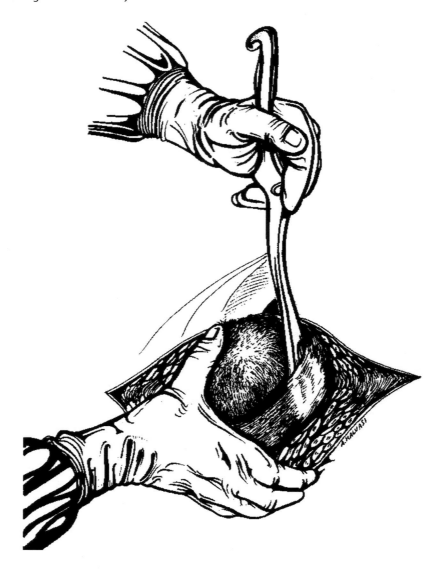

Figure 4.83 Once the right branch is freed, the operator uses the left branch as a lever to facilitate the extraction of the head.

Vacuum extractor

The use of an obstetric ventouse for fetal head extraction during a cesarean delivery was described for the first time by Solomons in 1962 and is an excellent alternative to the use of forceps [7].

After the uterine incision, the assistant generally stabilizes the head on the lower uterine breach and exerts a pressure on the uterine fundus. As in the vaginal delivery, the vacuum cup is carefully inserted inside the uterine breach (Figure 4.87).

The first operator places the ventouse on the presented part and applies an automatic vacuum suction (Figure 4.88) to carry out a test traction (Figure 4.89). The operator then pulls and rotates the fetal head following the movement with two left-hand fingers placed on the cup (Figure 4.90). The fetal head is then pulled in an upward direction so that the chin can emerge from the uterine breach (Figure 4.91) [8]. Once the head has emerged from the breach, the obstetrician releases the vacuum from the presented part by interrupting the negative pressure on the fetal head and releasing the suction mechanism on the soft tissues of the fetal head (Figure 4.92).

As mentioned, single-use vacuum extractors are currently used in many delivery rooms as they have many advantages over traditional extractors: they can be easily handled, are smaller compared to the traditional vacuum, the negative pressure on the fetal scalp can be modulated, the device can be released directly by the operator, and the materials are sterile and disposable (Figure 4.93).

There are several advantages to using the vacuum extractor during a cesarean delivery:

- The volume of the presented part is not increased.
- The head is not compressed.
- Damages or extensions of the uterine incision are infrequent.
- The head can be extracted at any level.

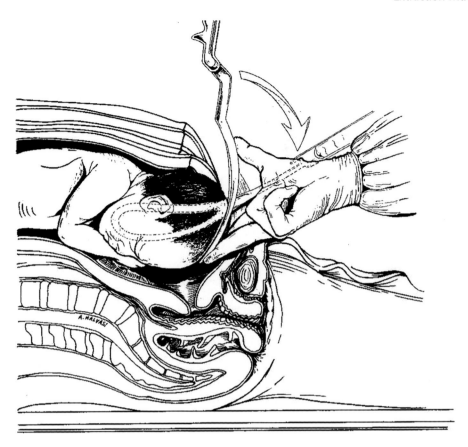

Figure 4.84 Sagittal section of a female pelvis, which shows the Naegele forceps inserted through the uterine breach and correctly applied, in a direct and symmetrical manner, on the fetal head. (Modified from Malvasi A, Di Renzo GC. *Ecografia intraparto ed il parto*, Bari, Italy: Editori Laterza; 2012.)

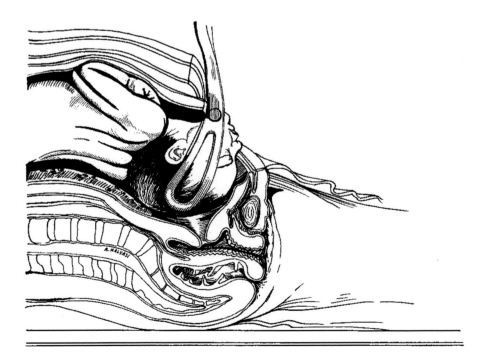

Figure 4.85 Sagittal section of a female pelvis, which shows the direct and symmetrical application of the branches of the Naegele forceps on the fetal head in the occiput posterior position.

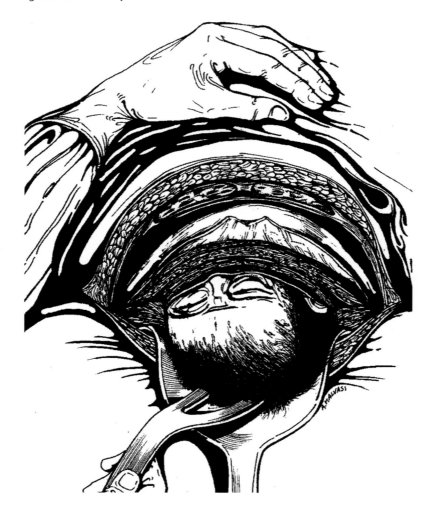

Figure 4.86 The operator uses only one branch of the forceps, placed between the fetal head and the Doyen retractor, in order to increase leverage; the operator exerts an external pressure on the uterine body to facilitate the disengagement of the presenting part.

- The vacuum can be applied at any level of the fetal head, even in the case of a not fully developed lower uterine segment.

The only disadvantage compared to forceps is the longer extraction time.

In 1973 Kobayashi introduced the plastic ventouse. Later, numerous soft and semirigid cups were manufactured, which contributed to the increase in use of the obstetric ventouse. Indeed, starting in the 1970s, the obstetric ventouse was the most widely used instrument in vaginal deliveries [9].

In certain cases, the new "soft" obstetric ventouses that improve the extraction of the fetal head are used even during cesarean delivery. An example is the "Kiwi" single-use ventouses of which there are two types: the OmniCup and the ProCup [10].

The ProCup (Figure 4.93) is based on the Malmstrom ventouse and is best indicated when the fetal scalp is positioned at the rima vulvae or in case of anterior occiput position.

The Kiwi OmniCup is suited for all fetal head positions including posterior asynclitism and lateral malposition. The Kiwi OmniCup is the most widespread, used in delivery rooms. It consists of a plastic cup inside which is a shaped sponge. The cup is connected to a flexible tube also made in plastic (Figure 4.94), connected to a manual graduated suction pump (*integral vacuum PalmPump*) with a quick-release button and a push-button bar that creates a vacuum in the cup. Once the cup is applied to the fetal scalp, the pressure needed to achieve the vacuum is indicated on the dynamic bar of the manual pump (Figure 4.95): clinical studies recommend a pressure between 450 and 600 mm Hg (green zone) and below 620 mm Hg (red zone).

The Kiwi OmniCup (Figure 4.96) allows for an easy and versatile application of a vacuum on the fetal scalp. Traction can be regulated even in case of contamination of the cup with amniotic fluid or blood.

Use the Bird concept (*Bird's "posterior cup" concept*) when applying the Kiwi to the occiput to achieve an optimal pulling force. The operator can thus extract

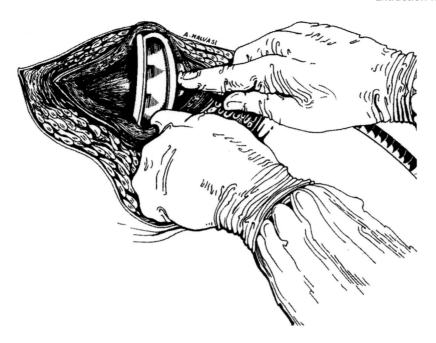

Figure 4.87 The operator inserts the vacuum cup inside the uterine breach in the same manner as during vaginal delivery—that is, the cup, as it is inserted, remains perpendicular to the centerline of the uterine breach.

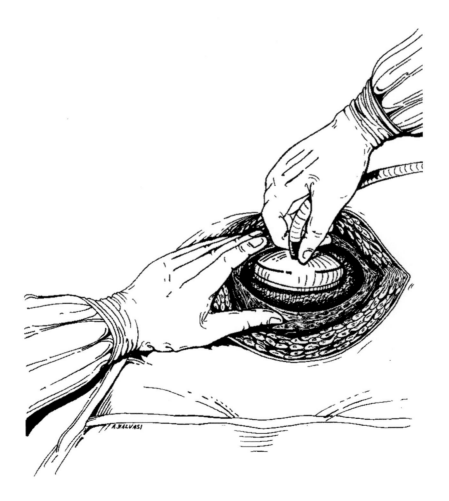

Figure 4.88 The operator positions the ventouse on the presenting part and applies the automatic suction of the vacuum extractor.

106 Fetal extraction during cesarean delivery

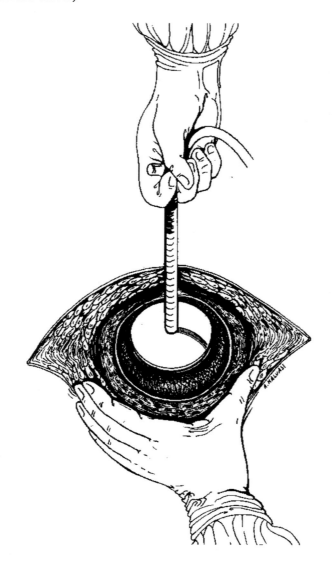

Figure 4.89 The operator pulls in order to test the cup's grip.

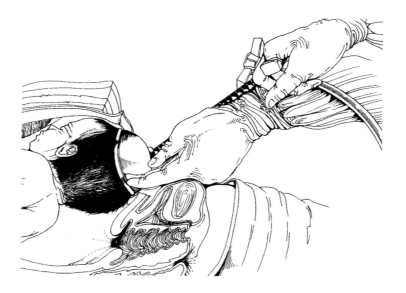

Figure 4.90 The operator pulls on the fetal head, with two fingers of the operator's left hand placed on the cup, as the head is rotated.

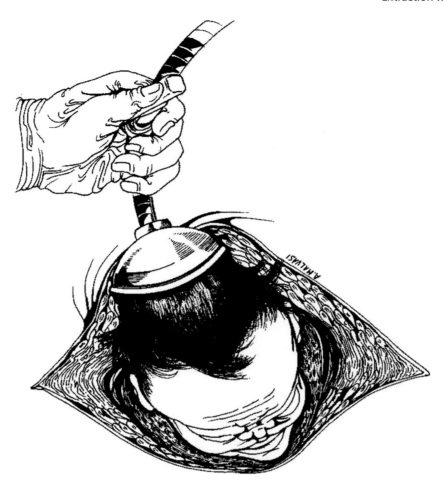

Figure 4.91 The obstetrician pulls on the fetal head in an upward direction so that the chin of the fetus can emerge from the uterine breach.

the presented part without detaching it from the pulling instrument. Unfortunately, the presented part is frequently malpositioned, especially in case of asynclitism and deflection. This complicates the application of the traditional vacuum. In cases such as these, the Kiwi OmniCup is practical, flexible, and does not cause trauma. It has thus proven to be better than traditional ventouses and can also be used for transverse and occiput posterior positions. This is especially true for a cesarean delivery in which the cup should be applied on any part of the scalp, except on the face and ears.

Literature contains comparative studies and meta-analyses on the application of both rigid and soft ventouses during vaginal delivery. There are, however, few references on the application of these instruments during a cesarean delivery [11].

Compared to vaginal delivery, soft ventouses reduce the risk of damage to the fetal scalp. However, it does not seem to reduce the more serious fetal lesions, such as subaponeurotic and intracranial hemorrhages. In addition, when applied outside the occiput, it has a higher risk of failure [12]. It seems therefore reasonable during a cesarean delivery to use soft ventouses for extractions in which the position of the fetal head is not especially difficult and in which a pulling force is sufficient.

To correctly apply the "soft" vacuum, once the lower uterine segment has been cut, start out by locating the fetal occiput so that the cup can be correctly applied on the fetal scalp. The operator then applies the cup on the presented part with the left hand and with the right hand maneuvers the manual pump to create the vacuum (Figure 4.97).

If the cup cannot be applied on the fetal occiput, the operator must position the cup as close as possible to the occiput (Figure 4.98). The pressure must be slightly higher than the standard pressure, and the traction must be prolonged and careful to avoid detachment of the device before the fetal head has been extracted (Figure 4.99).

The use of forceps or obstetric ventouse in a cesarean delivery depends on the experience of the operator and whether special cases are present, such as fetal malformations [13]. This practice is, however, not common. The forceps present a risk of facial and intracranial damages, whereas the risks posed by obstetric ventouses are not as severe. Literature, however, describes, in rare instances of

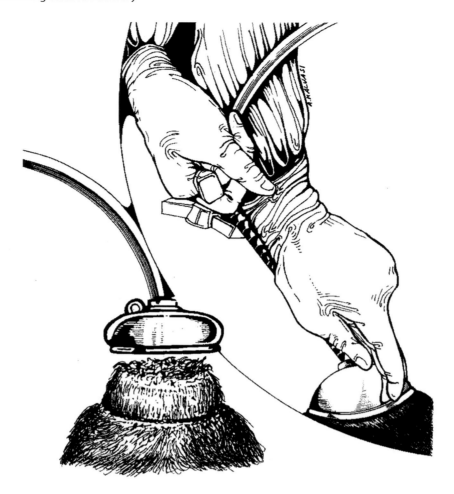

Figure 4.92 The operator releases the vacuum from the presenting part by reducing the negative pressure on the fetal head, which results in the swelling of soft tissues.

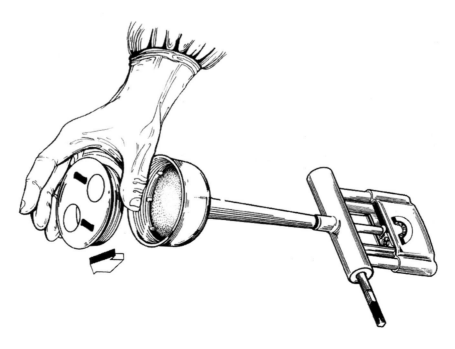

Figure 4.93 ProCup-type Kiwi ventouse.

Extraction with instruments 109

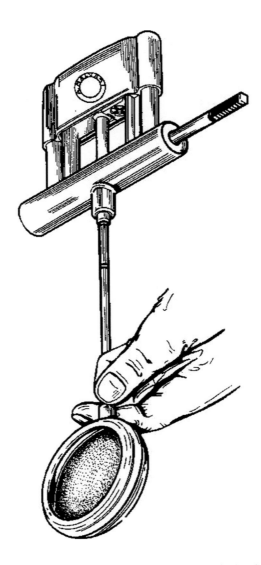

Figure 4.94 OmniCup-type Kiwi ventouse consisting of a plastic cup inside which is housed a shaped sponge; the cup is connected to a flexible plastic tube attached to a graduated manual suction pump.

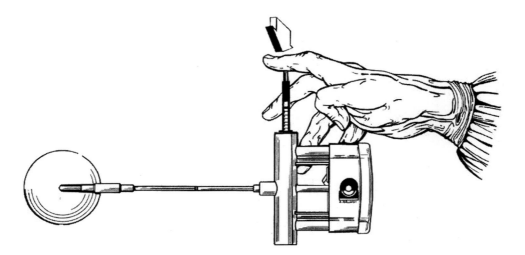

Figure 4.95 The pressure needed to create a vacuum on the fetal scalp is applied on the Kiwi OmniCup and is shown on a scale bar inserted in the manual pump: clinical studies recommend a pressure between 450 and 600 mm Hg (green zone) and in particular below 620 mm Hg (red zone).

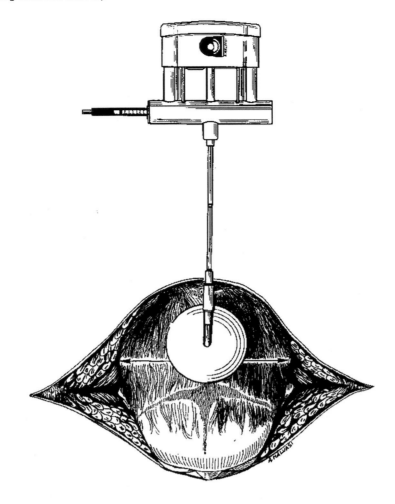

Figure 4.96 The Kiwi OmniCup should always be applied on the occiput to achieve the best pulling force, in accordance with the Bird concept.

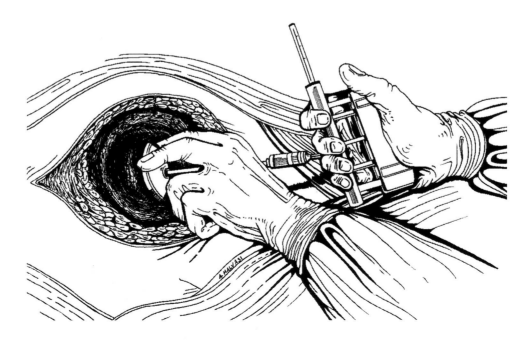

Figure 4.97 The single-use vacuum extractor cup can be easily applied on the fetal scalp due to its small size.

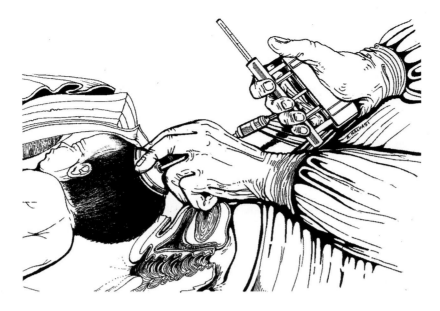

Figure 4.98 The operator exerts pressure and pulls by modulating the intensity.

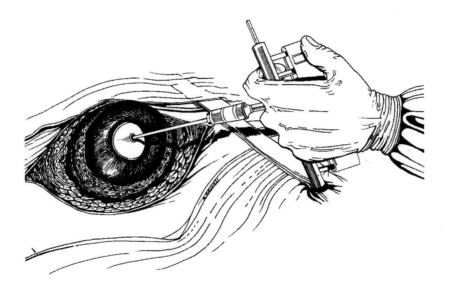

Figure 4.99 The operator employs a single-use vacuum extractor to disengage the fetal head from the uterine breach.

a vacuum applied during a cesarean delivery, intracranial hemorrhagic damage and, in particular, subaponeurotic, intraventricular, intracerebral, and subdural hemorrhages [14]. In particular, fetal damage of the dura mater results from repeated applications of the vacuum during particularly difficult extractions.

Conclusions

The cesarean delivery is an intervention that has been created to facilitate abdominal extraction of the fetus, which would otherwise be difficult or impossible through vaginal delivery.

Generally, the extraction is carried out manually by an operator who may be assisted by a "Kristeller" applied on the uterine fundus by the assistant.

However, in certain cases forceps and ventouses may prove useful in the extraction of the fetal head from the hysterotomy. Currently, a ventouse is preferred to forceps due to the fewer numbers of complications, especially to the fetus, that arise during their use [15].

As for the obstetric ventouse, the soft type is the most used as it causes less trauma on the fetal scalp. Although numerous studies in literature compare the use of rigid versus soft ventouse, only a few case reports describe the complications that arise following application of a ventouse during a cesarean delivery [16].

When determining whether these instruments can be used during a cesarean delivery, the operator, in the cost–benefit analysis, must consider the possible fetal complications that arise during use of these instruments [17].

On the other hand the emergency cesarean delivery, employed in the event of failure of both forceps and ventouse during vaginal delivery [18], is an extreme option that could harm the fetus [19–21].

REFERENCES

1. Cesarean delivery and postpartum hysterectomy. In: Cunningham FG, Gant NF, Leveno KJ, Gilstrap III LC, Hauth JC, Wenstrom KD, eds. *Williams Obstetrics*, 21st ed, Int ed.; 2002, Chapter 23:537–63.
2. Bofill JA, Lenki SG, Barhan S, Ezenagu LC. Instrumental delivery of the fetal head at the time of elective repeat caesarean: A randomized pilot study. *Am J Perinatol* 2000;17:265–9.
3. National Collaborating Centre for Woman's and Children's Health. *Cesarean delivery. Clinical Guideline.* London, UK: RCOG Press; April 2004.
4. Martella E, Quirino R. Operazioni ostetriche. In: Candiani GB, Danesino V, Gastaldi A, eds. *La clinica ostetrica e ginecologica*, II edizione, vol. 1, Ostetricia. Milan: Masson editore, 1996, capitolo 21, 817–65.
5. Zuspan FP, Quilligan EJ. *Douglas-Stromme Operative Obstetrics*, 5th ed. Norwalk, CT: Appleton and Lange; 1988.
6. Locksmith GJ, Gei AF, Rowe TF, Yeomans ER, Hankins GD. Teaching the Laufe-Piper forceps technique at caesarean delivery. *J Reprod Med* 2001;46:457–461.
7. Landy HJ, Zarate L, O'Sullivan M. Abdominal rescue using the vacuum extractor after entrapment of the aftercoming head. *Obstet Gynecol* 1994;84:644–6.
8. Nakano R. Use of the vacuum extractor for delivery of the fetal head at caesarean delivery. *Am J Obstet Gynecol* 1981;5:475–6.
9. Bercovici B. Use of vacuum extractor for head delivery at Cesarean delivery. *Isr J Med Sci* 1980;16(3): 201–3.
10. Vacca A. Vacuum-assisted delivery. *Best Pract Res Clin Obstet Gynaecol* 2002;16(1):17–30.
11. Dimitrov A, Pavlova E, Krŭsteva K, Nikolov A. Caesarean delivery with vacuum extraction of the head. *Akush Ginekol* (Sofiia) 2008;47(3):3–6.
12. Arad I, Linder N, Bercovici B. Vacuum extraction at cesarean delivery—Neonatal outcome. *J Perinat Med* 1986;14(2):137–40.
13. Akiyama Y, Moritake K, Maruyama N, Takamura M, Yamasaki T. Acute epidural hematoma related to cesarean delivery in a neonate with Chiari II malformation. *Childs Nerv Syst* 2001;17(4–5):290–3.
14. Clark SL, Vines VL, Belfort MA. Fetal injury associated with routine vacuum use during cesarean delivery. *Am J Obstet Gynecol* 2008;198(4):e4.
15. Boehm FH. Vacuum extraction during cesarean delivery. *South Med J* 1985;78(12):1502.
16. Fareeduddin R, Schifrin BS. Subgaleal hemorrhage after the use of a vacuum extractor during elective cesarean delivery: A case report. *J Reprod Med* 2008;53(10):809–10.
17. Clark SL, Vines VL, Belfort MA. Fetal injury associated with routine vacuum use during cesarean delivery. *Am J Obstet Gynecol* 2008;198(4):e4. doi:10.1016/j.ajog.2007.12.009.
18. Miot S, Riethmuller D, Deleplancque K, Teffaud O, Martin M, Maillet R, Schaal JP. Cesarean delivery for failed vacuum extraction: Risk factors and maternal and neonatal outcomes. *Gynecol Obstet Fertil* 2004;32(7–8):607–12.
19. Iffy L, Pantages P. Erb's palsy after delivery by Caesarean section. (A medico-legal keyplay a vexing problem). *Med Law* 2005;24(4):655–61.
20. Nikolov A, Veleva G, Nashar S, Markov P, Sluncheva B, Yarakova N Fracture of clavicle in newborns an attempt to make prognostics factors. *Akush Ginekol (Sofiia)* 2011;50(7):4–7.
21. Gardberg M, Leonova Y, Laakkonen E Malpresentations—Impact on mode of delivery. *Acta Obstet Gynecol Scand* 2011;90(5):540–2.

FURTHER READING

Pelosi MA, Apuzzio J. Use of the soft, silicone obstetric vacuum cup for delivery of the fetal head at caesarean delivery. *J Reprod Med* 1984;29(4):289–92.

Anomalous presentation

> … The mother and the fetus are in serious danger when a transverse situation is not resolved. This situation must therefore be considered "absolutely unfavourable"
>
> (Marzius H. *Trattato di Ostetricia*, 1953)

INTRODUCTION

In obstetrics the word "presenting" refers to the part of the fetus that initially encounters the maternal pelvis at the beginning of labor. In 95% of pregnant women, the presentation is cephalic, and the head of the fetus is at the entrance of the maternal pelvis.

Other presentations instead are defined as "anomalous." Anomalous presentations usually occur in twin pregnancies (which we will discuss at the end of the chapter) and frequently result in a cesarean delivery. Included among anomalous fetal situations are those in which the fetus is in the transverse situation—that is, the head is directed to the side of the mother and the buttocks are in the opposite direction.

Fortunately this situation defined as "transverse" is rare and occurs in less than 2% of all full-term pregnancies [1]. When the shoulder of the fetus is at the entrance of the pelvis, it is defined more commonly as "shoulder" presentation. In this case, vaginal delivery is impossible, as the fetus obviously cannot move through the maternal pelvis in a transverse position [2].

This occurs more frequently in pluriparous mothers and can at times have a serious complication, the prolapse of the funicle, as in the transverse situation the naval is close to the uterine orifice and the presenting part is high [3]. The transverse presentation of the fetus is an absolute indication for the completion of the cesarean delivery, as the fetus is horizontal, with high or low dorsum [1,4].

Below is a detailed explanation of fetal extraction in transverse presentation during a cesarean delivery.

FETUS IN A TRANSVERSE POSITION (SHOULDER PRESENTATION)

Whenever a fetus is in a transverse intrauterine position, its major axis is perpendicular to the major axis of the mother. The shoulder is located above the pelvic cavity with the head in one of the two iliac fossae and the breech in the contralateral side [1].

There are two types of transverse positions: anterior dorsal and posterior dorsal (Figure 4.100), both of which include two presentations: right shoulder and left shoulder. In order to determine the position of the fetus in transverse presentations, in addition to traditional abdominal palpations, it is recommended to perform an ultrasound examination before the cesarean delivery [5] so that the operator can prepare the proper extraction maneuvers (Figures 4.101 and 4.102). An ultrasound before a cesarean delivery is recommended due to the need to locate the placenta, which, when anterior, is likely to be encountered during the hysterotomy. An unstretched internal uterine segment in fact is "uninhabited" by any fetal part.

If the placenta is cut during the incision, it will bleed and may require version and fetal extraction maneuvers to be carried out quickly [6]. Therefore, it is best for them that the hand of the operator knows where to look for the fetal parts that were previously shown with ultrasound. In terms of fetal extraction, it is best to remember that the transverse position is more difficult for the operator compared to a cephalic and breech extraction (in all variant forms). The reason is that the transverse position stretches the longitudinal fibers of the myometrium in the transverse direction and therefore results in hypertonia (which in deliveries is generally referred to as "risk of uterine rupture") [7].

In the case of transverse position of the fetus, because most cesarean deliveries are carried out under regional anesthesia, it is important to determine with the anesthetist whether it is preferable and/or necessary to sedate the pregnant woman or even to perform general anesthesia [8].

Cesarean delivery for a fetus in transverse position must, obviously, be indicated during labor or outside of active labor when all preventive maneuvers for external version have failed. However, external version maneuvers may prove useful even during a cesarean delivery. These maneuvers may be performed by the operator to assist in the fetal version or by the assistant, in a coordinated manner, so as to preventively determine, for example, the movement of the cephalic extremity of the fetus [9,10].

If possible, before performing any traditional extraction maneuvers for the fetus in transverse position, the

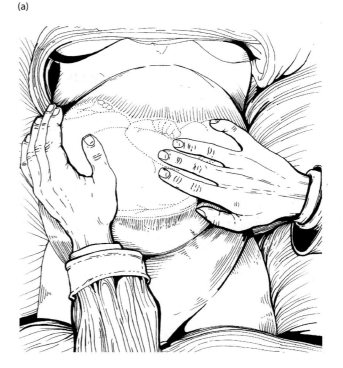

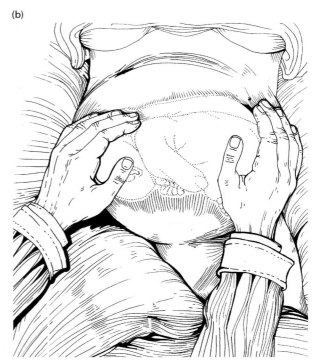

Figure 4.100 (a) Leopold maneuver in transverse presentation and inferior dorsum. (b) Anterior dorsum. (Modified from Malvasi A, Di Renzo GC. *Semeiotica Ostetrica*, Rome, Italy: CIC Edizioni Internazionali; 2012.)

position of the shoulder should be determined in order to avoid mistakenly grabbing the hands (Figures 4.103 through 4.105).

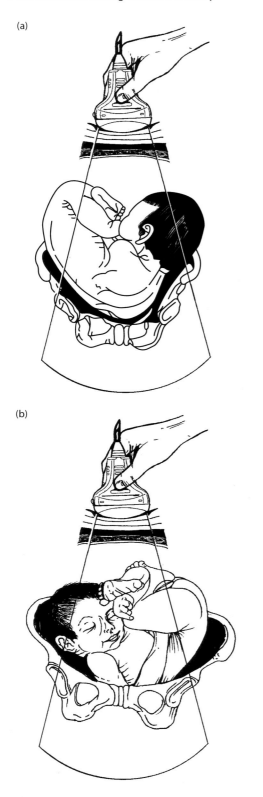

Figure 4.101 (a) Transverse presentation with head to the left and anterior dorsum. (b) Transverse position with head to the right and posterior dorsum. (Modified from Malvasi A, Di Renzo GC. *Ecografia intraparto ed il parto*, Bari, Italy: Editori Laterza; 2012.)

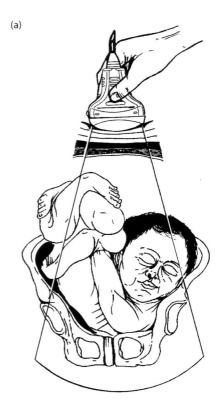

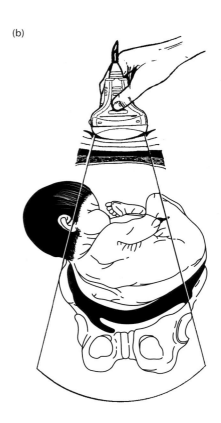

Figure 4.102 (a) Transverse presentation with head to the left and posterior dorsum. (b) Transverse position with head to the right and anterior dorsum. (Modified from Malvasi A, Di Renzo GC. *Ecografia intraparto ed il parto*, Bari, Italy: Editori Laterza; 2012.)

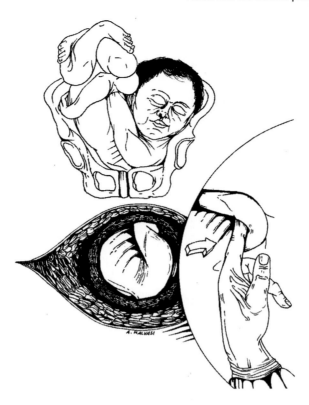

Figure 4.103 Transverse position with posterior dorsum and with head to the left (axillary space closed to the left). Through palpation of the axillary space closed on the side of the head, the operator can direct his or her hand toward the breech, avoiding the upper limb of the fetus.

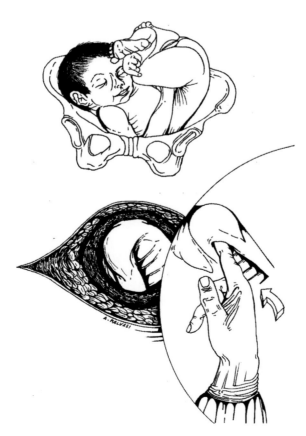

Figure 4.104 Transverse position with posterior dorsum and head to the right (axillary space closed at right).

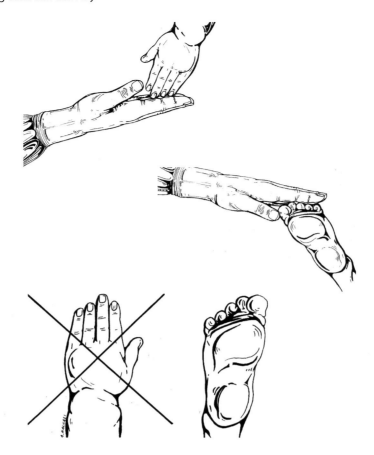

Figure 4.105 Maneuvers for locating the fetal hand and foot: the operator can feel the long and flexible fingers of the hand, whereas a foot is not as flexible and has short toes.

MANEUVERS FOR EXTRACTION OF THE FETUS IN TRANSVERSE POSITION DURING CESAREAN DELIVERY

The extraction of the fetus in transverse presentation requires a version maneuver that is more difficult, as the fetus is in a transverse, inferior dorsum position. In fact, it is necessary to reach back to the uterine fundus in order to locate the foot (Figure 4.106), grab it, bring it toward the uterine breach (Figure 4.107), and complete the extraction with both feet (Figure 4.108).

The extraction maneuvers for fetus with anterior dorsum are the following:

- After the hand has been inserted into the uterine breach and the feet have been located, carry out a maneuver similar to that of Pinard [11,12] to lower the lower fetal limb for an incomplete breech presentation, buttocks-only variant (Figure 4.109). If the fetus to be extracted is with the dorsum in an anterior position, the maneuver is more complex in that to reach the fetal feet a longer portion of the arm must be inserted. If possible the operator should grab both feet, otherwise he or she should grab the one foot that is easier to reach [12].
- Firmly hold onto the foot with the entire hand or, better yet, with the index and middle finger crossed on the fetal malleolus. If possible, grab the other foot with the third and fourth fingers. These maneuvers must be carried out with caution and proper timing, while taking into account that after the hysterotomy and rupture of the membranes the uterus tends to retract [13].
- After grabbing a foot or better yet both feet and bringing them to the uterine breach, the fetus will move toward a vertical position. If pulling on one foot is not concurrent with the descent of the other foot, then this other limb must be located. If there is difficulty in the version, the fetal head must be pushed back (with hand inserted in the uterus) in an attempt to bring the fetus to a vertical position in breech presentation. This verticalization maneuver [7–9] can be assisted by the second operator who pushes the head back toward the uterine fundus from the outside, while the operator extracts the fetus from the breach (Figures 4.110 and 4.111).
- Once the operator has grabbed the ankles of the fetus symmetrically, he must complete the extraction of the fetus in the same manner as in a complete breech presentation, foot variant (Figures 4.112 and 4.113).

In short, the operator must always perform the fetal version, for a fetus in a longitudinal position, by pulling in an external direction until the legs come out, and by

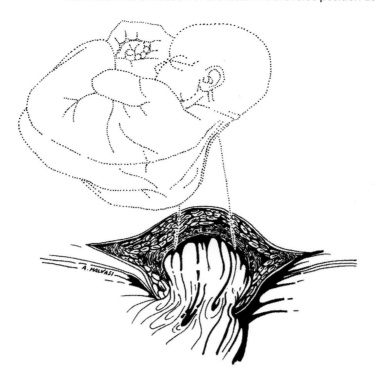

Figure 4.106 Transverse fetus with posterior dorsum: once the operator has reached inside the uterine cavity, he or she must search for the fetal foot and grab it.

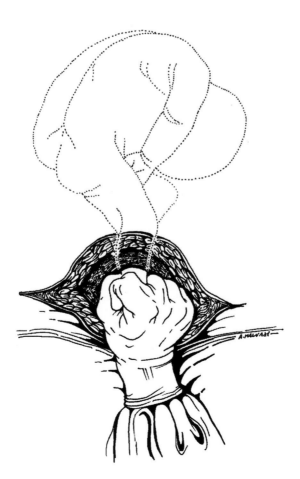

Figure 4.107 Once the foot has been grabbed, the obstetrician can perform the fetal version.

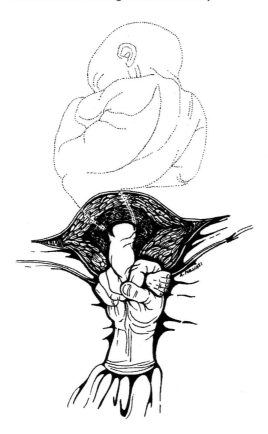

Figure 4.108 Once the version is performed, the operator can complete the fetal extraction.

completing the extraction as in a breech presentation [14]. However, these maneuvers are not always easy and may even prove to be especially difficult in cases of transverse position with lower dorsum, ruptured membranes, and wedged shoulder or, even worse, with "neglected shoulder" (Figure 4.114). This is a rare occurrence as the transverse position of the fetus can be evaluated and checked with ultrasound monitoring.

However, in case of premature rupture of membranes, for single or multiple births, with partial dilation of the uterine cervix, a "neglected shoulder" situation may occur. This anomalous presentation is a true obstetric emergency to be resolved with an emergency cesarean delivery. Further engagement of the shoulder would in fact make the fetal extraction more difficult. After a hysterotomy, the operator must use extreme skill and caution in disengaging the arm prolapsed into the vagina. It must be moved back up and reduced before the fetus can be extracted.

The entire maneuver is made more difficult due to uterine hypertonia caused by the stretching of the longitudinal muscles in the direction of the transverse fetus and by the possibility of uterine tears in the transverse direction (along the vessels).

It may become necessary to perform a "reverse T" uterine incision or, preferably, a longitudinal body incision (according to Sänger) or on the lower uterine segment (according to Krönig) [15].

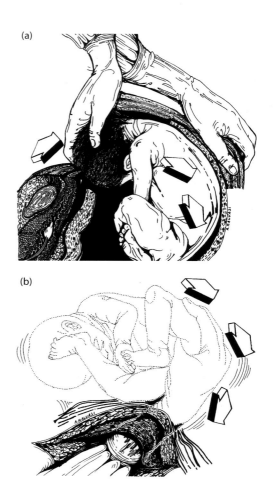

Figure 4.109 (a) After inserting the hand in the uterine breach and having located the feet, (b) perform a maneuver similar to that of Pinard to lower the lower fetal limb for an incomplete breech presentation, buttocks-only variant.

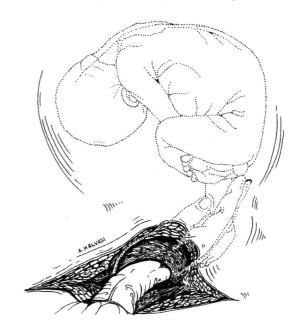

Figure 4.110 After inserting the hand in the uterine breach, gravity lower a fetal foot through the uterine breach.

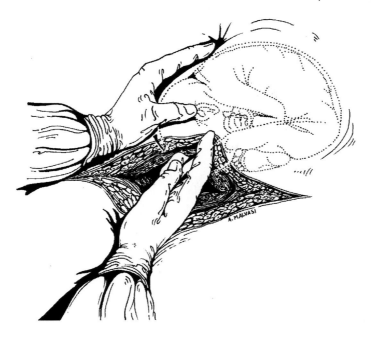

Figure 4.111 The operator moves the fetus toward a vertical position, pushes the head toward the uterine fundus, in mixed maneuvers.

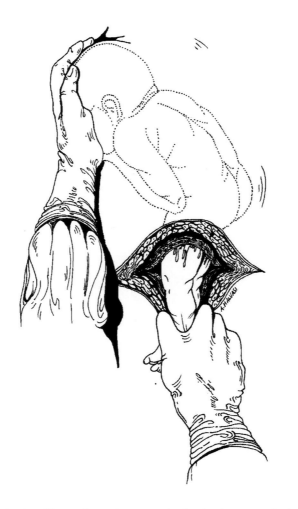

Figure 4.112 The operator grabs both ankles, judiciously moves the fetal axis to a vertical position before a breech extraction from the feet.

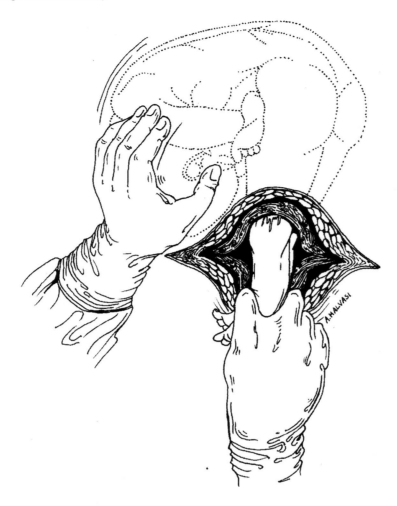

Figure 4.113 The operator extracts the fetus by exerting a slight and gradual traction and pushing, through external maneuvers, the head of the fetus from its original position toward the uterine fundus.

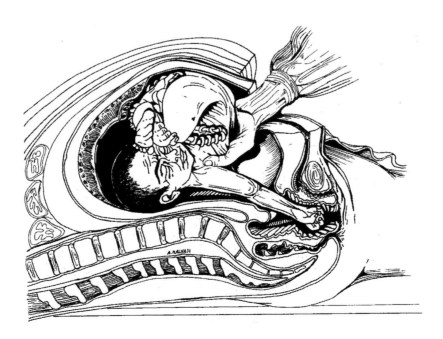

Figure 4.114 Sagittal section of full-term pregnant uterus during a cesarean delivery. The operator before the fetal extraction pulls the fetus up in order to recover the right upper limb prolapsed in the vagina.

Conclusions

Ultrasound is currently the gold standard in terms of diagnosis of transverse position of the fetus. Delivery is instead carried out with an elective cesarean delivery when the version of the fetus cannot be achieved through external maneuvers.

However, traditional semiotics at the opening of the uterine wall maintains its diagnostic validity. Palpation of the axillary space and differential palpation of hand and foot are of help for the subsequent extraction.

Fetal extraction in the transverse position is performed with internal version maneuvers similar to those performed vaginally.

The "neglected shoulder" is nowadays a rare occurrence, as the transverse position is monitored via ultrasound. However, when diagnosed it requires an emergency cesarean delivery. Careful attention must be paid during the reduction of the operator limb prolapsed into the vagina in order to prevent fetal lesions.

REFERENCES

1. Stitely ML, Gherman RB. Labor with abnormal presentation and position. *Obstet Gynecol Clin North Am* 2005;32(2):165–79.
2. Deep AA, Connell JN. Fetal mortality in persistent transverse presentation. *Obstet Gynecol* 1964;24:597–600.
3. Johnson CE. Transverse presentation of fetus. *JAMA* 1964;187:642–6.
4. Kawathekar P, Kasturilal MS, Srinivas P, Sudha G. Etiology and trends in the management of transverse lie. *Am J Obstet Gynecol* 1973;117(1):39–44.
5. Seffah JD. Maternal and perinatal mortality and morbidity associated with transverse lie. *Int J Gynaecol Obstet* 1999;65(1):11–15.
6. Chauhan AR, Singhal TT, Raut VS. Is internal podalic version a lost art? Optimum mode of delivery in transverse lie. *J Postgrad Med* 2001;47(1):15–18.
7. Pelosi MA, Apuzzio J, Fricchione D, Gowda VV. The "intra-abdominal version technique" for delivery of transverse lie by low-segment cesarean section. *Am J Obstet Gynecol* 1979;135(8):1009–11.
8. Shoham Z, Blickstein I, Zosmer A, Katz Z, Borenstein R. Transverse uterine incision for cesarean delivery of the transverse-lying fetus. *Eur J Obstet Gynecol Reprod Biol* 1989;32(2):67–70.
9. Haddad B, Abirached F, Calvez G, Cabrol D. Manual rotation of vertex presentations in posterior occipital-iliac or transverse position. Technique and value. *J Gynecol Obstet Biol Reprod (Paris)* 1995;24(2):181–8.
10. Phelan JP, Stine LE, Edwards NB, Clark SL, Horenstein J. The role of external version in the intrapartum management of the transverse lie presentation. *Am J Obstet Gynecol* 1985;151(6):724–6.
11. Henry GR. The management of transverse and oblique lie. *Ir Med J* 1974;67(13):359–62.
12. To WW, Li IC. Occipital posterior and occipital transverse positions: Reappraisal of the obstetric risks. *Aust N Z J Obstet Gynaecol* 2000;40(3):275–9.
13. Le Ray C, Serres P, Schmitz T, Cabrol D, Goffinet F. Manual rotation in occiput posterior or transverse positions: Risk factors and consequences on the cesarean delivery rate. *Obstet Gynecol* 2007;110(4):873–9.
14. Tam WH, Fung HY, Fung TY, Lau TK, To KF. Intrauterine growth retardation and transverse lie due to massive subchorionic thrombohematoma and overlying large subchorionic cyst. *Acta Obstet Gynecol Scand* 1997;76(4):381–3.
15. Boyle JG, Gabbe SG. T and J vertical extensions in low transverse cesarean births. *Obstet Gynecol* 1996;87(2):238–43.

FURTHER READING

Demol S, Bashiri A, Furman B, Maymon E, Shoham-Vardi I, Mazor M. Breech presentation is a risk factor for intrapartum and neonatal death in preterm delivery. *Eur J Obstet Gynecol Reprod Biol* 2000;93(1):47–51.

O'Leary JA, Cuva A. Abdominal rescue after failed cephalic replacement. *Obstet Gynecol* 1992;80(3 Pt 2):514–6.

Placental removal and uterine exteriorization techniques

ANTONIO MALVASI and GIAN CARLO DI RENZO

> …It is rare for the placenta to come off quickly and be detached with fingers. When strips of deciduous membranes remain adherent to the uterine wall they can be detached with fingers covered with sterile gauze…
>
> (A. Ribemont-Dessaignes, *Traité d'obstétrique*, 1923)

PLACENTAL REMOVAL

Placental removal and exteriorization maneuvers belong to the postpartum phase of a cesarean delivery (CD) and are accompanied by auxiliary maneuvers aimed at improving the postpartum and postnatal periods and reducing complications.

Placental removal (or the third stage of labor) is the period of delivery that goes from fetal expulsion and/or extraction to the delivery of placenta and membranes [1–3].

Placental removal can be seen as the phase between the second stage of labor and the stage of fetal separation from the placenta, which is the moment when the umbilical cord is cut (Figure 5.1).

Although placental removal in spontaneous delivery has been thoroughly studied, the literature has dedicated much less attention to placental removal in cesarean deliveries. One reason is the "routine" practice of manually removing the placenta in the course of a cesarean delivery. The placenta is manually extracted to reduce the third stage of labor or, more frequently, for the operator's convenience (Figure 5.2).

Manual removal of the placenta performed in the course of CD, however, does not have a clinical or scientific justification. In fact by examining the literature, including the not-so-recent items, one can see that Stoekel wrote in 1925, "wait until pain from manual placental removal appears and then obtain the expression of the placenta through the incision with the Credé's maneuver" [4].

The reluctance of obstetricians in the past to carry out manual placental removal during CD—as well as the decision to wait for spontaneous placental removal, or to squeeze the uterine fundus through the abdominal wall—was born from the need to reduce surgical maneuvers and therefore the likelihood of bacterial contamination of the uterine and abdominal cavities (Figure 5.3).

For that matter, Khan and Rogers have also shown that instrumental management of placental removal should only proceed with a careful traction on the umbilical cord after a prophylactic injection of oxytocin [5,6]. This same concept is confirmed by Merger who, in regard to the cesarean delivery technique, notes: "Sixth stage: expression of the placenta by squeezing the uterine fundus through the abdominal field, or normal placental removal through the uterine breach…" [7].

A more detailed description of placental removal during cesarean deliveries was described by Racinet and Favier, in their book titled *La Cesariènne*: "…if the cord has not been cut according to the Dunn technique, placenta detachment can be hastened by grasping the uterine fundus and gently massaging it so as to provoke uterine contractions: the placenta usually appears in the hysterotomy opening with its fetal side…." [8]. The free hand will then exercise a gentle traction on the cord to extract the placental mass (Figure 5.4). The membranes usually emerge from the uterine cavity without great difficulty, aided by the application of ring forceps to prevent them from being lacerated: if the cord is cut there is more time available for the spontaneous detachment of the placenta.

Remember that excessive traction force on the cord may cause a uterine inversion when the uterus is hypotonic. Inversion is almost always associated with strong adherence of the placenta to the decidua and, in such an event, the placenta appears voluminous. The obstetrician's external hand can also notice the characteristic vial bottom–shaped depression on the uterine fundus.

One should therefore proceed without haste (but without stalling) with the manual disengagement of the placenta, which can be favored by, usually uncomplicated, artificial placental removal (Figure 5.5).

An additional maneuver during placental removal is to extract the membranes with a "twisting maneuver" (Figure 5.6). This maneuver is an attempt to completely detach the membranes when they do not adhere to the underlying decidua. It should not be forgotten that, unlike spontaneous delivery, membranes in a CD are cut at the uterine segment level. The lower pole of the amnion–chorion sac, therefore, generally tends to remain in the lower part of the open uterine cavity. The "twisting maneuver" almost always detaches the entire amnion–chorion sac.

Therefore, despite the fact that "experience-based medicine" indicates that placental removal should occur spontaneously in the course of CD, often placenta is removed manually, without any real indication. (Note that pathological placental removal is discussed in another chapter of this book.)

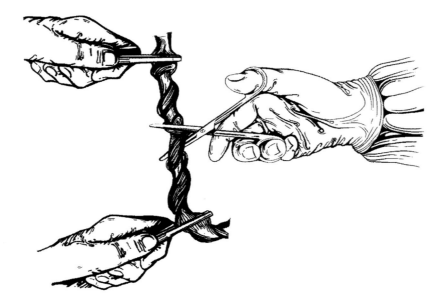

Figure 5.1 The umbilical cord is clamped with Kocher forceps and is cut off with straight Mayo scissors; this maneuver starts the third stage of labor.

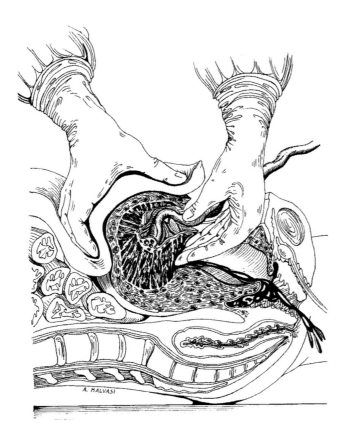

Figure 5.2 Manual removal of placenta in the third stage of labor in the course of a cesarean delivery. The technique is analogous to manual placental removal in spontaneous delivery: the hand is inserted through the lower uterine segment into the uterine cavity and feels the upper margin of the placental plate; the maternal side is gradually detached with the fingertips until the placenta with the membranes is extracted.

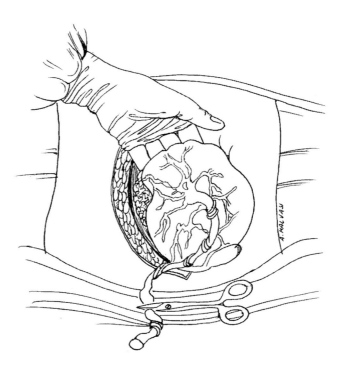

Figure 5.3 Manual placental removal in Sanger's traditional conservative cesarean delivery (modified by Berkeley and Bonney) was as follows: "fetal extraction must be followed by placental removal which can sometimes be achieved spontaneously, but more often needs to be preceded by squeezing with the Credé's maneuver or manually, while making sure that all membranes are detached from the inner surface of the uterus" [76].

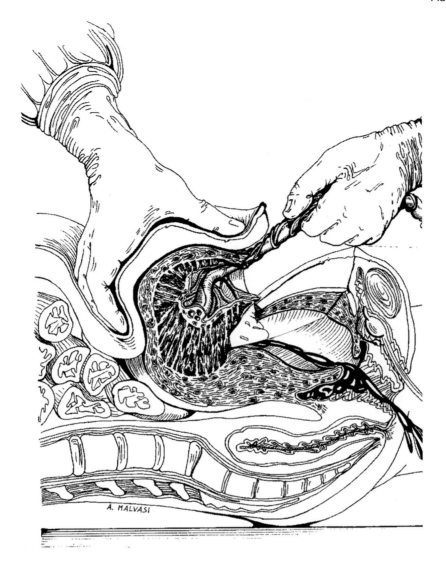

Figure 5.4 Spontaneous placental removal during cesarean delivery with Credé's technique and simultaneous careful traction on the previously clamped umbilical cord.

The method used during spontaneous placental removal in the course of CD, should not be different from the controlled traction on the umbilical cord that occurs during vaginal delivery. Spontaneous placental removal has, however, proven to be better than manual placental removal as the latter does not provide myometrial cells with the time necessary to contract and therefore determines an increased blood loss, as proven by a study from 2007 by Peña Marti [58] and by two Cochrane studies in 2008 [59,60].

Not only "experience-based medicine" but even "evidence-based medicine" has confirmed that spontaneous placental removal is preferable, whenever possible, to manual removal. In a review on *active management* of the third stage of labor, Prendiville et al. noted that manual placental removal is often associated with increased maternal blood loss (weighted mean difference of 79.33 mL, 95% confidence interval [CI], from 94.29 to 64.37) (Figure 5.7), postpartum hemorrhage of more than 500 mL (relative risk of 0.38, 95% CI, from 0.32 to 0.46) (Figure 5.8), and extension of the third stage of labor (mean difference measured in 9.77 minutes, 95% CI, from 10.00 to 9.53) [9]. *Active management* was also associated with maternal nausea (relative risk of 1.83, 95% CI, from 1.51 to 2.23), vomiting, and increased blood pressure, probably due to the use of ergometrine. Conversely, no advantages or disadvantages were noted in terms of neonatal outcomes [9].

In another Cochrane review, Carroli and Bergel, after confirming that manual placental removal represents an invasive procedure in spontaneous delivery that can result in bleeding, infections, and trauma of the maternal genital tract, concluded that the injection of saline solution associated with oxytocin could be the most suitable noninvasive method for favoring spontaneous placental removal in case of retained placenta [10].

In a further review, Wilkinson and Enkin evaluated several trials that compared manual placental removal methods in 224 women who underwent elective or emergency CD. The review showed how the manual removal

126 Placental removal and uterine exteriorization techniques

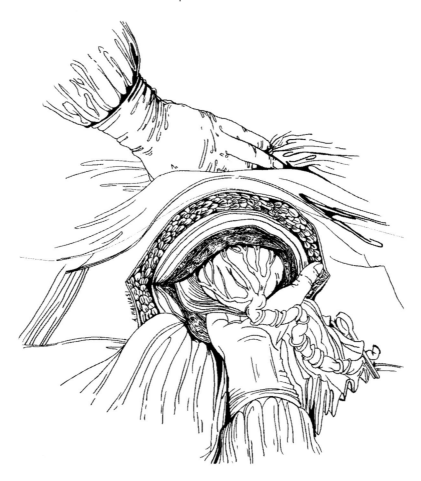

Figure 5.5 Completion maneuver of manual placental removal: the operator grasps the placenta from the bottom edge using both hands and completes the placental removal, without inserting the hands in the uterine cavity. (Modified from Di Renzo GC. *Trattato di Ostetricia e Ginecologia*, Rome, Italy: Verduci Editore; 2009.)

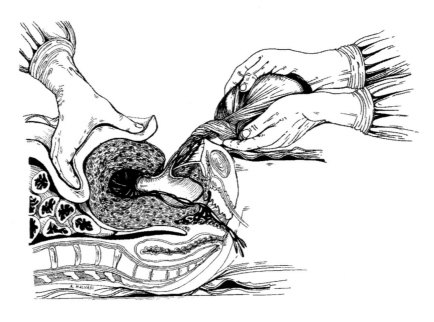

Figure 5.6 The "twisting maneuver" of the amnion–chorion membranes during placental removal.

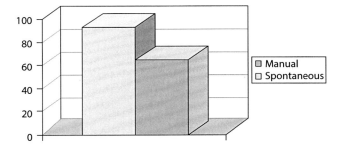

Figure 5.7 Assessment of blood loss after spontaneous placental removal. (From Prendiville WJ, Elbourne D, MacDonald, S: Active versus expectant management in the third stage of labour. (Cochrane review). *The Cochrane Library*. 2004. *Issue 3*. Copyright Wiley-VCH Verlag GmbH & Co. KGaA. Reproduced with permission.)

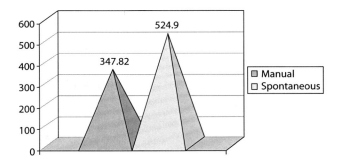

Figure 5.9 Evaluation of the incidence of endometritis after manual placental removal during a cesarean delivery. (From Wilkinson C, Enkin MW: Uterine exteriorization versus intraperitoneal repair at caesarean delivery (Cochrane review). *The Cochrane Library*. 2004. *Issue 3*. Copyright Wiley-VCH Verlag GmbH & Co. KGaA. Reproduced with permission.)

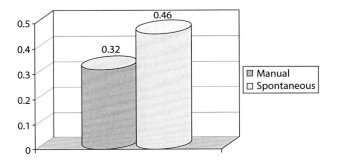

Figure 5.8 Evaluation of postpartum hemorrhage with manual placental removal. (From Prendiville WJ, Elbourne D, MacDonald, S: Active versus expectant management in the third stage of labour. (Cochrane review). *The Cochrane Library*. 2004. *Issue 3*. Copyright Wiley-VCH Verlag GmbH & Co. KGaA. Reproduced with permission.)

of the placenta was associated in a statistically significant manner with an increase in maternal blood loss (weighted mean difference of 436.35 mL, 95% CI from 347.82 mL to 524.9 mL) and a higher incidence of postpartum endometritis (odds ratio of 5.44, 95% CI, from 1.25 to 23.75) (Figure 5.9). This procedure also seemed to be associated, albeit in a manner that is not statistically significant, with an increase in fetal–maternal hemorrhages (odds ratio 2.19, 95% CI from 0.69 to 6.93) [11].

An important problem related to manual placental removal during a cesarean delivery is represented by an increase in endometritis. Magann et al. reported a significant increase in the rate of post-CD endometritis compared to the absence of manual placental removal (with only spontaneous placental removal, even with uterine exteriorization), or without uterine exteriorization (even with manual placental removal). The use of antibiotic prophylaxis, now a standardized obstetric practice, had however not been considered by the study [12].

Antibiotic prophylaxis, on the contrary, has proven to be a fundamental variable, as shown in the Cochrane review of Smaill and Hofmeyer. The review claims that antibiotic prophylaxis reduces endometritis by two-thirds to three-quarters and also reduces infection of the abdominal wall, to the point that antibiotic prophylaxis is recommended for patients undergoing both elective and nonelective CD [13].

McCurdy et al. also observed, in addition to a higher rate of endometritis, increased blood loss when the placenta was removed manually [14]. However, the incidence of endometritis in the course of CD is linked to several variables, including prolonged rupture of the membranes [15], number of intrapartum vaginal visits [16], prolonged labor [17], and the use of antibiotic therapy for membrane rupture [18].

Yancey et al., in a study conducted to evaluate contamination of surgical gloves during a CD, isolated staphylococci bacteria from the gloves of the first operator, immediately after extraction of the fetus, in 11 of 14 cases in which labor had already started. This incidence dropped to 1 in 11 cases when the woman was not in labor [19]. Starting from this data, Atkinson et al. carried out a randomized study on 634 pregnant women divided into four subpopulations. In the course of this study, a group of obstetricians manually removed the placenta without changing gloves after extracting the fetus. In another group the surgeon and the second assistant after extraction of the fetus wore new gloves and waited for spontaneous placental removal.

This study showed that the changing of surgical gloves could not be associated with a reduction in post-CD endometritis, and confirmed that manual placental removal is associated with an increased risk of endometritis in the postoperative period. In fact, postoperative endometritis was significantly more frequent in patients who underwent manual removal of the placenta (31% versus 22%, $p = 0.1$) (Figure 5.10), while changing gloves did not cause an increase in endometritis (relative risk of 1, with 95% CI, 0.79–1.3) [20].

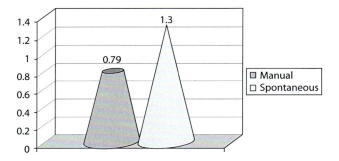

Figure 5.10 Evaluation of endometritis after manual removal of the placenta. (From Atkinson MW. et al., *Obstet Gynecol* 1996;87:99–102. With permission.)

Atkinson et al. thus commented their experience on the contamination of surgical gloves:

> [W]e assume that if contamination of the surgeon's gloves occurs due to direct contact with the cervical–vaginal flora during elevation of the fetal head from the maternal pelvis, then continuing to use these gloves could lead to contamination of the operative field and increase the risk of endometritis… however, after processing this data and that of other ambiguous elements regarding the entire population, changing gloves could not be significantly associated with the rate of endometritis. In those women with rupture of membranes an explanation for the lack of effect due to changing gloves could be the colonization that commonly occurs before the glove is introduced in the lower uterine tract. In this case changing gloves might not prevent bacterial contamination, whereas the type of placental removal would be the main factor of influence [20].

Cernadas et al. conducted an even more detailed study in which four groups of patients were considered: group A made up of 26 patients in which manual placental removal was performed without changing gloves, group B of 27 pregnant women in which placental removal was performed by expression (or squeezing) without changing gloves, group C of 27 women with the changing of gloves after manual removal of the placenta, and group D of 28 patients with a changing of gloves but only after placental expression.

Data were compared between groups that changed gloves with those that did not (groups A and B versus C and D) and between groups with manual placental removal and expression (groups A and C versus B and D): there were no statistically significant differences, respectively, for febrile morbidity (relative risk of 0.7, 95% CI, 0.3–1.4 and relative risk of 1.4 with 95% CI, 0.6–3.5) and endometritis (relative risk of 1.2, with 95% CI, 0.5–2.8 and relative risk 1.5, 95% CI:0.6–3.6) [21].

WIPING AND DILATATION OF THE CERVICAL CANAL

A complementary maneuver during placental removal is the inspection of the placenta and of the membranes. In the course of a CD the surgeon or assistant must check the morphology of the maternal side of the placenta to verify its completeness and integrity and to therefore exclude the presence of any remaining placental cotyledons in the uterine cavity (Figures 5.11 and 5.12).

The exploration of the uterine cavity with gauze after placental removal has been described since the beginnings of CD, as described by De Lee and Greenhill: "gauze pads are used to clean the uterine cavity, fragments of placenta and membranes are moved away and a large swab is placed in the open cavity which causes the uterus to rapidly contract" (Figure 5.13) [22]. Such a procedure might increase the risk of bacterial contamination and therefore the incidence of endometritis.

Magann et al., however, conclude that the removal of residues by wiping the uterine cavity versus not wiping, does not determine a significant reduction in the incidence of post-CD endometritis [23]. These authors enrolled in their study 614 patients who were subjected to wiping of the uterine cavity in the course of CD to remove residual placental and chorionic membranes, while in 616 patients this procedure was not adopted. The two groups shared the same demographic characteristics: maternal age, type of anesthesia, time before CD of rupture of membranes, use of intrauterine monitoring devices, type of skin incision, placental removal technique, blood loss, and operative times. The pregnant women received antibiotic prophylaxis consisting of 1 gram of first-generation cephalosporin administered by intravenous bolus injection after having cut the umbilical cord. Endometritis was determined on the basis of body temperature (38°C) measured on two occasions, 6 hours after the first 24 hours, with doughy uterine, as well as from malodorous lochia discharge.

The incidence of endometritis in this study is similar: 65 of 614 (10.5%) in the group with wiping versus 66 in the group without wiping (10.7%) (Figure 5.14) [23]. It can be speculated that the lower rate of endometritis after wiping is due to poor inoculation of bacteria in myometrium vessels "clipped" by the myometrial contraction following placental removal, which effectively reduces access of infectious agents.

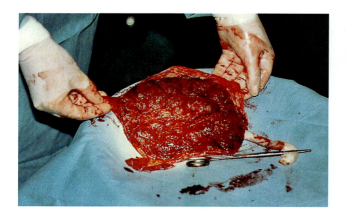

Figure 5.11 Maneuver for the inspection of the placenta and membranes after placental removal: the placenta is placed on the instrument nurse's table to be examined.

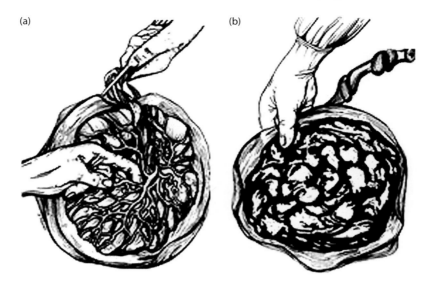

Figure 5.12 Examination of the (a) maternal side and of the (b) fetal side of the placenta after placental removal.

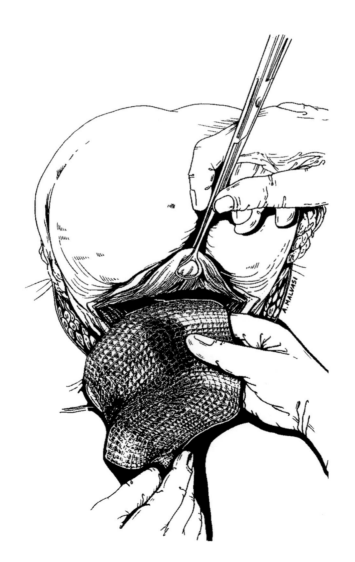

Figure 5.13 Wiping maneuver of the uterine cavity with gauze, performed to verify the complete removal of placenta and chorioamniotic material.

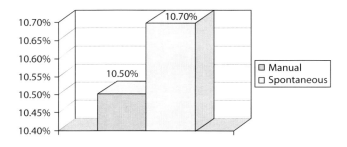

Figure 5.14 Incidence of endometritis with and without wiping of the post-cesarean delivery uterine cavity. (From Magann EF. et al., *J Matern Fetal Med* 2001;10:318–322. With permission.)

Wiping can be carried out in different ways, depending on the experience and convenience of the operator, with a cloth or better yet with a swab mounted on a ring (Figure 5.15) or Faure forceps. Moreover, the operating field near the hysterotomy can be cleaned with a suction cannula (Figure 5.16) to remove hematic material and thus facilitate surgical maneuvers. Gauze or swabs used for cleaning the uterine cavity can, however, be left inside. The same can be said for residual parts that, as Kazahov et al. state, can later be removed through hysteroscopy along with suture threads near the uterine scar area [24]. It is always recommended to use a pair of ring forceps to search for any conspicuous fragments of membranes that should be removed (Figure 5.17), while small residual pieces will be spontaneously reabsorbed in the puerperal period.

Another important maneuver is to inspect the area below the cesarean hysterotomy to verify the presence of the lower pole of the amniotic sac that may have adhered to the bottom of the uterine cavity. The persistence of a "cul de sac" that clogs the internal uterine orifice was already described by Proust and Charrierin: "depending on the case it may be advisable to check if a portion of the membranes has adhered to the lower uterine segment or to the internal uterine orifice of the neck" [25]. The membranes may be present due to the surgical incision of the anterior

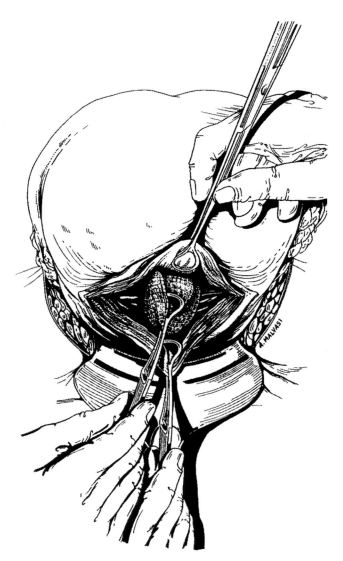

Figure 5.15 Wiping maneuver with a swab held by ring forceps.

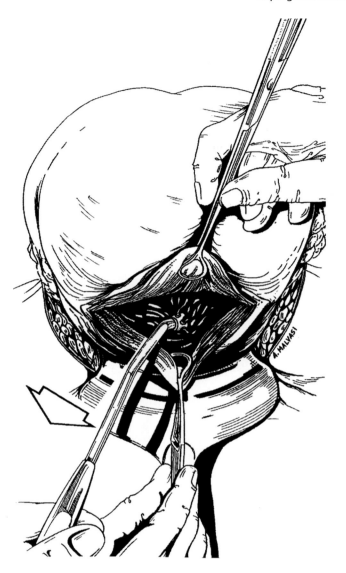

Figure 5.16 Removal from the uterine cavity, after placental removal, of residual amnion–chorion and membranes by mono-use aspirator cannula. These maneuvers reduce or avoid vaginal secretions with bacteria from the vagina to the uterine cavity.

wall of the amniotic sac, which can detach from the rest and remain in situ. This can, however, also be caused by particular adherences caused by a silent infection of the lower amniotic pole, which makes even forced removal difficult. A sign of the persistence of this unrecognized "cul de sac" is represented by an absence of lochia (Figure 5.18).

During iterative cesarean deliveries, or in patients in which labor has not started and in which, therefore, changes to the cervix have not yet occurred, some surgeons, after placental removal, choose to artificially dilate the cervical canal to facilitate lochia discharge. This maneuver can be performed digitally or instrumentally, with Hegar dilator [26] or forceps [27]. In fact Racinet and Favier commented on this maneuver in the following manner:

> [R]ather than performing this maneuver digitally, which constitutes a septic risk, we use a Hegar probe [Figure 5.19] or long forceps, such as the Jean-Louis Faure type, inserted along the entire length of the cervical canal and then opened along several diameters in order to dilate the canal…under exceptional circumstances we position a Foley catheter in the upper path; the expansion of the catheter balloon ensures lochia discharge in the first two or three days of puerperium [8].

Cervical canal dilation with open uterus can be achieved through the internal uterine orifice (Figure 5.20), making sure to change gloves to avoid bacterial contamination from the cervico-vaginal canal. It may be preferable to achieve dilation vaginally after the intervention (Figure 5.21), while checking, through the leaking of clots, the patency of the cervical canal with respect to lochia discharge.

Although no randomized studies support these maneuvers, they are commonly performed, even though they may result in post-CD endometritis. The cervical divulsion maneuver can also help in locating the internal

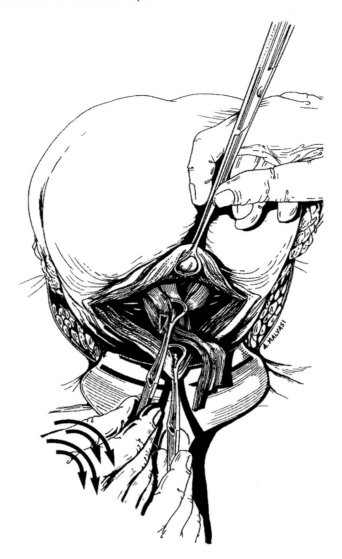

Figure 5.17 Removal from the uterine cavity, after placental removal, of residual amnion–chorion membranes by means of ring forceps.

uterine orifice and in determining the surgical anatomy of the area affected by hysterotomy. In fact, in the case of a repeated CD, it is common to notice a significant difference in thickness between the thick upper edge and the thin lower edge of the incision. The likelihood of this occurring increases with the thinness of the uterine segment and with the closeness of the incision to the cesarean scar. In such cases it is not uncommon for the operator to look for the internal uterine orifice and use it as a landmark, before starting to suture the hysterotomy incision.

UTERINE EXTERIORIZATION

The exteriorization of the uterus is a maneuver tied to the early history of CD and originates from the need, in times of puerperal infections, to isolate as much as possible the uterine viscera from the rest of the abdominal cavity. Uterine exteriorization was the fundamental surgical stage in the Gottschalk–Portes cesarean delivery technique, so named as it was created by Gottschalk in 1910 [28] and reintroduced by the Frenchman Portes [29] in 1924. Although completely outdated, it is worth mentioning to highlight all the postoperative difficulties that occurred in pre-sulfamide and pre-antibiotic times.

The intervention consisted of a CD with the Sanger technique [30]. This involves the longitudinal incision of the uterus in which the uterine viscera is exteriorized and then cut to extract the fetus. After placental removal, the exteriorized uterus is sutured together with the visceral and parietal peritoneum, thereby leaving the uterus exteriorized. Since the goal was to isolate the uterine body, a potential source of puerperal sepsis, after a week unless complications occurred the uterus was repositioned in the abdominal cavity.

Therefore, in the Sanger technique, in order to reduce contamination of the abdominal cavity, exteriorization came before fetal extraction: it was Leopold [31] who suggested uterine exteriorization should come after fetal extraction, which Sanger accepted (Figure 5.22).

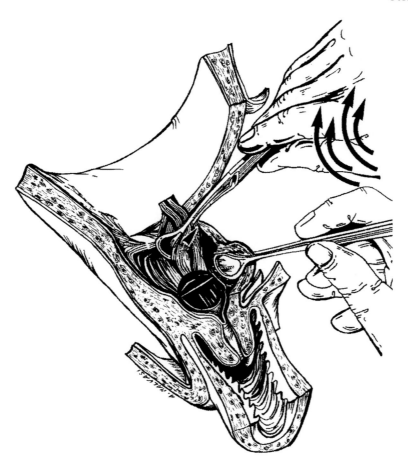

Figure 5.18 Removal with ring forceps of residual amnion–chorion membranes found at the bottom of the lower segment and that form a "cul de sac" that obstructs the lochia.

Paneuf [32] supported the Gottschalk–Portes intervention, at least in clearly infected cases in which exteriorization appeared at the time to be one of the few defenses against puerperal infection.

With the advent of the Munro–Kerr technique, Doerffler [33] suggested uterine exteriorization as a means to reduce the risk of peritoneal infection and to protect the abdominal cavity with waterproof sheets. This surgical CD maneuver was relegated to the past in the era of antibiotics, but has re-emerged since Michael Stark proposed it in the Misgav Ladach method [34]. However, as stated by Hershey and Quilligan, "the origin of the popular contemporary technique of extra-abdominal exteriorization of the uterus after childbirth and placental removal is not clear" [35].

The uterine exteriorization technique is simple and consists of inserting the operator's right hand through the laparotomy into the abdominal cavity and, with the same hand, exploring the uterine wall to make sure that there are no adherences to the omentum or intestine. The walls are also checked for uterine myomas and for the presence of ovarian cysts or formations that can increase the uterine volume and prevent exteriorization. Only then, in the absence of complications, can the uterus be extracted (Figure 5.23).

It is recommended in the case of adherences to not perform exteriorization to prevent lacerations, bleeding, and hematoma, especially if there are adherences with the uterine–ovarian plexus. In fact, in our experience there have been in two cases of vascular plexus injuries with hematoma, which required ovariosalpingectomy, while in three cases lacerations of the mesosigma occurred that required adequate hemostasis and surgical repair [36]. In the presence of large uterine myomas, exteriorization is not recommended because the increased volume of the uterus would make repositioning in the abdominal cavity difficult.

Uterine exteriorization has the immediate advantage of allowing an inspection of the exterior uterine wall, including the posterior surface of the uterus that is generally inaccessible in the traditional cesarean delivery technique without uterine exteriorization (Figure 5.24). In addition since the postpartum uterus "emerges" from the abdominal walls, all surgical maneuvers are facilitated. This is true in particular for the suture of the hysterotomy, which is "raised" from the uterovesical cavity which, at times, can be deep and narrow, especially in overweight patients.

Once the hysterotomy conditions are determined, the uterine corners are clamped and any substantial blood loss is stopped, the appendages can then be observed (Figure 5.25). Hershey and Quilligan carried out one of the first

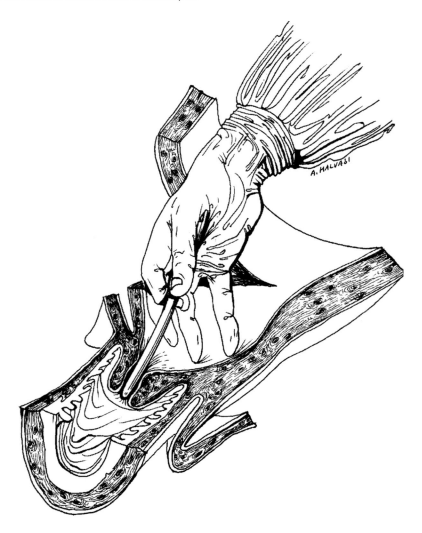

Figure 5.19 Dilation maneuver of the cervical canal from the internal uterine orifice with Hegar dilators (dilation up to six is sufficient), to ensure subsequent lochia discharge, in case of a particularly stenotic channel that cannot be dilated digitally.

evidence-based medicine studies on uterine exteriorization during a cesarean delivery [35]. The authors studied two randomized groups of patients: a group of 159 patients and another group of 149 patients. In the first group, the surgeon exteriorized the uterus after extraction of the fetus and placental removal and with a sterile cloth around the fundus, assisted the traction exerted by the assistant and facilitated the exposure of the lower uterine segment. In patients of the second group the uterus was sutured inside the peritoneum. χ^2 analysis between group 1 and 2 does not show a significant difference ($p > 0.5$), suggesting that the compared groups were similar [35].

Magann et al. studied 234 women divided into four groups: group I with spontaneous placental removal and in situ repair of the uterus, group II with spontaneous placental removal and uterine exteriorization, group III with manual removal of the placenta and no uterine exteriorization, and group IV with manual removal of the placenta and uterine exteriorization. The incidence of post-CD endometritis reported by the authors was greatest in group IV (32.45% of 71, $p = 0.003$) compared to group I (17.24% of 71), group II (12.30% of 71), and group III (13.18% of 71). The authors concluded that the association of manual placental removal and uterine exteriorization resulted in an increase in morbidity, hospitalization, and antibiotic consumption (Figure 5.26) [37].

Edi-Osage et al. in examining 194 women did not observe statistically significant differences in blood pressure, oxygen saturation, and hemoglobin concentration in the group with exteriorization compared to the one without exteriorization [38]. Vomiting developed in 10% of cases and reflected proper preoperative preparation of the patient. Pain, which reflected the adequacy of the type of anesthesia, occurred in 57% of cases during skin incision and significantly persisted in the exteriorized group up to the third postoperative day [38].

Wahab et al. in another randomized and controlled study carried out on 316 women found no statistically significant differences with regard to postoperative wound sepsis, hyperpyrexia, the need for blood transfusions, and days of hospitalization. The authors concluded that exteriorization with effective anesthesia is not associated in a

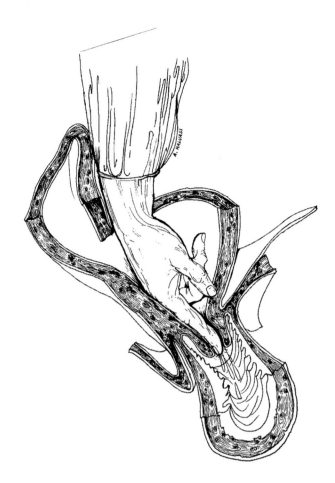

Figure 5.20 Dilation maneuvers of the cervical canal from above before uterine suture, to check adequate patency necessary for lochia discharge.

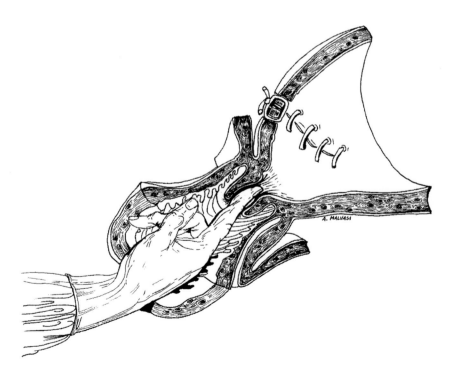

Figure 5.21 Probing maneuver and dilation of the cervical canal, performed vaginally upon completion of cesarean delivery, in order to verify patency or to improve patency in case of cervical tightness.

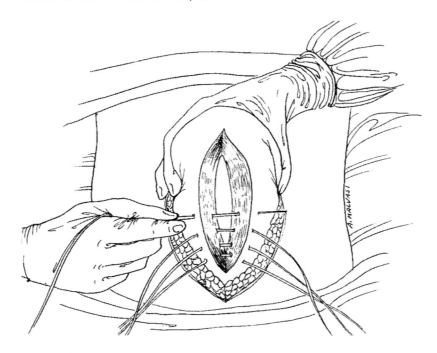

Figure 5.22 Suturing of the uterus after exteriorization with the traditional Sanger technique of Cesarean delivery, modified by Leopold, and by Berkeley and Bonney: "advantages of the fundal method with systematic exteriorization of the uterus consist of improved protection of the abdominal cavity from the possibility of contamination, as well as decreased blood loss during the sectioning of the uterine walls" [76].

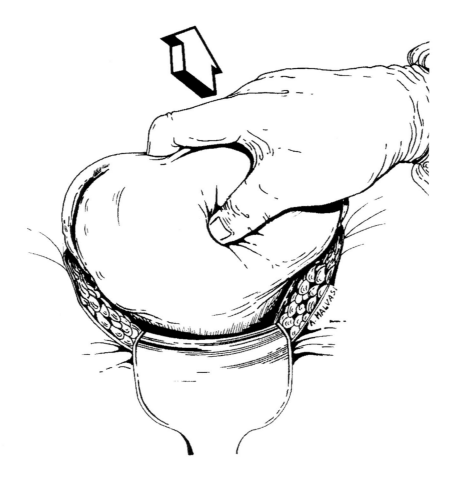

Figure 5.23 Extraction maneuver and uterine exteriorization after placental removal.

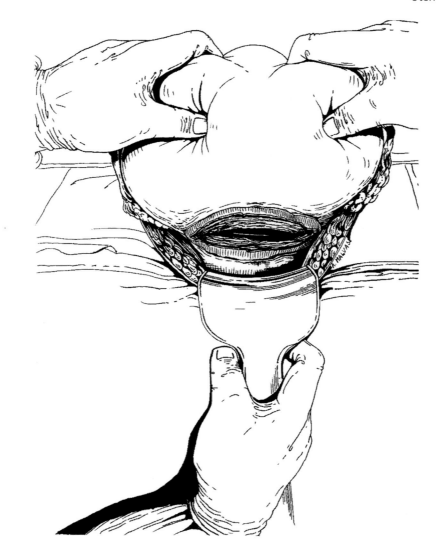

Figure 5.24 Inspection of the uterine breach after exteriorization and uterine massage.

statistically significant manner with any complications, but instead results in reduced intraoperative blood loss ($p < 0.05$) [39].

Wilkinson and Enkin in a Cochrane review [40] evaluated the effects of uterine exteriorization within the abdominal cavity, for both emergency and elective CD ($n = 486$). In this review exteriorization did not significantly reduce intraoperative blood loss [40]. On the contrary, exteriorization was associated with fewer days of postoperative fever (fever > 3 days, odds ratio 0.4, 95% CI, from 0.17 to 0.94) and, in a manner that is not statistically significant, with a reduction in infections [40]. Furthermore, when exteriorization was performed under locoregional anesthesia, there was an increased tendency toward nausea and vomiting. However, such symptoms, even under these conditions, were related to the type of anesthesia and, in particular, to the metameric level achieved.

Uterine exteriorization may result in a higher incidence of gas embolism, probably due to traction on the uterus increasing the caliber of the venous sinuses, and to the closeness of the hysterotomy to the heart, which increases the hydrostatic gradient, thus increasing the likelihood of gas embolism in the venous vessels [41]. The probability of venous embolism increases along with the time of uterine exteriorization. Therefore, if prolonged surgical times are expected, it is recommended to place the uterine viscera in axis and gently massage the plexuses so that the blood in the uterine–ovarian plexuses can circulate (Figure 5.27) [42].

A positive aspect of uterine exteriorization, especially in the case of hypotony or uterine atony, is the possibility of performing a "uterine massage" with both hands, more effective than when performed in situ. This allows for an improved view of uterine wall features, so that other causes of atony can be examined. For example, it is possible to wipe the uterine cavity to search for succenturiate or residual cotyledons, or myomas that might cause physiological postpartum uterine contraction.

In addition, in case of tubal ligation, exteriorization not only results in easier surgical maneuvers but also in a better control of surgical instruments that are near the

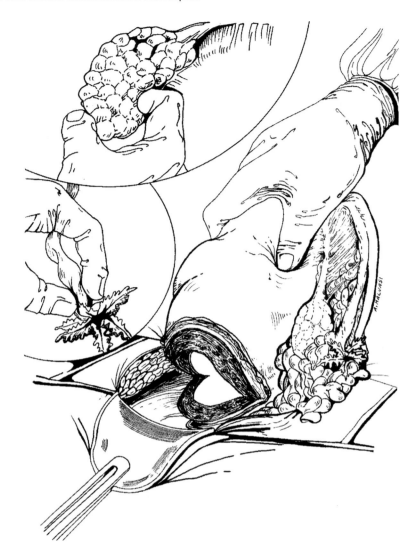

Figure 5.25 Inspection of the ovaries (top left) and tubes (bottom left) in the course of a cesarean delivery after uterine exteriorization.

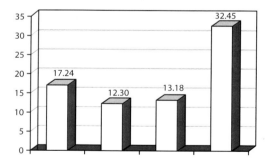

Figure 5.26 Incidence of post-cesarean endometritis in exteriorization and nonexteriorization and in replacement and nonreplacement of surgical gloves. Column 1, spontaneous placental removal and in situ repair of the uterus; column 2, spontaneous placental removal and uterine exteriorization; column 3 manual removal of the placenta and no uterine exteriorization; and column 4, manual removal of the placenta and uterine exteriorization. (From Magann EF. et al., *J Matern Fetal Med* 2001;10:318–322. With permission.)

congested uterine–ovarian plexus, thus avoiding accidental and dangerous damage to the aforementioned vessels.

However, uterine exteriorization is not always useful or practicable: in fact exteriorization in the presence of uterine myomas that increase uterine volume can prove to be difficult (Figure 5.28) or, in case of uterine–parietal or intestinal adherences, can cause bleeding due to lacerations in newly formed vessels.

Another maneuver that requires caution is the repositioning of the sutured uterus in the uterine cavity, to avoid potentially traumatic maneuvers on the uterine–ovarian venous plexuses.

Another interesting aspect of uterine exteriorization in the course of CD is the reduced use of laparotomy gauze. In addition, gauze that is used is more visible and controllable as it is found outside the abdominal cavity. On this matter Stark writes:

[P]ads are not useful inside the abdomen, as they have an abrasive effect on tissues and increase the risk of

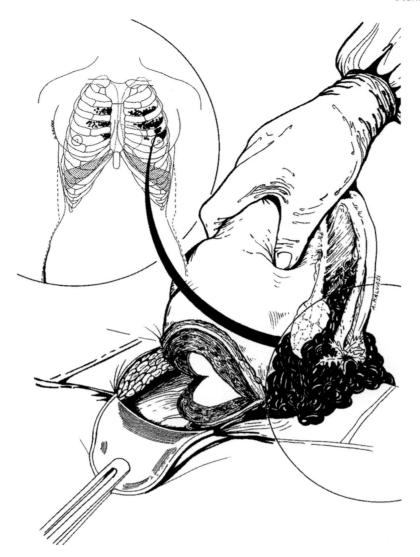

Figure 5.27 Congestion of the uterine–ovarian venous plexuses during uterine exteriorization in the course of cesarean delivery: uterine repositioning in the abdominal cavity must be preceded by uterine–ovarian venous decongestion. The image at top left shows pulmonary embolism, which fortunately has a low probability of occurring, resulting from uterine–ovarian venous congestion.

adherences, while reducing the beneficial effects of the antibacterial properties of the amniotic fluid. In addition, if the laparotomy pads are not inserted, there is no risk of leaving them inside!…. The excessive and meticulous removal of blood and amniotic fluid can cause peritoneal irritation and later on disturb the intestinal function [34].

Larsen et al. had in fact noted the antibacterial properties of human amniotic fluid [43], and Down et al. had observed the abrasive effect of laparotomy gauze on abdominal viscera [44].

The benefit of removing amniotic fluid, vernix caseosa, and hematic material is, however, a controversial topic, as demonstrated by the two cases of peritonitis from vernix caseosa following a cesarean delivery, as described by Davis et al. [45]. On the other hand, an ultrasound investigation conducted by Antonelli et al. showed that the persistence of fluids in the abdominal cavity after CD does not result in increased morbidity compared to patients without fluids. Therefore, a routine ultrasound examination of all patients who undergo a CD does not appear to be justified, but should instead be reserved to those patients who show signs of fever, the nature of which should be determined in the postoperative period [46]. However, as a result of the almost inevitable intraperitoneal collections, consisting of intraperitoneal fluid, amniotic fluid, blood clots, blood, and residual vernix caseosa, there is uncertainty on whether to perform antibiotic therapies on puerperal women in order to prevent infections.

Ultimately, the present state of the art suggests, as per Hofmeyer and Smaill [47], that penicillin or first-generation cephalosporin be used especially for the

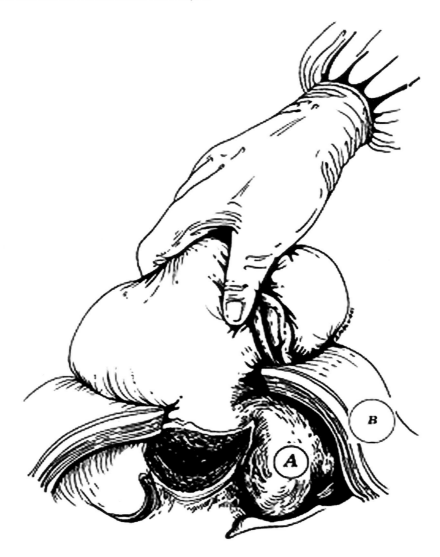

Figure 5.28 Failure to exteriorize the uterus during a cesarean delivery due to the presence of a subserous intramural myomas of the posterior wall (A) which blocks the uterus from emerging from the abdominal wall (B). The left fallopian tube and ipsilateral round ligament are hyperextended as they are trapped between the uterus and the abdominal wall.

prophylaxis of endometritis, in the preoperative phase in single dose or at the time of cord clamping. Smulian et al. instead state that there is no evidence that justifies the use of antibiotics in the postnatal period in the absence of overt infections [48].

An important aspect of "obstetric malpractice" tied to homeostasis control and cleansing of the lower abdominal cavity, is leaving surgical material, in particular laparotomy gauze, in the abdomen after a CD. As stated by Rajagopal and Martin [49], it is a ubiquitous and even fairly frequent, though preventable, medical error, which can be the cause of morbidity and, rarely, of mortality [50]. The materials found from previous cesarean deliveries and reported in the literature are varied: gauze [49], surgical sponges [51], fragments of gloves, or latex [52] accidentally left behind after surgery.

Ultrasound, which is useful for the often unrecognized diagnosis of these foreign bodies, achieves a sensitivity of 92% according to Davae et al. These diagnostic data are extremely important, considering the medicolegal implications [53]. However, radiographic examinations can unequivocally reveal the presence in the abdomen of laparotomy gauze thanks to marker wire, usually consisting of radiopaque material. Therefore, if unrecognized laparotomy gauze is suspected upon closure of the abdomen, an abdominal x-ray must be performed on the patient, followed by an appropriate radiographic report in case of medical-legal disputes involving the entire operating team.

This type of "medical malpractice" is especially relevant when it occurs in Italy, as these events, unlike in Anglo-Saxon countries, are criminally sanctioned (Art. 43 PC) [54].

The Misgav Ladach technique emphasizes simple and rapid surgical maneuvers in the course of CD (the "quick cesarean delivery"). However, the surgical times can be

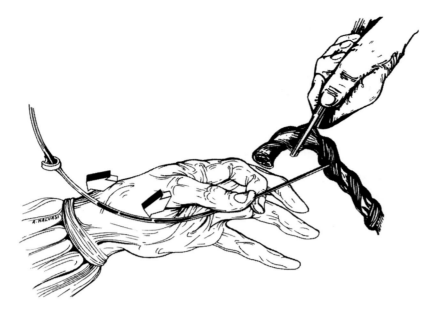

Figure 5.29 Sampling of placental blood from the umbilical cord, which is then sent to a transfusion center.

reasonably performed without unnecessary haste [34], because, as reported in a Cochrane review by Jorgensen et al., the postoperative course is mainly influenced by the type of analgesia rather used than by the surgical technique [55]. The authors, in fact, argue that the use of epidural analgesia in laparotomies reduces gastrointestinal paresis more than the systemic use of opioids.

In any case, all the problems associated with uterine exteriorization and repositioning have been analyzed in some studies: Siddiqui in 2007 and Coutinho in 2008 confirm that the exteriorization technique does not provide significant advantages other than a shorter operating time [56,57].

Nausea, vomiting, and tachycardia during cesarean delivery with spinal anesthesia and exteriorization, in addition to persistent postoperative pain, should prompt the surgeon to perform whenever possible an in situ uterine suture [56,57].

CORD BLOOD COLLECTION AND STORAGE TECHNIQUES

Immediately after birth the obstetrician will affix a clip in the vicinity of the newborn child, sever the cord, and deliver the baby to the neonatology team.

At this point the umbilical cord must be disinfected at the point of sampling in a distal position to the mother and, after removing the cap from the needle and clipping the tube downstream of the one to be used, the needle must be inserted into the cord.

Once the first part of the bag is filled, the obstetrician must clip the needle tube and perform the second sampling with another sterile needle near the maternal area until the blood flow stops.

Once the sampling is completed, the second tube connected to the needle will also be clamped and the bag containing the blood must be shaken in order to mix the anticoagulant inside. In addition, the preloaded vial in the extra pouch of the bag connected to the tube will be broken and squeezed so that the blood inside the tube can be retrieved.

At this point the bag tube can be definitively clamped, the superfluous tube can be cut and the needles can be removed following the disposal procedures. Two safety knots will then be tied on the tube before inserting it into the containers for transport to the Immunotransfusion Centre (Figure 5.29).

CONCLUSIONS

The scientific literature has discussed for years the benefits of spontaneous over manual placental removal in the course of a cesarean delivery [58–63].

Uterine suture can be performed with the uterus in the abdomen or with exteriorized uterus. Cochrane reviews do not report any differences between the two methods, although some authors report benefits with exteriorization, that include a reduction in the number of sutures and of surgery time [61–66]. Conversely, several important issues surrounding uterine exteriorization have been reported, among them pain and discomfort under locoregional anesthesia and in the postpartum period [67,68], which can be connected to drug type and dosage [69].

Uterine exteriorization may cause or contribute to serious, though rare, complications including pulmonary embolism [70].

Wiping the uterine cavity after placental removal is common technique, but the scientific literature contains little proof of validity of the method, with one author reporting no significant difference between performing and not performing wiping [23].

During placental removal, sampling of cord blood can be carried out upon the request of the patient, which is then sent to an immunotransfusion center for storage and preservation [71–75].

REFERENCES

1. Hermann A. Complicated third stage of labor: Time to switch on the scanner. (Editorial). *Ultrasound Obstet Gynecol* 2000;15:89–95.
2. Woo GM, Twickler DM, Stettler RW, Erdman WA, Brown CEL. The pelvis after cesarean delivery and vaginal delivery: Normal M R findings. *Am J R* 1993;161:1249–52.
3. Van Ham MA, Van Dongen PW, Mulder J. Maternal consequences of cesarean delivery. A retrospective study of intraoperative and postoperative maternal complications of cesarean delivery during a 10-years period. *Eur J Obstet Gynecol Reprod Biol* 1997;74:1–6.
4. Stoekel W. *Trattato di Ostetricia. Le operazioni ostetriche. Il taglio cesareo addominale.* Torino: U.T.E.T. Editore; 1925:967.
5. Khan GQ, John IS, Doerthy T, Sibai B. Controlled cord traction versus minimal intervention techniques in delivery of the placenta: A randomised controlled trial. *Am J Obstet Gynecol* 1997;177:770–4.
6. Rogers J, Wood J, Mac Candish R, Ayers S, Truesdale A, Elbourne D. Active versus expectant management of third stage of labour: The Hichingbrooke randomised controlled trial. *Lancet* 1998:351:693–9.
7. Merger R, Levy J, Melchior J. *Compendio di Ostetricia.* III Ediz. UTET- Masson & Cie; Torino-Parigi; 1972:Parte III: 920–40.
8. Favier M, Racinet C. *La Cèsarienne: Indications, techniques, complications.* Paris, France: Masson; 1984;73–75.
9. Prendiville WJ, Elbourne D, McDonald S. Active versus expectant management in the third stage of labour. (Cochrane review). In: *The Cochrane Library, Issue 3.* Chichester, UK: Wiley; 2004.
10. Carroli G, Bergel E. Umbilical vein injection for management of retained placenta (Cochrane review). In: *The Cochrane Library, Issue 3.* Chichester, UK: Wiley; 2004.
11. Wilkinson C, Enkin MW. Manual removal of placenta at caesarean section. (Cochrane review). In: *Cochrane Library, Issue 3.* Chichester, UK: Wiley; 2004.
12. Magann EF, Dodson MK, Harris RL, Floyd RC, Martin JN, Morrison JC. Does method of placental removal or site of uterine incision repair alter endometritis after cesarean delivery? *Inf Dis Obstet Gynecol* 1993;1:65–70.
13. Smaill F, Hofmeyr GL. Antibiotic prophylaxis for cesarean delivery (Cochrane review). In: *The Cochrane Library, Issue 3.* Chichester, UK: Wiley; 2004.
14. Mc Curdy CM, Magann EF, Mc Curdy CJ, Saltzman AK. The effect of placental management at cesarean delivery on operative blood loss. *Am J Obstet Gynecol* 1992;167:1363–7.
15. Cunningham FG, Hauth JC, Strong JD, Kappus SS. Infectious morbidity following cesarean delivery, comparison of two treatment regimens. *Obstet Gynecol* 1978;52:656–61.
16. Rehu M, Nilsson CG. Risk factors for febrile morbidity associated with cesarean delivery. *Obstet Gynecol* 1980;56:269–73.
17. Green SL, Sarubbi FA. Risk factors associated with post-cesarean delivery febrile morbidity. *Obstet Gynecol* 1977;49:688–90.
18. Kenyon S, Boulvain M, Nielson J. Antibiotics for preterm rupture of membranes. (Cochrane review). In: *Cochrane Library, Issue 3.* Chichester, UK: Wiley; 2004.
19. Yancey MK, Clark P, Duff P. The frequency of glove contamination during Cesarean delivery. *Obstet Gynecol* 1994;83:538–42.
20. Atkinson MW, Owen J, Wren A, Haulth JC. The effect of manual removal of the placenta on post-caesarean endometritis. *Obstet Gynecol* 1996; 87:99–102.
21. Cernadas M, Smulian JC, Giannina G, Ananth CV. Effects of placental delivery method and intraoperative glove chancing on postcesarean febrile morbidity. *J Matern Fetal Med* 1998;7:100–94.
22. De Lee JB, Greenhill JP. *Principi e Pratica dell'Ostetricia. Casa editrice Principato.* Chapter LXIII; Metodi di parto: Taglio Cesareo. Milano-Messina, 1954: 878.
23. Magann EF, Chauhan SP, Martin JN, Bryant KS, Bufkin L, Morrison JC. Does uterine wiping influence the rate of post-cesarean endometritis? *J Matern Fetal Med* 2001;10:318–322.
24. Kazahov BJ, Khankoev IM, Pererva VV. Results of histeroscopic method of foreign body removal out of uterus cavity. *J Am Assoc Gynecol Laparoscop* 1994;1(4, Part 2):S 16.
25. Proust R, Charrier J. *Precis de Tèchnique Opèratoire. Chirurgie de l'appareil genital de la femme.* Troisième. Partie. Cap. VII. Operation Cèsarienne. Paris, France: Masson et Cie Editeurs; 1992;291–6.
26. Gagliardi L, Cerruti G. Taglio cesareo. In: Ferrarsi G, ed. *Trattato di Tecnica Chirurgica. Ginecologica ed Ostetrica.* Torino: UTET Editore, 1986;1021–30.
27. Ragucci N. Taglio Cesareo. In: *Trattato Italiano di Ginecologia.* Vol. VI. Cap. CXXXVII, Istituto Geografico De Agostani, Novara. EDIPEM Editore 1976:127–50.
28. Portes L. La cesariènne suive d'exteriorization temporaire de l'uterus. *Gynecol Obstet* 1924;10:225.
29. Young JH. *The history of caesarean delivery.* London, UK: H.K. Lewis and Co. Ltd.; 1944:137–41.
30. Sanger M. Zur rehabilitirung bes classischen kaiserschnittes nebst eimen anhenge: Nachtridge zur geshichte der uterusnaht beim kaiserschnitte. *Arch F Gynaekol* 1882;19:370–99.
31. Leopold C. Ein Kaiserschnitt mit Uterusnht etc. *Arch F Gyn* 1882; Zur Vereinfachung und Naht des Kaiserschittes. *Arch F Gyn* 1889; Welche Stellung nimmt die Klassische Sectio caesarea etc. *Arch F Gyn* 1910.
32. Phaneuf LE. Caesarean delivery followed by temporary exteriorization of uterus: Portes operation. *Surg Gynecol Obstet* 1927;44:788.
33. Doerfler H. 30 Jhare Schnittbindung (Kaiserschnitt). *Munchen Med W Schr* 1929;76:2.

34. Stark M, Chavkin Y, Kupfersztain C, Guedj P, Finkel AR. Evaluation of combination of procedures in cesarean delivery. *Int J Gynecol Obstet* 1995;48:273–6.
35. Hershey DW, Quilligan EJ. Extraabdominal uterine exteriorization at cesarean delivery. *Obstet Gynecol* 1978;52:189–92.
36. Malvasi A, Vittori G, Martino V, Imparato E. Does the parietal peritoneum need to be closet at laparotomy? Second look laparoscopy for the adhesion evaluations. *Proceedings and Abstracts Book of World Meeting on Minimally Invasive Surgery in Gynecology*. Rome, Italy, 2003.
37. Magann EF, Washburne JF, Harris RL, Bass JD, Duff WP, Morrison JC. Operative procedure after cesarean delivery. *J Am Coll Surg* 1995;181;517–20.
38. Edi-Osagie EC, Hopkins RE, Ogbo V, Lockhat-Clegg F, Ayeko M, Akpala WO, Mayers FN. Uterine exteriorization at cesarean delivery: Influence on maternal morbidity. *Br J Obstet Gynecol* 1998;105:1070–8.
39. Wahab MA, Karantzis P, Eccersley PS, Russel IF, Thompson JW, Lindow SW. A randomized, controlled study of uterine exteriorization and repair at cesarean delivery. *Br J Obstet Gynecol* 1999;106:913–6.
40. Wilkinson C, Enkin MW. Uterine exteriorization versus intraperitoneal repair at caesarean delivery (Cochrane review). In: *The Cochrane Library, Issue 3*. Chichester, UK: Wiley; 2004.
41. Handler JS, Bromage PR. Venous air embolism during Cesarean delivery. *Reg Anesth* 1990;15:170–3.
42. Lowenwirt IP, Chi DS, Handwerker SM. Nonfatal venous air embolism during Cesarean delivery: A case report and review of the literature. *Obstet Gynecol Surv* 1994;49:72–76.
43. Larsen B, Davis B, Charles D. Critical assessment of antibacterial properties of human amniotic fluid. *Gynecol Obstet Invest* 1984;18:100–4.
44. Down RH, Whitehead R, Watts JM. Do surgical packs cause peritoneal adhesions? *Aust NZ J Surg* 1979;49:379–82.
45. Davis JR, Miller HS, Feng JD. Vernix caseosa peritonitis: Report of two cases with antenatal onset. *Am J Clin Pathol* 1998;109:320–3.
46. Antonelli E, Morales MA, Dumps P, Boulvain M, Weil A. Sonographic detection of fluid collections and postoperative morbidity following Cesarean delivery and hysterectomy. *Ultrasound Obstet Gynecol* 2004; 23:388–92.
47. Hoppkins L, Smaill F. Antibiotic prophylaxis regimens and drugs for cesarean delivery (Cochrane review). In: *The Cochrane Library, Issue 3*. Chichester, UK: Wiley; 2004.
48. Smulian JC, Potash SK, Lay YL, Scorza WE. Appropriateness of antibiotic use in the postpartum period. *J Matern Fetal Med* 2001;10:312–7.
49. Rajagopal A, Martin J, Gossypibom A. A surgeon's legacy: Report of a case and review of the literature. *Dis Colon Rectum* 2002;45:119–20.
50. Huep WW, Hermann K, Hesselmann J. Uterine foreign body and septic peritonitis after Cesarean delivery. *Ultrasound Med* 1982;3:142–4.
51. Silva Cs, Caetano Mr, Silva Ea, Falco L, Murta EF. Complete migration of retained surgical sponge into ileum without sign of open intestinal wall. *Arch Gynecol Obstet* 2001;265:103–4.
52. Confino E, Zbella E, Gleicher N. Abcess formation post cesarean delivery due to a piece of latex glove. *Int J Gynaecol Obstet* 1987;25:155–7.
53. Davae KC, Sofka CM, Di Carlo E, Adler RS. Value of power Doppler imaging and the hypoechoic halo in the sonographic detection of foreign bodies: Correlation with histopathologic findings. *J Ultrasound Med* 2003; 22:1309–13.
54. Harney DM. *Medical practice*. 3rd ed. Charlottesville, VA: The Michie Company; 1993.
55. Jorgensen H, Wetterslev J, Moiniche S, Dhal JB. Epidural local anaesthetics versus opioid analgesic regiments for postoperative gastrointestinal paralysis, ponv and pain after abdominal surgery (Cochrane review). In: *The Cochrane Library, Issue 3*. Chichester, UK; Wiley; 2004.
56. Siddiqui M, Goldszmidt E, Fallah S, Kingdom J, Windrim R, Carvalho JC. Complications of exteriorized compared with in situ uterine repair at cesarean delivery under spinal anesthesia: A randomized controlled trial. *Obstet Gynecol* 2007;110(3): 570–5.
57. Coutinho IC, Ramos de Amorim MM, Katz L, Bandeira de Ferraz AA. Uterine exteriorization compared with in situ repair at cesarean delivery: A randomized controlled trial. *Obstet Gynecol* 2008;111(3): 639–47. Erratum in: *Obstet Gynecol* 2008;112(1):188. Comment in: *Obstet Gynecol* 2008;112(1):183; author reply 183.
58. Blumenfeld Y, Caughey AB, Lyell DJ. Uterine exteriorization compared with in situ repair at cesarean delivery: A randomized controlled trial. *Obstet Gynecol* 2008;112(1):183.
59. Hema KR, Johanson R. Techniques for performing caesarean delivery. *Best Pract Res Clin Obstet Gynaecol* 2001;15(1):17–47.
60. Merchavy S, Levy A, Holcberg G, Freedman EN, Sheiner E. Method of placental removal during cesarean delivery and postpartum complications. *Int J Gynaecol Obstet* 2007:98(3):232–6.
61. Duff P. A simple checklist for preventing major complications associated with cesarean delivery. *Obstet Gynecol* 2010;116(6):1393–6.
62. Gün I, Ozdamar O, Ertuğrul S, Oner O, Atay V. The effect of placental removal method on perioperative hemorrhage at cesarean delivery; A randomized clinical trial [published online March 1, 2013]. *Arch Gynecol Obstet* 2013;288(3):563–7.
63. Dahlke JD, Mendez-Figueroa H, Rouse DJ, Berghella V, Baxter JK, Chauhan SP. Evidence-based surgery for cesarean delivery: An updated systematic review [published online March 1, 2013]. *Am J Obstet Gynecol* 2013;209(4):294–306.

64. Coutinho IC, Ramos de Amorim MM, Katz L, Bandeira de Ferraz AA. Uterine exteriorization compared with in situ repair at cesarean delivery: A randomized controlled trial. *Obstet Gynecol* 2008;111(3):639–47.
65. Gode F, Okyay RE, Saatli B, Ertugrul C, Guclu S, Altunyurt S. Comparison of uterine exteriorization and in situ repair during cesarean sections. *Arch Gynecol Obstet* 2012;285(6):1541–5.
66. Ezechi OC, Kalu BK, Njokanma FO, Nwokoro CA, Okeke GC. Uterine incision closure at caesarean delivery: A randomised comparative study of intraperitoneal closure and closure after temporary exteriorisation. *West Afr J Med* 2005;24(1):41–43.
67. Nafisi S. Influence of uterine exteriorization versus in situ repair on post-Cesarean maternal pain: A randomized trial. *Int J Obstet Anesth* 2007;16(2):135–8.
68. Siddiqui M, Goldszmidt E, Fallah S, Kingdom J, Windrim R, Carvalho JC. Complications of exteriorized compared with in situ uterine repair at cesarean delivery under spinal anesthesia: A randomized controlled trial. *Obstet Gynecol* 2007;110(3): 570–5.
69. Arzola C, Wieczorek PM. Efficacy of low-dose bupivacaine in spinal anaesthesia for Caesarean delivery: Systematic review and meta-analysis. *Br J Anaesth* 2011;107(3):308–18.
70. Stock RJ, Skelton H. Fatal pulmonary embolism occurring two hours after exteriorization of the uterus for repair following cesarean delivery. *Mil Med* 1985;150(10):549–51.
71. Elchalal U, Fasouliotis SJ, Shtockheim D, Brautbar C, Schenker JG, Weinstein D, Nagler A. Postpartum umbilical cord blood collection for transplantation: A comparison of three methods. *Am J Obstet Gynecol* 2000;182(1 Pt 1):227–32.
72. Surbek DV, Visca E, Steinmann C, Tichelli A, Schatt S, Hahn S, Gratwohl A, Holzgreve W. Umbilical cord blood collection before placental delivery during cesarean delivery increases cord blood volume and nucleated cell number available for transplantation. *Am J Obstet Gynecol* 2000;183(1):218–21.
73. Armson BA; Maternal/Fetal Medicine Committee, Society of Obstetricians and Gynaecologists of Canada. Umbilical cord blood banking: Implications for perinatal care providers. *J Obstet Gynaecol Can* 2005;27(3):263–90.
74. Gutman JA, Miller S, Kuenne S, Oppenheim J, Quinones R, Freed BM, Stark C, Zarlengo G. Cordblood collection after cesarean delivery improves banking efficiency. *Transfusion* 2011;51(9):2050–1.
75. Volpe G, Santodirocco M, Di Mauro L, Miscio G, Boscia FM, Muto B, Volpe N. Four phases of checks for exclusion of umbilical cord blood donors. *Blood Transfus* 2011;9(3):286–91.
76. Clivio I. Obstetric operations. In: *Trattato di Ostetricia*. Vol. III. Milan, Italy: F. Vallardi Edit; 1945:446–449.

Suture of uterine incisions

ANTONIO MALVASI and GIAN CARLO DI RENZO

> In 1769 Lebas from Mouilleron was apparently the first to suture the uterine wound. He was able to achieve this with only 3 sutures.
>
> (Pietro Gall, *The Abdominal Caesarean Delivery*, 1922)

HISTORICAL NOTES AND EVOLUTION

A reliable history of the uterine suture is reported by Piero Gall in *The Abdominal Caesarean Delivery*: "Suturing was performed with silk thread until the American Frank E. Polin (1852) began using silver thread to great effect. The use of silver thread was later adopted by John Parker (England) and Harris (United States). In 1872 Veit successfully applied in 2 cases catgut, which was already applied in surgery. By contrast Martin had 4 lethal outcomes due to faulty catgut preparation. This was therefore followed by a return to silver thread" (Figure 6.1) [1].

Mangiagalli writes: "while Martino D'Avanzo had in 1860 closed the uterine wound using the D'Apolito or 'mattress maker' suture, Lazzati in 1869 and Balocchi in 1872 made performed suture but with unfavourable outcome. A new page in the history of uterine sutures was written in 1873 by Olinto Grandesso-Silvestri, who successfully used an elastic thread" [2].

In the nineteenth century the focus was on the type of suture, as it was believed that complications derived from the type of material used.

Gall wrote:

> In general, the uterine incision, in women deliveryed a few days after a Caesarean delivery, was open: sutures would break, tearing the tissue and lochia discharge from the uterine cavity would cause lethal peritonitis. The actual cause of this was not due to a fault in the technique but to the presence of germs: whatever the material used and the method of preparation, the thread carried with it huge amounts of all kinds of infectious germs which could easily proliferate in the stitches and adjacent areas. Our colleagues of the time could not have realized this. In fact in their minds bacteriological infection did not exist and the first remedy that would logically come to mind would be to discourage the suture which was considered harmful per se [1].

On this matter Cazeaux wrote in 1845: "The uterus wound does not require precautions, other than it should be thoroughly cleansed. As to the wound of the abdominal walls the margins must be united by two or three stitches of an interlocking suture, while being careful to leave open space on the lower part for the discharge of abdominal fluids" [3].

On the same topic Scanzoni wrote: "Lauverjat's proposal to stop or prevent bleeding by suturing the uterine wall is needless and dangerous, since there evidently cannot be an advantage in suturing the relaxed organ, while suturing performed with walls that are contracted will result in the tearing of tissue as soon as relaxation occurs and the volume of the uterus grows. This in fact happened before my eyes to a patient I was operating in 1847. But even if this does not occur, this type of suture is not capable of stemming the bleeding in the uterine cavity" [4].

On the benefits of suturing the uterus, Vincenzo Balocchi in 1871 reported the following clinical consideration: "Should the uterine wound be sutured? In general when the incision is correctly executed and the uterus regularly contracts, the wound becomes so small that there is absolutely no need to suture it. Therefore most do not concern themselves with this but only with the ventral walls" [5].

At the time, puerperal necropsies revealed dehiscence of the uterine suture from infection and necrosis of the tissue, whereas autopsies of women who had died sometime after and not for reasons related to the cesarean delivery, instead showed the formation of large uterine adhesions to the abdominal wall.

These observations provided Pillore of Rouen (1854) with the justification for a uterine–abdominal suture that consisted of suturing the lower third of the uterine incision with the edges of the abdominal wall, while the upper two-thirds were sutured in a conventional manner. In his writings Gall came to these conclusions regarding uterine suture: "The uterine wound must be kept open to prevent blood and lochia discharge into the abdominal cavity and in particular to allow removal of threads which for the obstetricians of the time, were cause of serious concern and the subject of extremely heated debates" [1].

Lestocquoy, a surgeon from Arras, sutured the edges of the abdominal wall with the uterine wall even before it was cut to extract the fetus. Despite support from Braxton-Hicks and Martin, this uterine–parietal suture was soon disused in the few cases of maternal survival, because, in spite of surgical precautions, the necessary antisepsis was still absent.

In those days the mortality rate in cesarean deliveries from infections caused by suture materials was extremely high: the casuistry by Kaiser in the period between 1750 and 1839 showed a mortality rate in 338 cases of 62% for mothers and 30% for fetuses [6].

Gueniot reported a mortality rate that reached 100% in 40 cases performed in Paris before 1870 [7]. Similarly, Sparth reported that no cesarean delivery performed before 1877 at the Institute of Maternity of Vienna was successful [8]. It was this high mortality rate that led Edoardo Porro, on May 21, 1876, to perform the "utero-ovarian amputation" in addition to the cesarean delivery (Figure 6.2). The rationale behind the Porro intervention

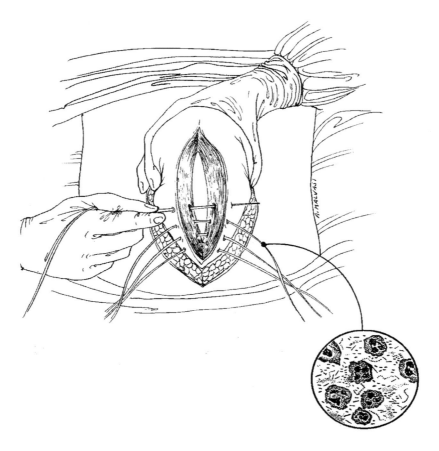

Figure 6.1 Contamination of suture threads by pathogenic germs during a cesarean delivery was a cause of maternal morbidity and mortality in the preantibiotic era.

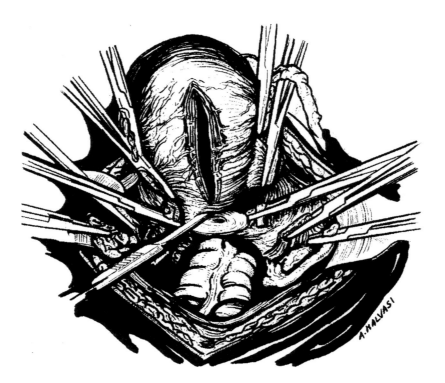

Figure 6.2 Utero-ovarian amputation by Edoardo Porro. (Modified from Porro, E. Della amputazione utero-ovarica come complemento di taglio cesareo. *Ann Univ Med* 1876;237.)

was well summarized later by Mangiagalli: "to remove a large fomite of infection, to ensure haemostasis, to make it impossible for secretions to spill into the peritoneal cavity, to benefit from monitoring and treating the surface of the remaining uterine stump, to sterilise the woman" [2].

Truzzi [9] reported that Porro after extracting the fetus and the placenta, exteriorized the uterus by applying a large iron wire mounted on a sturdy Cintrat snare at the level of the internal uterine orifice and after placing the constricting wire on the left ovary performed the amputation of the uterus 2 cm above the blocking noose. This was followed by vaginal–abdominal drainage through the Pouch of Douglas, the securing of the stump to the lower corner of the wound, the twisted suture of the abdominal walls with four stitches of silver thread, and the brushing of the stump with iron perchloride. The snare was left in situ, with the end between the legs of the woman who healed after a stormy puerperium.

Another historic date in the development of the cesarean delivery is the year 1882 when the German gynecologist Max Sanger (1853–1903) had the brilliant intuition to systematically close the uterine wall. Up until then it had been left open to overcome the two major dangers of the time: uterine hemorrhage and septic infection due to the passage of lochia in the abdominal cavity. This maneuver drastically reduced maternal mortality [10,11].

To distinguish it from Porro's "ablative" intervention that surgically induced sterility (as well as inducing a clinical, hormonal, and psychological condition typical of menopause), Sanger defined his cesarean delivery as "classical conservative" and it would become the typical intervention performed whenever childbirth by natural means was impossible.

Sanger was strongly in favor of a longitudinal incision along the anterior wall of the uterine body and suggested that the uterine breach be sutured in two layers. The first deeper layer brought the musculature closer without including the deciduous, with 8 or 10 silver thread stitches; the second more superficial layer, joined the edges of the serosa with 20–25 stitches using silk thread in a Lembert suture pattern (Figure 6.3).

Sanger's method found many supporters, such as Mangiagalli in Italy, but especially abroad with Porak and Daucourt in France, Eustache in Belgium, and Harris and Garrigues in the United States.

The suturing of the uterine wall, which was so heavily criticized and even opposed, became over time more important than the operation, as is evident from the words of the German Bumm (1924):

> Detach and extract the placenta and membranes. At this point the most important stage of the operation can start: the suturing of the uterine wall. One with experience will choose the intersecting suture and will prefer silver thread and silk over catgut, as it can be more safely sterilised, more easily handling and provides a final result that is not inferior. Even more important than the suture material is however the suturing technique. The stitches must be close to one another and cross the entire thickness of the wall, so that the two halves of the wound are brought into contact with each other. The

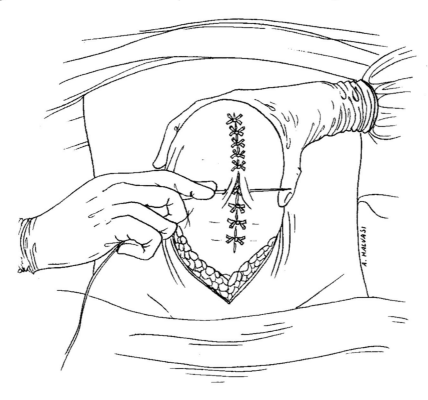

Figure 6.3 The corporeal longitudinal incision according to Sanger was followed by a double-layer suture: first layer with silver thread, second layer with silk thread.

needle penetrates near the edge of the peritoneum, exits from the decidua and continues in the reverse direction along the wall on the opposite side. ... Instead of using the intersecting suture, a more complete and accurate alignment can be achieved with a continuous suture, in layers, using catgut. One can start from the deepest layer of the wound, a second layer of suture is applied on the middle highly vascularised muscular layer. Lastly, the most superficial layer is aligned. Once the suture of the muscles is completed, it is recommended to add a continuous Lembert suture (seroserous) with thin silk, as done in intestinal sutures. It covers the knots of the interrupted stitches and achieves rapid adhesion of the aligned serous surfaces, which guarantees a good outcome. The sutured uterus is cleaned with sterile sodium chloride solution, and once the suture line is sprinkled with a solution of sublimate, the viscera is pushed deep into the cavity [12].

Table 6.1 presents various types of material used in hysterorrhaphy at the beginning of the last century.

During the same period, (1922) Proust and Charrier in France reaffirmed the hemostatic function of the uterine suture, which they also performed out in double layer. The deep layer was in silk (no. 2) with interrupted stitches, about 1.5 cm apart, which crossed the entire muscle and mucosa. The superficial layer was in catgut (no. 1), again with interrupted stitches, in which the needles passed through the intervals of the previous stitches, and ended with a peritoneal Lembert suture [13].

Walter Stoeckel, with regard to the "intraperitoneal" cesarean delivery, also carried out in 1925 a double-layer suture with a continuous superficial layer followed by the suture of the vesicouterine fold [14].

Some years later, De Lee and Greenhill in 1954 also emphasized that the suturing of the uterus represented the most important part of the intervention: starting from the upper end of the longitudinal incision they laid a first simple overlock layer that involved the thin layer of the musculature without including the mucosa (Figure 6.4). The second layer was of interrupted stitches, again in catgut (no. 1) and involved the muscle layer along its entire thickness (Figure 6.5).

The third layer, with interrupted stitches, included the peritoneum and the underlying musculature (Figure 6.6). The fourth layer included only the peritoneal prevesical surface with a simple continuous overlock suture [15].

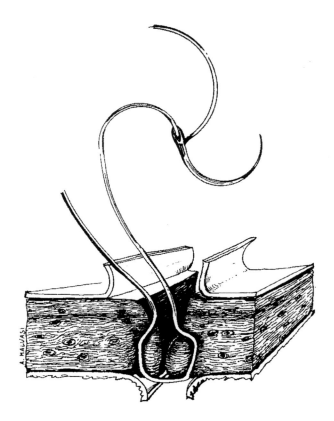

Figure 6.4 Cross section of the first layer of the longitudinal incision of the uterus according to De Lee and Greenhill: interrupted catgut stitches (no. 1) 1 cm apart without including the uterine mucosa.

Table 6.1 Various types of material used in hysterorrhaphy at the beginning of the last century

Thread used in the past in uterine sutures
Silk
Silver
Elastic thread
Iron wire[a]
Catgut

[a] Iron wire was employed by Porro on a Canard snare to close the uterine stump.

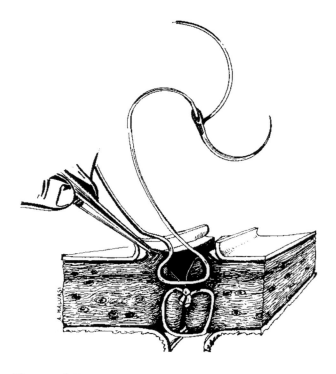

Figure 6.5 The second layer was always in catgut (no. 1), spacing the interrupted stitches about 1 cm apart, while being careful to not include in the suture the uterine wadding previously crammed into the cavity.

Current suturing techniques 149

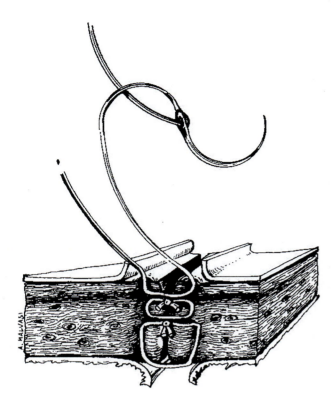

Figure 6.6 The third layer was done with stitches in catgut (no. 1), 0.5 cm apart and by juxtaposing the superficial layer of the muscle and the visceral peritoneum (which the authors called "fascia").

Potter and Elton, just as Johnson and Ober, used a single layer of interrupted silk stitches.

As time passed the incision in the longitudinal direction of the anterior wall of the uterus was performed less often compared to the low transverse incision on the lower uterine segment.

Martius performed a double-layer suture once the corners of the incision were sutured. The first layer consisted of interrupted catgut stitches (usually no. 1) 1.5 cm apart, excluding the mucosa; the second instead covered the first suture in a zig-zag pattern [16].

CURRENT SUTURING TECHNIQUES
General information

Some surgeons prefer exteriorizing the uterus when performing a cesarean delivery in order to facilitate the exposure and to quicken the suturing process.

This is particularly useful when there is major bleeding coming from one side of the incision, which is due to partial rupture of the uterine wall. This facilitates hemostasis as the maneuver decreases the loss of blood by stretching the uterine vessels.

Exteriorization appears to increase maternal discomfort and nausea, especially when the operation is performed in locoregional anesthesia. Exteriorization, however, seems to decrease the risk of infection [17] although a meta-analysis does not show which method is preferable (Figure 6.7) [18].

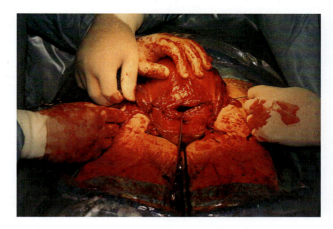

Figure 6.7 Suture of the cesarean hysterotomy with exteriorized uterus in which the corners have been sutured.

Usually uterine vessels lacerated at the corners of the uterine incision are sutured after placental extraction. It is always preferable to identify, clamp, and tie the bleeding vessels rather than to blindly perform a suture (Figures 6.8 and 6.9).

Some prefer to individually tie the corners of the hysterotomy with a single or double stitch, even when the hysterotomy is regular and has not spread laterally toward the uterine vessels.

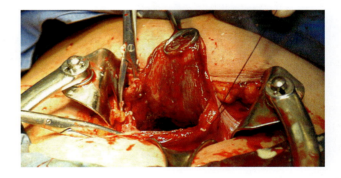

Figure 6.8 Individual suturing of the left corner of the uterine breach after placental removal.

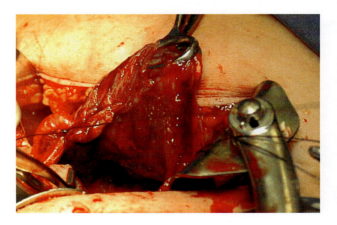

Figure 6.9 Suture of the right corner of the uterine breach.

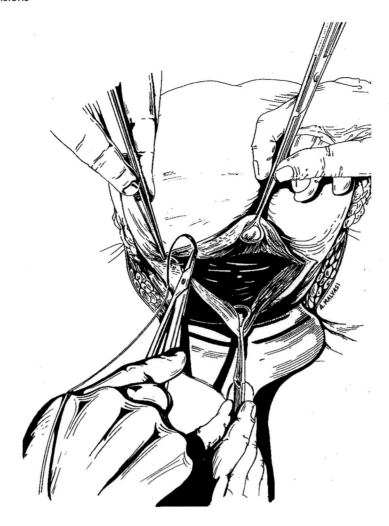

Figure 6.10 Transfixation of the lower right edge of the hysterotomy corner, while the apex is secured by an anatomical clamp and the curvature of the needle is directed outside the clamp prehension area.

The single suture of the corners is obligatory, in the presence of venous or arterial vessels with lateral lacerations, to better control the loss of blood and prevent hematomas that may appear in the parametrium. However, Stark considers this procedure unnecessary for the Misgav Ladach method. He starts with a 90-cm thread from the surgeon's side and performs a continuous suture ending on the side of the second operator.

Regardless of how the operator decides to carry out the uterine suture, corners should always be inspected to make sure that the entire uterine thickness is included in the suture stitch and that there are no areas without sutures [19]. Suturing the corners of a cesarean delivery hysterotomy is particularly important in terms of hemostasis. It is therefore recommended that the needle first enter one side and then the opposite side to make sure that the entire corner has been included in the stitch and that no bleeding areas were left outside the knot (Figure 6.10).

In this regard some obstetricians prefer to make sure that the corner is included in the suture by performing a double pass before knotting by means of interlocking threads. In particular, when the corner is "undermined," namely, the superficial part is less laterally extended than the inner or deep part of the corner, the stitch must come before the incision of the hysterotomy. In fact, in this case the suture stitch of the uterine corner must be applied more laterally, so as to include the apex of the corner that extends in depth with a beveled shape, and from which the bleeding can continue (Figure 6.11).

In cases such as these the suture-tying method is an important technique. It is performed behind the corner, which is stretched contralaterally with a ring forceps in order to include more tissue unaffected by the hysterotomy (Figure 6.12).

In order to achieve an anatomically correct closure of the margins of the wound, proper healing of the wound itself and good cicatrization for future pregnancies, as well as to not include the uterine mucosa in the suture (Figure 6.13), it is also important that the margins of the suture be firmly pushed together and that there is proper hemostasis by placing the stitches sufficiently far from the edge of the wound.

To correctly perform a hysterorrhaphy when suturing a uterine incision, various types of single-layer or

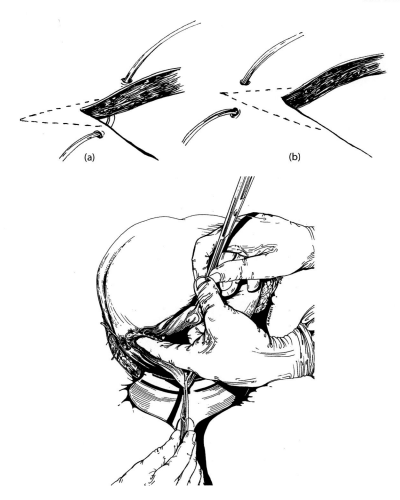

Figure 6.11 Inspection of the postcesarean hysterotomy with uterine exteriorization: the right corner extends laterally (at bottom) and the surgeon performs a maneuver to verify that the suture stitch has included the corner. The laceration of the corner has a beveled shape: at top left is the incorrect position (a) and at top right is the correct position (b) of the suture stitch, in which the stitch is applied further back and includes the apex of the corner.

multiple-layer sutures can be used, with continuous or interrupted sutures, as described in various studies in the literature (Figure 6.14).

The use of knotted stitches or numerous single or eight-pattern stitches does not represent a good technique. In rare cases it can be used to achieve hemostasis or, in certain cases, to tie large vessels laterally. Continuous sutures, instead, are widely used.

In 1992 Hauth performed a randomized study on the closure of the uterine breach in 906 women. Closure was achieved using a continuous single interlocking layer with chromic gut (no. 1) and CTX needle, as well as a double layer using the same thread, both continuous with interlocking first layer. In the conclusions the author recommended a continuous suture with single interlocking layer of the uterine breach in that, technically, it required less operative time and, from an outcome point of view, improved hemostasis, though with similar infectious complications [20].

The continuous suture in single layer does not preclude the possibility of subsequent labor of childbirth, as shown in a study on 292 women who underwent a previous cesarean delivery [21].

In 1993 Jelsema et al. tested the safety of closure of a continuous single nonlocking layer in 100 women (Figures 6.15 and 6.16) in comparison with a double layer with continuous first interlocking suture and continuous second inverted suture in 100 other women (Figures 6.17 and 6.18). It was also assumed that the nonlocking single layer could reduce ischemic vascular tissue damage and might, in theory, strengthen the uterine wall in the subsequent labor [22].

A current problem is represented by the suture of the hysterotomy, in a single or double simple layer, necessary to achieve a uterine scar with good structural characteristics. This allows for vaginal birth after cesarean (VBAC) delivery in a second pregnancy whenever indications make it viable (Figure 6.19).

Some years later Chapman et al. evaluated 164 women who had previously undergone a cesarean delivery, 83 with single-layer closure and 81 with double-layer closure with chromic catgut (no. 1). Of these, 19 had undergone

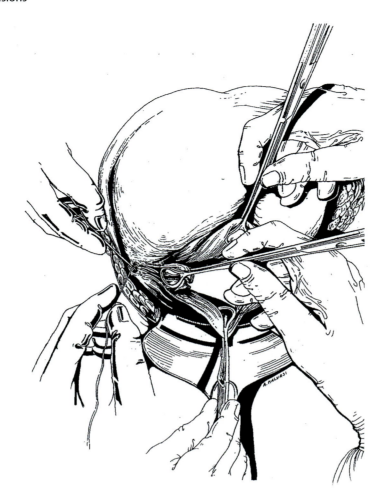

Figure 6.12 The connection can be perfected by suturing and tying the right uterine corner with a knot at the end while the assistant contralaterally stretches the corner.

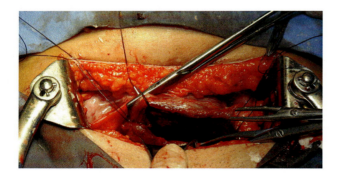

Figure 6.13 The suture of the uterine breach must respect the uterine mucosa, which should not be included in the suture. The needle should go through healthy tissue to ensure hemostasis and proper healing.

an elective cesarean delivery, while the other 145 underwent the labor of birth. In the conclusions the study authors asserted that the type of closure did not in any way affect the pregnancy that followed a cesarean delivery, and that no conclusions could be drawn on the incidence of dehiscence, given the limited number of cases. They hypothesized that

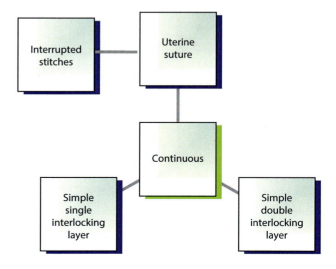

Figure 6.14 Chart showing the different uterine suturing methods during a cesarean section.

Current suturing techniques 153

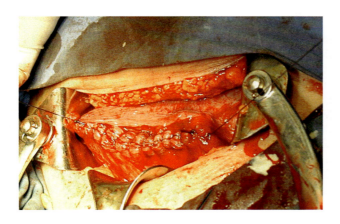

Figure 6.15 Simple continuous suture of the uterine breach, with uterus in situ (basically in the abdominal cavity).

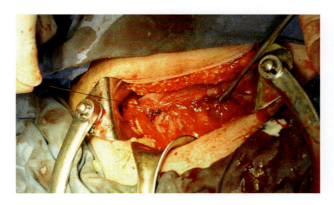

Figure 6.17 Continuous interlocking suture of the uterine breach with the uterus placed in the abdominal cavity.

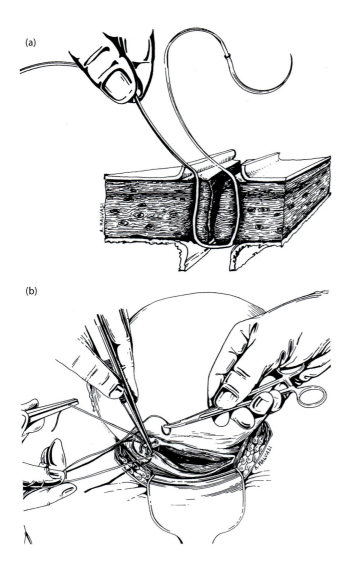

Figure 6.16 Simple continuous suture of the uterine incision with exteriorized uterus, (a) starting from the side of the assistant and excluding the uterine mucosa from the suture; (b) detail of the monolayer of the uterus that excludes the decidua.

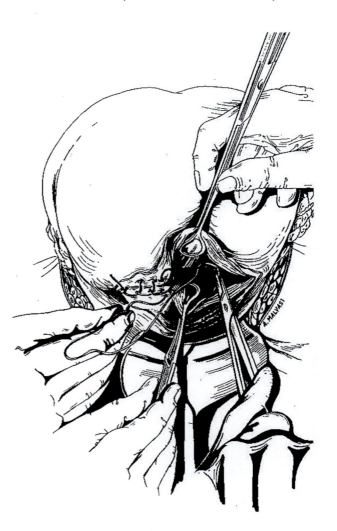

Figure 6.18 Interlocking uterine suture with exteriorized uterus.

over 2300 patients would have to be studied in order to obtain a statistical power of 80% (Figure 6.20) [23].

In 2004 Enkin and Wilkinson in evaluating the effects of the single-layer closure compared to the double-layer closure, considered only two trials that included 1006

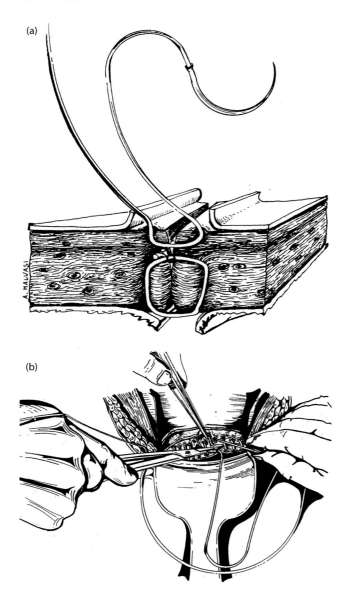

Figure 6.19 (a) Cross section that shows the double-layer suture, for both continuous and interrupted stitches. (b) Continuous double-layer suture of uterine breach.

women. They came to the conclusion that, except for a lower operative time, there were no substantial differences between the two types of closures with regard to the use of additional sutures, the incidence of subsequent puerperal endometritis, the decrease in hematocrit, and blood transfusions [24].

The same authors in 2008 confirmed their previous findings, stating that the only benefit of the single-layer suture compared to the double layer is the shorter operating time [25].

Ferrari et al. reached the same conclusions in a randomized study of 158 women in 2001. The continuous single interlocking suture with monocryl VS was compared to the continuous double-layer suture with catgut (no. 1) in 83 women with innovative cesarean and 75 with classic cesarean [26].

With regard to uterine rupture, Bujold et al. in 2002 observed 1980 women in labor after a previous cesarean delivery. They reported that a single-layer closure of the uterine breach increases the risk of uterine rupture by four times when compared with double-layer closure. In this study, chromic catgut had been used in 98% of cases and Vicryl in 2%; the suture was made with a single continuous interlocking layer; the single layer was used in 480 women, while in 1491 cases the hysterotomy was closed with a double layer.

According to data from a multivariate statistical analysis of risk factors, a time interval of less than 24 months between labor and a previous cesarean delivery was associated with an increased risk of uterine rupture (Table 6.2). The definition of uterine rupture included any type of dehiscence with extrusion of uterine content that resulted in surgical intervention [27].

In contrast to the above, a retrospective study by Durnwald and Mercer in 2003 evaluated the subsequent pregnancy of 768 women with previous cesarean delivery, 267 with single-layer suture and 501 with double-layer suture with Vicryl. The authors stated that the single-layer suture of the uterine breach did not increase the risk of uterine rupture in the subsequent pregnancy.

However, the authors reported a higher frequency of asymptomatic uterine dehiscence—that is, a defect of the myometrium with intact peritoneum in the group of women with a single layer, for whom dehiscence was 3.5% versus 0.7% [28].

Currently, there is no unanimous consensus in the scientific community as to which is the best way to close the uterine breach. Therefore, it would be appropriate to investigate the factors that affect the strength of the suture, in particular, the choice of materials, the technique, and the presence of postoperative infections.

After suturing the uterine incision, it is always necessary to provide hemostasis: any bleeding from superficial areas of the wound or from areas of application of the stitches is simply controlled with gauze or, when that is not sufficient, with an electric scalpel or by applying usually one or more 8 stitches.

Various suturing materials are employed in a hysterorrhaphy suture, and the most frequently used are summarized in Table 6.3. Some obstetricians consider the use of catgut appropriate especially in hemostatic sutures, due to its flexibility, though this material is no longer in use in Italy. New synthetic materials (e.g., polyglycolic acid such as Dexon and polyglactin such as Vycril) have, dimensions being equal, considerable advantages, as they are more resistant. This allows the surgeon to use thinner threads that are apparently stable even in the presence of infectious processes. Thin threads are an additional advantage in that larger suture threads can more actively stimulate phagocyte activity and may not be able to maintain their tension for a longer period of time than smaller-sized threads.

Braided polyglycolic acid threads or poliglecaprone sutures (Monocryl type) retain much of their

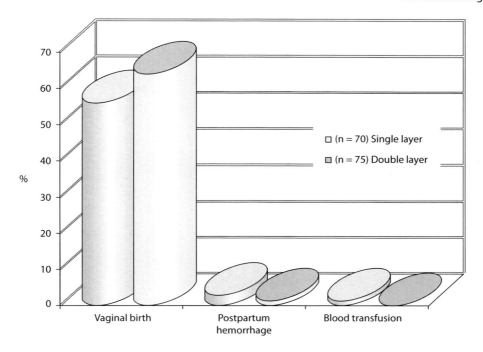

Figure 6.20 Percentage of vaginal births and hemorrhagic complications after a cesarean delivery with closure of the hysterotomy in single or double layer. (From Chapman SJ, Owen J, Hauth JC, *Obstet Gynecol* 1997;89:16–18. With permission.)

Table 6.2 Risk factors for uterine rupture

	Odds ratio	95% CI	*p* value
Single-layer closure	3.95	1.35–11.49	0.012
Interval between births ≤24	2.31	0.97–5.52	0.59
Weight at birth >4000 g	2.10	0.76–5.84	0.154
Use of epidural anesthesia	2.10	0.76–5.84	0.247
Previous vaginal childbirth	0.42	0.05–3.17	0.719

Source: From Bujold E et al., *Am J Obstet Gynecol* 2002;186:1326–30. With permission.

tensile strength for more than a month after surgery. New longer-lasting absorbable sutures (e.g., the new PDS polydioxanone or Maxon polyglyconate filaments) seem to be able to resist for periods up to 3 months. Because these sutures are able to remain in the tissue for a long time, the hysterotomy heals before they are absorbed, with less tissue reaction and consequently a more solid residual scar.

If the surgeon uses synthetic material, care should be taken to not damage the outer surface of the thread with forceps, needles, or loops, so that its resistance is not altered. In fact, special attention must be paid in continuous sutures, especially when hemostasis is performed with an electric scalpel, to not alter suture thread continuity, which could compromise the integrity of the suture. The synthetic threads must also be knotted several times, in general with a surgical knot followed by three successive knots.

After completion of the uterine suture the visceral peritoneum, whether it is sutured or not, should be inspected to verify hemostasis: in the presence of bleeding areas it is recommended to add one or more suture stitches for hemostatic purposes. Generally, these additional stitches are interrupted, single or double, and are placed transversely to the vessel in need of hemostasis. These stitches are particularly important in case of repeated cesarean delivery. In this case the thinness of the uterine breach needs needles and suture threads that are small in order to prevent tearing of the tissue in the suture (Figure 6.21).

The visceral peritoneum is left open but, at times, can be closed using a continuous suture (Figure 6.22) with a 3-0 absorbable monofilament (PDS or Maxon) that includes the uterine fascia in the peritoneal suture. Some surgeons include in a single layer the uterine muscle and the visceral peritoneum, in the single layer as well as in the double layer (Figure 6.23). There is no evidence on whether this suture is beneficial in terms of reduction of infections, morbidity, request for analgesia, or recovery of intestinal functionality [29–31]. The effect on the formation of adhesions is unclear, and conflicting data have been reported [29,32]. Another important aspect is the possible effects suturing the visceral peritoneum has on the quality of the uterine suture and therefore on its healing, so that the scarring area of the lower uterine segment in the event of a VBAC delivery can properly heal [33].

Once this phase of the intervention is completed and hemostasis is achieved, the adnexa are inspected and

Table 6.3 Summary of the most used suture materials in hysterorrhaphy during a cesarean delivery

			Suture threads used in a cesarean delivery			
Name	**Origin**	**Biology**	**Chemical structure**	**Morphology**	**Loss of tensile strength**	**Complete absorption**
Catgut	Natural	Absorbable	Protein	Twisted multifilament	8 days	30 days
Chromic catgut	Natural	Absorbable	Protein	Twisted multifilament	18 days	30 days
Vicryl	Synthetic	Absorbable	Glycolic or lactic acid (polyglactin)	Braided multifilament	20 days	90 days
Prolene	Synthetic	Not absorbable	Polypropylene	Monofilament	—	—
Dexon, Sorbifil	Synthetic	Absorbable	Polyglycolic acid	Braided multifilament	14 days	90–119 days
Monocryl	Synthetic	Absorbable	Poliglecaprone	Monofilament	14 days	90 days
PDS	Synthetic	Absorbable	Polydioxanone	Monofilament	40 days	180 days
Maxon	Synthetic	Absorbable	Polyglyconate	Monofilament	40 days	240 days
Nylon, Nyfil	Synthetic	Not Absorbable	Polyhexamethylene-adipamide	Braided multifilament	—	—

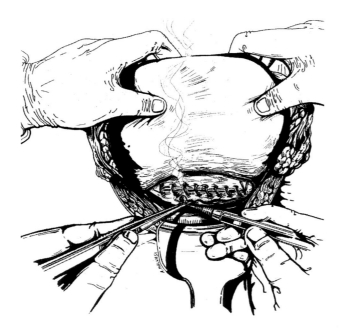

Figure 6.21 Electrocoagulation control of hemostasis by electric scalpel in the area of the simple continuous uterine suture.

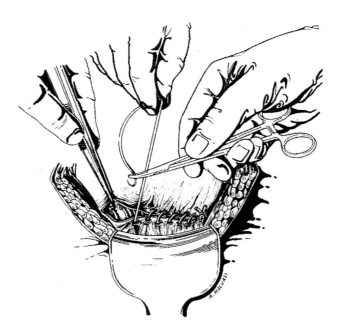

Figure 6.22 Simple continuous suture starting from the top by the assistant surgeon of the visceral peritoneum.

blood and amniotic fluid are removed from the abdominal cavity with a vacuum or with damp swabs. Irrigation for cleansing purposes of the abdominal cavity with physiological solution does not reduce maternal morbidity more than antibiotic prophylaxis [34].

At the end of the intervention, before proceeding to systematically close the abdominal wall, the laparotomy gauze and the surgical instruments in the operating field must be carefully counted.

If the uterus has been exteriorized, care must be taken when repositioning it in the abdominal cavity, being careful to avoid damaging the uterine–ovarian venous plexuses against the abdominal walls (Figure 6.24).

CONCLUSIONS

Uterine sutures have undergone several changes over the years with respect to the suture material and to the type of uterine incisions performed.

A hysterorrhaphy in the course of a cesarean delivery can be performed in double or single layer, even though the scientific literature leans toward a simple continuous suture in single layer [35,36], which has also been tested in experimental studies on animal models [37,38].

Some authors maintain the equivalence of the single- and double-layer techniques [38]. Others advocate the use of the double layer, especially when the pregnant women must be subjected to VBAC delivery, in order to reduce the risk of uterine rupture [39].

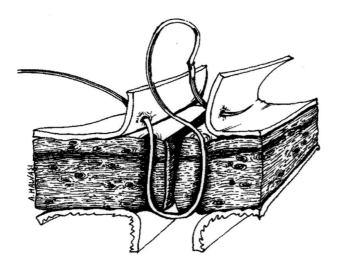

Figure 6.23 Suture of the myometrium and, simultaneously, of the visceral peritoneum "mass closure cesarean delivery technique" in cross-delivery.

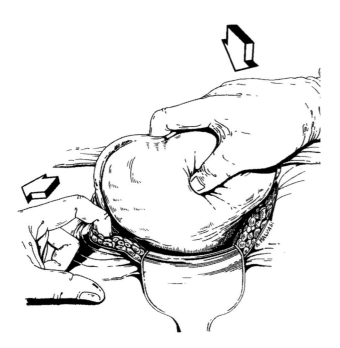

Figure 6.24 Repositioning the exteriorized uterus in the abdominal cavity, while paying attention to the uterine–ovarian plexus (the hand on the left laterally widens the laparotomy breach in order to introduce the adnexum and the uterine–ovarian plexus).

An important aspect concerns sutures performed with continuous rather than interrupted stitches, in which generally benefits are reported for the first technique [40].

A hysterorrhaphy can also be performed with particular materials, such as staples or clips, although the literature does not report any difference in perinatal morbidity with the use of devices or sutures [41–43].

A comparison between autosutures and traditional sutures does not show differences in intraoperative blood loss but does show an increase in surgical time [44].

A subject that remains open to debate (but which most authors are in favor of) is the nonsuturing of the visceral peritoneum. This is done to prevent the formation of a surgical pocket in which hematic residues, edema clots, and, at times, puruloid material can gather, which can then cause puerperal complications [45–49].

On the contrary, during a repeated cesarean delivery, in the presence of an adherent vesicouterine fold and a thin lower uterine segment, a direct incision of the lower uterine segment, without detaching the peritoneum, followed by a suturing of the visceral peritoneum together with the myometrium is advantageous [50,51] This technique is called MCM (mass closure method) [52], and is a modification of the Misgav Ladach method [53].

REFERENCES

1. Gall P. *Il Taglio Cesareo Addominale. Studio storico-clinico.* Bologna, Italy: Cappelli; 1922:39–41.
2. Mangiagalli L. Le più recenti modificazioni del taglio cesareo. *Ann Ost e Gin* 1912;1883–84.
3. Cazeaux P. *Trattato di Ostetricia Teorico-Pratica. Versione italiana dei Dottori Ernesto Begni e Niccolò Martini.* Firenze: Tipografica sopra le Logge del Grano, Part 4, Chapter VI (Dell'Operazione Cesarea), 1845:796–804.
4. Scanzoni von Lichtenfels FW. *Lehrbuch der Geburtshilfe.* Vienna:L. W. Seidel;1867.
5. Balocchi V. *Ostetricia (per gli studenti Medicina e Chirurgia e gli Esercenti).* IV Edizione, Milano: presso Ernesto Oliva Librajo Editore, 1871:824.
6. Kaiser O. *De Eventu Deliveryis caesareae.* Copenhagen, 1841.
7. Gueniot A. De l'operation cesarienne a Paris e des modifications qu'elle comporte dans son execution. Paris: Delahaye, 1870.
8. Spaeth F. Ein Fall von cervikalem Kaiserschnitt. *Zentrlbl. f. Gyn* 1908;20.
9. Truzzi. L'operazione cesarea Porro. Nel *XXV Anniversario, Volume Giubilare, Officina Poligrafica Romana.* Roma, Italy;1901.
10. Sanger M. *Der Kaiserschnitt bei Uterusfibromen nebst vergleichender Methodik.* Leipzig, Germany: Engelmann;1882.
11. Hem E, Bordhal PE. Max Sanger—Father of the modern caesarean delivery. *Gynecol Obstet Invest* 2003;55:127–9.
12. Bumm E. *Trattato Completo di Ostetricia.* IV Edizione italiana sulla 13 tedesca a cura del Prof. Cesare Merletti. Milano, Italy: Società Editrice Libraria; 1924; II: 514–6.
13. Proust R, Charrier J. *Chirurgie de l'Appareil Genital de la Femme.* 5th ed. Paris, France: Masson et Cie; 1922:291–6.

14. Stoeckel W. Il Taglio Cesareo. In: Bertone G, ed. *Trattato di Ostetricia*. Milano, Italy: Unione Tipografico-Editrice Torinese (UTET); 1925:963–71.
15. De Lee JB, Greenhill JP. Metodi di parto—Taglio Cesareo. In: Vitulano D, ed. *Principi e Pratica dell'Ostetricia*. Milano-Messina, Italy: Casa Editrice Giuseppe Principato; 1954:872–907.
16. Martius H., Martius G. Parto Cesareo Addominale. In: *Operazioni Ostetriche. Traduzione dalla X edizione tedesca a cura del Prof. Giuseppe Vecchietti*. Rome, Italy: SEU; 1971:144–56.
17. Wilkinson C, Enkin MW. Uterine exteriorization versus intraperitoneal repair at caesarean section. *Cochrane Database Syst Rev* 2000;CD000085.
18. Jacobs-Jokhan D, Hofmeyr GJ. Extra-abdominal versus intra-abdominal repair of the uterine incision at caesarean section (Review). *Cochrane Database Syst Rev* 2004;(4):CD000085.
19. Stark M, Chavkin Y, Kupferzstain C, Guedj P, Finkel AR. Evaluation of combination of procedures in caesarean delivery. *Int J Gynecol* 1995;48:273–6.
20. Hauth JC, Owen J, Davis RO. Transverse uterine incision closure: One versus two layers. *Am J Obstet Gynecol* 1992;167:1108–11.
21. Tucker JM, Hauth JC, Hodgkins P, Owen J, Winkler CL. Trial of labor after a one- or two-layer closure of a low transverse uterine incision. *Am J Obstet Gynecol* 1993;168:545–6.
22. Jelsema RD, Wittingen JA, Vander Kolk KJ. Continuous, nonlocking, single-layer repair of the low transverse uterine incision. *J Reprod Med* 1193;38:393–6.
23. Chapman SJ, Owen J, Hauth JC. One versus two-layer closure of a low transverse cesarean: The next pregnancy. *Obstet Gynecol* 1997;89:16–18.
24. Enkin MW, Wilkinson C. Single versus two layer suturing for closing the uterine incision at caesarean section. *Cochrane Database Syst Rev* 2004;(2):CD000192.
25. Enkin MW, Wilkinson CS. Withdrawn: Single versus two layer suturing for closing the uterine incision at Caesarean delivery. Cochrane *Database Syst Rev* 2008;16(3):CD000192.
26. Ferrari AG, Frigerio LG, Candotti G, Buscaglia M, Petrone M, Taglioretti A, Calori G. Can Joel-Cohen incision and single layer reconstruction reduce cesarean delivery morbidity? *Int J Gynaecol Obstet* 2001;72:135–43.
27. Bujold E, Bujold C, Hamilton EF, Harel F, Gauthier RJ. The impact of a single layer or double layer closure on uterine rupture. *Am J Obstet Gynecol* 2002;186:1326–30.
28. Durnwald C, Mercer B. Uterine rupture, perioperative and perinatal morbidity after single-layer and double-layer closure at cesarean delivery. *Am J Obstet Gynecol* 2003;189:925–9.
29. Bamigboye AA, Hofmeyr GJ. Closure versus non closure of the peritoneum at cesarean delivery. *Cochrane Database Syst Rev* 2003;CD000163.
30. Cheong YC, Bajekal N, Li TC. Peritoneal closure. To close or not to close. *Hum Reprod* 2001;16:1548.
31. Bamigboye AA, Hofmeyr GJ. Non-closure of peritoneal surfaces at caesarean delivery—A systematic review. *S Afr Med J* 2005;95(2):123–6.
32. Lyell D, Caughey A, Hu E, Daniels K. Peritoneal closure at primary cesarean delivery decreases adhesion formation. *Am J Obstet Gynecol* 2004;189:S61.
33. Koutsougeras G, Karamanidis D, Chimonis G, Gottas N, Polydorou A, Elmaziz Ch, Chatzidis B. Evaluation during early puerperium of the low transverse incision after cesaran delivery through vaginal ultrasonography. *Clin Exp Obstet Gynecol* 2003;30(40):245–7.
34. Harrigill KM, Miller HS, Haynes DE. The effect of intra-abdominal irrigation at cesarean delivery on maternal morbidity: A randomized trial. *Obstet Gynecol* 2003;101:80.
35. Dodd JM, Anderson ER, Gates S. Surgical techniques for uterine incision and uterine closure at the time of caesarean delivery. *Cochrane Database Syst Rev* 2008;16(3):CD004732.
36. CAESAR study collaborative group. Caesarean delivery surgical techniques: A randomised factorial trial (CAESAR). *BJOG* 2010;117(11):1366–76.
37. Gül A, Simşek Y, Uğraş S, Gül T. Transverse uterine incision non-closure versus closure: An experimental study in sheep. *Acta Obstet Gynecol Scand* 2000;79(10):813–7.
38. Gül A, Kotan C, Uğraş S, Alan M, Gül T. Transverse uterine incision non-closure versus closure: An experimental study in dogs. *Eur J Obstet Gynecol Reprod Biol* 2000;88(1):95–9.
39. Bujold E, Goyet M, Marcoux S et al. The role of uterine closure in the risk of uterine rupture. *Obstet Gynecol* 2010;116(1):43–50.
40. Walsh CA. Evidence-based cesarean technique. *Curr Opin Obstet Gynecol* 2010;22(2):110–5.
41. Enkin MW, Wilkinson C. Single versus two layer suturing for closing the uterine incision at Caesarean delivery. *Cochrane Database Syst Rev* 2007;18(3):CD000192.
42. Hohlagschwandtner M, Chalubinski K, Nather A, Husslein P, Joura EA. Continuous vs interrupted sutures for single-layer closure of uterine incision at cesarean delivery. *Arch Gynecol Obstet* 2003;268(1):26–28.
43. Wilkinson C, Enkin MW. Absorbable staples for uterine incision at caesarean delivery. *Cochrane Database Syst Rev* 2007;18(3):CD000005.
44. Dodd JM, Anderson ER, Gates S. Surgical techniques for uterine incision and uterine closure at the time of caesarean delivery. *Cochrane Database Syst Rev* 2008;16(3):CD004732.
45. Malvasi A, Tinelli A, Tinelli R, Rahimi S, Resta L, Tinelli FG. The post-cesarean delivery symptomatic bladder flap hematoma: A modern reappraisal. *J Matern Fetal Neonatal Med* 2007;20:709–14.

46. Malvasi A., Tinelli A, Stark M. Il taglio cesareo:confronto tra tecniche chirurgiche. In: Di Renzo, GC, ed. *Trattato di Ginecologia e Ostetricia*. Rome, Italy: Verduci Editore; 2009:1453–1475.
47. Malvasi A, Tinelli A, Hudelist G, Vergara D, Martignago R, Tinelli R. Closure versus non-closure of the visceral peritoneum (VP) in patients with gestational hypertension—An observational analysis. *Hypertens Pregnancy* 2009;28:290–9.
48. Malvasi A, Tinelli A, Farine D, Rahimi S, Cavallotti C, Vergara D, Martignago R, Stark M. Effects of visceral peritoneal closure on scar formation at cesarean delivery. *Int J Gynaecol Obstet* 2009;105:131–5.
49. Malvasi A, Tinelli A, Tinelli R, Cavallotti C, Farine D. The diagnosis and management of post-cesarean delivery hemorrhagic shock. *J Matern Fetal Neonatal Med* 2008;21:487–91.
50. Malvasi A, Tinelli A, Pacella E. Mass closure of visceral peritoneum at cesarean delivery. A proposal method. *J Matern Fetal Neonatal Med* 2010;23:345–6.
51. Babu K, Magon N. Uterine closure in caesarean delivery: A new technique. *N Am Med Sci* 2012;4(8):358–61.
52. Malvasi A, Farine D, Stark M, Cavallotti C, Tinelli A. Adesions and one layer suture in cesarean delivery. *J Matern Fetal Neonatal Med* 2010;23(Suppl 1):48.
53. Malvasi A, Tinelli A, Stark M. Stark or Misgav Ladah cesarean delivery. In: Eyal Sheiner, ed. *Cesarean Delivery: Procedures, Complications and Recovery. Part. II. Procedures.* New York, NY: Nova Science; 2012:Chapter 7.

FURTHER READING

Madsen K, Grønbeck L, Rifbjerg Larsen C, Østergaard J, Bergholt T, Langhoff-Roos J, Sørensen JL. Educational strategies in performing cesarean delivery. *Acta Obstet Gynecol Scand* 2013;92(3):256–63.

Tulandi T, Al-Jaurodi D. Non closure of peritoneum: A reappraisal. *Am J Obstet Gynecol* 2003;189:609.

Optimal cesarean delivery of the twenty-first century

MICHAEL STARK

INTRODUCTION

Many surgeons tend to adhere to traditions. Most of them will follow methods taught to them by their teachers, who learned them from their own teachers.

The first successful cesarean delivery as described in the modern era was performed by Ferdinand Kehrer on September 25, 1881, in Meckelsheim, Germany [1]. He performed the operation in the house of the patient, while the abdomen was illuminated by an oil lamp. He used a midline incision, and in the following years, along with the development of anesthesia, hygiene, and sterility, many surgeons followed a similar technique until 1897, when Johannes Pfannenstiel introduced the transverse incision as an alternative [2].

For many years both the transverse and the longitudinal incisions were used for cesarean deliveries, and as each department adhered to its own traditions, no comparative studies were published until 1971, when Mowat and Bonnar showed that there is significantly less wound dehiscence when a transverse incision is performed [3].

Similar to the abdominal incision, many other steps in cesarean delivery are also the outcome of local traditions, and very few of these steps have been examined by comparative studies.

Cesarean delivery seems to be a unique operation not just because of its role in obstetrics but also because, while endoscopic alternatives exist for most of the other abdominal operations, it seems that except for very few conditions—like emergencies—the cesarean delivery will be the only indicated laparotomy remaining in the future. Therefore, it is very important that each step used in cesarean delivery is examined for its necessity, and if it is found essential, the optimal way of performing this step should be defined.

When in 1983 I became the Medical Director and Head of Obstetrics and Gynecology of the Misgav Ladach General Hospital in Jerusalem I noticed that cesarean deliveries were performed by different obstetricians, all of them experienced surgeons, in different ways. Each one used different steps and instruments, and even the positioning of the patient was different. As I already used to evaluate other operations for their way of performance, I decided to analyze the cesarean delivery together with the culture around it by examining every step for its necessity and for its optimal way of performance. This was a process that was carried out not without resistance as many of the emerged ideas happened to be in contradiction to the existing local traditions. However, when the process was completed and the results of the first studies were introduced at the International Federation of Gynecology and Obstetrics (FIGO) conference in Montreal in 1994 [4], the method was taken as an example for a structured operation by the Mother and Child Unit of the University of Uppsala in Sweden, and they distributed the way it was described in more than 100 countries through written information, workshops, and videos.

The distribution of information by a well-known university hospital was probably meant as a provocative act, and it gave many obstetricians all over the world the opportunity to initiate comparative studies. However, all these studies showed the benefits of this method over traditional methods, although different studies showed different benefits for reasons that will be explained later.

PLACING THE PARTURIENT

These days, it is usual to encourage the partner of the parturient to accompany her during birth and also during cesarean delivery. The cesarean delivery should be perceived by the partner as nontraumatic as possible. For many years I made it a habit to have a playback of classical music inside the operation room and to reduce the noise of the monitors to the necessary minimum. I found this habit to create a relaxed atmosphere for the family and also for the medical staff, which sometimes works under pressure. As we seek to promote a healthy bonding between mother and baby, it is advised to leave one hand of the mother free, so she will be able to touch or hold the baby after the delivery and even during the closure of the abdomen, given there is no medical reason to treat the baby.

A Trendelenburg position is helpful because the intestines do not enter the operation field and the access to the lower segment of the uterus is easier, but it should not be too steep as it can become uncomfortable to the mother. The legs of the parturient should be parallel to each other; if they are extended, the suturing of the fascia becomes difficult. It is advised to remove the curtain between the mother's head and the abdominal wall [5]. Thus, she can see the baby while it is born. It is impossible for her to see the inside of the abdomen anyhow. The department of obstetrics at the Charité university hospital in Berlin has started using this method with a lot of enthusiasm on the side of the parturients. However, this has generated much criticism, again probably to prevailing traditions.

The surgeon should relate to the mother during the surgery, and reassure her in order to help her keep her confidence. Unless there is a clinical indication, the baby should be left in the operation room with the mother and be taken with her when she leaves. It is advised that the examination by the pediatrician be carried out in the presence of the parents.

ANESTHESIA

In the past, most cesarean deliveries were carried out under general anesthesia. Today general anesthesia is still used in case of an emergency. However, the state of the art these days is to perform cesarean deliveries under epidural or spinal anesthesia or a combination of both (Figure 7.1). The use of local anesthesia assists the bonding as the mother is aware of the delivery process. Leaving the epidural catheter for the first hours after the delivery enables top-ups preferably with 2% lidocaine 20 mL plus epinephrine 100 mµg and fentanyl 100 mµg [6] to relieve the postoperative pain. It was found that when using this method, due to its short duration, 2% Mepivacaine is optimal and enough when local anesthesia is given [7].

ABDOMINAL INCISION

The prevailing methods are the longitudinal and transverse incisions. The transverse incision seems superior over the longitudinal one concerning wound dehiscence [3]; however, handling the uterus, abdominal inspection, and delivering the baby seemed to be easier when the longitudinal one was used compared to the Pfannenstiel incision.

The Pfannenstiel incision was challenged by Joel Cohen. He was convinced that the transverse incision is superior over the longitudinal incision when performing abdominal hysterectomy, and even safer. He suggested a different, innovative way for transverse laparotomy.

In 1972, I met Joel Cohen for the first time on the stairs of the second Gynecological Department in Vienna. I already knew who he was, and I plucked up courage and approached him to introduce myself, and so our contact started, which would later, in 1976, lead to me being accepted to work in his department. Originally South African, and an extremely talented surgeon, he had original ideas in any aspect of surgical technique, mainly in oncological surgery. He had his own way to follow the ureter and open the ureteric canal when performing Wertheim operation, which he did with very few instruments using stretched peritoneum sutured to the skin rather than metal retractors. He also had very original and interesting ergonomic ideas using a steep Trendelenburg position and placing the instrument tray over the head of the patient, which enabled the surgeon to pick up the instruments himself.

In the year we met he published his first book *Abdominal and Vaginal Hysterectomy* [8], in which he suggested an innovative and original way of laparotomy by cutting the fascia above the linea arcuata.

At this anatomical level the fascia moves freely over the recti muscles. Before being exposed to Joel Cohen's ideas, I used to open the abdomen using the Pfannenstiel incision. Doing so, I had to bluntly separate the fascia from the muscles. Reading Joel Cohen's book I assumed that opening the fascia above the linea arcuata and stretching the muscles without necessity to separate them from the fascia would be less traumatic than opening the fascia below this line. As it happened before, Joel Cohen's idea to open the abdomen at this level was used by him and his disciples but at that time it was not subjected to any comparative study. We took the challenge, and indeed, we could show that opening the fascia above the linea arcuata reduced febrile morbidity dramatically [9].

The longitudinal structures of the abdomen, like blood vessels and the straight muscles, have a lateral sway, like strings on a musical instrument. One can easily stretch them laterally given it is done far away from their insertion through their tendons to the pubic bone. The innervation is segmental anyhow, and when one estimates the location of the blood vessels, hemostasis can be superfluous. I have been using the modified Joel Cohen incision for over 35 years for nearly every indicated laparotomy and rarely used any kind of hemostasis.

It is important to plan the first incision parallel to the Langer skin lines, which are easy to show up if one stretches the estimated planned lateral incision point to

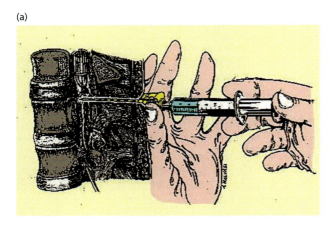

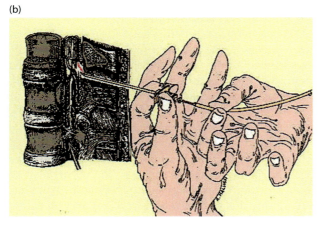

Figure 7.1 (a and b) Combined spinal epidural in cesarean delivery. (From Di Renzo GC. *Trattato di Ginecologia e Ostetricia*. Rome, Italy: Verduci Editore, 2009. With permission.)

Abdominal incision 163

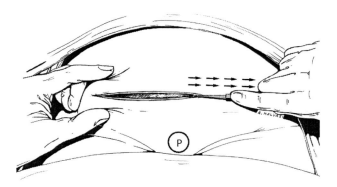

Figure 7.2 Skin incision made in a straight line about 3 cm below an imaginary line between spinae iliacae anterior and superior.

the side, and to mark the site of the planned incision. The first cut is made in a straight line about 3 cm below an imaginary line connecting both spinae iliacae anteriores superiores (Figure 7.2). Here is the place to say that the optimal position for a right-handed surgeon is on the right side of the parturient. It is easier to deliver the head of the baby with your more sensitive hand, avoiding unnecessary extensions and bleedings. When you stand on the right side of the parturient while suturing the uterus after the delivery, the tip of the needle points away from the bladder, which helps avoid injuries. Of course, left-handed surgeons should stand on the parturient's left side.

The first incision should only cut the cutis until the fat tissue becomes visible. There are no major blood vessels in the cutis itself, and the superficial epigastric vessels are embedded in the fat tissue but never in the central line (Figure 7.3). Therefore, the incision of the fat tissue can be

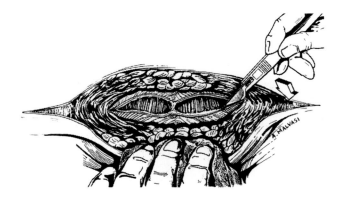

Figure 7.4 Therefore, the incision of the fat tissue can be deepened in the midline without causing any bleeding followed by a small transverse incision to the fascia (5–7 mm) until the underlying muscle becomes visible. (Modified from Malvasi A et al., Rome, Italy: CIC Edizioni Internazionali; 1997.)

deepened in the midline without causing any bleeding followed by a small transverse incision to the fascia (5–7 mm) until the underlying muscle becomes visible (Figure 7.4). Straight blade scissors with round tips are now inserted into the opening, one blade below the fascia and the other above. The scissors' blades are opened 3–4 mm while they are pushed laterally above the muscle and below the blood vessels once to the left and once to the right until the desired opening size of the fascia is achieved (Figure 7.5). Once the fascia is open the surgeon inserts two fingers between the recti muscles and stretches the fascia caudally and cranially (Figure 7.6). This enables the assistant and later the surgeon to insert the index and middle fingers below the recti muscles and stretch the muscles together with the blood vessels as lateral as necessary (Figure 7.7).

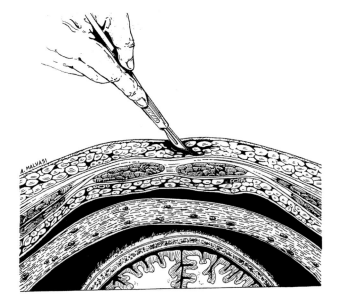

Figure 7.3 Central inclusion of the fat tissues because of superficial epigastric vessels embedded in the fat tissue in the central line.

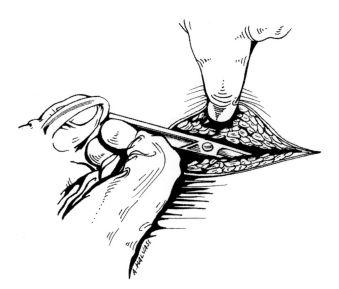

Figure 7.5 The scissors' blades are opened 3–4 mm while they are pushed laterally above the muscle and below the blood vessels once to the left and once to the right until the desired opening size of the fascia is achieved.

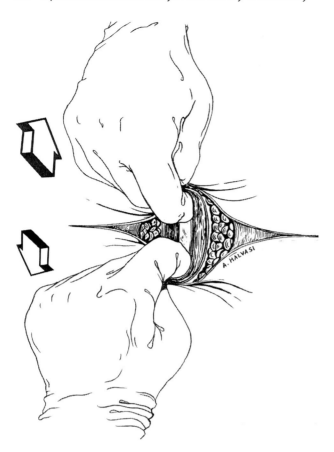

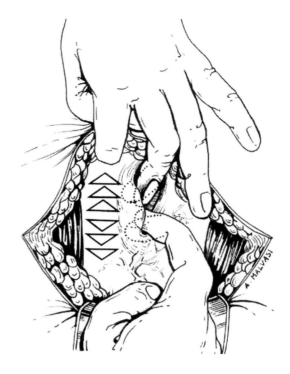

Figure 7.6 Once the fascia is open the surgeon inserts two fingers between the recti muscles and stretches the fascia caudally and cranially.

Many cesarean deliveries are performed as an emergency. When you are in a hurry and using sharp instruments to open the peritoneum, you might unintentionally damage the urine bladder or other underlying structures. Therefore, the more optimal way is to open the peritoneum by gently stretching it repeatedly until a hole appears, and then by stretching the opening up and down, the peritoneum will open transversely [10] (Figure 7.8).

Figure 7.8 Many cesarean deliveries are performed as an emergency. When you are in a hurry and using sharp instruments to open the peritoneum, you might unintentionally damage the urine bladder or other underlying structures. Therefore, the more optimal way is to open the peritoneum by gently stretching it repeatedly until a hole appears, and then by stretching the opening up and down, the peritoneum will open transversely.

For many years, I avoided with very few exceptions the usage of abdominal towels, and not just because they can be forgotten in the cavity. It was shown that the usage of abdominal packs causes adhesions [11].

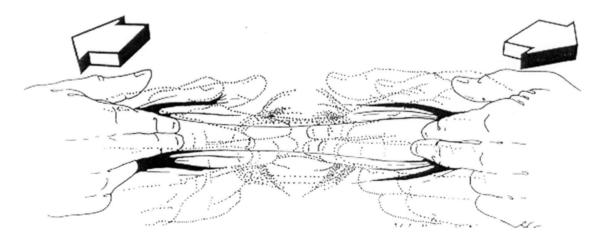

Figure 7.7 This enables the assistant and later the surgeon to insert the index and middle fingers below the recti muscles and stretch the muscles together with the blood vessels as lateral as necessary. (Modified from Malvasi A et al., Rome, Italy: CIC Edizioni Internazionali; 1997.)

Whatever the reasons for postoperative adhesions may be, certainly the abdominal bags play a big role here, even if just for their abrasive effect [12]. The deep Trendelenburg position is not popular among anesthesiologists but usually makes the usage of abdominal packs unnecessary. Blood clots can and should be removed with the surgeon's palm, fluid blood if not contaminated should be left intraperitoneal as it will be absorbed back into the system within a couple of hours as happens in hemodialysis [13].

REPEATED CESAREAN DELIVERY

After any laparotomy the tissue can react with fibrosis and adhesions. The described method is not different in this respect, and although fewer adhesions were reported when leaving the peritoneum open, there are cases where fibrotic tissue might cause difficulties when entering the abdomen, even though adhesions after cesarean deliveries seem to be a unique group, as in a prospective study no correlation was found between the severity of the adhesions and the postoperative clinical symptoms. Adhesions resulting from previous operations usually do not have any clinical significance [14].

In a study the described method was successful in 100%, 80%, and 65.6% of patients with no, one, and multiple previous cesarean deliveries, respectively [15]. In this study no information is given concerning the standardization of this method, and maybe different surgeons used different variations. However, I completely agree that with increased numbers of cesarean deliveries the difficulties might increase, and it is highly suggested that only experienced surgeons should be present in repeated operation.

There is no reason to change the technique in repeated operations. Trying to avoid difficulties by returning to the Pfannenstiel incision will not solve the problem because the fibrosis can be extended all the way to the os pubis.

Due to the fibrosis more traction power is needed to achieve the optimal opening of the abdominal wall.

To achieve it, I recommend doing the traction with four fingers rather than two. The index and middle fingers of the right hand of both the surgeon and the assistant should be placed below the recti muscles. The index and middle fingers of their left hands should be placed over the two fingers of the right hand. Now, traction can be done (Figure 7.9). The reason is that if two hands make the traction side by side, the surgeon tends to separate them from each other while pulling. The blood vessels have a lateral sway, but they do not have length elasticity. You can remove them to the side but traction will tear them. As a result unnecessary bleeding will occur.

THE DELIVERY

In 1924 John Martin Munro Kerr (1868–1960) described the transverse lower incision of the uterus in contrast to the prevailing longitudinal incisions [16].

Histologically, in the upper part of the uterus muscle tissue prevails, whereas in the lower segment fibrous tissue does. Opening the uterus in the lower segment will cause less damage to the uterine wall, and therefore it makes sense to open the plica, push it down, and open the uterus transversely in the lower segment. The plica can be opened using a transverse incision by scalpel above the bladder and pushing the plica down with two fingers (Figure 7.10). It is a good practice to use a nontraumatic hand retractor to facilitate access to the lower segment. The lower segment is opened in the midline first superficially with the scalpel, and usually the anterior wall of the lower segment can be penetrated with pressure of the inserted index finger (Figure 7.11). Now, the thumb of the right hand of the surgeon is inserted into the uterus, pushing to the left, and the left index finger to the right. In the last weeks of a pregnancy the lower segment of the uterus is evolved. The direction of the fibers becomes transverse, and therefore doing extensions using both fingers separates the lower

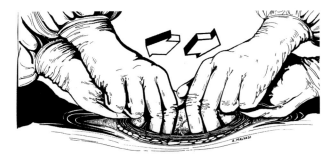

Figure 7.9 To achieve it, I recommend doing the traction with four fingers rather than two. The index and middle fingers of the right hands of both the surgeon and the assistant should be placed below the recti muscles. The index and middle fingers of their left hands should be placed over the two fingers of the right hand. Now, traction can be undertaken.

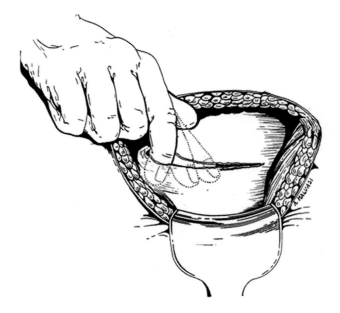

Figure 7.10 The plica can be opened using a transverse incision by scalpel above the bladder and pushing the plica down with two fingers.

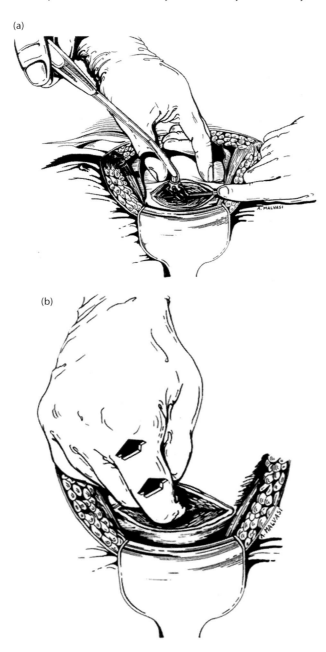

Figure 7.11 (a) The lower segment is opened in the midline first superficially with the scalpel; (b) usually the anterior wall of the lower segment can be penetrated with pressure of the inserted index finger.

segment in a minimally traumatic way, thus causing very little bleeding.

Comparing my own experiences using the Pfannenstiel incision and the modified Joel Cohen incision, I find the delivery of the baby much easier with the latter. Usually it is easy to deliver the baby in a spontaneous delivery with the assistance of the palm of the right hand exerting slight pressure on the fundus. When I was using the Pfannenstiel incision forceps were often needed, and in breech delivery often a further extension of the incision—sometimes with sharp instruments—became necessary. The location of the

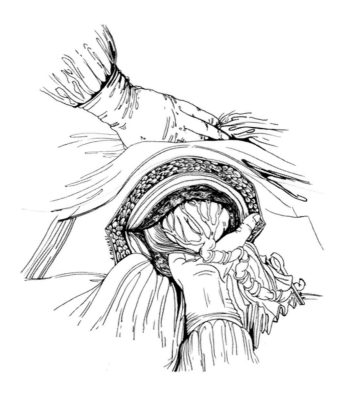

Figure 7.12 Spontaneous assisted delivery of the placenta.

high transverse incision enables a more extended opening due to the free movement of the muscles under the fascia. In other gynecological operations the same incision enables an optimal access to the lateral site of the pelvis as needed for lymphadenectomy, and it is even easier than when using longitudinal incision of the abdomen using retractors.

Except for a Fritsch or a similar retractor no other retractor was ever necessary when using this abdominal incision, also for other indications like oncological operations.

Spontaneous assisted delivery of the placenta is the optimal way. It was shown that manual removal of the placenta increases significantly the blood loss [17] (Figure 7.12).

A towel should only be used if remaining cotyledons or membranes are suspected.

Exteriorization of the uterus enables better vision and the manual contraction of the uterus, facilitates its suturing, and makes the inspection of the ovaries easier. Exteriorization of the uterus involves less bleeding than when sutured inside the abdomen [18] (Figure 7.13).

Despite occasional intra-operative pain due to inadequacy of the anesthesia, exteriorizing the uterus during CS is considered a valid option [19]. It is important to examine the ovaries before closing the abdomen in order to make sure that ovarian pathologies like dermoid cysts are not left behind.

CLOSURE OF THE UTERUS

Many ways to close the uterus have been described. Traditionally, it has been done with two layers, sometimes

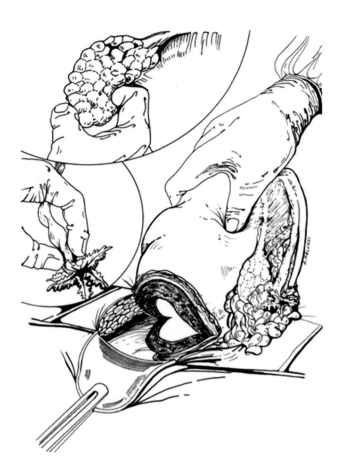

Figure 7.13 Uterine and adnexal examination.

continuously, sometimes with single knots, or with combinations of both. Some are placing hemostatic sutures on the lateral aspects of the opening, all following local traditions.

In 1973 Csúcs recommended for the first time a single-layer closure [20]. When he performed hysterosalpingographies a few weeks after surgery, less sacculations were demonstrated, and therefore it was assumed that the scars would be stronger when using one layer.

Believing it is so, I have used only single-layer closure for many years. My own reasoning is that the uterus contracts immediately after birth, even in the first hours. After 6 weeks the uterus usually returns to its size as it was before the pregnancy. The lower segment contracts together with the uterus. The sutures cannot follow the diminishing in size of the uterus and therefore probably disturb the natural healing. The more sutures are placed, the more foreign-body reaction and therefore theoretically weaker scars will be the result. In order to avoid extra sutures I developed the habit of using huge needles—80 mm in diameter—which enable closure of the uterus with very few stitches and therefore a minimum of suturing material is left behind.

There are studies supporting single-layer suturing that maintain there are stronger scars and less ruptures in the following pregnancies [21], while others claim the opposite [22]. A Cochrane study could not show any disadvantage in using single-layer suturing and confirmed a shorter operation time [23] (Figure 7.14).

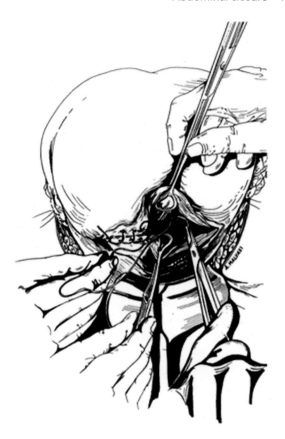

Figure 7.14 Uterine single-layer suture.

After a detailed examination of the articles I am certain that only standardized methods enable comparative studies and not just for cesarean deliveries [24]. Very often we come across meta-analyses that do not include detailed descriptions of the methods used in the different hospitals. Of course, I will again start suturing the uterus with a double layer should a standardized method prove the superiority of double-layer over single-layer suturing.

ABDOMINAL CLOSURE

A similar situation can be found concerning the question of closure versus nonclosure of the peritoneal layers. In 1980 Harold Ellis from the Westminster Hospital in London published his data showing the closure of the peritoneum during laparotomy is not necessary. His reasoning was that, unlike the skin, the peritoneum cannot be sutured end to end, that sutures cause adhesions, and that if the peritoneum is left open a new one will emerge from the coelom cells within days [25].

As I was convinced of these ideas I started leaving the peritoneum open as early as in 1980, and I have done so until today, and in any abdominal operation including laparoscopies. I was able to show that in repeat cesarean deliveries significantly less adhesions were found [26]. A similar discussion emerged in the literature among those who believe that leaving the peritoneum open causes more [27] or less adhesions [28]. My reasoning for continuing leaving the peritoneum open can be found in the literature [24], and again, only standardized methods can be compared to each other. If it is unknown which methods were used, what were the indications for the cesarean delivery, whether or not abdominal packs were used, etc., it is impossible to reach a reasonable conclusion.

Because towels are not used, blood clots can be removed manually. Fluid blood does not have to be suctioned because in short time it will be completely absorbed, as happens with peritoneal dialysis [29].

As both peritoneal layers are left open, the next step is the closure of the fascia (Figure 7.15). It is done with continuous suturing, starting from the surgeon toward his assistant. Thus the surgeon's hand will not cross the hands of the assistant, and the surgeon is responsible for keeping the tension of the suturing material. The first knot should be placed below the fascia, and to do so the needle is inserted first from inside the lower part of the fascia, taking both layers with it, then going from outside the upper part inside, and knotting the suture below the fascia. This will prevent a subcutaneous knot, a focus for reaction and pain. The skin can be closed in various ways, and there is no convincing study comparing intracuticular to single knots, although staples were preferred by women over single knots [30]. The studies relate to the Pfannenstiel incision and not to the modified Joel Cohen incision [31]. Usually, no hemostasis in the abdominal wall is needed. However, once in a while a small collection might occur. Therefore it is important to enable spontaneous drainage in the first hours after the operation. If just a few stitches are placed, it is more likely that no seromas or hematomas collect under the skin due to the possibility for free drainage between the stitches. The more experienced the surgeon is, the less stitches are needed. The optimal way is placing one stitch in the middle and two laterally. With experience one learns where to put the lateral ones in order to get a good adaptation. It is recommended to use the largest skin needle and to go through the subcutis in order to avoid free open spaces.

Most mothers experience pain at the suture level in the days after surgery. The reason is that the skin reacts to the trauma by swelling. The suture material is nonelastic, and therefore the skin is pinched. After 48 hours the lateral stitches can be removed, which is followed by immediate pain relief. Some surgeons find it helpful to place Heaney clamps between the stitches for 5 minutes in order to receive a good adaptation. Once in a while, due to specific circumstances or the surgeon's lack of experience more stitches are needed. Even in these cases the lateral stitches can and should be removed after 48 hours.

AFTER THE OPERATION

Recovery after surgery is individual. Early mobilization is of advantage mainly in overweight women [32]. The main reason for the possibility for early mobilization as compared to the Pfannenstiel method is the nontraumatic separation of the fascia from the recti muscles, as was shown also by the significantly lower febrile morbidity rate as documented in one of our first studies [33]. It is not unusual that mothers undergoing this method a couple of hours after surgery can move freely, bend down, and look after their babies, which makes this operation as similar as possible to a normal birth. As no towels are used and due to the size of the uterus there is nearly no exposure of the intestines, there is no reason for abstinence of fluids after surgery, and the mother can drink freely as long as she was operated on with epidural anesthesia or when she is

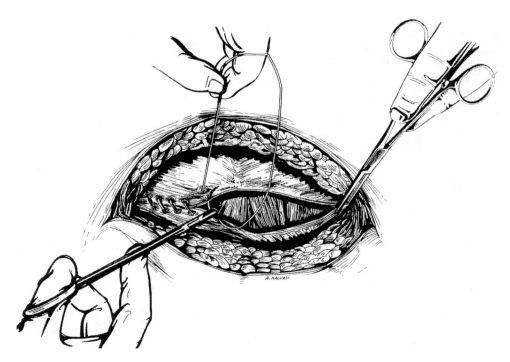

Figure 7.15 Continuous suture of the fascia.

completely awake after general anesthesia [34,35]. A birth is a happy family event, and therefore, if the physical conditions allow it, the partner and the baby should stay in the same room with the mother.

SCIENTIFIC EVALUATION OF THE DESCRIBED METHOD

This method was presented for the first time during the FIGO conference in Montreal, Canada, in 1994 [36]. It was scientifically evaluated again in the University Hospital of Uppsala, Sweden, which showed significant benefits over traditional methods [37]. As mentioned before, the mother and child unit of the University of Uppsala distributed films and written descriptions to more than 100 countries. The acceptance was overwhelming, and soon peer-reviewed publications appeared. Only standardized surgical methods give us the opportunity to compare outcomes of operations carried out in different hospitals and by different surgeons. This is true in all departments as well as in meta-analyses [24]. This explains why in the evaluation of this method very often different outcomes are documented. Generally, all the publications until now have shown benefits over any kind of traditional cesarean deliveries. There is one publication reporting eventuation after the operation [38]. However, as far as we know eventuation happens after any kind of laparotomy, but they are not usually reported in the literature. Probably because of the differences and variations it is interesting to see that while all publications report benefits over traditional methods, each publication highlights other benefits. Examples are benefits concerning costs [39], the need for pain killers [40], the duration of the operation [41], the time until the beginning of mobilization [42], and the amount of blood loss [43]. It seems that not only the described method but also the method used for control groups vary due to local differences. Therefore, it will be necessary to conduct future comparative studies using standardized surgical methods for both our described method and the control groups.

This method is now in use in many countries around the globe. The reasons are not just the improved outcome, early mobilization, and early hydration, but also the fact that only 10 instruments and usually only three stitching materials are necessary. This is important everywhere but definitely in countries with limited resources. Our group conducted surgical courses in countries like Burkina Faso and Senegal, and we could see the immediate and enthusiastic application. The principles of minimalism work for any surgery, as for example, the vaginal hysterectomy [44].

THE DANGERS OF OVERUSED CESAREAN DELIVERIES

In the last decade there has been a tendency all over the world to increase the rate of cesarean deliveries. It rose from 2.1% in 1931 in Germany [45] to more than 30% in the United States [46].

There are many reasons for this dramatic increase: The fear of court cases, the misinterpretation of the monitoring or missing knowledge of the physiological birth, the acceptance of cesarean delivery on demand through scientific publications [47], and certainly also the availability of easier and modified surgical methods like the one described here.

Homo sapiens is the only species that developed methods to assist the physiological birth process. We know that more than 4000 years ago midwifery was a recognized profession. The main reason for the need of birth assistance is the relatively big size of the human head compared to the pelvic size [48]. This similarity of diameters is due to the bipedalism of the *Homo sapiens*, which results in a narrow pelvis and the evolution of a big brain.

In the past, in case of disproportion between the size of the head and the pelvis, the result was the death of both mother and baby. Evolution arranged delivery that is conducted and initiated by the newborn itself [49] in such a way that vaginal birth is possible. However, as a result human babies are dependent. In comparison to most mammals, which very shortly after birth are able to find themselves the mother's nipples and are able to walk instantly, the human baby needs months and years until independency. In these days, where a dramatic rise in the rate of cesarean deliveries is occurring, the question arises: What will be the future of generations born by cesarean delivery [50]?

When the size of the head and pelvis are no longer a limiting factor, the normal evolution of our species concerning the timing of a physiological birth might change. The genetic message will get lost, and it is not improbable that in the future, physiological characteristics of *Homo sapiens* might change. The changes happen much faster than we believe. The average height of adults has increased [51]. This could be due to nutrition and environmental as well as other factors. Blue eyes and lactose tolerance are features of the human species that did not exist 10,000 years ago [52]. If the size of the head or the diameter of the pelvis, due to repeated cesarean deliveries along the generations, will not be an evolutionary factor, there will not be any reason for restricted pregnancy time. It is possible that the longevity of the placenta will change. Longer pregnancies will become possible and as a result babies will be born more mature.

Even the shape of the head might change. The shape of the head is a result of the need during labor. The relatively long neck enables the movements and rotation during the passage through the different levels of the pelvis. The narrow pelvis serves as the optimal bipedal gate of our species. The female pelvis is wider than the male pelvis because it also functions as the birth channel. If this function is no longer used, the female pelvis might become narrow over the generations. It is not improbable that the shape of the neck will change as well. The shape of the baby's neck enables the rotations in the birth channel which are followed by the shoulders. The result of generations born by cesarean delivery might be therefore longer pregnancies, a larger head, a shorter neck, and a narrow pelvis.

I strongly support the idea that any intervention should be based on a correct indication. In order to prevent an excessive use of cesarean deliveries I worked with a system in the hospital that prescribed that every cesarean delivery should be reported to the senior gynecologist, who was able to contact his senior, present the case, and get permission to perform the operation. With this system only the indicated cesarean deliveries were performed. There is no justification for any operation, even if its method is optimal, if the indication was not correct.

REFERENCES

1. Lurie S, Glezerman M. The history of cesarean technique. *Am J Obstet Gynecol* 2003;189(6):1803–6.
2. Pfannenstiel J. Über die Vorteile des suprasymphysären Faszienquerschnitts für die gynäkologische Koliotomien, zugleich ein Beitrag zu der Indikationsstellung der Operationswege. *Samml Klin Vortr Gynäkol* 1897;68–98 (*Klin Vortr NF Gynäk* 1900; 97:268).
3. Mowat J, Bonnar J. Abdominal wound dehiscence after caesarean section. *Br Med J* 1971;2(5756):256–7.
4. Stark M. Technique of caesarean section: Misgav Ladach method. In: Popkin DR, Peddle IJ, eds. *Women's Health Today. Perspectives on Current Research and Clinical Practice. Proceedings of the XIV World Congress of Gynecology and Obstetrics, Montreal.* New York, NY: Parthenon; 1994:81–5.
5. Smith J, Plaat F, Fisk NM. The natural caesarean: A woman-centred technique. *BJOG* 2008;115(8):1037–42.
6. Balaji P, Dhillon P, Russell IF. Low-dose epidural top up for emergency caesarean delivery: A randomised comparison of levobupivacaine versus lidocaine/epinephrine/fentanyl. *Int J Obstet Anesth* 2009;18(4):335–41.
7. Meininger D, Byhahn C, Kessler P et al. Intrathecal fentanyl, sufentanil, or placebo combined with hyperbaric mepivacaine 2% for parturients undergoing elective cesarean delivery. *Anesth Analg* 2003;96(3):852–8.
8. Joel Cohen SJ. *Abdominal and Vaginal Hysterectomy. New Techniques Based on Time and Motion Studies.* London, UK: William Heinemann Medical Books; 1972.
9. Stark M, Finkel AR. Comparison between the Joel-Cohen and Pfannenstiel incisions in cesarean delivery. *Eur J Obstet Gynecol Reprod Biol* 1994;53(2):121–2.
10. Stark M. In the era of "non-closure of the peritoneum," how to open it? (Not every simple method is optimal, but every optimal method is simple). *Acta Obstet Gynecol Scand* 2009;88(1):119.
11. Schwemmle K. Causes for adhesions in the abdomen. *Langenbecks Arch Chir Suppl II Verh Dtsch Ges Chir* 1990:1017–21.
12. Down RH, Whitehead R, Watts JM. Why do surgical packs cause peritoneal adhesions? *Aust N Z J Surg* 1980;50(1):83–85.
13. Almeida PB, Pinheiro da Costa BE, Figueiredo AE et al. Erythrocyte L-arginine uptake in peritoneal dialysis patients changes over time. *Adv Perit Dial* 2007;23:48–50.
14. Stark M, Hoyme UB, Stubert B et al. Post-cesarean adhesions—Are they a unique entity? *J Matern Fetal Neonatal Med* 2008;21(8):513–6.
15. Bolze PA, Massoud M, Gaucherand P et al. What about the Misgav-Ladach surgical technique in patients with previous cesarean deliveries? *Am J Perinatol* 2013;30(3):197–200.
16. Dunn PM. Professor Munro Kerr (1868–1960) of Glasgow and caesarean delivery. *Arch Dis Child Fetal Neonatal Ed* 2008;93(2):F167–9.
17. Wilkinson C, Enkin MW. Manual removal of placenta at caesarean section. *Cochrane Database Syst Rev* 2007;3:CD000130.
18. Wahab MA, Karantzis P, Eccersley PS et al. A randomised, controlled study of uterine exteriorisation and repair at caesarean section. *Br J Obstet Gynaecol* 1999;106(9):913–6.
19. Edi-Osagie ECO, Hopkins RE, Ogbo et al. Uterine exteriorisation at caesarean section: Influence on maternal morbidity. *BJOG* 1998;105:1070–8.
20. Csúcs L, Kött I, Solt I. Mono-layer sutures of uterine incision in cesarean delivery based on clinical experience and animal experiments. *Zentralbl Gynakol* 1972;94(34):1121–6.
21. Ghahiry A, Rezaei F, Karimi Khouzani R et al. Comparative analysis of long-term outcomes of Misgav Ladach technique cesarean delivery and traditional cesarean delivery. *J Obstet Gynaecol Res* 2012; 38(10):1235–9.
22. Hudic I, Bujold E, Fatusic Z et al. Risk of uterine rupture following locked vs unlocked single-layer closure. *Med Arh* 2012;66(6):412–4.
23. Enkin MW, Wilkinson C. Single versus two layer suturing for closing the uterine incision at Caesarean section. *Cochrane Database Syst Rev* 2007;3:CD000192.
24. Stark M. Optimised meta-analysis should be based on standardised methods. *BJOG* 2011;118(6):765–6; author reply 766.
25. Ellis H. Internal overhealing: The problem of intraperitoneal adhesions. *World J Surg* 1980; 4(3):303–6.
26. Stark M. Clinical evidence that suturing the peritoneum after laparotomy is unnecessary for healing. *World J Surg* 1993;17(3):419.
27. Shi Z, Ma L, Yang Y et al. Adhesion formation after previous caesarean section—A meta-analysis and systematic review. *BJOG* 2011;118(4):410–22.
28. Nabhan AF. Long-term outcomes of two different surgical techniques for cesarean. *Int J Gynaecol Obstet* 2008;100(1):69–75.
29. Kang GW, Jang MH, Hwang EA et al. Comparison of peritoneal dialysis and hemodialysis after kidney transplant failure. *Transplant Proc* 2013; 45(8):2946–8.
30. Aabakke AJ, Krebs L, Pipper CB et al. Subcuticular suture compared with staples for skin closure after cesarean delivery: A randomized controlled trial. *Obstet Gynecol* 2013;122(4):878–84.

31. Feese CA, Johnson S, Jones E et al. A randomized trial comparing metallic and absorbable staples for closure of a Pfannenstiel incision for cesarean delivery. *Am J Obstet Gynecol* 2013;209(6):556.e1–556.e5.
32. Loubert C, Fernando R. Cesarean delivery in the obese parturient: Anesthetic considerations. *Womens Health (Lond Engl)* 2011;7(2):163–79.
33. Stark M, Chavkin Y, Kupfersztain C et al. Evaluation of combinations of procedures in cesarean delivery. *Int J Gynaecol Obstet* 1995;48(3):273–6.
34. Mulayim B, Celik NY, Kaya S et al. Early oral hydration after cesarean delivery performed under regional anesthesia. *Int J Gynaecol Obstet* 2008;101(3):273–6.
35. Guedj P, Eldor J, Stark M. Immediate postoperative oral hydration after caesarean section. *Asia Oceania J Obstet Gynaecol* 1991;17(2):125–9.
36. Stark M. Technique of caesarean section: Misgav Ladach method. In: Popkin DR, Peddle IJ, eds. *Women's Health Today. Perspectives on Current Research and Clinical Practice. Proceedings of the XIV World Congress of Gynecology and Obstetrics, Montreal.* New York, NY: Parthenon; 1994:81–85.
37. Darj E, Nordström ML. The Misgav Ladach method for cesarean delivery compared to the Pfannenstiel method. *Acta Obstet Gynecol Scand* 1999;78(1):37–41.
38. Fournié A, Madzou S, Sentilhes L et al. Two observations of evisceration after caesarean section performed according the so-called Stark procedure. *Gynecol Obstet Fertil* 2008;36(12):1211–3.
39. Moreira P, Moreau JC, Faye ME et al. Comparison of two cesarean techniques: Classic versus Misgav Ladach cesarean. *J Gynecol Obstet Biol Reprod (Paris)* 2002;31(6):572–6.
40. Fatušić Z, Hudić I, Sinanović O et al. Short-term postnatal quality of life in women with previous Misgav Ladach caesarean section compared to Pfannenstiel-Dorffler caesarean section method. *J Matern Fetal Neonatal Med* 2011;24(9):1138–42.
41. Naki MM, Api O, Celik H et al. Comparative study of Misgav-Ladach and Pfannenstiel-Kerr cesarean techniques: A randomized controlled trial. *J Matern Fetal Neonatal Med* 2011;24(2):239–44.
42. Belci D, Kos M, Zoricić D et al. Comparative study of the "Misgav Ladach" and traditional Pfannenstiel surgical techniques for cesarean delivery. *Minerva Ginecol* 2007;59(3):231–40.
43. Hofmeyr JG, Novikova N, Mathai M et al. Techniques for cesarean delivery. *Am J Obstet Gynecol* 2009;201(5):431–44.
44. Stark M, Gerli S, Di Renzo GC. The importance of analyzing and standardizing surgical methods. *J Minim Invasive Gynecol* 2009;16(2):122–5.
45. Stark L. Auswertung von 1000 Anstaltsgeburten. *Monatsschrift für Geburtshilfe und Gynäkologie* 1931:LXXXIX. Heft 3.
46. Osterman MJ, Martin JA. Changes in cesarean delivery rates by gestational age: United States, 1996–2011. *NCHS Data Brief* 2013;124:1–8.
47. Schindl M, Birner P, Reingrabner M et al. Elective cesarean delivery vs. spontaneous delivery: A comparative study of birth experience. *Acta Obstet Gynecol Scand* 2003;82(9):834–40.
48. Fathalla MF. How evolution of the human brain shaped women's sexual and reproductive health. *Reproductive Biology Insights* 2013;6:11–18.
49. Marton IS. Foetal adrenal steroids—Initiation of human parturition. *Acta Physiol Hung* 1988;71(4):557–9.
50. Odent M. Wie steht es um die Zukunft einer durch Kaiserschnitt entbundenen Zivilisation. In: Stark M, ed. *Der Kaiserschnitt S.* Munich, Germany: Elsevier; 2009:396–411.
51. Wurm H. History of the determination body height from skeletal findings (body height determination for men). The proposed methods of body height determination from skeletal findings since the middle of the 20th century. *Gegenbaurs Morphol Jahrb* 1985;131(3):383–432.
52. Cochran G, Harpending H. *The 10,000 year explosion. How civilization accelerated human evolution.* New York, NY: Basic Books, 2009.

Fibroids and myomectomy in cesarean delivery

ANDREA TINELLI and ANTONIO MALVASI

INTRODUCTION

Uterine fibroids or myomas are the most common pelvic tumors in women. The occurrence of these tumors in the reproductive age group is 25%–40% [1].

Uterine myomas are observed more frequently in pregnancy with an estimated incidence of 2%–4%, because many women are delaying childbearing to their late thirties or early forties, the time of greatest risk for myoma growth [2]. Uterine myomas are commonly encountered in women older than 30 years [1,2], and their growth is related to exposure to circulating estrogens levels. The prevalence of leiomyomas among pregnant women ranges from 0.1% to 3.9% [3–7]. The effective rate of uterine myomas in pregnancy is unknown; however, they are associated with numerous pregnancy-related maternal and fetal complications, including spontaneous abortion, preterm labor, placental abruption, postpartum hemorrhage, and high rate of cesarean deliveries [8].

Complications in pregnancy, labor, and delivery occur almost twice as frequently among women diagnosed with uterine myomas than in those without [3–6]. Literature suggest high rate of cesarean delivery in women with myomas up to 58.3% [9].

In fact, in a population-based series of women who delivered singleton, live infants in Washington, Coronado et al. [9] observed from 1987 to 1993 an independent association between uterine leiomyomas and abruptio placentae, fetal malpresentation, dysfunctional labor, and breech presentation. The authors found an increased risk of 58% for cesarean delivery (CD) among 2065 women with uterine myomas, compared to 17% in 4243 women without myomas (odds ratio [OR] 6.39, 95% confidence interval [CI] 5.46–7.5). Some of the excess risk may be related to biased detection of myomas during CD. Conversely, the aforementioned complications of abruption, dysfunctional labor, and breech presentation are usually managed by CD, indicating that the increased risk is probably related to the leiomyomas.

And, if CD is the worldwide most common obstetric operation [10], it is mandatory to consider the possibility of being faced with the necessity of having to remove, necessarily and properly, a myoma during CD or, in other cases, to delivery by an iterative CD on a previous myomectomy.

CONSEQUENCES OF MYOMAS IN PREGNANCY

The medical literature has reported an increasing rate of myomectomies during CD in the past decade, even for the use of ultrasonography that has improved diagnostic capability of detecting myomas in pregnancy (Figure 8.1) [11]. In view of these, it is mandatory to frequently use ultrasonography to detect either fetal well-being or myoma growth and dislocation. Myomas can be asymptomatic or associated with serious complications, and the overall risk of major complications can reach 71% [2,3].

Less common complications of myoma in pregnancy are disseminate intravascular coagulation, cervical pregnancy, spontaneous hemoperitoneum, uterine inversion, and urinary retention in the first trimester. According to the literature, fetal complications related to myoma in pregnancy included limb reduction anomalies and head and body deformities related to fetal compression [1,5–7,9].

Operations on the uterus during the CD, except for excision of pedunculated myomas, are traditionally discouraged for the aforementioned reasons, as uncontrolled and profuse bleeding that may lead to severe anemia, puerperal infection, and an unwanted hysterectomy.

Uterine fibroids, a part of the risk of spontaneous abortion, preterm labor, placental abruption, and postpartum hemorrhage, have been associated with a 10%–40% obstetric complication rate pre-labor, and adverse obstetric outcomes during and after delivery [4,5,9,12].

The greatest risks of cesarean myomectomy frequently result from lack of knowledge of uterine myoma presence during unexpected or scheduled CD, or from a wrong knowledge of myoma dislocation. Myomas lead to dystocia as tumor previa or, when located in the lower uterine segment (LUS), they cause extreme difficulty during closure of the hysterotomy while leaving the fibroid in situ.

Also, for the above reasons, myomectomy performed during pregnancy still remains a risky operation.

Later, with the accumulated experience and lack of major complications, coupled with the fact that no evidence-based contraindications could be found in the literature, we were inspired to develop our own technique and to use it also for large fibroids that were located remotely from the LUS.

UTERINE-MODIFIED ANATOMY AND PHYSIOLOGY WITH MYOMAS IN PREGNANCY

Pregnancy induces profound anatomical and physiological changes to uterus and vascularization, all factors to consider before starting an operation in pregnancy. So, once diagnosis of myoma is confirmed by ultrasonography,

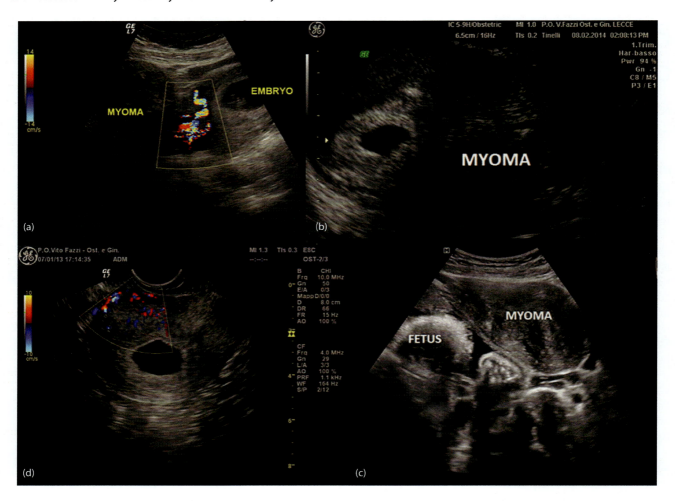

Figure 8.1 Ultrasonographic scan of myomas during pregnancy: (a) a pedunculated myoma of 10 cm in a pregnant woman at 6 weeks of pregnancy, with the echo Doppler enhancing peripheral myoma vascularization; (b) a posterior subserous corporal myoma of 3 cm of diameter at 5 weeks of pregnancy; (c) an anterior fundal intracorporeal myoma in patient at 5 weeks of pregnancy; and (d) a myoma previo at 22 weeks of pregnancy.

management of myoma encountered during CD poses a therapeutic dilemma: how can myomas be better managed during pregnancy, labor, and delivery? For example, consider myomas located near the LUS. In such cases, and in order to deliver the baby, the obstetrician is faced with the emergency decision of making the incision through or near the myoma, removing it, or choosing the classical incision to deliver the baby while avoiding cutting through or near the myoma.

The surgeon has to make decisions if myomectomy is really needed during CD or should be delayed until some months have passed from delivery.

During pregnancy, uterine enlargement involves marked hypertrophy of the muscle cells and a progressive increase in the uteroplacental blood flow ranging from approximately 450 to 650 mL/min near term [12,13]. This increased blood flow is mediated primarily by means of vasodilatation. The uterine artery diameter doubles by 20 weeks' gestation, and concomitant mean Doppler velocimetry is increased eightfold [14]. Thus, any surgical procedure performed on or around the uterus has the potential of causing severe hemorrhage, and for this reason, uterine myomectomy during CD has consistently been discouraged, in the past years, as a risky procedure.

In cases of a small pedunculated subserous fibroid attached to the uterus with a small pedicle (Figure 8.2), myomectomy is relatively easy, with forcipressure (Figure 8.2a), cut (Figure 8.2b), and suturing of the myoma pedicle (Figure 8.2c).

On the contrary, resection of an intramural myoma is inadvisable and contraindicated during CD by some obstetric textbooks [15,16], for the risk of profuse uncontrolled bleeding that could lead to hysterectomy. Authors remark that myomas often undergo a remarkable involution after delivery, and they may even become pedunculated, making myomectomy (if necessary) easier and safer as a postpartum intervention than at the time of CD [16,17]. Furthermore, because of bizarre nuclear changes at pathologists' examination, myomas enucleated during pregnancy or delivery can often be confused with leiomyosarcoma, thus leading to unnecessary anxiety and fear.

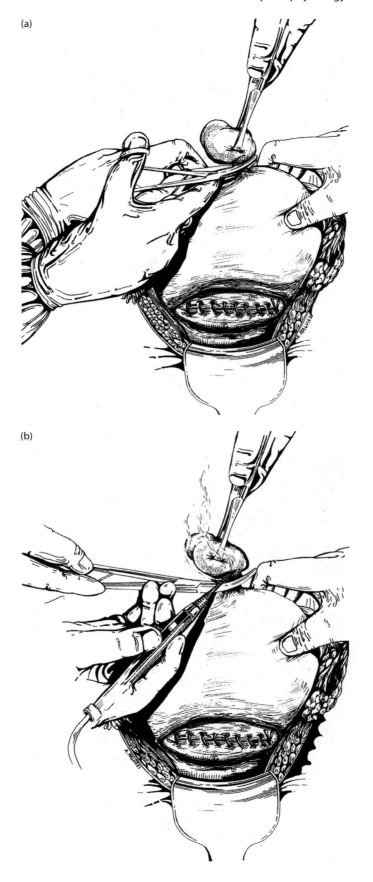

Figure 8.2 The figures represent a cesarean myomectomy in a pregnant woman 38 weeks after hysterorraphy. The myoma is fundal and pedunculated: (a) forcipressure of myoma pedicle; (b) cut of myoma pedicle. (*Continued*)

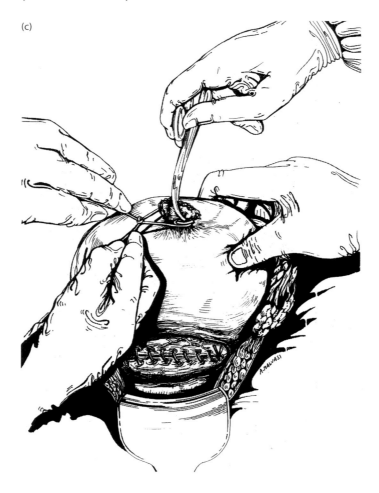

Figure 8.2 (*Continued*) The figures represent a cesarean myomectomy in a pregnant woman 38 weeks after hysterorraphy. The myoma is fundal and pedunculated: (c) suturing of myoma base.

In the scientific literature data and recent, larger studies indicate myomectomy during CD or even during pregnancy is probably a safer procedure than previously believed.

LITERATURE ON CESAREAN MYOMECTOMY

In 1989, Burton et al. [6] were probably the first to report the procedure of a myomectomy during pregnancy and CD. They reviewed an 8-year experience with surgical management of leiomyomata during pregnancy at the Los Angeles County Women's Hospital, California. Five women underwent exploratory laparotomy only, six had a myomectomy during pregnancy, and three had a hysterectomy; one patient aborted after surgery. Thirteen other women had incidental myomectomies at cesarean delivery; one of these had an intraoperative hemorrhage. No other complications occurred.

During 1997–2001, Ben Rafael et al. [18] prospectively evaluated the surgical outcome of a planned myomectomy during CD in cases where the fibroids were known to be large enough to require surgery at a later stage, or when the fibroid led to malpresentation. Investigated parameters at the outcome were type of anesthesia, type of incision, intraoperative blood loss, need for blood transfusion, intra- or postoperative complications, and length of hospital stay. Thirty-nine myomas were removed from 32 patients in 15 elective and 17 emergency procedures. Indications for CD were obstetrical (breech presentation, more than one previous CD, among others) in most cases. Indications in the other women included three cases of myomas causing dystocia as tumor previa, one suffering from a degenerative myoma and intractable pain, and two who had undergone previous myomectomies with uterine cavity penetration. Ninety percent of the myomas were subserous or intramural, and 10% were submucous. The average size (largest dimension) was 6 cm (1.5–20), with 26 myomas measuring >3 cm, and 11 >6 cm. Four CDs (12.5%) were classical, and the rest were low segmental. Most of the operations were performed under regional anesthesia (spinal block). The differences in hemoglobin and hematocrit levels before and 12 hours after the operation were significantly lower in patients who underwent cesarean myomectomies, compared to women who underwent CD without a myomectomy ($p < 0.05$), yet only four patients required a blood transfusion. Two patients underwent repeated surgery: one with two large myomas and excessive bleeding, and the other because of a subcutaneous hematoma. No hysterectomy was required.

Six patients had postpartum fever (18.7%). The average duration of hospitalization was 5.7 days, with five patients requiring more than 6 days of hospitalization. There was no correlation between complications or duration of hospital stay and patient age, gravidity, parity, or indication for CD [18].

Michalas et al. [19] performed a myomectomy on a 31-year-old primigravida during the 15th week of pregnancy due to a large, 23 cm diameter myoma. At the 39th week of pregnancy, during the CD, eight fibroids obstructing the lower part of the uterus were removed. There were no maternal or fetal complications.

Celik et al. [20], in his study conclusions, reported that myomectomy could also be safe if performed during pregnancy. Five pregnant women with myomas requiring surgical removal because of severe pain underwent a myomectomy at a median gestational age of 17.8 ± 3.4 weeks. The mean size of the myomas was 14 ± 3.8 cm. No major surgical and postoperative complications were observed, and all pregnancies continued to term.

Reporting surgical experiences of the last century, other authors reported their experience with cesarean myomectomies, as did Hsieh et al. [21] who retrospectively reviewed 47 incidental cesarean myomectomies. The procedure added only 11 minutes to the operating time, 112 mL to the operative blood loss, and extended the hospital stay by about 1.5 days. There was no wound infection or serious morbidity.

Dimitrov et al. [22] conducted a prospective study in Bulgaria to evaluate a myomectomy during CD as "a routine method." Their study group included 21 cases that underwent myomectomies during CD, and were compared to a control group of 162 consecutive CDs without having undergone myomectomies. They found that a myomectomy during CD increased hemorrhage by 10%. Analysis of the cases with severe hemorrhage showed that they were related to other placental disorders (abruptio placentae and placenta previa) as the main cause of the increased blood loss. There were no postoperative complications.

Omar et al. [23] reported two cases with large, uterine myomas, situated in the anterior aspect of the lower segment, complicating pregnancy at term. A myomectomy in both instances facilitated delivery of the fetus through the lower segment, making vaginal delivery in subsequent pregnancies possible.

Brown et al. [24] from Jamaica retrospectively analyzed the records of 32 women: 16 underwent cesarean myomectomy and were compared to 16 cases of CD chosen as the first normal CD occurring after each cesarean myomectomy. The myomectomy was always performed after delivery of the fetus and after administration of oxytocin. Diluted oxytocin was also injected into the capsule overlying the myoma to help achieve hemostasis. The results indicated that the patients who underwent a cesarean myomectomy were significantly older ($p < 0.0001$), but there was no statistical difference in parity between the two groups. The median number of myomas found was two (range: 1–6). The mean blood loss was similar between the two groups: 403 ± 196 mL in the myomectomy group versus 356 ± 173 mL in the regular CD. No significant difference between the groups was observed in relation to hemoglobin levels, need for blood transfusion, febrile morbidity, or hospital stay.

Ehigiegba et al. [25] prospectively assessed the intra- and postoperative complications of cesarean myomectomies in 25 pregnancies. Patients with known fibroids were required to provide their consent for a possible cesarean myomectomy. Leiomyomas in the anterior uterine wall (cervical, body, or fundal) were removed through the CD incision when possible, otherwise other incision(s) were performed. Nineteen patients (76%) underwent emergency CD after trial of labor, and six (24%) had elective CD. A total of 84 fibroids were removed. In most women there were only one to two leiomyomas, but in one patient 22 myomas were extracted; 57% of the myomas were intramural, 35.7% subserous of which only 1% was pedunculated. Anemia was apparent in 60% of patients, but only five patients (20%) required blood transfusion. No case necessitated hysterectomy. Three patients (12%) had subsequent pregnancies, two of whom had normal vaginal deliveries and one underwent a repeat CD.

The largest report by Roman and Tabsh [26] compared the results of cesarean myomectomies to "no touch" CD. They retrospectively evaluated 111 women who underwent a cesarean myomectomy and 257 women with documented fibroids who underwent CD alone. The two groups were similar with respect to median age, median parity, median gestational age, and median size of the fibroids. Most patients in both groups underwent low transverse incision CD. In 86% of the patients the fibroids were incidental findings, while in the rest symptoms such as pain, dystocia, and unusual appearance of the myoma dictated its removal. The incidence of hemorrhage in the study group was 12.6%, compared with 12.8% in the control group ($p = 0.95$). There was also no statistically significant increase in the incidence of postpartum fever, operating time, and length of postpartum stay. The size of fibroid did not appear to affect the incidence of hemorrhage. After stratifying the procedures by type of fibroid removed, intramural myomectomy was found to be associated with a 21.2% incidence of hemorrhage, compared with 12.8% in the control group, but this difference was not statistically significant ($p = 0.08$). No patient in either group required hysterectomy or embolization following the operation. A similar study by Kaymak et al. [27] on 40 patients undergoing a cesarean myomectomy compared to 80 patients with untouched myomas during CD also showed that performing a myomectomy during CD does not increase the surgical and postoperative complication rate [26].

Although all these above-mentioned studies and reports indicate a good outcome after a cesarean myomectomy, or even after performing a myomectomy during pregnancy, one should remember that hemorrhage can still occur and lead to grave consequences.

Exacoustos et al. [4] reported nine myomectomies performed during cesarean delivery. Of these, three were complicated by severe hemorrhage, necessitating hysterectomy. The authors emphasized the role of various ultrasound findings in identifying women at risk for myoma-related complications: the size of the myoma, its position, location, relationship to the placenta, and echogenic structure.

Several studies have described techniques that can minimize blood loss at cesarean myomectomy, including uterine tourniquet [28], bilateral uterine artery ligation [29], and electrocautery [30].

However, the majority of the mentioned literature indicates that a myomectomy performed at the time of CD should not increase the risk of hemorrhage and postoperative fever or should not prolong hospital stay. In fact, cesarean myomectomy was stated as a feasible and safe procedure when performed by an experienced surgeon [24–27].

Pedunculated subserous myomas can be safely removed even if of large size (Figure 8.3). Subserous and intramural myomas that are located at the LUS can and probably should be removed and not bypassed by performing a classical incision (Figures 8.4 and 8.5).

Performing an elective myomectomy from other uterine locations should be considered with caution, because most of these myomas will nevertheless involute to an insignificant size during puerperium. Meticulous attention to hemostasis,

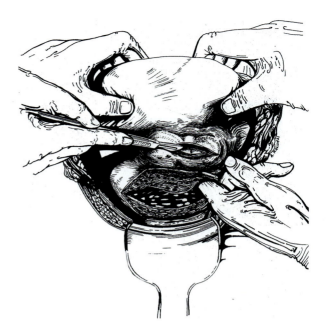

Figure 8.4 Incision of the uterine wall overlying the myoma, in the upper portion of the lower uterine segment.

enucleation using sharp dissection with Metzenbaum scissors, and adequate approximation of the myometrium and all dead spaces to prevent hematoma formation can increase the safety of the procedure. Despite the lack of prospective and randomized studies, the retrospective investigations clearly show that the old dictum that discouraged cesarean myomectomy should be reassessed. Women with known myomas undergoing elective or emergency CD should be properly informed in order to obtain their consent for the option of performing a cesarean myomectomy.

TRADITIONAL TECHNIQUE OF CESAREAN MYOMECTOMY

The operation should be performed, at least at the outset, by a gynecologist who is proficient in myomectomies on nongravid uteri [31]. After newborn delivery, the hysterotomy is chosen to allow the maximal myoma exposure for its removal and the minimal myometrial damage for hysterorrhaphy. Myomectomies could be performed through a transversal or vertical incision, depending on attitude and preferences of the surgeon.

In case of myomas located near hysterotomy, an interlocked suture is temporarily placed on the edge of the cesarean uterine incision without closure. In such cases, myomectomies are preferably performed from the edge of the CD incision (for myomas located near the lower uterine segment). This also facilitates working from within the uterine cavity or from the outer part of the uterus without significant bleeding from the cesarean incision. In case of fibroids located far from the CD incision, myomectomies are preferably performed by making new incisions above the myomas, in instances where they are located in a site remote from the CD incision.

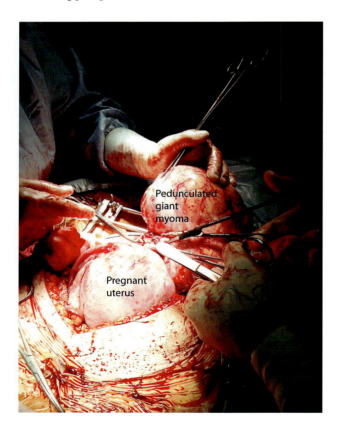

Figure 8.3 Myomectomy during cesarean delivery in a pregnant woman of 37 weeks with preterm rupture of membranes and preterm labor, with a left cornual pedunculated myoma of 16 cm diameter.

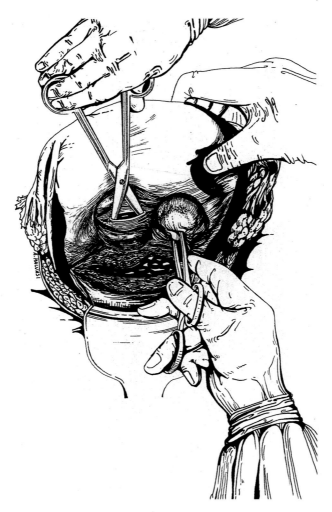

Figure 8.5 Cautious dissection, by Metzenbaum scissors, of myometrial fibers overlying the myoma.

Surgeons always perform the myoma dissection from myometrium using a sharp Metzenbaum scissor. Intravenous oxytocin drip is generally given after enucleation of the fibroid (some surgeons prefer also during myomectomy). No tourniquet is used by many surgeons as routine; however, this may be used to control unexpected bleeding. Suturing of the fibroid base is traditionally performed by using two layers of interrupted sutures, and a baseball-type suture is used for the serosa as a third layer [31,32].

One important issue with myomectomy is controlling blood loss from the raw myoma beds after they have been excised. Blood loss is generally estimated from suction aspiration, and from weighing mops, swabs, and drapes used during surgery. Several techniques to reduce blood loss have been studied and reported. A randomized trial comparing vasopressin and saline injected into the serosa prior to the uterine incision showed that vasopressin is extremely effective for decreasing blood loss. In this study, 50% of patients receiving saline required transfusion, while none of those in the vasopressin group required transfusion (13% versus 5% decrease in hematocrit values) [33].

To reduce bleeding after cesarean myomectomy, some surgeons sometimes place tourniquets around the uterus. This is usually performed, especially in the case of placenta accreta [34,35], by making a window in the broad ligament at the level of the internal cervical os bilaterally and passing a Foley catheter or red rubber catheter through the windows and around the cervix and then tightening it with a clamp to constrict the uterine vessels. In combination with this, vascular clamps are generally placed on the utero-ovarian ligaments [36].

Two randomized trials compared vasopressin and tourniquet use after myomectomy.

In 1996, Fletcher et al. showed that vasopressin was associated with less blood loss and lower risk of either transfusion or blood loss of more than 1 L [37].

In 1993, Ginsberg et al. [38] noted no statistically significant difference between the groups, although their study was much smaller. Study results very clearly suggest that vasopressin (usually 20 U in 50–100 mL normal saline) should be injected routinely prior to making the incision in the wall of the uterus. Whether additional use of a tourniquet further decreases blood loss remains unclear. After dilute vasopressin has been injected, an incision is made through the wall of the uterus into the myoma. Once the plane between the myometrium and myoma has been defined, it is dissected bluntly and sharply until the entire fibroid is removed. As many fibroids as possible are removed through a single incision. Once the fibroids have been removed, the defect is closed in layers with delayed absorbable suture [38].

Proper placement of the incision side is frequently overlooked but is important.

Tulandi et al. [39] studied 26 women with uteri larger than 6–8 weeks' size in 1993. Abdominal myomectomies were performed, followed by a second-look laparoscopy 6 weeks later. Patients with incisions in the posterior wall of the uterus had a much higher likelihood of significant adhesions as measured by percentage with adhesions or American Fertility Society (AFS) adhesion score compared with patients with incisions in the fundus or anterior wall of the uterus [39].

INTRACAPSULAR CESAREAN MYOMECTOMY

Myoma pseudocapsule is a neurovascular bundle or fibrovascular network attached the fibroids, which separates the fibroids from the normal myometrium. At ultrasonographic exam, myoma pseudocapsule appears as a white ring around the fibroid, and at echo Doppler check, it appears as a "ring of fire" (Figure 8.6), even in pregnancy (Figure 8.7).

It has been shown that the pseudocapsule not only has similar architecture to the normal myometrium, but also contains different neurofibers and neuropeptides. Consequently, a pseudocapsule damage during myomectomy surely negatively impacts successive on myometrial healing, although a variety of factors may affect the postoperative healing. Therefore, the excision of a fibroid in daily clinical practice should be done inside the pseudocapsule separating this vascular network (Figure 8.8) [40,41].

After the development of well-detailed technique, the intracapsular myomectomy, successfully performed during laparoscopy in nonpregnant women with single or multiple fibroids [42,43], authors decided to study their methods of myomas removal during CD, exploring its outcomes.

During the years 2005–2011, my international research group and I [44] prospectively evaluated the surgical outcome of intracapsular myomectomy during CD, in university-affiliated hospitals, by a prospective case-control study on 68 patients who underwent intracapsular cesarean myomectomy, compared with a control group of 72 patients with myomatous pregnant uterus who underwent cesarean delivery without myomectomy.

All operations were performed by gynecologists proficient in intracapsular myomectomies on nongravid uteri, and by CD by Stark's method, under regional anesthesia.

A routine intracapsular cesarean myomectomy was then done for all anterior fibroids—cervical, body, or fundal—using the same cesarean incision where possible, or utilizing other incisions, when necessary.

Each intracapsular cesarean myomectomy was performed after LUS closuring. A linear incision was made over the uterine serosa direct to the myoma by a scalpel or a monopolar electro-scalpel at low wattage (≤30 watt), gradually until the opening of the pseudocapsule (Figure 8.9),

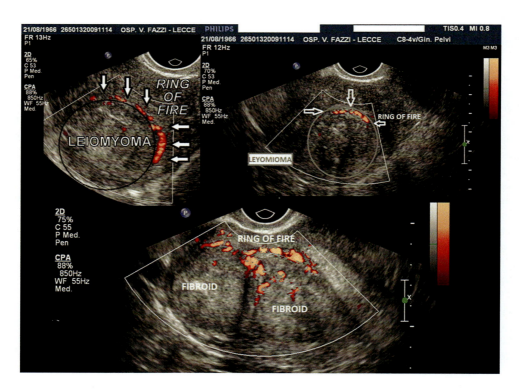

Figure 8.6 Ultrasonographic scan of myomas, by echo Doppler shows the pseudocapsule surrounding myoma, appearing as a "ring of fire."

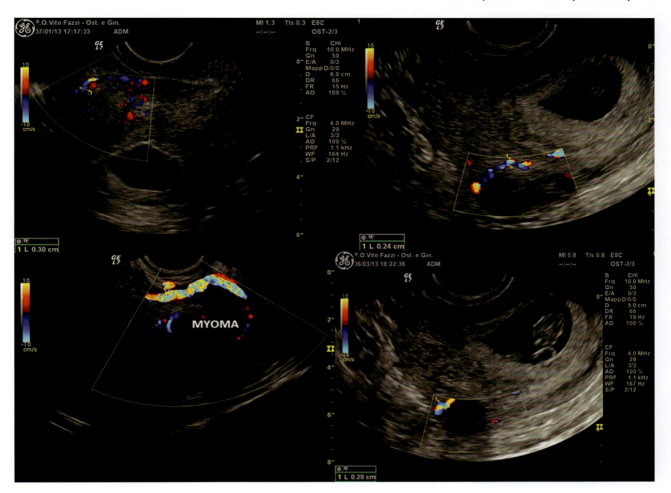

Figure 8.7 Ultrasonographic scan of myomas in pregnancy shows myoma pseudocapsule as a "ring of fire," by echo Doppler scan.

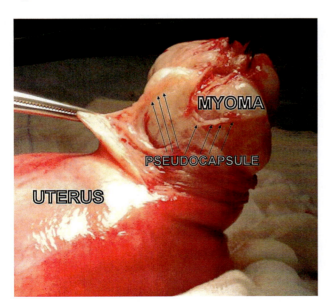

Figure 8.8 A myoma removal by intracapsular cesarean myomectomy; the image highlights the gentle dissection of pseudocapsule surrounding myoma during its enucleating. (The arrows indicate the myoma pseudocapsule.) (From Tinelli A et al. *J Matern Fetal Neonatal Med* 2014;27(1):66–71. With permission.)

enabling the relatively bloodless plane between the pseudocapsule and its myoma to be entered (Figure 8.10). Once the surface of the myoma was reached and its fiber bridges freed, the myoma was hooked (Figure 8.11) and extracted from its capsule (Figure 8.12), also by traction and pushing down the capsule using sharp Metzenbaum scissors. The hemostasis during intracapsular cesarean myomectomy was always reached by gentle low wattage coagulation (≤30 watt) of pseudocapsule vessels, with minimal blood loss. Then, 10 units of intravenous oxytocin drip was given as standard to all patients to control bleeding, after enucleating the fibroid.

For myomas located near LUS, we temporarily changed the operational steps: after completion of the CD, an interlocked suture is temporarily placed on the edge of the cesarean uterine incision without closure. Then we performed intracapsular cesarean myomectomies from the edge of the cesarean incision. This also facilitates working from within the uterine cavity or from the outer part of the uterus without significant bleeding from the CD incision. After that, in case of other myomas far from LUS, surgeons make a new incision above the myoma in instances where they were located in a site remote from the CD incision.

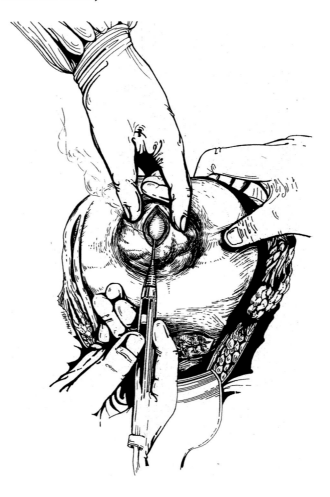

Figure 8.9 A linear incision is made over the uterine serosa direct to the myoma by a scalpel or a monopolar electro-scalpel at low wattage, gradually until opening the myoma pseudocapsule.

Suturing of the fibroid base was routinely performed by using two layers of interrupted absorbable sutures (1-0 caliber Vicryl) and a baseball-type suture was used for the serosa, using a continuous absorbable suture (2-0 or 3-0 caliber Vicryl), as a third layer (Figures 8.13 through 8.16). Pelvic irrigation was done with saline solution. Postoperatively, oxytocin infusion was continued for 12–24 hours in parallel with normal saline infusion.

Seventy-two control subjects were randomly selected among pregnant women with myomas undergoing CD without myomectomy, at the same institutions and during the same period, and CD indications were breech presentation, more than one previous CD, and CD on demand. These women did not receive cesarean myomectomy because they refused this operation, and both myomectomy and control groups were similar in terms of characteristics without statistical differences.

Removed myomas were generally subserous or intramural: 48 subserous, 14 intramural, and six pedunculated. Of these, 12 had multiple sites myomas (17.6%), but we tried to use the same hysterotomy for neighboring fibroids.

Sites of myoma removal were fundal in 37 women (54.4%), corporal in 22 (32.3%), and peri-low uterine segment in nine women (18.7%), where we temporarily changed the steps of the operation in five women. The average myoma size was 8 cm (1.5–20), in 40 women, with eight myomas measuring 4–6 cm, 14 myomas between 10 and 12 cm, and >13 cm in six patients.

The difference in blood chemical and surgical outcome in intracapsular cesarean myomectomy was nonstatistically significant ($p > 0.05$) (Table 8.1).

During the postoperative course, five patients had postpartum fever of 38.8°C, on average, for two consecutive days after surgery (7.3%); the blood culture did not show any bacteria, and patients were treated by broad-spectrum antibiotics. The average duration of hospitalization of intracapsular cesarean myomectomies was 5 days, with six patients requiring more than 5 days of hospitalization (8.8%); these five patients felt too weak to be discharged, so they preferred to stay in the hospital an extra day.

There was no correlation between complications or duration of hospital stay and patient age, gravidity, parity, or indication for CD.

None of the patients underwent repeated surgery after intracapsular cesarean myomectomy and no hysterectomy was required after intracapsular cesarean myomectomy.

Authors' data show no difference between the intracapsular cesarean myomectomy group and the control group,

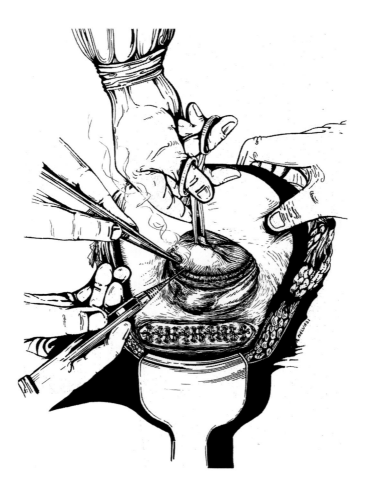

Figure 8.10 The electro-scalpel proceeds in cutting, helped by myoma contra traction, enabling entrance to the relatively bloodless plane between the pseudocapsule and its myoma.

in terms of pre- and postoperative hemoglobin values, mean change in hemoglobin values, incidence of intraoperative hemorrhage, frequency of blood transfusion, and of postoperative fever. The only two parameters that affect negatively the group submitted to intracapsular cesarean myomectomy are the duration of the operation and the length of hospital stay.

Because obstetricians are often confronted with fibroids while performing CD and face the dilemma of how they should be managed, considering the cost–benefit of our study, the authors affirm that the intracapsular cesarean myomectomy procedure can be performed with some confidence, without affecting adversely the postoperative course and clinical outcomes.

CONCLUSION

In conclusion, performing additional surgical procedures on the uterus, such as cesarean myomectomy, was relatively considered contraindicated for many years. Nevertheless, this dictum was not based on evidence, but rather on conjectural experience, which discouraged cesarean myomectomies with the exception of small pedunculated fibroids. Some medical literature, however, indicates that cesarean myomectomies are probably safe if performed for justified indications, by experienced surgeons, and by using meticulous tissue-handling techniques in order to avoid serious or life-threatening complications. There is the benefit of one surgery rather than two operations, as only one scar is produced. These situations are a challenge to the obstetrician and carry a legal dilemma because the patients need to be adequately informed, prior to surgery, in regard to size and location of the myoma during CD, and the possible complications to which a concomitant enucleation may lead. To be successful any operation always needs adequate patient preparation, careful surgical planning, and correct intra- and postoperative management of complications.

CONFLICT OF INTEREST

The author certifies that there is no actual or potential conflict of interest in relation to this article and he reveals any financial interests or connections, direct or indirect, or other situations that might raise the question of bias in the work reported or the conclusions, implications, or opinions stated—including pertinent commercial or other sources of funding for the individual author(s) or for the associated department(s) or organization(s), personal relationships, or direct academic competition.

184 Fibroids and myomectomy in cesarean delivery

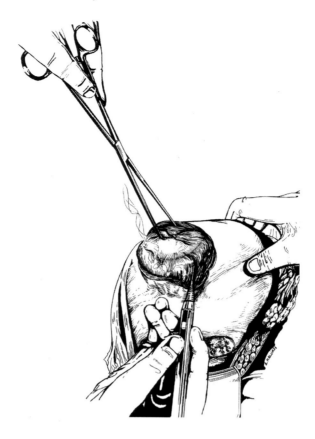

Figure 8.11 Traction on the myoma with Collins forceps, while the operator cuts the pseudocapsule bridges anchoring the uterine myoma to the myometrium.

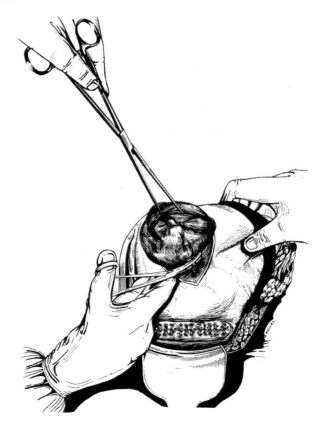

Figure 8.12 Clamping of the vessels supplying blood to the myoma, while running a cautious but firm traction on the myoma.

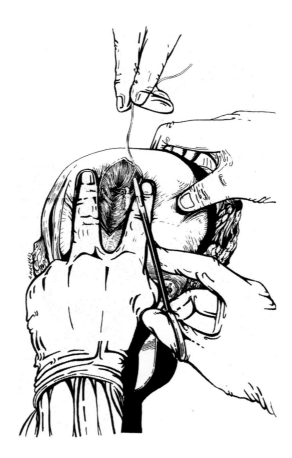

Figure 8.13 Deep hysterorrhaphy where the myoma was enucleated (the myoma bed): needle insertion into the deep myometrial layer.

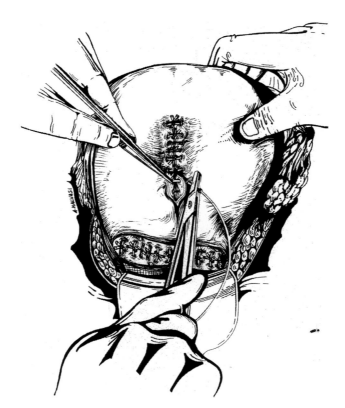

Figure 8.14 Technique of longitudinal hysterorrhaphy: closure of the uterine serosa overlying the myoma bed.

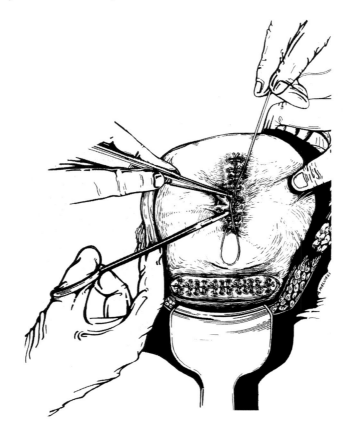

Figure 8.15 Synthesis of uterine serosa: needle piling, by separate stitches, into the suture midline.

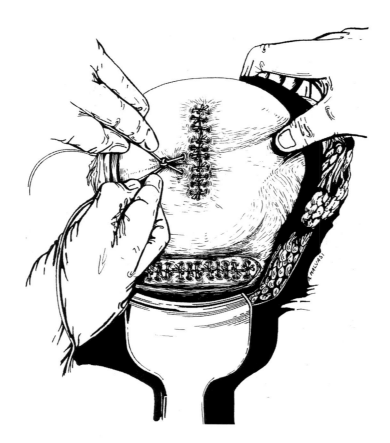

Figure 8.16 Synthesis of uterine serosa: safety knotting of the wire tips, in the center of the longitudinal uterine incision.

Table 8.1 Blood tests and outcome differences among intracapsular cesarean myomectomy (ICM) and cesarean deliveries, as control group

	Cesarean myomectomy (CM): 68 patients	Control group (CS): 72 patients	p value
Preoperative hemoglobin values (g/dL) (mean ± S.D.)	12.1 ± 1.5	11.8 ± 1.3	NS
Postoperative hemoglobin values (g/dL) (mean ± S.D.)	10.6 ± 1.8	10.2 ± 1.4	NS
Mean change in hemoglobin values (g/dL)	1.5 ± 0.3	1.6 ± 0.1	NS
Incidence of intraoperative hemorrhage (>1 L of blood)	3 (4.4%)	4 (5.5%)	NS
Frequency of blood transfusion	4 (5.8%)	4 (5.5%)	NS
Frequency of postoperative fever	5 (7.3%)	3 (4.1%)	NS
Duration of operation (minutes) (mean ± S.D.)	50.5 ± 19.2	41.6 ± 8.2	>0.05
Length of hospital stay (days) (mean ± S.D.)	5.0 ± 1.4	4.4 ± 0.7	>0.05

Source: From Tinelli A et al. *J Matern Fetal Neonatal Med* 2014;27(1):66–71. With permission.
Note: S.D.: standard deviation; NS: nonsignificant.

REFERENCES

1. Novak ER, Woodruff JD. *Myoma and Other Benign Tumours of the Uterus, Novaks' Gynecologic and Obstetric Pathology with Clinical and Endocrine Relations.* Philadelphia, PA: W.B. Saunders; 1979: 795–801.
2. Ouyang DW. Obstetric complications of fibroids. *Obstet Gynecol Clin North Am* 2006;33:153–69.
3. Rice JP, Kay HH, Mahony BS. The clinical significance of uterine leiomyomas in pregnancy. *Am J Obstet Gynecol* 1989;160:1212–6.
4. Exacoustos C, Rosati P. Ultrasound diagnosis of uterine myomas and complications in pregnancy. *Obstet Gynecol* 1993;82:97–101.
5. Katz VL, Dotters DJ, Droegemueller W. Complications of uterine leiomyomas in pregnancy. *Obstet Gynecol* 1989;73:593–6.
6. Burton CA, Grimes DA, March CM. Surgical management of leiomyomata during pregnancy. *Obstet Gynecol* 1989;74:707–9.
7. Hasan F, Arumugam K, Sivanesaratnam V. Uterine leiomyomata in pregnancy. *Int J Gynaecol Obstet* 1991;34:45–48.
8. Vergani P, Locatelli A, Ghidini A, Andreani M, Sala F, Pezzullo JC. Large uterine leiomyomata and risk of cesarean delivery. *Obstet Gynecol* 2007;109:410–4.
9. Coronado GD, Marshall LM, Schwartz SM. Complications in pregnancy, labor, and delivery with uterine leiomyomas: A population-based study. *Obstet Gynecol* 2000;95:764–9.
10. Zizza A, Tinelli A, Malvasi A, Barbone E, Stark M, De Donno A, Guido M. Caesarean section in the world: A new ecological approach. *J Prev Med Hyg* 2011;52(4):161–73.
11. Pei-Chun M, Yin-Chen J, I-De W, Chien-Han C, Wei-Min L, Cherng-Jye J. A huge leiomyoma subjected to a myomectomy during a cesarean delivery. *Taiwan J Obstet Gynecol* 2010;49(2):220–2.
12. Edman CD, Toofanian A, MacDonald PC, Gant NF. Placental clearance rate of maternal plasma androstenedione through placental estradiol formation: An indirect method of assessing uteroplacental blood flow. *Am J Obstet Gynecol* 1981;141:1029–37.
13. Kauppila A, Koskinen M, Puolakka J, Tuimala R, Kuikka J. Decreased intervillous and unchanged myometrial blood flow in supine recumbency. *Obstet Gynecol* 1980;55:203–5.
14. Palmer SK, Zamudio S, Coffin C, Parker S, Stamm E, Moore LG. Quantitative estimation of human uterine artery blood flow and pelvic blood flow redistribution in pregnancy. *Obstet Gynecol* 1992;80: 1000–6.
15. Cunningham FG, Leveno KL, Bloom SL, Hauth JC, Gilstrap LC III, Wenstrom KD, eds. Abnormalities of the reproductive tract. In: *Williams Obstetrics.* 22nd ed. New York, NY:McGraw-Hill Medical; 2005.
16. Ludmir J, Stubblefield PG. Surgical procedures in pregnancy. In: Gabbe SG, Niebyl JR, Simpson JL, eds. *Gabbe: Obstetrics: Normal and Problem Pregnancies.* 4th ed. Philadelphia, PA: Churchill Livingstone; 2002:613.
17. Haskins RD, Haskins CJ, Gilmore R, Borel MA, Mancuso P. Intramural leiomyoma during pregnancy becoming pedunculated postpartally. A case report. *J Reprod Med* 2001;46:253–5.
18. Ben-Rafael Z, Perri T, Krissi H, Dekel A, Dicker D. Myomectomy during cesarean delivery-time to reconsider. In: Ben-Rafael Z, Diedrich K, Dudenhausen J-W, Mettler L, Schnider HPG, Shoham Z, eds. *Controversies in Obstetrics, Gynecology, and Infertility.* Berlin: Oren Publisher; 2003:352–6.
19. Michalas SP, Oreopoulou FV, Papageorgiou JS. Myomectomy during pregnancy and caesarean section. *Hum Reprod* 1995;10:1869–70.
20. Çelik C, Acar A, Çiçek N, Gezginc K, Akyürek C. Can myomectomy be performed during pregnancy? *Gynecol Obstet Inv* 2002;53:79–83.
21. Hsieh TT, Cheng BJ, Liou JD, Chiu TH. Incidental myomectomy in cesarean delivery. *Changgeng Yi Xue Za Zhi* 1989;12:13–20.

22. Dimitrov A, Nikolov A, Stamenov G. Myomectomy during cesarean delivery. *Akush Ginekol (Sofia)* 1999;38:7–9.
23. Omar SZ, Sivanesaratnam V, Damodaran P. Large lower segment myoma. Myomectomy at lower segment cesarean delivery. A report of tow cases. *Singapore Med J* 1999;40:109–10.
24. Brown D, Fletcher HM, Myrie MO, Reid M. Caesarean myomectomy—A safe procedure. A retrospective case controlled study. *J Obstet Gynaecol* 1999;19(2):139–41.
25. Ehigiegba AE, Ande AB, Ojobo SI. Myomectomy during cesarean delivery. *Int J Gynecol Obstet* 2001;75:21–35.
26. Roman AS, Tabsh KM. Myomectomy at time of cesarean delivery: A retrospective cohort study. *BMC Pregnancy Childbirth* 2004;4:14–17.
27. Kaymak O, Ustunyurt E, Okyay RE, Kalyoncu S, Mollamahmutoglu L. Myomectomy during cesarean delivery. *Int J Gynecol Obstet* 2005;89:90–93.
28. Kwawukume EY. Cesarean myomectomy. *Afr J Reprod Health* 2002;6:38–43.
29. Sapmaz E, Celik H, Altungul A. Bilateral ascending uterine artery ligation vs. tourniquet use for hemostasis in cesarean myomectomy. A comparison. *J Reprod Med* 2003;48:950–4.
30. Cobellis L, Florio P, Stradella L, Lucia ED, Messalli EM, Petraglia F, Cobellis G. Electro-cautery of myomas during caesarean section—Two case reports. *Eur J Obstet Gynecol Reprod Biol* 2002;102:98–99.
31. Wallach EE. Myomectomy. In: Thompson JD, Rock JA, eds. *Te Linde's Operative Gynaecology*. New York, NY: JB Lippincott; 1992:647–62.
32. Song D, Zhang W, Chames MC, Guo J. Myomectomy during cesarean delivery. *Int J Gynaecol Obstet* 2013;121(3):208–13.
33. Frederick J, Fletcher H, Simeon D et al. Intramyometrial vasopressin as a haemostatic agent during myomectomy. *Br J Obstet Gynaecol* 1994;101(5):435–7.
34. Huijgen QC, Gijsen AF, Hink E, Van Kesteren PJ. Cervical tourniquet in case of uncontrollable haemorrhage during caesarean section owing to a placenta accreta. *BMJ Case Rep* 2013 April 22;2013.
35. Ikeda T, Sameshima H, Kawaguchi H, Yamauchi N, Ikenoue T. Tourniquet technique prevents profuse blood loss in placenta accreta cesarean delivery. *J Obstet Gynaecol Res* 2005;31(1):27–31.
36. DeLancey JO. A modified technique for hemostasis during myomectomy. *Surg Gynecol Obstet* 1992;174(2):153–4.
37. Fletcher H, Frederick J, Hardie M, Simeon D. A randomized comparison of vasopressin and tourniquet as hemostatic agents during myomectomy. *Obstet Gynecol* 1996;87(6):1014–8.
38. Ginsburg ES, Benson CB, Garfield JM et al. The effect of operative technique and uterine size on blood loss during myomectomy: A prospective randomized study. *Fertil Steril* 1993;60(6):956–62.
39. Tulandi T, Murray C, Guralnick M. Adhesion formation and reproductive outcome after myomectomy and second-look laparoscopy. *Obstet Gynecol* 1993;82(2):213–5.
40. Tinelli A, Malvasi A, Hurst BS et al. Surgical management of neurovascular bundle in uterine fibroid pseudocapsule. *JSLS* 2012;16:119–29.
41. Malvasi A, Cavallotti C, Morroni M et al. Uterine fibroid pseudocapsule studied by transmission electron microscopy. *Eur J Obstet Gynecol Reprod Biol* 2012;162:187–91.
42. Tinelli A, Hurst BS, Hudelist G et al. Laparoscopic myomectomy focusing on the myoma pseudocapsule: Technical and outcome reports. *Hum Reprod* 2012;27:427–35.
43. Tinelli A, Malvasi A, Hudelist G, Cavallotti C, Tsin DA, Schollmeyer T, Bojahr B, Mettler L. Laparoscopic intracapsular myomectomy: Comparison of single versus multiple fibroids removal. An institutional experience. *J Laparoendosc Adv Surg Tech A* 2010; 20(8):705–11.
44. Tinelli A, Malvasi A, Mynbaev OA, Barbera A, Perrone E, Guido M, Kosmas I, Stark M. The surgical outcome of intracapsular cesarean myomectomy. A match control study. *J Matern Fetal Neonatal Med* 2014;27(1):66–71.

FURTHER READING

Shavell VI, Thakur M, Sawant A, Kruger ML, Jones TB, Singh M, Puscheck EE, Diamond MP. Adverse obstetric outcomes associated with sonographically identified large uterine fibroids. *Fertil Steril* 2012; 97(1):107–10.

Management of placenta previa and/or accreta

GRAZIANO CLERICI and LAURA DI FABRIZIO

Abnormal placentation is one of the major causes of maternal and fetal morbidity and mortality [1,2]. This condition is associated with high demands on health resources [2], and it can be a cause of life-threatening antepartum and/or postpartum hemorrhage [3].

Placental abnormalities can be diagnosed by ultrasound and often necessitate cesarean delivery. These abnormalities can be divided into two groups:

- Placental morphological and placental insertion site abnormalities
- Abnormalities of the placental parenchyma

Abnormalities of placental morphology are found in about 15% of physiological at term pregnancies, and in the majority of cases they are the consequence of a defect of placental implantation or of a malfunction of the placental localization.

The main anatomical and clinical frameworks are

- Placenta previa
- Placenta accreta

PLACENTA PREVIA

Placenta previa is a disorder of implantation, in which the placenta is inserted partially or wholly in the lower uterine segment. This condition is commonly associated with different degree of accretism in the myometrium.

From a clinical point of view, it can be the cause of a sudden and painless bleeding in the third trimester, as a result of small detachments. Other complications may include premature rupture of membranes and prolapsed umbilical cord, placental abruption, acute and chronic fetal anemia, and prematurity.

According to the last guideline of the Royal College of Obstetricians and Gynecologists (RCOG), placenta previa can be classified as major previa if the placenta lies over the internal cervical os, or minor or partial previa if the leading edge of the placenta is in the lower uterine segment but not covering the cervical os (Figure 9.1).

However, a recent "Executive Summary Report" of the Ultrasound Fetal Imaging Workshop in 2014 [4] suggests to simplify the traditional classification considered very confusing. So the panel agreed to a revised classification eliminating the classical terms "partial" and "marginal" and only retaining the terms "placenta previa" and "low-lying placenta." In particular they suggest that if the placental edge is 2 cm or more from the internal os, the placental location should be reported as normal. If the placental edge is less than 2 cm from the internal os but not covering it, the placenta should be labeled as low-lying and a follow-up ultrasonography is recommended at 32 and 36 weeks of gestation. Only if the placental edge covers completely the internal cervical os, the placenta should be labeled as "placenta previa" that requires the same transvaginal ultrasonographic follow-up at 32 and 36 weeks of gestation as suggested for the low-lying placenta.

The increasing incidence of cesarean deliveries combined with the increasing maternal age represent important risk factors for placenta previa and/or accreta [2], as well as smoking, grand multiparity, recurrent miscarriage, low social class, and infertility treatment [3,5].

Taipale et al. [6] reported an incidence of placenta previa at term varying from 0.2% to 1.2%, depending on the diagnostic method used.

Diagnosis of placenta previa

The ultrasound has substantially changed the semiotics of placenta previa. According to the RCOG guidelines, routine ultrasound of the second trimester should include placental localization.

As noted by Becker et al. [7], in fact, viewing placental insertion in early gestational ages allows to plan the correct timing of delivery and to limit the complications related to this disease.

Transvaginal ultrasound is currently the "gold standard" for the diagnosis of the localization of the placenta (Figure 9.2). It has been demonstrated that it is an accurate and safe diagnostic tool to confirm the suspected diagnosis of placenta previa by transabdominal scan [7] (Figure 9.3).

Oppenheimer et al. [8] showed that 90% of low-lying placentas diagnosed by ultrasound during the second trimester will "migrate" in a normal location at term of pregnancy, but it has been demonstrated that if the placenta is posterior or if there has been a previous cesarean delivery, this is less likely [9].

It is well known that placental pathologies can simultaneously present both anomalies of the placental insertion (placenta previa) and of placental implantation (placenta accreta); women with a history of previous cesarean delivery have a higher risk of both these conditions. In these cases it is recommended to perform antenatal sonographic imaging complemented by magnetic resonance imaging (MRI) to individuate women at real risk of placenta accreta.

The antenatal sonographic imaging includes associated techniques such as grayscale, color Doppler, and three-dimensional power Doppler (which are able to highlight

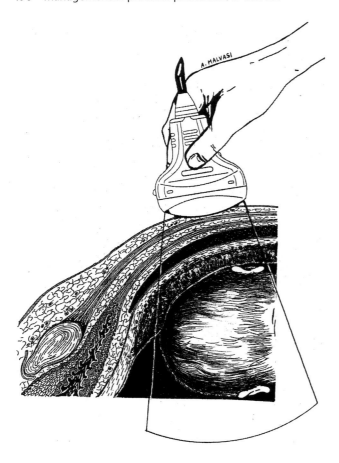

Figure 9.1 Longitudinal transabdominal two-dimensional sonographic section in uterus at term of placenta previa.

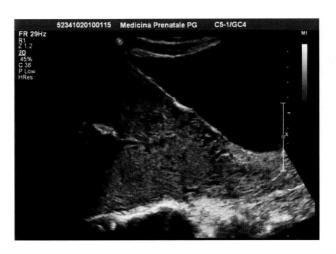

Figure 9.3 Placenta previa sonographic transabdominal view.

the vascularization not only in relation to the internal uterine orifice, but also in the context of the myometrium) [2].

Management of placenta previa

The RCOG guidelines in the management of placenta previa recommend in the third trimester to counsel the woman about the risks of preterm delivery, obstetric hemorrhage and the possible indication for blood transfusion and hysterectomy [2].

About half of the cases of placenta previa will not have antepartum bleeding, but in the cases of women with antepartum bleeding/hemorrhage, management will depend on the degree of bleeding and gestational age [3].

Tocolysis, for treatment of bleeding in these patients, may be useful in selected cases, but the use of prophylactic

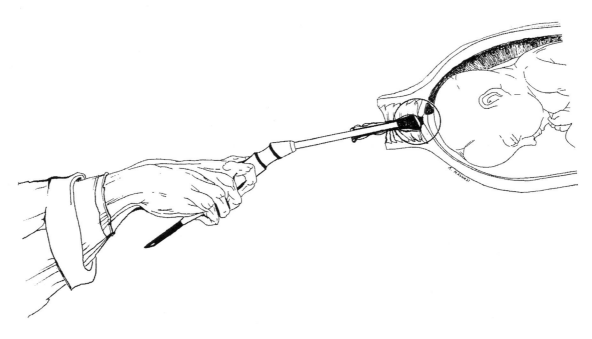

Figure 9.2 Transvaginal longitudinal ultrasonographic section in uterus at term of central placenta previa. (Modified from Malvasi A, Di Renzo GC. *Semeiotica Ostetrica*, Rome, Italy: CIC Edizioni Internazionali; 2012.)

tocolytics to prevent bleeding has not been demonstrated to have benefits. Conservative management is possible in case of low bleeding and if the fetus is not mature.

Mode of delivery

In accordance with the Italian Guidelines (Italian National Institute of Heath–National System of Guidelines [SNLG-ISS]) on cesarean delivery (January 2012), placenta previa represents an indication for cesarean delivery and must be performed in a tertiary-level hospital to manage possible fetal–maternal emergencies, in order to reduce perinatal/maternal mortality and morbidity [10] (Figure 9.4).

However, it is demonstrated that a trial of vaginal delivery is appropriate if the placental edge is at least 2 cm away from the internal os (Figure 9.5) and, moreover, according to the most recent scientific literature [11], more than two-third of women with the placenta edge to cervical os distance of >10 mm deliver vaginally without increased risk of hemorrhage [11]. So the distance of ≥11 mm from the placental edge to the cervical os can be considered a new cutoff for safely admitting a patient to a trial of labor [11]. According to the relationship of placental edge and the internal cervical os and to the degree of the eventually present/previous bleeding, the time of cesarean delivery can be modulated prior to 38 weeks, taking into account the possibility of inducing fetal lung maturity by the administration of corticosteroids.

Also, RCOG guidelines recommend cesarean delivery if the placental edge is less than 2 cm from the internal os in the third trimester. Moreover, in the case of previous cesarean delivery, the risk of massive hemorrhage and hysterectomy is higher, and cesarean delivery should be performed in a unit with a blood bank and facilities for high-dependency care [2].

A cesarean delivery in the case of placenta previa needs an expert team of obstetricians and anesthetists.

In patients with placenta previa maneuvers of dissection of the visceral peritoneum require care and attention because of the presence of dilated blood vessels that, if discontinued, can be a cause of bleeding, so that the subsequent incision of the lower uterine segment can be compromised (Figure 9.6).

If the incision of the uterus is transverse, it is important to know if the placenta is anterior or posterior. If anterior, it may be possible to go through the placenta or to define

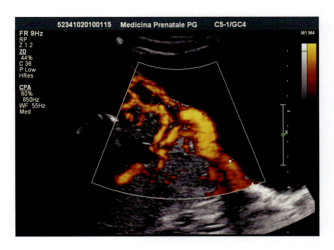

Figure 9.5 Doppler of the chorionic plate vessels in central placenta previa. In these cases, cesarean delivery at 38 weeks is recommended.

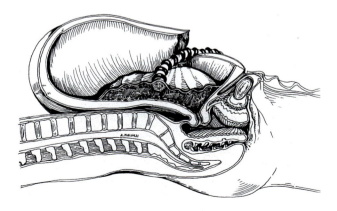

Figure 9.4 Anatomic longitudinal section of the uterus at term with posterior placenta previa during cesarean delivery after birth delivery.

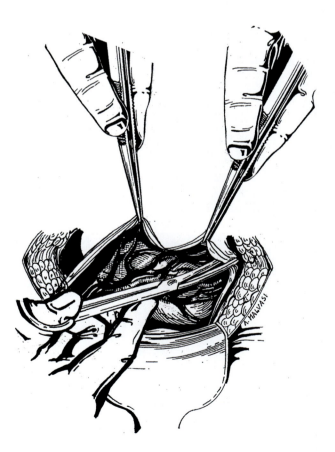

Figure 9.6 Incision of visceral peritoneum with Mayo scissors at cesarean delivery to avoid placental vessels of the lower uterine segment.

the placental edge going through the membranes above or below the placenta [3,12].

In the case of anterior low-lying placenta, in fact, there is a variable risk of bleeding at the moment of the incision of the lower uterine segment. In these cases, the placenta is between the uterine incision and the fetal presenting part. When the operator reaches the maternal side of the placenta inserted on the lower uterine segment, the loss of blood is caused, and it can be reduced by going through the placenta manually and quickly until the amniotic sac and the presenting part are reached, or by digitally punching the placenta to the membranes (Figure 9.7).

If the placenta previa is posterior and with a lateral insertion (minor previa), there are generally few problems both for the extraction and the afterbirth (Figure 9.8).

If the placenta previa is posterior but lies over the internal cervical os (major previa), instead, there are few problems during the fetal extraction, but it can often cause problems of bleeding due to the insertion of the placenta in the lower uterine segment. In these cases, intraoperative conservative treatment could be required.

The risk and the incidence of postpartum hemorrhage following placental removal is high, also because the lower segment is less muscular and occlusion of the sinuses of the placental bed can be inadequate, even without histological confirmation of placenta accreta [3,12,13]. Other procedures may be necessary to control bleeding (i.e., hemostatic balloon, uterine artery ligation, hemostatic sutures). If conservative methods are not enough to stop bleeding, hysterectomy is necessary.

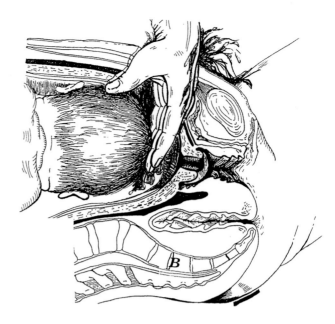

Figure 9.8 Manual fetal head extraction during cesarean delivery in marginal placenta previa.

PLACENTA ACCRETA

One of the most dreadful complications of placenta previa is its association with accretism, an abnormal attachment of the placenta to the myometrium. This pathological condition is characterized by the invasion of placental trophoblast into the endometrium beyond the Nitabuch layer due to a defect in the decidua basalis. If the trophoblast invades the myometrium or the serosa, placenta is defined as increta or percreta, respectively.

Any procedure or factor that produced a uterine scar (i.e., previous septostomy, curettage, myomectomy) is a risk factor for this condition, but prior cesarean delivery is the most important factor for placenta accreta [1], followed by placenta previa, advanced maternal age, grand multiparity, and Asherman syndrome [3]. Lachman et al. [14] assessed the frequency of the placenta accreta as 1:1420 deliveries.

Diagnosis of placenta accreta

The importance of making an antenatal diagnosis of placenta accreta is that it allows an appropriate timing of the delivery in order to minimize the potential maternal and neonatal risks.

The diagnosis of placenta accreta is very difficult, and its confirmation is possible only through pathological diagnosis. Already Hudon et al. [15] argued the importance of ultrasound in the diagnosis of placenta accreta. Especially, transvaginal ultrasound is considered a safe and complete tool to examine the lower uterine segment [16].

According to the last American Congress of Obstetricians and Gynecologists (ACOG) committee's opinion about placenta accreta, a normal placental attachment is characterized by the presence of a hypoechoic limit between the placenta and the myometrium.

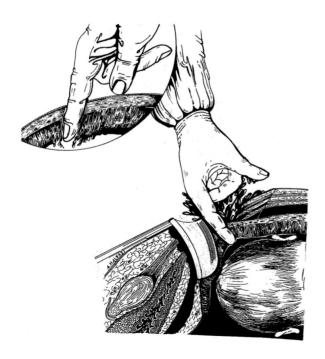

Figure 9.7 Going through the placenta manually and quickly until the amniotic sac and the presenting part are reached, or digitally punching through the placenta to the membranes.

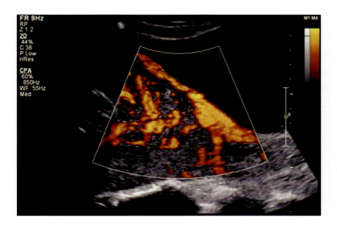

Figure 9.9 Angio mode 3D reconstruction of the chorionic plate vessels in placenta previa.

Finberg and Williams [17] showed that the use of two-dimensional (2D) ultrasound in the diagnosis of placenta accreta is based on the absence of a hypoechoic area normally interposed between myometrium and placenta. Catanzarite et al. [18] have proposed the use of color Doppler for the diagnosis of placenta accreta, and Jauniaux et al. [19] reported that the presence of hypoechoic lacunas in the context of the myometrium is strongly suggestive for the diagnosis of placenta accreta in its various degrees. Levine et al. [20] and Chou et al. [21] reported the usefulness of the color Doppler 2D with a variable sensitivity from 82.4% to 100% and a specificity between 92% and 96.8% in the diagnosis of placenta accreta; Shih et al. [22] and Chou et al. [23] also reported good diagnostic possibilities with three-dimensional (3D) power Doppler, even in the early stages of pregnancy (Figure 9.9).

The presence of an increasing number of placental lacunae is now considered the most predictive ultrasonographic sign of placenta accreta. However, other ultrasonographic signs are considered suggestive of placenta accreta (thinning of the myometrium overlying the placenta, loss of retroplacental "clear space," protrusion of the placenta into the bladder, increased vascularity of the uterine serosa–bladder interface, and turbulent blood flow through the lacunae on Doppler ultrasound) [16].

MRI is considered an additional tool to ultrasound, especially useful in cases of ambiguous findings, and it is particularly useful in cases of posterior placenta. Regarding the possible use of gadolinium contrast to delineate the placental surface related to the myometrium, it has been demonstrated to have no effects on the fetus [24], but the American College of Radiology recommends to avoid the use of this intravenous contrast [25] (Figure 9.10).

Management of placenta accreta

In the case of patients with abnormal placental insertion, the preparation and the performance of cesarean delivery are certainly more challenging than in the case of "simple" placenta previa [26]. Women with these placental pathologies, in fact, should be transferred to a tertiary perinatal care center, where a multidisciplinary team (anesthesiologist, obstetrician, pelvic surgeon, gynecologic oncologist, intensivist, maternal–fetal medicine specialist, neonatologist, hematologist, interventional radiologist), blood products and a neonatal intensive care unit are available to manage these high-risk patients [1,27].

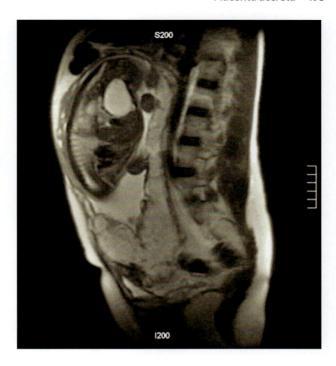

Figure 9.10 Placenta previa MRI mid-sagittal view.

It is important to make the patient aware that this is a life-threatening condition and that there is a possibility of demolitive operation in case of failure of conservative methods [28], with the acquisition of presurgical informed consent, due to the possibility of needing to perform a hysterectomy after the cesarean delivery to control the hemorrhage [29,30].

The timing of the delivery should be different depending on individual circumstances, but it has been demonstrated that both maternal and neonatal outcomes are high in case of delivery at 34 weeks of gestation. The administration of antenatal corticosteroid should be individualized, as well as the choice of the type of anesthetic techniques, because both the general type and the regional one have been shown to be safe [16].

Surgical technique

After the diagnosis of placenta accreta and the identification of the site of placental insertion, the hysterotomy should be done on a placenta-free region. Sometimes this means to do it in the fundal or posterior wall of the uterus [1]. The choice of a midline vertical incision may be considered for higher exposure if hysterectomy becomes necessary [16]. After the delivery of the baby, the placenta should not be removed [1]. The decision to leave the placenta in situ is made to avoid severe hemorrhagic morbidity [16]. Uterotonic drugs should be administrated to avoid uterine atony and to reduce possible bleeding. At this point, if there is an intraoperative confirmation of placenta accreta, it should be quickly decided to proceed with hysterectomy. In this case, the hysterotomy incision should first be closed. If the placental invasion is through the anterior uterine wall to the bladder, during hysterectomy, a dissection between the bladder and the uterus/placenta is required (sometimes it is necessary to perform a cystotomy) [1]. The decision to perform a subtotal hysterectomy is related to the presence and to the amount of bleeding from the surface of the cervix [1,16]. After the removal of the uterus and placenta, the entire pelvis should be inspected.

A possible alternative approach includes ligating the cord close to the fetal surface, removing the cord, and leaving the placenta in situ. The outcome of this approach is unpredictable (possible later hysterectomy), so it could be performed only if the patient has a high desire for future fertility and if there is a hemodynamic stability [16].

Conservative management

In order to allow future fertility and to reduce morbidity related to peripartum hysterectomy, a conservative management can be taken into consideration. Independently of the type of approach used, in all these cases, when the uterus is closed after delivery, the placenta is left in situ. The possible conservative strategies are: pelvic artery embolization, administration of methotrexate, application of hemostatic sutures (Figure 9.11), pelvic devascularization and application of balloon tamponade [1,16].

Proposed protocol to manage postpartum hemorrhage

The frequent association between placenta previa and accretism is related to a greater maternal morbidity and mortality due to the higher risk of postpartum hemorrhage (PPH), which is the leading cause of maternal death worldwide. In addition to death, serious morbidity may follow.

The treatment of massive PPH can be summarized in two points: replacing circulating blood volume to maintain perfusion and tissue oxygenation and stopping the bleeding by treating the causes or using surgical procedures.

Treatment options of PPH during cesarean delivery provide conservative management: uterotonic drugs, external compression with specific uterine sutures (B-Lynch, Hayman, Cho), intrauterine packing (Figure 9.12) and selective devascularization by ligation (Figure 9.13) or embolization of the uterine arteries or of the internal iliac arteries in relation to the amount of bleeding and to the success of procedures to reduce bleeding. Failure of these options requires hysterectomy.

Uterine compression sutures and balloon tamponade can be combined to apply pressure synergistically to both surfaces of the myometrium (the "sandwich" approach), and this procedure has been described as effective in cases of persistent uterine atony and massive hemorrhage.

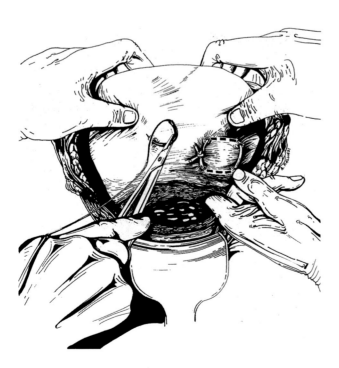

Figure 9.11 Hemostatic sutures of lower uterine segment during cesarean delivery with anterior placenta previa-accreta.

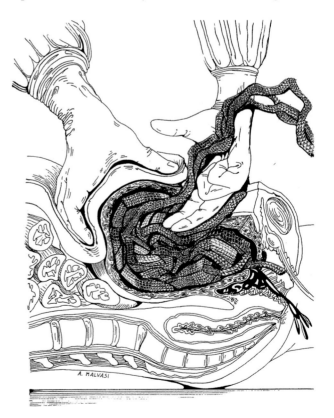

Figure 9.12 Anatomical sagittal section of the uterus at term after placenta-previa delivery and intrauterine packing to stop uterine bleeding.

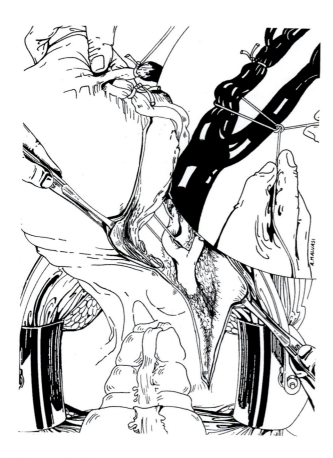

Figure 9.13 Posterior view of the uterus after placenta previa removal and right iliac artery ligation. If this surgical treatment is ineffective, cesarean hysterectomy should be mandatory.

We have experienced a specific conservative management protocol to treat patient undergoing cesarean delivery with PPH in cases of placenta previa major and/or accreta, based on clinical findings, sonography and MRI, planned at 32–34 weeks of gestation. Our conservative approach is characterized by a philosophy of liberal use of resources and treatment options/devices with the contemporary involvement of all professionals in a multidisciplinary approach.

The multidisciplinary team includes gynecologists, anesthesiologists, interventional radiologists, blood bank, central laboratory, midwives and, in a few cases, urologists and general surgeons.

The main aspects of this organizational model are as follows:

- Extensive information and discussion with the patient and the couple of issues related to risk factors
- The presence of interventional radiologists in the surgery room
- Temporary clamping of uterine vessels before placental delivery
- Systematic association of B-Lynch suture and Bakri-balloon application ("sandwich" approach)

According to this protocol, the patient is adequately hydrated during the 4 hours before intervention (1000 mL of saline solution 4 hours before the surgery and 1000 mL 1 hour before) and wears support stockings. Central venous catheter (CVC) is applied before surgery. Cells separator, four blood bags (two ready for use and two in standby) and portable digital angiography must be available in the operating room. A radiolucent operating table, medical thermal blankets and lead aprons are used for the procedure. Positioning of the graduate sterile bag is aimed at the evaluation of the blood loss during cesarean delivery.

The protocol for management of PPH used in our institution can be briefly summarized as follows:

1. Preliminary prophylactic transfemoral/transhumeral catheterization using 5 French catheter: this is the only step that is not applied in case of urgency and/or emergency.
2. Delivery of the fetus, administration of oxytocics (carbetocine) within 1 minute, temporary clamping of uterine arteries by ring forceps, followed by placental delivery.
3. Multiple square endouterine hemostatic sutures. Their application (on the anterior or posterior uterine wall) is related to the prevalent site of bleeding.
4. Preparation of B-Lynch compressive sutures.
5. Application of hydrostatic balloon (Bakri balloon) and partial filling with 30–60 mL of saline solution.
6. Hysterorrhaphy.
7. Repositioning of uterus with:
   a. Hydrostatic balloon inflation with a maximum of 400 mL (depending on the size of the uterus)
   b. B-Lynch ligature, followed by further inflation of 100 mL of saline solution in the Bakri balloon (Figure 9.14).

   When necessary, especially in case of previous cesarean delivery, application of surgical sealants.

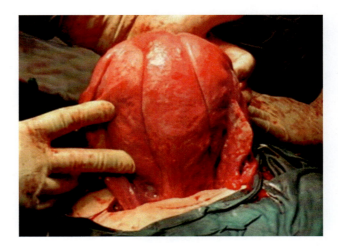

Figure 9.14 Posterior view of complete B-Lynch technique during cesarean delivery in placenta previa-accreta.

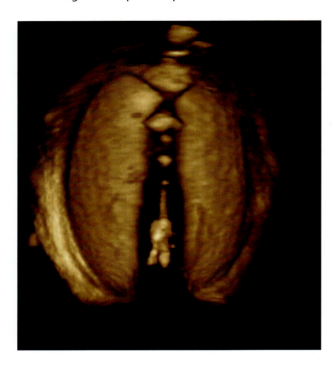

Figure 9.15 3D reconstruction of Bakri balloon in uterine cavity in combined technique B-Lynch and Bakri balloon application in placenta accreta.

8. If these maneuvers fail, the next step is the devascularizing ligature/selective embolization of the uterine arteries.
9. If all the above described procedures fail, hysterectomy.

Monitoring of maternal hematologic parameters is carried out 24 hours before cesarean delivery and 2 hours after the procedure, then every 2–4 hours for the following 24 hours, in relation to clinical conditions/blood loss and, finally, at 48 hours.

Blood transfusion is performed if the hemoglobin values are less than 7 g/dL and the hematocrit values are less than 21%.

The Bakri balloon is removed 24 hours after delivery after rectal administration (30 minutes before) of 400 mcg misoprostol as uterotonic drug (Figure 9.15).

REFERENCES

1. Perez-Delboy A, Wright JD. Surgical management of placenta accreta: To leave or remove the placenta? *BJOG* 2014;121(2):163–9.
2. Royal College of Obstetricians and Gynecologists (RCOG). Placenta Praevia, Placenta Praevia Accreta, and Vasa Praevia: Diagnosis and Management (Green-top 27), 2011.
3. Oxford Desk Reference. In: Arulkumaran S, Regan L, Papageorghiou AT, Monga A, Farquharson DIM, eds. *Obstetrics and Gynecology*. Oxford, UK: Oxford University Press; 2011, p. 402.
4. Reddy UM, Abuhamad AZ, Levine D, Saade GR. Fetal imaging. *J Ultrasound Med* 2014;33:745–57.
5. Makhseed M, el-Tomi N, Moussa M. A retrospective analysis of pathological placental implantation site and penetration. *Int J Obstet Gynecol* 1994;47:127–34.
6. Taipale P, Hiilesmaa V, Ylostalo P. Transvaginal ultrasonography at 18–23 weeks in predicting placenta previa in delivery. *Ultrasound Obstet Gynecol* 1998;12:422–5.
7. Becker RH, Vonk R, Mende BC, Ragosch V, Entezami M. The relevance of placental location at 20–23 gestational weeks for prediction of placenta previa at delivery: Evaluation of 8650 cases. *Ultrasound Obstet Gynecol* 2001;17:496–501.
8. Oppenheimer L, Holmes P, Simpson N, Dabrowsky A. A diagnosis of low-lying placenta: Can migration in the third trimester predict outcome? *Ultrasound Obstet Gynecol* 2001;18:100–2.
9. Oyelese Yl, Catanzarite V, Prefumo F, Lashley S, Schachter M, Tovbin Y, Goldstein V, Smulian JC. Vasa previa: The impact of prenatal diagnosis on outcomes. *Obstet Gynecol* 2004;103(5 Pt 1):937–42.
10. Ministero della Salute. *Taglio cesareo: Una scelta appropriate e consapevole—Seconda parte*. Rome, Italy: Ministero della Salute, SNLG-ISS; 2012.
11. Vergani P, Ornaghi S, Pozzi I et al. Placenta previa: Distance to internal os and mode of delivery. *Am J Obstet Gynecol* 2009;201:266.e1–5.
12. James DK, Steer PJ, Weiner CP, Gonik B. *High Risk Pregnancy: Management Options* (Expert Consult - Online and Print), 4th ed.; 2010, p. 1038.
13. Cunningham FG, Leveno KJ, Bloom SL, Hauth JC, Rouse DJ, Spong CY, eds. *Williams Obstetrics*, 23rd ed. New York, NY: McGraw-Hill.
14. Lachman E, Mali A, Gino G, Burnstein M, Stark M. Placenta accrete with placenta previa after previous caesarean sections a growing danger in modern obstetrics. *Harefauh* 2000;16:628–31.
15. Hudon L, Belfort M, Broome D. Diagnosis and management of placenta percreta: A review. *Obstet Gynecol Surv* 1998;53:509–17.
16. American College of Obstetricians and Gynecologists, Committee on Obstetric Practice (ACOG). *Committee opinion. Placenta Accreta*. Number 529. July 2012. Washington, DC: ACOG.
17. Finberg HJ, Williams JW. Placenta accrete: Prospective sonographic diagnosis in patients with placenta previa and prior caesarean section. *J Ultrasound Med* 1992;11:333–43.
18. Catanzarite VA, Stanco LM, Schrimmer DR, Conroy C. Managing placenta previa/accreta. *Contemp Ob Gyn* 1996;41:66–95.
19. Jauniaux E, Toplis P, Nicolaides K. Sonographic diagnosis of a non-previa placenta accreta. *Ultrasound Obstet Gynecol* 1996;7:58–60.
20. Levine D, Hulka CA, Ludmir J, Li W, Edelman RR. Placenta accrete: Evaluation with color Doppler US, Power Doppler US, and MR imaging. *Radiology* 1997;205:773–6.

21. Chou MM, Ho ESC, Lee YH. Prenatal diagnosis of placenta previa accrete by transabdominal color Doppler ultrasound. *Ultrasound Obstet Gynecol* 2000; 15:28–35.
22. Shih JC, Cheng WF, Shyu MK, Lee CN, Hsieh FJ. Power Doppler evidence of placenta accrete appearing in the first trimester. *Ultrasound Obstet Gynecol* 2002;19:623–5.
23. Chou MM, Tseng JJ, Ho ESC. The application of three-dimensional color power Doppler ultrasound in the description of abnormal uteroplacental angio-architecture in placenta previa percreta. *Ultrasound Obstet Gynecol* 2002;19:625–7.
24. Webb JA, Thomsen HS, Marcos, SK. The use of iodinated and gadolinium contrast media during pregnancy and lactation. Members of Contrast Media Safety Commettee of European Society of Urogenital Radiology (ESUR). *Eur Radiol* 2005;15:1234–40.
25. Kanal E, Barkovich AJ, Bell C et al. ACR blue ribbon panel on MR safety. *AJR Am J Roentgenol* 2007;188: 1447–74.
26. Bręborowicz GH, Markwitz W, Gaca M et al. Conservative management of placenta previa complicated by abnormal placentation. *J Matern Fetal Neonatal Med* 2013;26(10):1012–5.
27. Timmermans S, van Hof AC, Duvekot JJ. Conservative management of abnormally invasive placentation. *Obstet Gynecol Surv* 2007;62(8): 529–39.
28. Chan BC, Lam HS, Yuen JH, Lam TP, Tso WK, Pun TC, Lee CP. Conservative management of placenta praevia with accreta. *Hong Kong Med J* 2008; 14(6):479–84.
29. Rahman J, Al-Ali M, Qutub HO, Al-Suleiman SS, Al-Jama FE, Rahman MS. Emergency obstetric hysterectomy in a university hospital: A 25-year review. *J Obstet Gynaecol* 2008;28(1):69–72.
30. Omole-Ohonsi A, Olayinka HT. Emergency peripartum hysterectomy in a developing country. *J Obstet Gynaecol Can* 2012;34(10):954–60.

The proactive use of balloons for management of postpartum hemorrhage in cesarean delivery

YAKOV ZHUKOVSKIY

The matter of vital importance in obstetrical hemorrhage management is timely recognition of its severity [1]. But clinical estimation of blood loss, especially in cesarian delivery (CD), is notoriously imprecise. In spite of routine uterotonics administration, major obstetric hemorrhage is common, even in women who seem at low risk [2]. Besides we should remember that the blood loss in CD may be partially or even completely concealed [3]. And any surgeon can get into a situation of finding a pool of blood under the patient only after finishing the operation and removing surgical drapes.

In our opinion there are *objective reasons* for CD hemorrhage complications. These reasons originate from the existent technique of CD. After the uterine repair a surgeon becomes unable to keep basic surgical rules. He cannot provide complete intrauterine hemostasis, prevent blood clot accumulation in the cavity, and obliterate dead space in the wound. When the uterine incision is stitched, the uterine cavity immediately turns into dead space under the uterine seam. And this dead space may harbor both concealed bleeding and blood clot accumulation. Intrauterine clots as well as retained parts of placenta are well-known causes of hemorrhage. So the concealed blood loss often results in dramatic delay in recognition of its severity and ill-timed treatment [4,5].

As main complications start in the uterine cavity after the stitching of the hysterotomic incision, a consequential reaction is to do something before the closure of the wound to avoid these problems. One easily comes to the idea of *uterine cavity temporal occlusion*, until clotting all potentially bleeding vessels. This occlusion should be reversible, noninvasive, and atraumatic. After this maneuver the uterus should be left unaffected, without any bleeding and blood clots and with proper lochia discharge.

Our idea of this uterine occlusion is to occupy the cavity immediately after emptying the uterus with an easy expandable thin-walled silicon balloon.

But the secure placement of an expanding inflated balloon inside the newly incised and stitched uterus is possible only when we obey some clear, strict demands. The balloon should

- Be easily and safely placed into the uterus via the incision.
- Provide minimal sufficient pressure on the uterine wall during the whole procedure to avoid overstretching the newly stitched incision.
- Occupy entirely the whole cavity, covering all potentially bleeding vessels.
- Be easily removed per vias naturalis after its usage.

Having revised all existent methods and balloon models, we could not find the ones that would meet all the mentioned demands. So we had to create our own method and our own kit for uterine cavity balloon occlusion (UCBO).

THE CORE OF THE METHOD AND THE DEVICE FOR ITS IMPLEMENTATION

The basic idea of the method uses the principle of connected vessels to fill the balloon to gravity.

One of the vessels is a thin-walled easily expandable *intrauterine balloon*, and the second is a *tank* placed at the required height above the balloon level. Both vessels are connected with a rather wide tube that stays *constantly open* during the whole procedure. It allows the solution to flow freely back and forth between the balloon and the tank (Figure 10.1). Filling the balloon using the principle of connected vessels (Figure 10.2) gives numerous crucial clinical benefits, as the surgeon is able to

- Maintain constant required pressure in the cavity that constantly changes its size.
- Use the appropriate filling solution volume for any individual case.
- Occupy the whole cavity covering all the potentially bleeding vessels without interfering with the spontaneous contractile activity of the uterus.
- Receive visual information about uterine activity by the changing level of solution in the tank.
- Decide precisely when it is time to remove the balloon.
- Leave the cavity without bleeding and clots.
- Provide proper cavity drainage in the postoperative period.

THE ABDOMINAL INSERTION TECHNIQUE OF OUR BALLOON CATHETER

The essential point of the UCBO method is correct placement of the balloon in the cavity via hysterotomic incision. There are three steps to follow:

1. Insert the deflated balloon into the cavity.
2. Stitch the incision.
3. Fill the balloon using the principle of connected vessels.

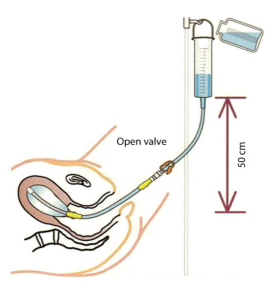

Figure 10.1 The principle of connected vessels activated (solution passing freely).

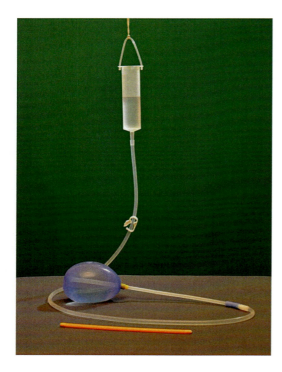

Figure 10.2 Uterine balloon filled due to gravity. The orange thin plastic stick is the Probe-Plug.

The axial tube of the balloon catheter should be inserted through the incision, into the cervix and vagina, and then outside the patient's body.

But sometimes it is a challenging task to find the internal cervical ostium from the inside of the uterine cavity without any visual control. To noticeably simplify this step, we created an auxiliary tool specially designed for retrograde insertion of the balloon catheter. We named this tool "Probe-Plug." It has no analogs among existent obstetric balloon sets.

The Probe-Plug is an orange plastic stick: its length is 25 cm and its diameter is 5.5 mm. It is flexible and soft enough to avoid perforation or trauma of the uterus during the insertion, and rigid enough to allow the internal cervical ostium to be found easily without visual control. So by this auxiliary tool we easily penetrate the cervical canal and move the Probe-Plug further into the vagina (Figure 10.3). Then we connect the balloon catheter to the proximal end of the Probe-Plug and move them together through the vagina until the deflated balloon base comes into contact with the internal cervical ostium (Figure 10.4).

In some cases we may use the Probe-Plug as a plug for saving the solution in the balloon when we attach the vaginal balloon catheter.

After repair of the uterus (Figure 10.5) we start filling the intrauterine balloon. For this we remove the Probe-Plug and connect the catheter to the tank pre-filled with the warm solution placed half a meter above the patient. Turning on the connecting tube we start filling

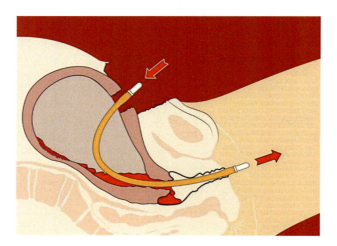

Figure 10.3 Probe-Plug passing through the cervical canal.

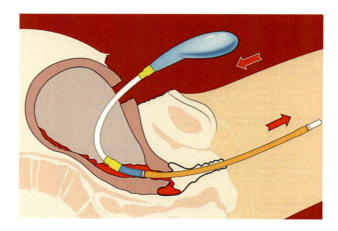

Figure 10.4 The balloon catheter placement by means of the Probe-Plug.

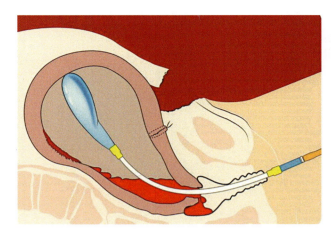

Figure 10.5 Appropriate placement of the balloon after stitching of the incision.

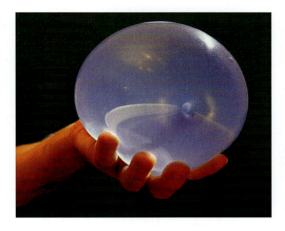

Figure 10.7 Now the balloon contains 1700 mL and remains soft enough.

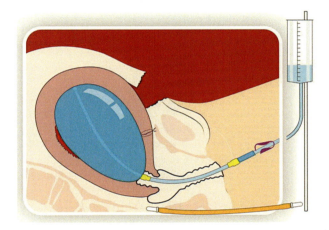

Figure 10.6 The whole cavity secure occlusion.

the balloon. Filling is over when the level of solution in the tank has become stable. This indicates that the cavity is totally occupied with the balloon, and we precisely know the magnitude of the predetermined pressure (Figure 10.6).

Filling to the gravity implies that the balloon is quite large. It needs very low pressure for its expanding and easily receives up to 1700 mL of solution (Figure 10.7). Its task is only to hold the solution within the uterine cavity and to prevent escape of the solution into the vagina and fallopian tubes. While the connecting tube stays open during the procedure, the balloon is able to react spontaneously on uterine contraction by changing its volume. Adjusting the height of the tank allows selection of any required pressure on the uterine wall for any individual case.

The first cases of application revealed that achievement of intrauterine hemostasis requires surprisingly low pressure (10–15 mm Hg). Our early experience revealed that even just a touch of uterine wall with the balloon is enough to achieve a preventive effect.

In rare cases of blood leakage over the balloon, we can arrest bleeding by raising the tank to increase the pressure.

But there we can encounter the problem of protruding the balloon from the uterus. The expulsion of the balloon may interrupt the procedure. Thus we may have a problem of holding the uterine balloon in its place.

INCREASING THE EFFECTIVENESS OF THE METHOD WITH VAGINAL BALLOON CATHETER USAGE

Today's recommendations to prevent the protruding of the balloon by packing the vagina with gauze cannot be estimated as an acceptable solution. The method of making sufficient counterpressure for holding the balloon in the cavity and conducting proper blood loss monitoring in the case of ongoing bleeding seems to not be realistic.

If we have managed to keep the expanding balloon in the uterine cavity, we will be able to arrest any bleeding, as we can always create external pressure exceeding the internal arterial blood pressure in the bleeding vessel. Even a temporal hemostasis is vitally important to give time for a clinician, but in most cases we can achieve the completed one.

So we had to create an additional vaginal balloon catheter. Its purposes are to hold the uterine balloon in the cavity and at the same time make it possible to detect uterine bleeding.

The vaginal catheter is an independent module that can be freely coaxially attached to the intrauterine balloon when we need to hold it within the cavity (Figure 10.8a). The uterine balloon should be deflated a little to fit the cavity and avoid protruding. Only after this may we start using the vaginal balloon. Being deflated, the vaginal balloon catheter is placed up close to the base of moderately inflated intrauterine balloon (Figure 10.8b). Then the vaginal balloon is filled with 120–150 mL of solution (Figure 10.8c). Thus the vaginal module is safely fixed in the upper part of the vagina, adjoining the bottom side of the intrauterine balloon. Any possibility of intrauterine balloon prolapse into the vagina during its refilling even with an open cervix is absolutely excluded.

Due to the fact that the inner diameter of the axial tube of the vaginal catheter is 19 mm, and the external

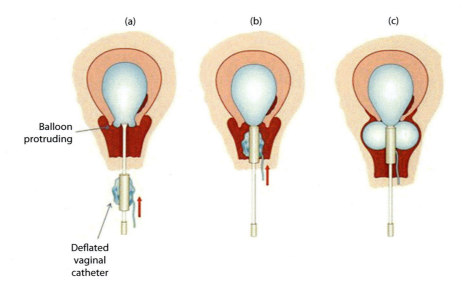

Figure 10.8 (a–c) Assembling the uterine and vaginal balloons.

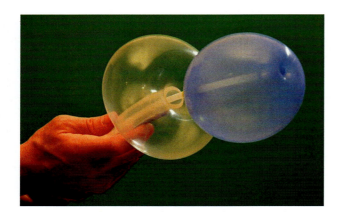

Figure 10.9 Uterine and vaginal balloon catheters assembled (note the gap between axial tubes).

diameter of the uterine catheter axial tube is 7 mm, there is a gap of about 12 mm between the two coaxial placed axial tubes (Figure 10.9). The gap allows blood and even clots to run freely out in case of uterine bleeding. Thus a surgeon is capable of evaluating the effectiveness of applying this method. Also it is guaranteed that there is no concealed bleeding in any segment of the birth canal, because this space is fully occupied with the uterine and vaginal balloons.

INDICATIONS FOR THE UCBO

Because we regard UCBO as a prophylactic measure, then we have to decide to what group of patients it is addressed. Usually obstetricians start application of a balloon for the patients who are at high risk of hemorrhage in CD.

Before the closure of the uterine incision, a surgeon encounters the dilemma of whether he or she should use this unique transitory access to the uterine cavity for UCBO or not. At this crucial moment nobody in the world is able to recognize the case with oncoming problems [6].

And when complications start after closure of the incision, any surgeon regrets his denial to use a balloon, as he has to fight a "near-miss" situation.

The only obstacle for wide UCBO application is a surgeon's subconscious fear to waste the balloon, having no evident indications for its usage. But we know well that only about one-third of postpartum hemorrhage (PPH) cases have identifiable risk factors [7]. The natural desire to "save money" in this case appears to be most misleading. In reality, wide preventive usage of the method gives huge economic effect, as more and more often we manage to prevent "near-miss" cases, and each of them costs $50,000–$70,000 for medical budget. Costs of treatment for cases with severe maternal outcomes significantly exceed the expenses on wide usage of UCBO.

The summarized calculation of expenses after method implementation in the Tyumen region of the Russian Federation has revealed a $1.3 million budget saving during 1 year [8].

Thus, we cannot find reasonable contraindications for this proactive management of CD.

Results

An intrauterine balloon provides direct pressure on the bleeding vessel, and for 100% efficiency we need only to create appropriate pressure.

Therefore, theoretically, the efficiency of our UCBO should be close to 100%. Actually it exceeds 95%. In cases where the vascular system of the uterus was intact, the technique almost always works.

Retrospective analysis of rare cases requiring surgical intervention showed that the integrity of the vascular system of the uterus had been broken (uterine laceration, retained lobule of placenta accreta, congenital diseases of the uterine vessels, etc.).

Processing the results, we found a dramatic reduction in postpartum endometritis cases [8]. This leads us to a new understanding of infectious complication pathogenesis in CD.

Endometritis

Bacterial colonization of the uterine cavity is detected in 94% of postpartum patients, but only a small fraction actually develop the infection. Other factors different than colonization play their part in pathogenesis [9].

In our opinion the role of blood clots trapped in the cavity of the uterus is underestimated. Particularly in CD there are conditions predisposing this accumulation of nonviable tissue inside the uterus. During the operation the blood usually collects in the cavity and its discharge is impeded. Contractive function of the incised uterus is insufficient, drainage of the cavity is poor, and the cervix frequently is closed. The pathological contents stored in the uterus are inaccessible after closure of the incision. This inviable tissue trapped in the uterus very soon becomes a nutrient medium for microbial growth.

It is a well-known clinical fact that after the evacuation of these contents the recovery is quickly achieved.

And one more fact that confirms the role of inviable tissue in the cavity as a cause of inflammatory process development is that there were practically no cases of endometritis in the group of our UCBO preventive application patients. In our opinion, this could be possible because we prevented the accumulation of pathological contents by the balloon occlusion. After the removal of the deflated balloon, we leave the cavity dry and clean with proper drainage (Figure 10.10).

Discussion

Once retained products and genital tract trauma have been excluded, an obstetrician has only four options to provide intrauterine hemostasis:

- Uterotonic medications
- Intrauterine balloon
- Uterine artery ligation/embolization
- Uterine compression sutures

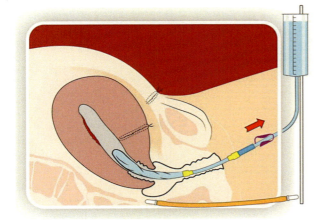

Figure 10.10 The deflated uterine balloon removal from the recovering uterus.

Uterotonics

Some data show that 10%–21% of women fail to respond to treatment with conventional uterotonics [10].

Retrospective analyses of PPH cases and severe maternal outcomes showed that uterotonics were applied in nearly 93% [7].

When giving uterotonic therapy, the clinician usually counts on a sufficient amount of muscle tissue being ready to respond, but in a number of cases (lower segment placentation, cicatricial changes of myometrium, etc.) the uterine source of hemorrhage does not have enough myometrial tissue to compress bleeding vessels. In such cases uterotonics usage appears to be unsuccessful [11].

But when the uterotonics fail the bleeding can be arrested with the intrauterine balloon.

Uterine artery ligation/embolization

This technique may be helpful to arrest corpus uteri hemorrhage, but it often fails in case of low segment bleeding. This failure can be explained by the fact that the low part of the uterus receives blood from a highly interconnected system, so after bilateral uterine arterial ligation, the uterine blood flow is compensated for by the presence of rich anastomoses between the internal pudendal anastomotic branches and the uterine artery [12].

But when the uterine artery ligation/embolization fails, the bleeding can be arrested with the intrauterine balloon.

Uterine compressing sutures

The data on the effectiveness of uterine compressing sutures are rather controversial: the declared failure rate ranges from 25% to 50% [13,14].

Compression sutures are generally more risky than vessels ligation. The most common complications involve variations of uterine ischemic necrosis. Some of them are potentially life threatening; others jeopardize any further scope for pregnancy [15]. A case of total uterine necrosis was reported, following which a hysterectomy was done [16].

There are many other unique complications: closure of the uterine cavity with blood entrapment resulting in infection, synechia of varying degrees, uterine deformation, pyometra, peritonitis, pelvic adhesions, erosion into the lower segment of the uterus, etc. [17–25].

And in order to avoid these flaws of the method, we are again forced to use the intrauterine balloon by combining it with sutures. We modified the well-known technique of "uterine sandwich" [25] but made it much safer.

The main idea is to prevent excessive injuring pressure of surgical thread and to shorten the duration of the compression.

In our case the sutures are not tightly knotted over a partially filled intrauterine balloon. After this we finally fill the balloon using the principle of connecting vessels to select minimal sufficient myometrium compression between the external knotted sutures and internal balloon expanding. Our method implies that the compression continues for quite a short period of time (about 2 hours), only until hemostasis is achieved. Then, by deflating the balloon we release the tightness of the sutures. This allows us to cease the compression of the myometrium and to encourage earlier restoration of its perfusion.

Finally having reviewed all four options to arrest PPH, we have to confess that the intrauterine balloon is the most actionable measure among the others.

But our priority is to avoid invasive methods where possible, so we have started to use "the intrauterine balloon plus the vaginal balloon" technique instead of "the intrauterine balloon plus the sutures." We hold the intrauterine balloon in place by the vaginal balloon, instead of doing it with sutures as it was in the previous technique. By now we have already had promising results in combined application of uterine and vaginal balloons.

CONCLUSIONS

Hemorrhage and infectious complications of CD do not depend fully on the proficiency of the surgeon due to anatomical and functional features of the organ that undergoes surgery. Pharmacological agents are not efficient in a certain number of cases.

The uterine incision is made for an absolutely different purpose. And this access into the cavity lasting for only a few minutes is a precious accidental gift for a surgeon. Evidently the right decision is not to miss this chance to take certain effective preventive measures.

The UCBO fully complies with the basic principles of surgery.

Clotting all potentially bleeding vessels by proactively covering the entire inner uterine surface with a silicon film proves to be an efficient way to prevent basic CD complications.

UCBO application allows an obstetrician to lay aside pharmacological and surgical measures for managing hemorrhagic and infectious CD complications.

REFERENCES

1. Gary Cunningham F, Leveno KJ, Bloom SL et al., eds. *Williams Obstetrics*, 24th ed. New York, NY: McGraw-Hill Medical; 2014:781.
2. Sheehan SR, Montgomery AA, Carey M, McAuliffe FM, Eogan M, Gleeson R, Geary M, Murphy DJ; ECSSIT Study Group. Oxytocin bolus versus oxytocin bolus and infusion for control of blood loss at elective caesarean section: Double blind, placebo controlled, randomised trial. *BMJ* 2011;343:d4661.
3. Knight M, Callaghan WM, Berg C et al. Trends in postpartum hemorrhage in high resource countries: A review and recommendations from the International Postpartum Hemorrhage Collaborative Group. *BMC Pregnancy Childbirth* 2009;9:55.
4. Kayem G, Kurinczuk JJ, Alfirevic Z, Spark P, Brocklehurst P, Knight M, U.K. Obstetric Surveillance System (UKOSS). Uterine compression sutures for the management of severe postpartum hemorrhage. *Obstet Gynecol* 2011;117(1):14–20.
5. Fleming D, Gangopadhyay R, Karoshi M, Arulkumaran S. Maternal deaths from Major Obstetric Hemorrhage in the UK: Changing evidence from the confidential enquiries (1985–2011). In: Sir Arulkumaran S, Karoshi M, Keith LG, Lalonde LG, B-Lynch C, eds. *A Comprehensive Textbook of Postpartum Hemorrhage*. 2nd ed. London, UK: Sapiens; 2012:163.
6. Antony KM, Dildy GA 3rd. Postpartum hemorrhage: The role of the Maternal-Fetal Medicine specialist in enhancing quality and patient safety. *Semin Perinatol* 2013;37(4):246–56.
7. Sheldon WR, Blum J, Vogel JP, Souza JP, Gülmezoglu AM, Winikoff B, WHO Multicountry Survey on Maternal and Newborn Health Research Network. Postpartum haemorrhage management, risks, and maternal outcomes: Findings from the World Health Organization Multicountry Survey on Maternal and Newborn Health. *BJOG* 2014;121(Suppl 1):5–13.
8. Zhukovskiy YG, Kukarskaya II. Preventive abdominal application of Zhukovskiy Balloon in Cesarean section in a series of 289 cases. *Fourth International Symposium MSRM NESA*; September 19–21, 2014, Greece. Book of Abstracts, 44.
9. Berghella V, eds. *Obstetric Evidence-Based Guidelines*, 2nd ed. London, UK: Informa Healthcare; 2012:247.
10. Mousa HA, Cording V, Alfirevic Z. Risk factors and interventions associated with major primary postpartum hemorrhage unresponsive to first-line conventional therapy. *Acta Obstet Gynecol Scand* 2008;87(6):652–61.
11. O'Grady JP, Gimovsky ML, Bayer-Zwirello LA, Giordano K, eds. *Operative Obstetrics*, 2nd ed. New York, NY: Cambridge University Press; 2008:163.
12. Palacios-Jaraquemada JM, García Mónaco R, Barbosa NE, Ferle L, Iriarte H, Conesa HA. Lower uterine blood supply: Extrauterine anastomotic system and its application in surgical devascularization techniques. *Acta Obstet Gynecol Scand* 2007;86:228–34.
13. Kayem G, Kurinczuk JJ, Alfirevic A et al. Uterine compression sutures for the management of severe postpartum hemorrhage. *Obstet Gynecol* 2011;117(1):14.
14. Gary Cunningham F, Leveno KJ, Bloom SL et al., eds. *Williams Obstetrics*, 24th ed. New York, NY: McGraw-Hill Medical; 2014:818.
15. Begum J, Pallave P, Ghose S. B-lynch: A technique for uterine conservation or deformation? A case report with literature review. *J Clin Diagn Res* 2014;8(4):OD01–OD03.
16. Friederich L, Roman H, Marpeau L. A dangerous development. *Am J Obstet Gynecol* 2007;196:92.
17. Ochoa M, Allaire AD, Stitely ML. Pyometria after hemostatic square suture technique. *Obstet Gynecol* 2002;99:506.

18. Alouini S, Coly S, Megier P et al. Multiple square sutures for postpartum hemorrhage: Results and hysteroscopic assessment. *Am J Obstet Gynecol* 2011:205(4):335.
19. Gottlieb AG, Pandipati S, Davis KM et al. Uterine necrosis. A complication of uterine compression sutures. *Obstet Gynecol* 2008:112:429.
20. Joshi VM, Shrivastava M. Partial ischemic necrosis of the uterus following a uterine brace compression suture. *BJOG* 2004;111:279.
21. Treloar EJ, Anderson RS, Andrews HG et al. Uterine necrosis following B-Lynch suture for primary postpartum haemorrhage. *BJOG* 2006:113:486.
22. Pechtor K, Richards B, Paterson H. Antenatal catastrophic uterine rupture at 32 weeks of gestation after previous B Lynch suture. *BJOG* 2010;117:889–91.
23. Akoury H, Sherman C. Uterine wall partial necrosis following combined B-Lynch and Chi-square sutures for the treatment of primary postpartum hemorrhage. *J Obstet Gynaecol Can* 2008;30:421–4.
24. Grotegut CA, Larsen FW, Jones MR, Livingston E. Erosion of a B-Lynch suture through the uterine wall: A case report. *J Reprod Med* 2004;49:849–52.
25. Danso D, Reginald P. Combined B-lynch suture with intrauterine balloon catheter triumphs over massive postpartum haemorrhage. *BJOG* 2002;109(8):963.

Exceptional situations after cesarean delivery and postpartum hemorrhage

JOSÉ M PALACIOS-JARAQUEMADA

INTRODUCTION

After the introduction of anesthesia and antisepsis, cesarean was considered a safe procedure for the mother and the fetus. Nowadays, it is one of the most common surgical procedures in obstetrics. But as happens with other medical techniques, cesarean delivery is not a procedure free from complications, and while many of them are uncommon, they can be severe and even life threatening [1]. Some cesarean complications usually provide time to be solved, but others, particularly those related to hemorrhage, do not. Placental blood flow at term is about 600–1000 mL/min; for this reason, some problems related with postpartum hemorrhage can modify the maternal hemodynamic state in a short time [2].

Other cesarean complications are difficult to diagnose, even with the current technology or in fully equipped hospitals. This group of problems may remain hidden until the obstetrician realizes that something is wrong. Sometimes diagnosis comes too late or implies the use of surgical maneuvers not habitual for obstetricians.

In this chapter we explain the common and uncommon cesarean complications mainly associated with postpartum hemorrhage [3], their diagnoses, and the simplest solutions for them. Due to the poor results in many cases, medical quotations are scarce or inexistent. Therefore, most of this text is based on my over-23-year personal experience in the treatment of these complications.

UNEXPECTED PLACENTA ACCRETA DURING PLACENTAL DETACHMENT

Focal invasions

An unexpected finding of placenta accreta during cesarean may be solved by different methods. In general, options depend on medical experience, surgical skills, and hospital resources. For this reason, there is not a unique or ideal treatment for all of them, but preventing massive or uncontrollable bleeding must be the primary aim. Unpredicted diagnosis of abnormal placentation after cesarean incision is not a common event. Today, it is possible to perform a correct diagnosis of abnormal placentation in most cases; clinical knowledge of risk factors in addition to the high sensitivity and specificity of ultrasound signs [4] allow us to detect 90%–95% of cases. In cases of doubt associated with the clinical practice or imaging studies, magnetic resonance imaging (MRI) performed in trained centers is an excellent tool to define the diagnosis. But even today, some cases of abnormal placentation may remain undiagnosed, even after two or three ultrasound studies (Figure 11.1).

We must remember that medical imaging studies are operator dependent, and mistakes by human factors need to be considered [5]. We must realize that this threat is possible, real, and that it happens in both developed and underdeveloped countries.

Because most cases of abnormal placentation are associated with placenta previa or lower placentation, visualization of engorged vessels or dark blue tissue protruded by the uterine segment during cesarean is highly suggestive of abnormal placentation (Figures 11.2 and 11.3). This suspicion is especially important in patients with previous cesarean or other uterine scars, such as those secondary to myomectomies (Figure 11.4) or D&C [6]. When the physical aspect of the lower segment is suspicious, the obstetrician could ask for help, or choose to perform a hysterotomy outside the invaded area (usually in the uterine fundus), or ask for help to attempt a resective conservative procedure (Figure 11.5a–c). Crossing the placenta, delivering the baby, and performing a quick hysterectomy is a very dangerous option without the possibility of turning back if bleeding is difficult to control (Figure 11.6).

In typical cases, unexpected abnormal placentation is suspected when the placenta is retained after a standard cesarean. Normally, after the fetus is delivered we need to wait some minutes for spontaneous placental detachment. But, if after this time and gentle cord traction or manual maneuvers nothing happens, we must suspect abnormal placentation. In these cases, increasing cord traction could end up in an acute uterine inversion or placental abruption with active bleeding; for this reason, it is recommended to move the uterus outside the abdomen to identify an adherent area. When the entire uterus is exposed, firm cord traction modifies the myometrium surface making the area with placental invasion clear. Because the only possibility to separate the myometrium and the adherent placenta is to cut between the two tissues (placenta and myometrium), we need to perform a simple technique to avoid consecutive bleeding of the placental bed. One of the simplest methods is to introduce two U stitches 2 cm outside the abnormal placentation area (horizontal and vertical) with absorbable suture number 1 (which includes all myometrial thickness) and then to perform a tight surgeon's knot. Then, detach the placenta manually up to the adherence area and carefully cut with electrocautery between the placenta and the myometrium. In general, this hemostatic method is enough to separate the uterus from the placenta without bleeding. However, if some residual bleeding is detected, using simple X stitches is

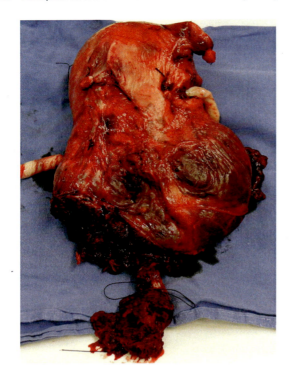

Figure 11.1 Hysterectomy piece of massive placenta percreta with parametrial invasion. One day before the surgery, the patient was diagnosed a placenta previa by three ultrasounds made in a reference center. By chance, the patient asked for a new ultrasound in another center and a diagnosis of massive placenta percreta was made. MRI was performed on the same day and confirms the diagnosis and also a parametrial invasion by axial slices. Obstetric background: 29 years old, one previous cesarean + IVF (in vitro fertilization).

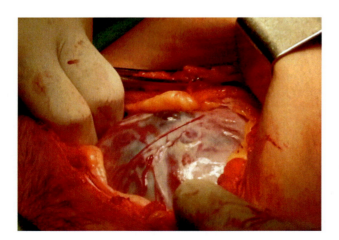

Figure 11.2 Unexpected placenta accreta during cesarean. Presence of newly formed vessels of dark blue tissue on the uterine segment is highly suggestive of abnormal placentation. Obstetric background: First pregnancy, no other antecedents were declared at that time. After cesarean she admitted two D&C for abortions at 9 and 14 weeks.

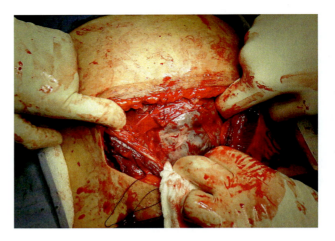

Figure 11.3 Unexpected placenta accreta–percreta. Obstetric background: 33 years old, one previous cesarean, one D&C + embolization by cesarean scar pregnancy (10 weeks). Three ultrasounds negative for abnormal placentation (placenta previa).

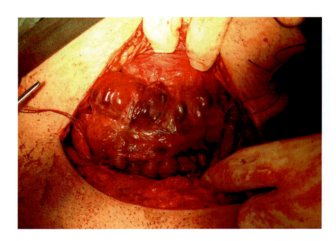

Figure 11.4 Unexpected placenta percreta during cesarean. Obstetric background: 35 years old, the patient had a laparoscopic myomectomy (5 cm) 3 years before she became pregnant. Ultrasound during pregnancy informed anterior placenta. Due to the clear segmental area below invasion, the obstetrician decided to perform a lower hysterotomy. The placenta was detached without additional bleeding, although anterior defect of plenty of newly formed vessels is evident, it was not touched or repaired.

probably the simplest option to stop any remaining blood loss. I particularly recommend covering the endouterine adhesive area with a double sheet of Surgicel and then fix it in place with two stitches of absorbable 000 suture. This material (regenerated cellulose) reduces the possibility of secondary endometrial adhesions, and it disappears in a couple of weeks.

According to personal experience, these types of focal placental adhesions are posterior and habitually the consequence of D&C for abortions. It is common in some countries that women avoid commenting on this episode

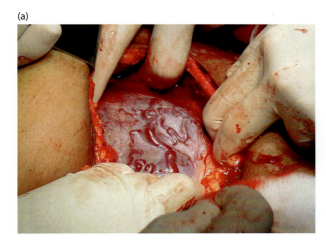
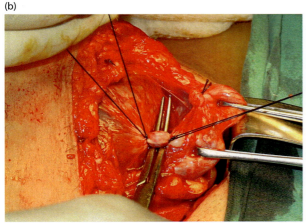
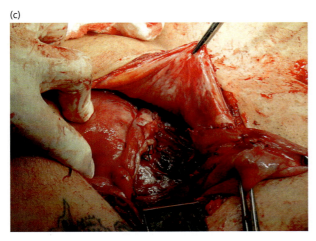

Figure 11.5 (a) Unexpected placenta accreta during cesarean. Obstetric background: 26 years old, one previous cesarean and one D&C by abortion made 3 months after cesarean. According to the patient's desire of future pregnancy, the obstetrician called for help to attempt a one-step conservative surgery for abnormal placentation. (b) Two Allis clamps pull up the bladder to identify and cut, between ligatures, all newly formed vessels between the uterus and the bladder. (c) Final aspect of one-step conservative surgery for abnormal placentation. All invaded tissues and the entire placenta were removed before uterine reconstruction. The procedure was made by Pfannenstiel incision.

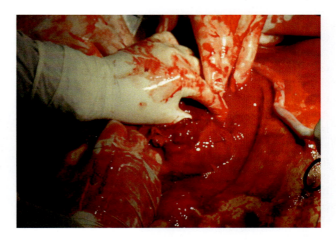

Figure 11.6 After crossing the placenta to deliver a baby, secondary bleeding by invaded tissues may be very difficult to control.

to their obstetrician, because they consider that this procedure was performed a long time ago, and most of them prefer to forget this event.

Massive hidden invasions

Unexpected and massive placental invasions may happen in patients with simple total occlusive placenta previa. In general, these cases have a clinical background of multiple cesareans, D&C, or curettage, but auxiliary diagnosis did not show or did not recognize signs of abnormal placentation. Always remember that association of multiple cesareans or curettage in patients with placenta previa is a recognized clinical high-risk factor for abnormal placentation, even after two or three negative ultrasounds. Although ultrasound is highly sensitive to suspect or to make a diagnosis of placental invasion, the method is operator dependent, and the results may differ according to experience or training. For this reason, to think that everything is fine after a negative ultrasound in high-risk patients may be a mistake [7]. Although it is uncommon nowadays, a frightening and life-threatening situation may occur when the obstetrician detaches the placenta and massive bleeding floods the pelvis in a few seconds. The scenario may range from continuous bleeding from the placental bed to a massive hemorrhage from multiple vessels. In the first case, we have time to compress the placental bed strongly, call for help, or attempt to use one of the standard uterine hemostatic procedures such as compression sutures, embolization, vessel ligatures, or perform a hysterectomy as a last resort. In the second case, when the bleeding is massive, acute, and uncontrollable, accurate measures to stop the bleeding need to be taken immediately because we can lose the patient in a few minutes [8,9]. To understand the real dimension of this problem, we need to remember that placental blood flow at term is about 800–1000 mL/min. During normal placental detachment, myometrium contraction provides the first hemostasis mechanism, which is absent in cases of abnormal placentation due to the myometrial thinning. When abnormal placentation is posterior and low, physical signs are not as evident as for anterior invaded placenta; in these cases myometrial weakening in addition to abnormal placentation make it possible for you to detach part or the entire uterus during placental detachment, a situation that usually turns the bleeding uncontrollable within seconds. Although the standard and automatic obstetric response is to perform an immediate hysterectomy, this is almost always a bad choice. To practice a hysterectomy under massive hemorrhage in a patient with distorted anatomy is almost always a recipe for disaster. In these cases, there is no time to call for help, to ask for blood, or to ask for the radiologist, and chaos occurs within a few minutes while the patient loses all her blood. It is completely understandable that it is not common to find papers that mention this type of complications.

A practical solution for this unusual but real complication is to compress the abdominal aorta immediately [2]. The uterus must be quickly exteriorized outside the abdomen, while a surgical exposure moves the intestines upward and the aortic division is instantaneously accessible to compress against the promontory. Internal aortic compression provides an excellent proximal control to the pelvis, because it occludes with one simple maneuver the iliac internal, external, and femoral anastomotic components [10]. Then, it is strongly recommended to call for help and take time to recover from this event; interventional radiologists can use an aortic balloon by femoral route [11,12] without fluoroscopy if necessary. If an interventional radiologist is not available, the use of aortic cross clamping is also highly efficient [13]. Abnormal placentation team members or available skilled doctors must be called immediately. During the waiting time, intensive care unit (ICU) doctors and anesthesiologists request blood and other elements to stabilize the hemostatic and hemodynamic state. Aortic compression or occlusion may be kept up for 60–90 minutes without problems; this time is usually enough to receive help. When abnormal placental invasion has destroyed a wide area of the myometrium, a total hysterectomy to reduce late hemorrhagic complications is frequently performed. But remember that in these cases, total hysterectomy is a big challenge even for trained obstetricians, and the procedure's complexity should not be underestimated.

SUBPERITONEAL EXTENSION OF HYSTEROTOMY

On some occasions, during macrosomic or difficult fetal extraction, the hysterotomy edges may extend and produce myometrial or unintentional uterine vessel injuries. When vessels are damaged above the peritoneal reflection, bleeding is shown as hemoperitoneum; but if the tear is extended under this, the myometrial edge may remain hidden and be a possible cause of complications. As happens in upper vaginal tears, bleeding in subperitoneal spaces can be self-limiting or produce a large retroperitoneal hematoma. Nevertheless, and as a general rule, when hypotension or hemodynamic deterioration appears without evident cause after cesarean, we need to think of pelvisubperitoneal or retroperitoneal bleeding. Remember

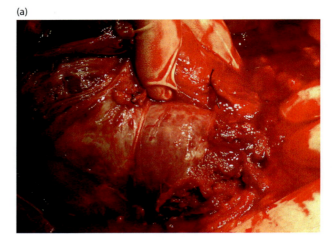

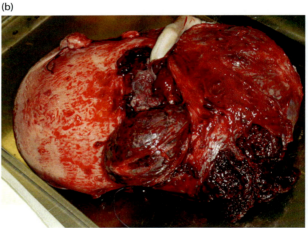

Figure 11.7 (a) Uterine aspect after delivering the baby through the placenta. Then, the obstetrician decided to perform a hysterectomy, but unexpected bleeding in the parametrial invasion was impossible to stop with standard measures. Aortic compression was made until the vascular surgeon performed an aortic cross clamping to do the hysterectomy. (b) Hysterectomy specimen of Figure 11.7a. Lower right parametrial invasion was evident during dissection. We must know (before starting a hysterectomy) that this procedure could be very difficult to perform, even for trained teams. If we have some doubts according to experience, surgical skills, or hospital resources, the safest option is to deliver the baby through a safe area (uterine fundus) to then leave the placenta in situ and close the uterus.

that in these cases ultrasound may be negative even in the presence of large volumes of blood; and that in cases of clinical doubt on stable patients, a computed tomography (CT) scan is preferred (Figure 11.7a and b).

Due to the proximity among the ureter, the uterine artery, and the cervix, suturing the low extension of hysterotomy can be technically difficult, especially in the presence of active bleeding [14]. There is a tendency to avoid dissecting this area, partly for lack of confidence, or to prevent further damage. Ureteral identification is strongly recommended before performing tissue repair (Figure 11.8a–c). If uterine vessels are injured, they can be sutured

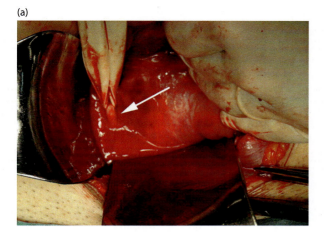
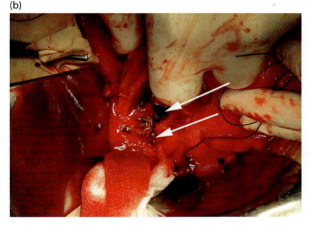
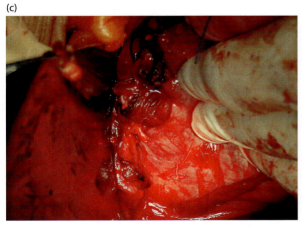

Figure 11.8 (a) Ureteral identification before repairing a subperitoneal extension of hysterotomy (white arrow). Patient: one cesarean. Fetal extraction was difficult due to weight (4500 g). Placental detachment was normal. After 2 hours, postpartum bleeding by atonic uterus was detected. Medical treatment was ineffective, and uterine curettage was successful to stop the bleeding. Two hours later, the uterus lost tonus and PPH started again. Laparotomy was performed and only a small hematoma was detected in the anterior left parametrial area. (b) After ureteral identification, suture of lower extension of hysterotomy is exposed below the peritoneal reflection (white arrows). (c) After repairing the hysterotomy tear by simple stitches, the uterine tonus was restarted.

without risk of devascularization, because the lower anastomotic system replaces blood flow immediately [10].

PERSISTENT BLEEDING IN PLACENTA PREVIA

Due to the special features of the lower segment, such as myometrial thickness, tissue structure, and development of its vessels, placental implantation in the lower segment is different from other uterine areas, and it is more likely to bleed after placental detachment. Myometrial compression of spiral arteries is weak or not as efficient as in the uterine body, and it is a usual cause of postpartum bleeding. Published cases describe complications such as hysterectomy [15] or even death [16] in cases of persistent bleeding for placenta previa; for this reason, it is very important to describe an easy and efficient bleeding control to be performed by all obstetricians.

When the placenta covers the lower uterine segment, it may be necessary to cross the placenta to deliver the baby [17], a maneuver that usually causes additional hemorrhage. If the bleeding is not promptly controlled, it may result in coagulopathy [18] or other severe complications in a short time. Therefore, a rational approach in cases of placenta previa is first to avoid bleeding and then to provide an easy and accurate control of hemorrhage. In cases of lower placentation, access to the upper part of the vagina and lower uterine segment is almost always necessary for accurate bleeding control in the lower uterus. Although this access is only possible after a wide retrovesical dissection, it nevertheless allows correct vascular control and the use of hemostatic compression techniques [19]. This maneuver is not commonly practiced in obstetrics, and some may have concerns about bladder damage or unwanted bleeding. Safe retrovesical dissection, though, is possible using simple techniques. After a correct and complete dissection of the vesicouterine space, bleeding control can be carried out by manual compression of the lower uterus or with the use of a simple rubber drainage tube tied around the cervix. Although most obstetricians can quickly transect an underlying placenta, the use of modified hysterotomy is a good alternative in cases of placenta previa. This procedure, originally published by Ward [20], starts with a hysterotomy carried out to prevent any initial damage to the placenta. The obstetrician's hand is inserted between the myometrium and the placenta, and partial abruption is created before membranes are ruptured to deliver the newborn through the uterine incision. After the baby is delivered, most of the placenta is still attached in the lower segment; hence, additional bleeding is prevented. Then, the placenta is manually detached and an oxytocic drug administered at the same time. In cases of excessive bleeding, the uterus is exteriorized outside the pelvic cavity and the isthmic portion tightened with one hand above the cervix immediately to stop the blood loss. As a second treatment line, an additional oxytocic drug is recommended, along with manual compression of the placental bed with a laparotomy pad. If these measures are not effective after 15 minutes, the use of lower-compression sutures is recommended. But not all compression sutures have the same effect, because their effectiveness depends on the skill of the surgeon and on the source of bleeding (uterine irrigation areas) [19]. Compression sutures such as B-Lynch, Pereira, or Hayman compress the uterine body, and consequently they act over the uterine branches, but they are less effective, or ineffective, for bleeding originating in the lower segment or cervix (pelvisubperitoneal pedicles). The B-Lynch procedure has been combined with the concomitant use of an intrauterine balloon to increase the pressure over the lower segment and the cervix [21]. However, excessive compression using two methods simultaneously could be a cause of uterine necrosis [22]. As multiple vessels supply the lower segment, it is quite difficult to identify specific vessels one by one. Therefore, the compression square suture described by Cho achieves hemostasis of a specific area, regardless of how many vessels supply this sector. In workshops, B-Lynch showed a novel and specific compression suture for the lower segment; this technique is very easy and will probably represent a new and easy alternative for these cases. The procedure is not published yet, but it prevents one possible problem of the Cho compression suture, because it does not occlude the uterine drainage. When the vesicouterine space is open, the placement of compression sutures is probably the most effective and easiest procedure to stop bleeding in the lower uterus [23,24].

HIDDEN UTERINE RUPTURE
Pelvisubperitoneal hematomas

Previous uterine surgeries, such as myomectomies, abortions, D&C, or septum resection could produce an undetected lack of myometrial strength. These conditions are known predisposing causes for uterine rupture in labor or cesarean delivery [25,26]. If uterine rupture happens, injured tissues are visible during cesarean, but a small group could be left hidden under the peritoneal reflection. Although the damaged area is almost always visible to repair by simple stitches, small defects may remain unnoticed, healing by secondary intention. However in some cases, the injured area may begin to bleed, slowly but continuously when uterine tonus is reduced. The bleeding may stop, be self-limiting, or start again and cause serious complications. When bleeding is originated below peritoneal reflection it is usually evident because it produces metrorrhagia, or it might expand through pelvisubperitoneal or retroperitoneal spaces, which turns diagnosis difficult at initial stages [27].

When hemorrhage is continuous, the blood finds the route with the least resistance (such as the fat of pelvisubperitoneal spaces), and it is a cause of hypotension within 2 or 3 hours after cesarean. Clinical and ultrasound examination are commonly negative, unclear, or not conclusive, even in the presence of large volumes of blood. This contradiction may occur because postpartum ultrasound is usually performed over the hypogastrium area, while the hematoma expansion is extended over the pelvic floor or the retroperitoneum. In case of clinical doubt, CT is indicated because it is the quickest and most accurate method to detect extraperitoneal collections. When CT is indicated, ask especially for a coronal reconstruction. This series makes it easier to understand the size of the hematoma in relation to the abdomen.

Frequently, unexplained hypotension in the presence of negative physical and ultrasound examination is misinterpreted as underestimated blood loss during cesarean; consequently, blood and fluid reposition is habitually prescribed. But if a second episode of hypotension happens, it is doubtlessly proof of undetected bleeding. Volume and fluid replacement must be quickly provided to improve an acid–base state before stopping the bleeding. If embolization is available, remember that the time from the clinical decision until the procedure is done is about 1 or 2 hours; in addition, embolization of infraperitoneal vessels is completely different than embolization of the uterine arteries. Access to the uterine arteries is made through the anterior division of iliac internal arteries, while lower uterine or vaginal vessels habitually arise from the pudendal internal arteries, which are branches of the posterior division of the iliac internal artery [10]. This difference implies different skills, complexity, and time for the second group. If laparotomy is your first option, remember that subtotal hysterectomy is not a solution at all, because the source of bleeding originates below peritoneal reflection. To perform a hysterectomy in these cases causes clinical deterioration by hemodynamic shock and acidosis, a consequence of the blood loss during the procedure and of the blood inside the myometrial sinus, estimated between 2 and 3 L [28]. Even if you discover a large retroperitoneal hematoma, please remember that the origin of the bleeding is below the peritoneal reflection; otherwise, other kinds of uterine ruptures are expressed as hemoperitoneum. Posterior dissection of the bladder and ureteral identification are mandatory in order to guarantee the best anatomical access, but mainly to avoid unwanted complications [29]. According to personal experience, the hard part of the procedure is access and dissection, because almost always the injured area is quickly repaired with two or three stitches.

BLADDER AND URETERAL INJURY

Although cesarean is usually performed above the bladder dome, adhesions as consequences of previous surgical uterine procedures such as cesareans [30] or myomectomies could modify the smooth plane between the bladder and the uterus, and be more tense and prone to injury. Also, during delivery of a macrosomic or heavy newborn, obstetric maneuvers could damage the bladder unintentionally [31]. Due to its strong muscular structure, the bladder is an organ easy to repair with few surgical considerations. At first, we need to dissect the posterior bladder wall to have easy access, and to explore the injured area correctly. Before repairing the bladder injury, it is necessary to know that dissection must provide a clear vision of the two tear edges; this technical detail is very important because bladder tissue usually folds itself during suture,

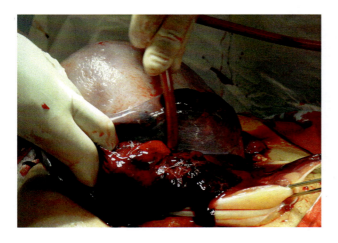

Figure 11.9 Infraperitoneal and retrovesical hematoma secondary to hidden uterine rupture. Obstetric background: 41 years old, two previous cesarean and uterine lower myomectomy performed 2 months after a current pregnancy. Emergency cesarean was performed at 38 weeks for intensive lower pain and mild metrorrhagia. During cesarean a partial dehiscence of cesarean scar was discovered with 200 mL of free abdominal blood. After placental detachment, the uterus appeared normal without any evidence of abnormal bleeding. Ninety minutes later, the arterial pressure dropped suddenly (80/60) without physical evidence of bleeding. Ultrasound study showed a large retrovesical hematoma and a laparotomy was indicated. After hematoma drainage, a subperitoneal uterine rupture was exposed. The right cervical artery was ligated and the uterine tear was repaired with three stitches.

and injured edges tissues could be left hidden. If the injury is anfractuous, do not doubt to cut the borders to find vital tissue to perform an improved suture. It is recommended to perform bladder suture with 000 absorbable materials, extramucosal, and one-layer technique. It is practical to start by the borders and wait to tighten until all sutures are in place. Then, it is recommended to check the indemnity of the suture [32] to detect any urine leak by Foley infusion of methylene blue or sterile milk until the bladder is almost filled (Figure 11.9).

Ureteral injury during cesarean is not a common event, mainly because the hysterotomy is performed far away from the ureter. But in some circumstances, especially during active bleeding, quick attempts to stop the bleeding may produce an unwanted ureteral injury [32]. When myometrial tears are sutured under the peritoneal reflection, there is a real risk of ureteral entrapment because of the close relations between lower uterine elements and the ureter. There are two main mechanisms to produce ureteral injury during cesarean, by entrapment or by cutting [33], and both may remain unnoticed immediately after cesarean. When injuries are recognized and repaired intraoperatively, they can immediately bring satisfactory surgical results and fewer complications. If surgical entrapment is diagnosed during surgery, it is recommended to release the stitches and evaluate the extent of possible damage.

Multiple ureteral knots in a short segment may result in subsequent fistula or fibrosis; for this reason, placement of a double J catheter or similar is recommended to avoid further complications. Ureteral cutting is not a common cesarean injury and may be a cause of unspecific postoperative states. In general the abdomen is distended, but peritoneal irritation is not always evident. If the ureter was cut partially, diagnosis could be difficult to perform without auxiliary diagnostic methods. On the other hand, ureteral entrapment is a cause of early and recurrent back pain. When these symptoms appear after cesarean or other gynecologic surgeries, ureteral ligature or entrapment must be suspected. Delayed diagnosis [33,34] requires individualized treatment based on the patient's condition and the length of delay.

SUMMARY

Uncommon situations can happen during cesarean delivery, and they may end up causing serious complications or even death. Knowledge of these mechanisms and their solutions is strongly recommended for all obstetricians.

REFERENCES

1. Chazotte C, Cohen WR. Catastrophic complications of previous cesarean delivery. *Am J Obstet Gynecol* 1990;163(3):738–42.
2. Palacios-Jaraquemada JM. *Abnormal Invasive Placenta*. Berlin, Germany: DeGruyter; 2012:93–94.
3. Blanchette H. The rising cesarean delivery rate in America: What are the consequences? *Obstet Gynecol* 2011;118(3):687–90.
4. Bowman ZS, Eller AG, Kennedy AM et al. Accuracy of ultrasound for the prediction of placenta accrete. *Am J Obstet Gynecol* 2014;211(2):177e1–7. doi:10.1016/j.ajog.2014.03.029
5. Farina R, Sparano A. Errors in sonography. In: Romano L, Pinto A, eds. *Errors in Radiology*. Milan, Italy: Springer-Verlag Italia; 2012:79–85.
6. Abuhamad A. Morbidly adherent placenta. *Semin Perinatol* 2013;37(5):359–64.
7. Sivasankar C. Perioperative management of undiagnosed placenta percreta: Case report and management strategies. *Int J Womens Health* 2012;4:451–4.
8. Abbas F, Talati J, Wasti S et al. R. Placenta percreta with bladder invasion as a cause of life threatening hemorrhage. *J Urol* 2000;164(4):1270–4.
9. Vettraino I, Graham C, Shyken J et al. Placenta percreta: A case of maternal death. *J Matern Fetal Med* 1993;2:276–8.
10. Palacios-Jaraquemada JM, García-Mónaco R, Barbosa NE et al. Lower uterine blood supply: Extrauterine anastomotic system and its application in surgical devascularization techniques. *Acta Obstet Gynecol Scand* 2007;86(2):228–34.
11. Masamoto H, Uehara H, Gibo M et al. Elective use of aortic balloon occlusion in cesarean hysterectomy for placenta previa percreta. *Gynecol Obstet Invest* 2009;67(2):92–95.

12. Paull JD, Smith J, Williams L et al. Balloon occlusion of the abdominal aorta during caesarean hysterectomy for placenta percreta. *Anaesth Intensive Care* 1995;23(6):731–4.
13. Chou MM, Ke YM, Wu HC et al. Temporary cross-clamping of the infrarenal abdominal aorta during cesarean hysterectomy to control operative blood loss in placenta previa increta/percreta. *Taiwan J Obstet Gynecol* 2010;49(1):72–76.
14. Lee JS, Choe JH, Lee HS et al. Urologic complications following obstetric and gynecologic surgery. *Korean J Urol* 2012;53(11):795–9.
15. Jin R, Guo Y, Chen Y. Risk factors associated with emergency peripartum hysterectomy. *Chin Med J (Engl)* 2014;127(5):900–4.
16. Alchalabi H, Lataifeh I, Obeidat B et al. Morbidly adherent placenta previa in current practice: Prediction and maternal morbidity in a series of 23 women who underwent hysterectomy. *J Matern Fetal Neonatal Med* 2014;27(17):1734–7.
17. Xiaojing J, Ying W, Khan I. Clinical analysis of 322 cases of placenta previa. *J Med College PLA* 2009;24:366–9.
18. Palacios-Jaraquemada J, Fiorillo A. Conservative approach in heavy postpartum hemorrhage associated with coagulopathy. *Acta Obstet Gynecol Scand* 2010;89:1222–5.
19. Palacios-Jaraquemada JM. Efficacy of surgical techniques to control obstetric hemorrhage: Analysis of 539 cases. *Acta Obstet Gynecol Scand* 2011;90:1036–42.
20. Ward CR. Avoiding an incision through the anterior previa at cesarean delivery. *Obstet Gynecol* 2003;102:552–4.
21. Patacchiola F, D'Alfonso A, Di Fonso A et al. Intrauterine balloon tamponade as management of postpartum haemorrhage and prevention of haemorrhage related to low-lying placenta. *Clin Exp Obstet Gynecol* 2012;39(4):498–9.
22. Lodhi W, Golara M, Karangaokar V et al. Uterine necrosis following application of combined uterine compression suture with intrauterine balloon tamponade. *J Obstet Gynaecol* 2012;32(1):30–31.
23. Palacios-Jaraquemada JM. Caesarean section in cases of placenta praevia and accreta. *Best Pract Res Clin Obstet Gynaecol* 2013;27(2):221–32.
24. Penotti M, Vercellini P, Bolis G et al. Compressive suture of the lower uterine segment for the treatment of postpartum hemorrhage due to complete placenta previa: A preliminary study. *Gynecol Obstet Invest* 2012;73(4):314–20.
25. Turgut A, Ozler A, Siddik Evsen M et al. Uterine rupture revisited: Predisposing factors, clinical features, management and outcomes from a tertiary care center in Turkey. *Pak J Med Sci* 2013;29(3):753–7.
26. Kiseli M, Artas H, Armagan F et al. Spontaneous rupture of uterus in mid trimester pregnancy due to increased uterine pressure with previous laparoscopic myomectomy. *Int J Fertil Steril* 2013;7(3):239–42.
27. Bienstman-Pailleux J, Huissoud C, Dubernard G et al. Management of puerperal hematomas [in French]. *J Gynecol Obstet Biol Reprod (Paris)* 2009; 38(3):203–8.
28. Henrich W, Surbek D, Kainer F et al. Diagnosis and treatment of peripartum bleeding. *J Perinat Med* 2008;36:467–78.
29. Baggish MS, Karram MM. *Atlas of Pelvic Anatomy and Gynecologic Surgery*. Philadelphia, PA: W.B. Saunders; 2001:204–13.
30. Gasim T, Al Jama FE, Rahman MS et al. Multiple repeat cesarean deliveries: Operative difficulties, maternal complications and outcome. *J Reprod Med* 2013;58(7–8):312–8.
31. Shazly SA, Elsayed AH, Badran SM et al. Abdominal disimpaction with lower uterine segment support as a novel technique to minimize fetal and maternal morbidities during cesarean delivery for obstructed labor: A case series. *Am J Perinatol* 2013;30(8):695–8.
32. Rao D, Yu H, Zhu H et al. The diagnosis and treatment of iatrogenic ureteral and bladder injury caused by traditional gynaecology and obstetrics operation. *Arch Gynecol Obstet* 2012;285(3):763–5.
32. Ustunsoz B, Ugurel S, Duru NK et al. Percutaneous management of ureteral injuries that are diagnosed late after cesarean delivery. *Korean J Radiol* 2008;9(4):348–53.
33. Davis JD. Management of injuries to the urinary and gastrointestinal tract during cesarean delivery. *Obstet Gynecol Clin North Am* 1999;26:469–80.
34. Rajasekar D, Hall M. Urinary tract injuries during obstetric intervention. *Br J Obstet Gynaecol* 1997;104(6):731–4.

Dystocia and intrapartum ultrasound in cesarean delivery

GIAN CARLO DI RENZO, CHIARA ANTONELLI, IRENE GIARDINA, and ANTONIO MALVASI

INTRODUCTION

Dystocia is defined as a difficulty in the progression of labor or in the completion of delivery, usually secondary to abnormalities of the cervix, uterus, fetus, or of the mother's pelvis, that may contribute individually or in combination.

A common cause of dystocia is cephalopelvic disproportion, characterized by a disparity between the size of the maternal pelvis and the fetal head, which therefore precludes vaginal delivery (Figures 12.1 and 12.2). An early diagnosis of this condition—that is, prior to the onset of labor—is difficult. Another common cause of dystocia is a slower than normal progression (abnormal progression of the fetus) or the complete stoppage of the presenting part (failure to progress) in the birth canal. Both of these labor abnormalities can only be diagnosed when the expectant mother is in the active phase of labor (Figure 12.3).

There are, moreover, alterations of labor produced by inadequate uterine contractility; these are called dynamic or uterine dystocias. Alterations of labor due to the fetus are called fetal dystocias. In assessing fetal dystocias, in order to have an early detection of labor alterations, and to prevent an erroneous diagnosis of dystocia, a key role is played by the modern obstetrician, who will adapt his or her own obstetric skills and semiotic training to the variability inherent in labor and delivery.

ULTRASOUND AND DYSTOCIA

In order to diagnose certain dystocias during labor it is essential to use ultrasound, a diagnostic tool commonly found in every hospital and outpatient care setting. In fact, ultrasound, used in either the first or second stage of labor to determine the position of the fetal head, can be useful in determining whether the delivery will be carried out spontaneously or will require surgical intervention (Figure 12.4).

In evaluating the fetal position one must take into account the position and dimensions of the fetal head. Before childbirth it would therefore be beneficial to estimate the weight of the fetus in each patient. An assessment of the fetal size by ultrasound is, however, often inaccurate, due to the extreme subjectivity of the ultrasound measurement (±10%).

It is difficult to make a diagnosis of dystocia in the first stage of labor, unless the patient is in the active phase characterized by adequate uterine contractile activity.

Fetal abnormalities, such as hydrocephalus, omphalocele, and soft tissue swelling may also hinder labor. Fetal ultrasound should, however, be taken into consideration as an auxiliary, yet fundamental, diagnostic method when abnormal presentations or positions are suspected, and when there is no progression of the presenting part.

Anomalies of labor may, however, also be secondary to pelvic defects, though before attributing dystocia to pelvic defects, insufficient uterine contractile activity and fetal dystocia should be considered as factors that inhibit the progression of labor.

In the West or in the "industrialized societies," pelvic bone diameters may represent a limiting factor in the completion of vaginal delivery of a fetus in a cephalic presentation, though not to the same degree as in underdeveloped countries where bone anomalies are present.

One last aspect, no less important than others in the context of dystocias, is prolonged labor.

ULTRASOUND AND POOR FETAL POSITIONS

The use of intrapartum ultrasound (Figure 12.5) to evaluate the position of the fetal head during labor, has proven to be useful and reliable, especially in confirming the diagnosis of fetal head malposition, suspected at times during the obstetric visit [1]. Although it is not yet part of the obstetric routine, this diagnostic tool has the potential to determine the position of the fetus in a much more accurate way than basic clinical tools.

It is important to have precise tools to evaluate abnormal positions of the fetal head. Such abnormalities may be predictive of a difficult delivery, thereby greatly decreasing the chances that the childbirth will be carried out vaginally, and at the same time increasing the possibility of a cesarean delivery. The evaluation of the position of the fetal head by ultrasound is performed with longitudinal and transverse scans [2].

INTRAPARTUM ULTRASOUND PROCEDURE

An ultrasound description of the fetal head position in the suprapubic transverse scan is based on the identification of the structures of the interhemispheric line: cavum septum pellucidum, cerebral falx, thalami, and cerebellar hemispheres (Figure 12.6). In addition, the position of the fetal head is based on the identification of the anterior and posterior cranial structures: orbits, nasal arches, and cervical tract of the column (Figures 12.7 and 12.8).

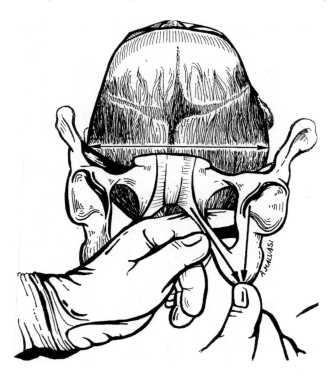

Figure 12.1 Digital examination of the left ischial–pubic bone in outlet restricted pelvis, during the second labor stage with the occiput-posterior position of the fetal head.

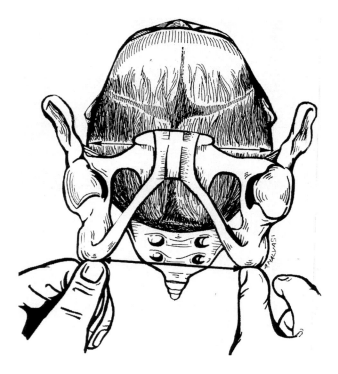

Figure 12.2 Digital examination of the pelvic outlet in the narrow and asymmetric pelvis, during dystocic second labor stage, with the fetal head in the occiput posterior position.

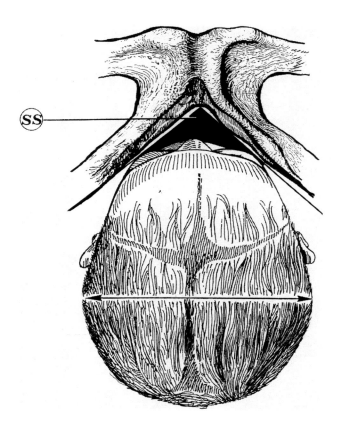

Figure 12.3 The two black lines under the symphysis limit the subpubic arch. The subsymphysary space (SS) is shown in the second stage of labor, with the fetal head in the occiput posterior malposition. The transverse line on the fetal head indicates the biparietal diameter.

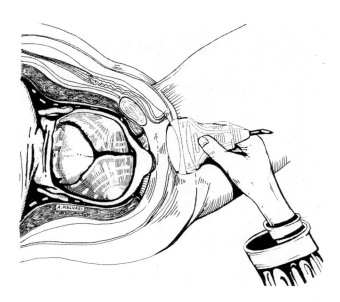

Figure 12.4 Ultrasound evaluation, with translabial technique, of the fetal head position in the second stage of labor. The intrapartum sonography shows the caput succedaneum and the molding, normal anatomical modifications during labor.

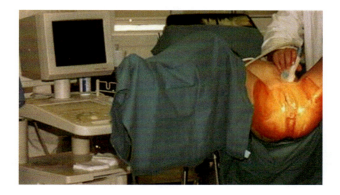

Figure 12.5 Intrapartum ultrasound evaluation in the second stage of labor.

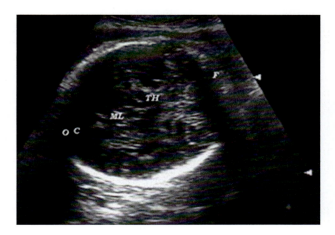

Figure 12.6 Intrapartum ultrasound evaluation in the second stage of labor of a fetus in a cephalic position, in right occiput posterior position.

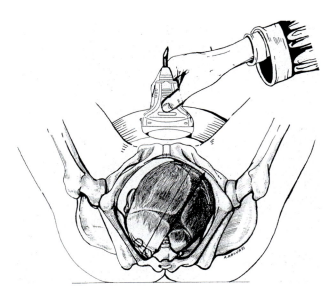

Figure 12.7 Transabdominal intrapartum ultrasonography, during the second labor stage, with fetal head in left occiput anterior position and anterior right asynclitism. (The circle represents the "squint sign.")

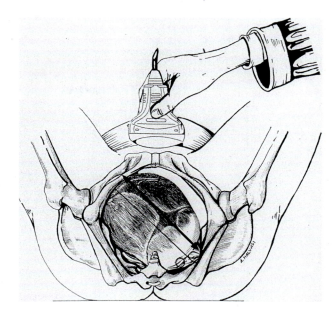

Figure 12.8 Transabdominal intrapartum ultrasonography, during the second labor stage, with the fetal head in right occiput anterior position and anterior left asynclitism. (The circle represents the "squint sign.")

Many technicians, obstetricians, and gynecologists believe that the position of the fetal head, assessed by evaluating the topography of the fetal fontanels and of the pelvic landmarks can, as in the past, be detected with a simple obstetric visit. However, the literature clearly indicates that the opposite is true: the obstetric visit is often inaccurate even in very experienced hands.

The smoothing of the cervix and the level of the presenting part in relation to the ischial spines can influence the accuracy of the vaginal examination. The intrapartum ultrasound can instead overcome these obstacles and provide a means to more accurately assess the position of the fetal head. Intrapartum ultrasound can therefore document the presence of a dystocic labor so that either a vaginal delivery or a cesarean delivery can be carried out.

SCIENTIFIC ROLE OF INTRAPARTUM ULTRASOUND

Some scholars, such as Akmal [3], assert that the likelihood of a cesarean delivery can be established during the early stages of labor by using ultrasound to determine the occiput anterior or posterior position (Figure 12.9) of the fetal head.

Regardless of the risk factors and causes that lead to the occiput anterior or posterior position of the fetal head, Gardberg et al. [2] reported that 68% of occiput posterior positions are caused by malrotation from the initial occiput anterior position, and 32% of the occiput posterior positions are present at the beginning of labor.

This theory has been challenged by Akmal et al. [3,4] who believe that the majority of occiput posterior positions are not due to malrotation of the fetal head during

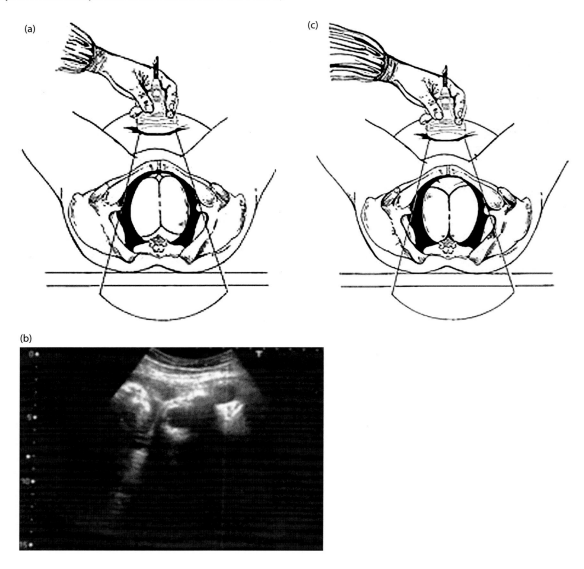

Figure 12.9 Intrapartum ultrasound diagnosis of vertex presentation: (a) the sacral rotation of the occiput; (b) with corresponding ultrasound; and (c) Occiput anterior position.

the descent of the fetus in the birth canal, but instead to a persistent occiput posterior position of the head from the beginning of labor. Rotation of the fetal head is highly unlikely when labor begins in occiput posterior. In fact, the persistence of the fetal head in this position prevents rotation, resulting in persistent occiput posterior position. All this was observed by performing serial ultrasound examinations during labor at 3–5 cm of cervical dilatation, 6–9 cm dilatation, and 10 cm of dilatation, finding probabilities, respectively, of 70%, 91%, and 100% of giving birth in occiput posterior position.

Traditionally, the position and level of the fetal head have been evaluated during the visit to the obstetrician or with Leopold maneuvers. More recently it has been proposed to use ultrasound in the delivery room [5,6]. Katanozaka et al. [7] had, however, already proposed the use of ultrasound during labor to determine the obstetric conjugate, arguing that ultrasound is safer and more effective. Numerous studies have shown that the accuracy of obstetric visits in determining the exact position of the fetal head is not optimal and, specifically, that this type of assessment is too subjective and therefore conditioned by the experience of the operator [8–10].

Sherer et al. [8] on 102 patients in the first stage of labor, reported that the position of the fetal head, determined by digital exploration, matches the position determined by ultrasound in only 47% of cases. The same evaluation performed on 112 patients in the second stage of labor had a percentage of 61% [9]. Kreiser et al. [11] on 44 patients reported a matching rate of 70% between the obstetric visit and ultrasound evaluation in the second stage of labor (Figure 12.10). In a larger study conducted on 496 women Akmal [10] reports that the position of the fetal head cannot be determined in 34% of cases, and that even when the position can be defined it differs in 52% of cases from the position determined by ultrasound.

Scientific role of intrapartum ultrasound 219

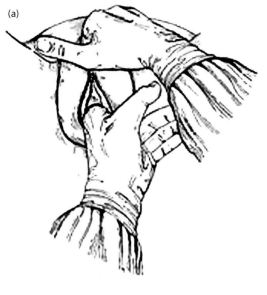

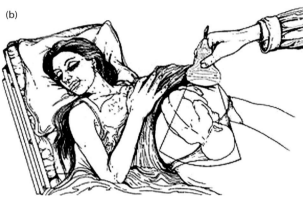

Figure 12.10 (a) The traditional vaginal exploration during childbirth labor is increasingly being supplemented with intrapartum ultrasound (b) to assess the position of the fetal head.

Chou et al. [12] in 2004 reported that the use of transabdominal ultrasound, combined with transperineal ultrasound, is more reliable in defining the position of the fetal head than the sole obstetric visit in the second stage of labor, with a statistically significant difference of 71.6% with a visit compared to 92% with ultrasound.

Souka et al. [13] on 148 patients in active labor, reported that it is impossible to determine the position of the fetal head with a visit to an obstetrician in 60.7% of cases in the first stage of labor, and in 30.8% in the second stage of labor, and with an accuracy rate compared to ultrasound of 31.28% in the first stage and 65.7% in the second stage.

Uguwumadu, in his "opinion" on "intrapartum sonography," confirms that in dystocic labor the inevitable error that occurs in a traditional obstetrician visit is greater than in eutocic labor. In fact the swelling in childbirth, greater during dystocia, results in fetal sutures and fontanels, used to determine the position of the fetal head, that are less palpable [1]. This is especially true for malpositions

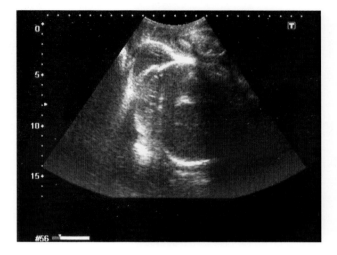

Figure 12.11 Ultrasound view showing "caput succedaneum" in sagittal translabial section scan during the second stage of dystocic labor.

of the fetal head, which in order to be diagnosed by vaginal examination require palpation of the fetal sutures and fontanels.

One of the more frequent fetal head anomalies during labor is asynclitic positions (Figures 12.11 through 12.13), which, especially during prolonged labors, may not be recognized due to swelling that prevents the anatomical landmarks (sagittal suture and anterior and posterior fontanels) from being detected. In these cases the intrapartum ultrasound settles the diagnostic doubt by evaluating the position and symmetry of the orbital cavities and of the spinal column in relation to the ultrasound scan plane (Figures 12.14 and 12.15) by identifying the orbit that is closer to the wave front (also known as the "squint sign"). Generally, an asynclitism occurs in flat pelvises that force the fetal head to bend forward or backward in an attempt to overcome

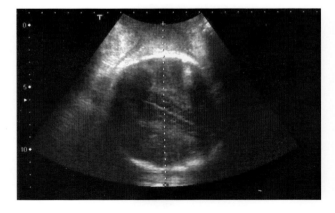

Figure 12.12 Ultrasound view showing internal rotation, in sagittal translabial section scan during the second stage of dystocic labor. Internal rotation is a difficult diagnosis with vaginal digital examination, especially in dystocic labor; in contrast translabial ultrasound makes this a simple diagnosis, through evaluation of the angle of internal rotation evaluation.

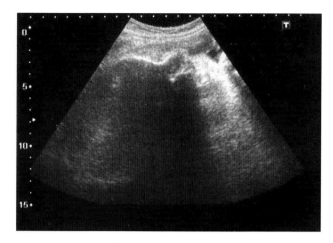

Figure 12.13 Translabial intrapartum ultrasound sagittal scan of the fetal head in the occiput posterior position, during the second stage of labor.

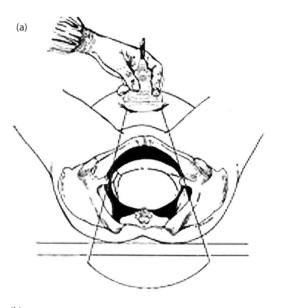

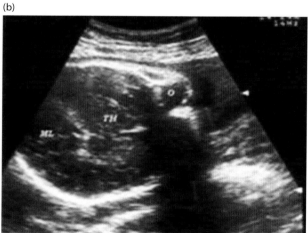

Figure 12.14 (a) Ultrasound assessment of posterior fetal asynclitism with (b) ultrasound image: median line (ML), thalami (TH), and orbit (O), "squint sign."

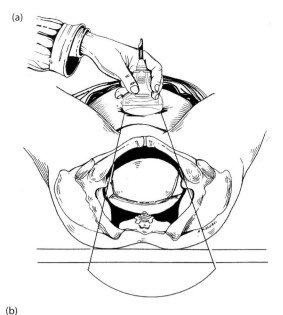

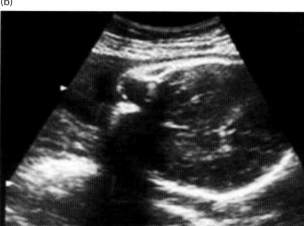

Figure 12.15 (a) Ultrasound assessment of anterior fetal asynclitism, and (b) ultrasound image with "squint sign." (Modified from Malvasi A, Di Renzo GC. *Ecografia Intrapartum*, Bari, Italy: Editori Laterza; 2010.)

the obstacle. Typically, the head engages in a posterior asynclitism, more rarely in an anterior asynclitism.

Ultrasound during childbirth labor not only allows for a more accurate diagnosis of the position of the fetal head in the birth canal, but often leads to an early diagnosis of dystocia. This allows for better planning of the operative delivery, avoiding unnecessary maternal and fetal complications. For example, the disengagement of the fetus in an occiput posterior position (Figures 12.16 and 12.17) requires a prolonged second stage and, oftentimes, surgical delivery. Therefore, the occiput posterior diagnosis, in relation to the completion of delivery, is appropriately assessed in case of uniparous or multiparous female.

Then, if a vaginal delivery is decided upon for a vertex presentation and occiput posterior position, the position of the fetal head that allows for optimal application of forceps and vacuum extractor will be known.

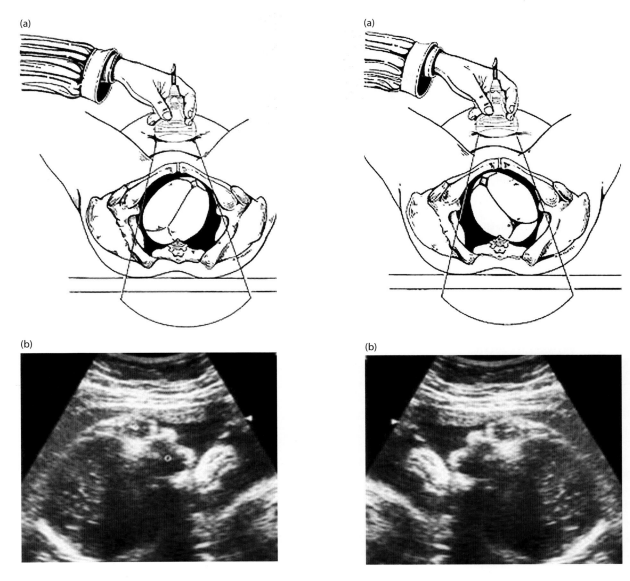

Figure 12.16 (a) Ultrasound evaluation of vertex presentation, right occiput posterior position. (b) Corresponding ultrasound (O, orbits).

Figure 12.17 (a) Ultrasound evaluation of vertex presentation, left occiput posterior position. (b) Corresponding ultrasound.

If instead a laparotomy is decided upon for the delivery, it would be ineffective or harmful to extend the dystocic labor. Difficulties include extracting the fetal head wedged in the birth canal, injuries to the bladder (the bladder is extra pelvic and is compressed by the fetal head), or a need for surgical reconstruction of the lower dystocic uterine segment, ultra stretched and at times sacculated by the abnormal position of the fetal head.

Ponkey et al. [14] reported the maternal outcome for occiput posterior delivery compared to occiput anterior. In this cohort study on 6434 births, the overall incidence of occiput posterior position was 5.5%, with an incidence of 7.2% for nulliparous women and 4% for multiparous women, a statistically significant difference ($p < 0.001$).

The persistence of the occiput posterior position, in relation to the occiput anterior position, has a statistically significant association with low maternal height, previous cesarean deliveries, the extension of the first (48.3% versus 30.3%) and second stage (53.3% versus 18.1%) of labor, respectively, of more than 12 hours and 2 hours, increased consumption of oxytocin needed to increase uterine contractility, epidural analgesia, the increase in assisted vaginal deliveries (24.6% versus 9.4%), chorioamnionitis (4.7% versus 1.1%), third- and fourth-degree perineal tears (18.2% versus 6.7%), cesarean deliveries (37.7% versus 6.6%), excessive blood loss (13.6% versus 9.9%), and postpartum infections (0.8% versus 0.1%).

Reithmuller et al. [15] also report in a retrospective study on 210 births in persistent occiput posterior, that even though the prognosis of the occiput posterior position was good, the anterior position is preferable. This is due to the improved maternal and neonatal outcome in terms of infections, and to the lower amount of damage to the maternal perineal tissues, as use of the vacuum extractor in the anterior position is limited.

The application of the vacuum extractor is closely linked to a correct assessment of the position of the fetal head. Any deflection of the fetal head could result in the detachment of the suction cup and in increased neonatal morbidity. The application of a vacuum extractor on a deflected occiput increases by four to five times the likelihood of failure, whereas its application on occiput posterior or lateral doubles the chances of failure [16]. If the fetal head is deflected at the time of application of the vacuum extractor, the probability of a low Apgar (below 6) increases by 3.2 times, that of severe trauma of the scalp by 5.2 times and the probability of hospitalization in a neonatal intensive care unit by 12 times.

The lateral and posterior positions are the most difficult to diagnose during an obstetric visit and, according to the literature, these situations occur more frequently with epidural analgesia. Therefore it is important to use ultrasound in the operative delivery in labor with analgesia [17].

THE ROLE OF INTRAPARTUM ULTRASOUND AND THE OUTCOME OF DELIVERY

The diagnosis of malposition from a traditional obstetric visit has limitations. For this reason it is important to improve the diagnosis with an objective instrumental method, such as the ultrasound [18]. This is especially true when an operative delivery is expected, as is recommended by the Canadian Society of Obstetrics and Gynaecology.

The diagnosis of occiput posterior position also assumes importance in predicting the outcome of the induction. In fact, in 2004 Rane et al. [20] reported that ultrasound evaluation of occiput posterior position of the fetal head, the posterior cervical angle, and the maternal BMI are parameters that can predict the outcome of the induction better than the Bishop score.

A greater accuracy in the diagnosis of posterior occiput position in the early stages of labor, and at the induction of labor, would lead to a reduction in maternal and fetal morbidity, which is possibly linked to an increase in cesarean sections, though it remains to be quantified. In spite of the occiput posterior position being the most common fetal malpresentation encountered by obstetricians, there is little information about it in the literature. Between 10% and 20% of fetuses are in occiput posterior positions at the beginning of labor. During labor, in most cases, they turn spontaneously toward the occiput anterior. Nonetheless, approximately 5% of total births occur in occiput posterior.

Epidural analgesia, performed at 5 cm dilation, and in particular with the fetal head still "high," has been associated with an increase in fetal head malposition (occiput posterior and occiput transverse positions) during childbirth [2]. It has been hypothesized that, due to the interruption of a series of events determined by epidural analgesia pertaining to the dynamics of delivery, there is a reduction in the intensity of the maternal thrust. These events contribute to reducing the duration of labor in the expulsion stage, with the possible inhibition of the Ferguson reflex and motor blockade of the abdominal and pelvic muscles.

The vertical position of women in labor was also investigated within the context of dystocias, in terms of its effects on instrumental deliveries and cesarean deliveries during the second stage, on patients with epidural analgesia. There is however insufficient data in the literature demonstrating significant benefits of the vertical position in the second stage.

TIMING OF INTRAPARTUM ULTRASOUND

Last, in the context of the diagnosis of dystocia and the timing of ultrasound applied to labor, special attention should be paid to the lengthening of the cervical dilatation time and the progression of the fetal head, with resulting extension of the first and second stages of labor. In fact, it would seem that the cervical dilatation and fetal head descent periods have changed from those reported by Friedman in the 1950s, as some studies report an extension, even of several hours, of the average duration of labor, both with and without analgesia.

The cervical dilatation curve has characteristics that are different from the old Friedman curves, in which the transition to intermediate dilations in the active phase of labor was much sharper than in Zhang's modern cervicometric curves. This is important, as many labors that are absolutely normal, in an analysis of the progression of labor according to the curves of Friedman, appear dystocic. These "dynamic" or "pharmacological" dystocias can be attributed to epidural analgesia.

An analysis of the literature leads to the conclusion that it cannot be determined whether epidural analgesia increases or decreases the incidence of cesarean deliveries. Instrumental deliveries have however increased. An important factor that influences morbidity, therefore, is the increase in cesarean deliveries and the extension of the first stage of labor, which becomes significant for the second stage. With regard to the extension of the second stage of labor, a multivariate analysis of the risk factors significantly associated with an arrest of fetal descent, shows that epidural analgesia is clearly not a major factor. Furthermore, the duration threshold tolerated in primiparae has been raised by the American College of Obstetricians and Gynecologists (ACOG) from 2 to 3 hours.

The amount of time epidural analgesia in labor can prolong the active phase compared to the original Friedman curves has been quantified as 1 hour. The study by Zhang has, however, shown how the current population has markedly different Friedman curves. Cervical dilation occurs more slowly in the active phase: 5.5 hours on average compared to 2.5 hours in the original Friedman curve. The results of this study indicate that there is, in common practice, a substantially different pattern of labor progression than the original Friedman study, due in part to a high percentage of pregnant women making use of oxytocin and epidural analgesia. Consequently, the criteria that determine whether labor continues or stops may also be too restrictive.

In terms of halting the administration of analgesia, when dilatation is complete, so as to not affect labor, the length of the second stage would seem to be drug dependent, though not capable of influencing neonatal outcome.

INTRAPARTUM ULTRASOUND AND MEDICO-LEGAL ASPECTS

Last, the possible medico-legal role of intrapartum ultrasound must not be overlooked. The ever-increasing medico-legal litigation in our country has in fact made it appropriate to establish an accurate diagnosis of dystocia. Additional and reliable documentation on the progress of labor could provide, in the event of maternal and fetal complications, further shelter from any claims.

The traditional partogram results from subjective obstetric visits and is, as demonstrated in the literature, scarcely reliable. An intrapartum ultrasound evaluation with photographic documentation can instead ascertain, with a wide margin of safety, the position of the fetal head in labor and whether it is eutocic or dystocic, thereby legitimizing subsequent obstetric management.

It must be noted that it is important to have, especially in light of possible medico-legal litigation, a safe and effective tool, such as the intrapartum ultrasound, to diagnosis the fetal head position for all labors at risk of dystocia (including those where analgesia is used).

CONCLUSIONS

To date, external and internal pelvimetry maneuvers allow an assessment of the pelvic fetus proportion or disproportion and, therefore, of whether the delivery will be eutocic or dystocic.

All pelvimetric maneuvers are affected by the subjective evaluation of the examiner, which, in addition to the substantial number of other fetal and maternal variables and anthropomorphic and individual variations, results in a diagnosis that is scarcely reliable.

The determination of fetal weight has not improved the diagnosis of dystocia or the fetal outcome.

The need for an objective determination of the level of the presenting part, of the cervical dilatation, and of the rotation of the fetal head has led to various studies. In particular, the diagnosis of the fetal head position with obstetric intrapartum ultrasound has proven to be more specialized as well as more sensitive. Various studies have reported the results of the comparison between vaginal examination and ultrasonography in the diagnosis of the position of the head [4,5].

In terms of asynclitism, ultrasound allows for a more reliable diagnosis, because dystocic labor produces swelling and therefore renders the sutures, as well as the fetal fontanels, less palpable. These in fact are the landmarks from which the location of the fetal head in the birth canal can be determined.

The same can be said for the sacral rotation of the occiput. Here vaginal evaluation is hampered by the swelling of the delivery, whereas a transabdominal ultrasound examination easily reveals the anterior position of the orbits and the posterior position of the vertebral column occiput.

Even in regard to the management of delivery, in case of instrumental vaginal delivery, intrapartum ultrasound allows for a more accurate application of the forceps and of the suction cup. This is especially true for the latest single-use cups that, if not positioned appropriately, can easily give way due to the low negative pressure (lower than that of the traditional vacuum).

Last, all documentation needed in case of medicolegal litigation, and which proves the need for an operative delivery, should be attached to the medical record.

REFERENCES

1. Ugwumadu A. The role of ultrasound scanning on the labor ward. (Opinion). *Ultrasound Obstet Gynecol* 2002;19:222–4.
2. Gardberg M, Laakkonen E, Salevaara M. Intrapartum sonography and persistent occipital posterior position: A study of 408 deliveries. *Obstet Gynecol* 1998;91:746–9.
3. Akmal S, Tsoi E, Howard R, Osei E, Nicolaides KH. Investigation of occipital posterior delivery by intrapartum sonography. *Ultrasound Obstet Gynecol* 2004;24:425–8.
4. Akmal S, Tsoi E, Nicolaides KH. Intrapartum sonography to determine fetal occipital position: Interobserver agreement. *Ultrasound Obstet Gynecol* 2004;24:425–8.
5. Sherer DM, Onyeije CI, Bernstein PS, Kovacs P, Manning FA. Utilization of real time ultrasound on labor and delivery in an active academic teaching hospital. *Am J Perinatol* 1999;16(6):303–7.
6. Malvasi A, Brizzi A, Cecinati A, Martino V. Marcatori di distocia nel parto in analgesia epidurale. Simposio satellite ESRA 2002 "obiettivo sala parto di eccellenza" Asti 20 Novembre 2002, 53–60, CD-ROM.
7. Katanozaka M, Yashinaga M, Fuchiwaki K, Nagata R. Measurement of obstetric conjugate by ultrasonic tomography and its significance. *Am J Obstet Gynecol* 1999;180:159–62.
8. Sherer DM, Miodovnik M, Bradley KS, Langer O. Intrapartum fetal head position I: Comparison between transvaginal digital examination and transabdominal ultrasound assessment during the active stage of labour. *Ultrasound Obstet Gynecol* 2002;19:258–63.
9. Sherer DM, Miodovnik M, Bradley KS, Langer O. Intrapartum fetal head position II: Comparison between transvaginal digital examination and transabdominal ultrasound assessment during the second stage of labour. *Ultrasound Obstet Gynecol* 2002;19:264–8.
10. Akmal S, Tsoi E, Kametas N, Howard R, Nicolaides KH. Intrapartum sonography to determine fetal head position. *J Matern Fetal Neonat Med* 2002;12:172–7.

11. Kreiser D, Schiff E, Lipitz S et al. Determination of fetal occiput position by ultrasound during the second stage of labor. *J Matern Fetal Med* 2001;10:283–6.
12. Chou MR, Kreizer D, Taslimi MM, Druzin ML, El Sayed Y. Vaginal versus ultrasound examination of fetal head position occipital position during the second stage of labor. *Am J Obstet Gynecol* 2004;191:521–4.
13. Souka AP, Haritos T, Basayiannis K, Noikokyri N, Antsaklis A. Intrapartum ultrasound for the examination of the fetal head position in normal and obstructed labor. *J Matern Fetal Neonatal Med* 2003;13:59–63.
14. Ponkey SE, Cohen AP, Heffner LJ, Lieberman E. Persistent fetal occiput posterior: Obstetric outcome. *Obstet Gynecol* 2003;101:915–20.
15. Reithmuller D, Teffaud O, Eyraud JL, Sautiere JL, Schaal JP, Maillet R. Maternal and fetal prognosis of occipital-posterior presentation. *J Gynecol Obstet Biol Reprod* 1999;28:41–47.
16. Mola GD, Amoa AB, Edilyong J. Factors associated with success or failure in trials of vacuum extraction. *Aust N Z J Obstet Gynecol* 2002;42:35–39.
17. Malvasi A, Brizzi A, Cecinati A, Martino V. Analgesia epidurale in travaglio di parto e valutazione ecografica: Studio prospettico. *Atti LXXVIII congr. SIGO-XLIII AOGOI-AGUI*. Rome, Italy: CIC Edit. Intern.; 2002:211–8.
18. Sherer DM, Abulafia O. Intrapartum assessment of fetal head engagement: Comparison between transvaginal digital and transabdominal ultrasound determinations. *Ultrasound Obstet Gynecol* 2003;21(5):430–6.
19. Rane SM, Guirgis RR, Higgins B, Nicolaides KH. The value of ultrasound in the prediction of successful induction of labor. *Ultrasound Obstet Gynecol* 2004;24:538–49.

FURTHER READING

Van den Hof M, Demianczuk N. Society Canadian obstetrics and gynaecology: Guideline for ultrasound in labour and delivery. *J Soc Obstet Gynecol Can* 2001;23(5):431–2.

Dystocia and cesarean delivery

New perspectives in the management of labor and the prevention of cesarean delivery

ANTONIO MALVASI, GIAN CARLO DI RENZO, and ELEONORA BRILLO

INTRODUCTION

Cesarean deliveries have been constantly increasing worldwide, with a percentage in the United States of almost 29.1% [1]: this has been a record increase, higher by 6% from the national rate of the previous year [2]. Brazil is among the countries in which the greatest number of cesarean deliveries have been performed: percentages close to 80% were reached some years ago [3].

This steady increase is in marked contrast with the published guidelines regarding the optimal rate: World Health Organization (WHO) guidelines, since 2000, have recommended that the rate should not exceed 15%. Unfortunately, this figure has been consistently disregarded, especially in the industrialized countries.

This is linked to a number of reasons, ranging from social factors to the frequency of medical comorbidities: the extremely low acceptance of maternal and fetal risks during labor and delivery, combined with concerns about pelvic injury, fear of pain, and availability of the procedure, have led to a small but increasing number of women requesting the cesarean delivery without any medical indication [4].

In a survey carried out in the center of which one of the authors (EB) is director, the Department of Obstetrics and Gynaecology at Mount Sinai Hospital in Toronto (Canada), 42% of the women interviewed would undergo more than one cesarean delivery to avoid possible damages to the newborn infant [5]. Another study conducted in the United Kingdom found that 38% of women would undergo an elective cesarean delivery [6].

The fact that even well-informed patients chose this option shows that the perceived risks from elective cesarean deliveries are much lower than those regarding fetal distress during labor.

CESAREAN DELIVERY AND SOCIOLOGICAL ASPECTS

In the United Kingdom, the risk of death by elective cesarean delivery is lower than the risk of dying while attending a weekend football match, as stated by Nichols Fisk.

Another element that has contributed to the increase in cesarean deliveries and that deserves attention is the hesitancy displayed in complex obstetric situations. This results in physicians and staff choosing to immediately perform a cesarean delivery instead of continuing with procedures that would lead to a spontaneous delivery. It has in fact been demonstrated that obstetricians who have incurred an "obstetric failure" with medico-legal repercussions, have later recorded a higher rate of cesarean deliveries compared to the period prior to the event [7]. Nowadays, even in the absence of such a negative and extraordinary event, in order to prevent a statistically possible outcome, many obstetricians prefer a cesarean delivery. In fact, in many countries, obstetricians are aware of the possible medico-legal consequences resulting from an unsatisfactory childbirth management outcome, in terms of protracted, costly, and traumatic legal experiences.

Physiological and behavioral changes of the human species can also be held responsible for the increased rate of cesarean deliveries: the frequency of women bearing their first child at a later age compared to the past (over the age of 35), which has proven to be linked to a significant increase in cesarean deliveries, is on the rise [8]. Bad nutritional habits are also a contributing factor. For example, the percentage and degree of obesity in North America and other countries is increasing along with cesarean deliveries [9]. In fact, a review of the global statistics on the major causes of cesarean deliveries shows an increased frequency of medical and surgical indications, including extreme obesity, diabetes, and high blood pressure, as well as previous pelvic surgery, such as myomectomy.

Among the causes of cesarean deliveries in developed countries are social phenomena, such as an increase in the frequency of diabetes mellitus (including all the type I and II subcategories, in addition to gestational diabetes [10]), as well as of macrosomic fetuses [11] in subjects with a substantial increase in pelvic adiposity. Obesity is in fact also associated with an increased rate of unengaged fetal head in primaparae. These phenomena have numerous social, political, and health-care consequences, many of which lead, as mentioned, to an increase in the frequency of cesarean deliveries. Whereas in the previous century, with regard to the tendency of giving birth late in life, most primaparae had an unengaged fetal head in late gestation, some studies have shown that the frequency of delivery with an unengaged head at the onset of labor is 43%–78% [12–14]. This may also justify changes in the standard labor curves, as in the Zhang curve [15] that is longer than the original Friedman curve [16].

CESAREAN DELIVERY AND INDICATIONS

The new indications for a cesarean delivery include all the breech deliveries [17] that previously were performed

Table 13.1 Classification of cesarean deliveries (CD) in 10 groups, according to Robson

Nulliparous/Pluriparous	Presentation	Type of labor
Nulliparous	Single fetus in cephalic presentation	Spontaneous, ≥37 weeks
Nulliparous	Single fetus in cephalic presentation	Induced or cesarean delivery after labor, ≥37 weeks
Pluriparous (excluding prior cesarean delivery)	Single fetus in cephalic presentation	Spontaneous, ≥37 weeks
Pluriparous (excluding prior cesarean delivery)	Single fetus in cephalic presentation	Induced or cesarean delivery after labor, ≥37 weeks
Prior cesarean delivery	Single fetus in cephalic presentation	No labor, ≥37 weeks
All breech presentations	—	—
All breech presentations (including prior cesarean delivery)	—	—
All pluriparae (including prior cesarean delivery)	—	—
All malpresentations (including prior cesarean delivery)	—	—
All cephalic presentations (including prior cesarean delivery)	—	≤36 weeks

Source: Robson M, *Fetal Matern Med Rev*, 12(1), 23–39, 2001.

vaginally, multiple births as a result of infertility treatments [18], previous hysterotomy in the 18 months prior to gestation, and the closure of the uterus wall with a single layer. With regard to childbirth after a cesarean delivery (vaginal birth after cesarean [VBAC]), fears of dire medicolegal consequences can be an indication for an iterative and programmed cesarean delivery or for inducing early labor.

In any case, the frequency of cesarean deliveries during active labor is progressively increasing.

Robson classified the reasons for a cesarean delivery, which comprise 10 mutually exclusive groups, as shown in Table 13.1: three countries and many institutions have adopted this classification system [19]. Data emerging from the use of this classification show that the groups that contribute most to the increase in cesarean deliveries are primiparous women at term with vertex presentation or in induced or spontaneous labor. The third major group includes women with previous uterine scar, the majority of which is admitted as primiparous in labor.

CESAREAN DELIVERY AND SUBSEQUENT DELIVERY

In North America the rate of VBAC is decreasing. The frequency of labor pain has also significantly dropped. The rate of VBAC has decreased annually from 28% in 1996 to less than 10% in 2004 [1].

In contrast to the above, it is interesting to observe that the frequency of induced labor is increasing in developed countries. In fact, in the United States it has increased by 125% from 1989, when a percentage of 20.5% of all births was registered for the first time, to 2001. In fact, the need for induced labor has increased by 68% in this time period [20]. Robson has shown that this group of induced women shows a higher percentage of cesarean deliveries compared to those with spontaneous labor [19].

An analysis of the literature reveals that the most common reason for cesarean deliveries in primiparae is nonprogressive labor [20]. This indication relates to approximately 80% of cesarean deliveries, while only 1%–2% of all cesarean deliveries are caused by fetal distress [21].

LIMITATIONS IN THE CURRENT MANAGEMENT OF LABOR

Limitations in the current management of labor that can lead to an increase in the rate of cesarean deliveries can be divided into

- Limitations in the physician's ability to evaluate the progress of labor
- Use of inadequate protocols, with the acquired information, regarding the appropriate management of labor

Reliable data indicate that human fingers are far from being accurate in evaluating the important parameters of labor progress, with the exception of engagement, position of fetal head, and cervical dilatation.

Engagement of the fetal head in the birth canal

This definition describes the position of the lower portion of the fetal head in relation to the ischial spines of the female pelvis.

The ability of clinicians to assess the engagement of the presenting part (Figure 13.1) was evaluated with a pelvic model. The results of the study were clearly insufficient, with a failure to diagnose engagement in 36%–80% of cases. Even when asked to define the head of the fetus as high, medium, or low, there were inaccuracies in judgment in 34% of the cases [22]. In addition, clinical experience did not in any way improve the ability of clinicians to accurately determine the real position of the fetal head in the female pelvis.

A potential bias of this study was the definition used for the engagement of the fetal head. One study has shown that

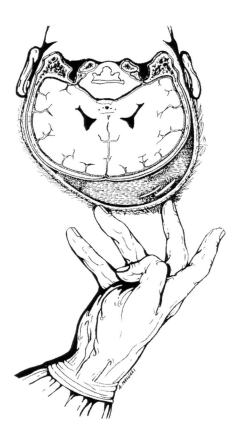

Figure 13.1 The caput succedaneum represents the most important obstacle in dystocic labor of fetal head position diagnosis. It reduces the accuracy of digital palpation of the sutures and fontanels. (Modified from Malvasi A, Di Renzo GC. *Ecografia intraparto ed il parto*, Bari, Italy: Editori Laterza; 2012.)

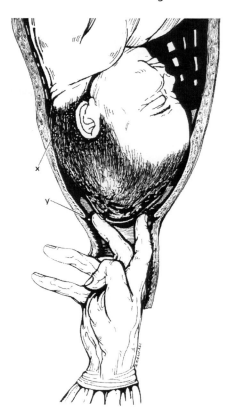

Figure 13.2 During the first stage of labor, small cervical dilatation reduces the accuracy of digital palpation of the sutures and fontanels (y, the inferior limit of lower uterine segment; x, the superior limit of lower uterine segment). (Modified from Malvasi A, Di Renzo GC. *Ecografia intraparto ed il parto*, Bari, Italy: Editori Laterza; 2012.)

243 female obstetric students from four university obstetric clinics employed four different definitions of head engagement during labor [23]. In order to settle this question, some clinicians have used the American College of Obstetrics and Gynecology (ACOG) classification, which measures the engagement in centimeters, while others still use the old system of dividing the pelvis into thirds (thus defining the station in a ratio from 1 to 3). However, in the previous study clinicians also did not agree on the obstetric moment in which the fetal head enters the pelvis: some obstetricians defined engagement as the moment in which the presenting part reaches the ischial spines, while others defined it as when the biparietal diameter reaches that level.

The result of this confusion in obstetric terminology is four definitions for the engagement of the presenting part. The most striking aspect of this disagreement in terminologies was that obstetric students themselves were not aware of their disagreement in defining the engagement.

Position of the fetal head

Very few studies have evaluated the accuracy of digital examination in the evaluation of the position of the fetal head in labor. Evaluation of the position of the fetal head during labor is traditionally determined vaginally, by locating the sagittal suture and anterior and posterior fontanels of the fetus in relation to the diameters of the pelvis.

In dystocic labor, birth swelling renders the fontanels and fetal sutures scarcely tangible, and thus digital examination has limitations in terms of evaluating the position of the fetal head, and hence in terms of diagnostic judgment (Figure 13.2).

Clinical evaluation of the position of the fetal head by digital examination during active labor can be easily compared to the position of the fetal head viewed by ultrasound in labor. Sherer et al. [24] observed a correct evaluation with obstetric visit in only 40% of cases. Akmal et al. [25] compared these two methods of determining the position of the fetal head: the occiput transverse position was correctly identified in only 54% of cases (Figure 13.3).

Cervical dilation

There is no universal standard applicable for the evaluation of cervical dilation. There are, however, studies that evaluate the ability to determine cervical dilation by comparing the digital examination of two examiners or the evaluation of an examiner on a cervical model (Figure 13.4). Research comparing two examiners in an obstetric examination has shown that usually there is a variability of 1–2 cm of

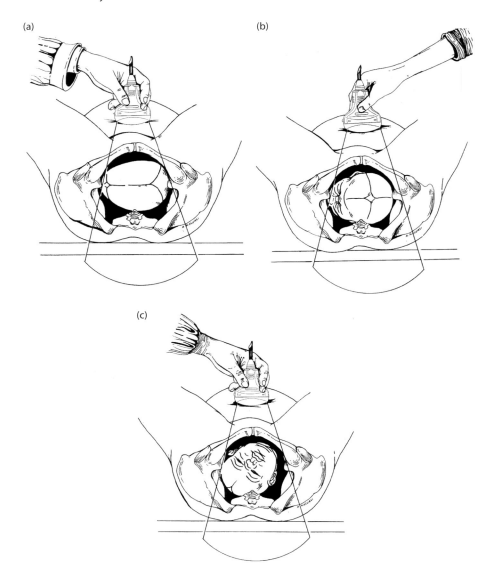

Figure 13.3 Images of intrapartum ultrasound: (a) vertex presentation, left occiput transverse position; (b) frontal presentation; (c) face presentation (easily diagnosed vaginally by palpation of the face). (Modified from Malvasi A, Di Renzo GC. *Ecografia intraparto ed il parto*, Bari, Italy: Editori Laterza; 2012.)

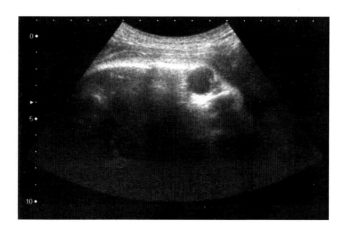

Figure 13.4 Translabial ultrasound shows a right deep transverse occiput position that required cesarean delivery.

dilation in the vaginal examination evaluation, although this variability can go up to 6 cm [26]. Studies with cervical models have shown that the accuracy of clinicians in evaluating cervical dilation within 1 cm was only about 50% [27,28].

Tufnell showed that digital examinations from a single observer were appropriate only 33% of the time, suggesting that even repeated examinations by a single clinician provide a variable value. The authors of this study conclude that an examiner who believes to have correctly estimated cervical dilation, usually either overestimates or underestimates it.

Problems with digital examination, for example, include the poor accuracy of the examination in relation to the speed of labor: human fingers are able to determine differences of at most 1–2 cm. In the dilation of the active phase of labor it takes on average 2 hours to achieve a change

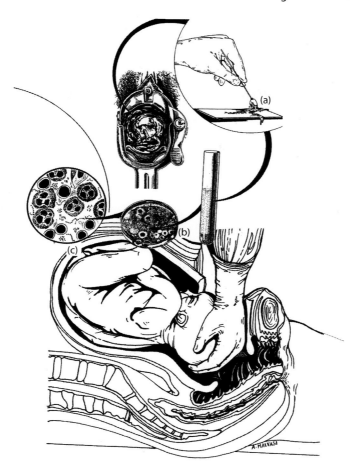

Figure 13.5 Fresh vaginal bacteriological examination: (a) culture, (b) presence of bacteria-cocci (c) in the course of pregnancy. (Modified from Malvasi A, Di Renzo GC. *Semeiotica Ostetrica*, Rome, Italy: CIC Edizioni Internazionali; 2012.)

of dilation that exceeds this value; more frequent examinations presumably increase the inaccuracy of the digital examination.

There is also the additional risk of causing infections with a vaginal examination (Figure 13.5). In the presence of rupture of membranes, vaginal examinations are linked to an increased risk of chorioamnionitis [29], which is why clinicians must choose between gathering more information about the dilation and the evolution of the labor or increasing the risk of infections.

There is also the cervix parameter, seen as a dynamic organ. Cervical dilatation during the active phase of labor is stimulated by contractions. During a contraction the cervix dilates and subsequently retracts. In one of our experiments we have shown that this effect is more than 1 cm in 50% of contractions and can reach 4 cm [30]. Therefore, it is important to document whether the vaginal examination has been carried out during or between contractions. Additionally, the cervix has its own degree of elasticity. In order to assess the cervical dilation with greater accuracy, the fingers of examiners must try to stretch the cervix as much as possible in a latero-lateral sense. Dilatation is achieved when fingers obtain a counterpressure produced by the plasticity of the cervix.

We have data that demonstrate how the uterine cervix is further extended by a few millimeters during a vaginal examination.

There are also obstetric dogmatic assertions: a dogma, never put to the test yet always considered a truthful statement, is that full dilatation of the cervix is at 10 cm. This can be quite inaccurate. For example, in preterm labor the cervix can accommodate the fetal head at a lower level of dilatation. Moreover, even in full labor, complete dilatation is a function of the full circumference of the fetal head, which can be quite variable.

INSUFFICIENT ALGORITHMS FOR THE MANAGEMENT OF LABOR

It therefore seems clear that obstetricians have little ability to scientifically determine certain key events in labor. The only obstetric event that seems to be documented with sufficient accuracy is the time and date of birth. Other events of labor, including the beginning and the achievement of full dilation, are usually defined retrospectively.

Patients often have difficulty determining when contractions become painful, due to the subjective perception of pain, and to what often seems to be premature labor or completion of gestation but is actually false labor or a prodromal event. In the same way that it is difficult to make the diagnosis of early labor, it is equally difficult to define the active phase, which, again, is usually determined retrospectively. The assessment of full dilatation of the uterine cervix through bimanual examination implies that this event occurs at a specific time, between the obstetric visit and the previous evaluation.

An important factor in the decision-making process is the occurrence of nonprogressive labor, determined by a limited progression in the dilation of the cervix between two visits. Generally, the time necessary to ensure an expansion between one visit and the next is between 1 and 4 hours.

Similarly, the speed of labor is hard to define, because it is based on inaccurate and, above all, subjective measurements that are not collected in real time by an accurate instrument.

Letic has calculated that, considering only the error committed during the visit in the evaluation of the cervical dilation, there would be an incorrect assessment of the evolution of labor in 33% of cases with an interval of 2 hours, and in 11% of the cases in 4 hours [31]. This is due to the fact that there are no individual dilation curves in childbirth labor but only standard curves, which in most cases are misleading.

Cervical dilation curves or partograms describe the cervical dilation and the descent of the presenting part, but not the position of the head. A vaginal examination is hardly reliable as it is a subjective evaluation. However, the resultant curves of a partogram are similarly unreliable, both in the labor of primiparae as well as of multiparae, in which different variables come into play.

As mentioned, the more recent curve of labor is Zhang's [15], which appears quite different from that described by Friedman more than 60 years ago [16]. The differences result from the fact that Friedman's curve was conceived about 30 years before the one by Zhang. These in fact reflect the fetal and maternal anthropomorphic mutations in industrialized populations.

The use of oxytocin to induce or increase the labor of childbirth creates problems on how to interpret labor itself, as this drug is used in about 50% of all labors. An additional and more complex problem inherent in an oxytocin-controlled delivery concerns the disagreements in protocols regarding the use of oxytocin. There are, in fact, various recommended regimes, dosages, and increments in dosages. In this regard, there are fundamental differences among the various study protocols. For example, many North American protocols support the reduction in the administration of oxytocin when the patient experiences tachysystole, with more than five contractions in 19 minutes [32], whereas the active management of labor in Ireland has no limitations. There is also a lack of clarity about when to reduce or suspend administration of oxytocin. One study has demonstrated that when a dilation of 5 cm is achieved, the dose of oxytocin can be reduced appreciably, as significant contractions are no longer necessary, and would serve only to maintain contractile activity [33].

The inherent problem with all these protocols and clinical studies is that oxytocin has a short half-life of only 1–5 minutes and its administration can be dosed and alternated, minute by minute. Given the current state of knowledge we do not have a good feedback mechanism for modulating the use of oxytocin, as feedback with dilation and/or descent of the presenting part is at intervals of hours, rather than minutes.

We now discuss the innovative ability to evaluate dilation of the uterine cervix by means of an instrumental measurement of the cervical dilation, defined as cervicometry.

THE INVENTION OF CERVICOMETERS AND INITIAL ATTEMPTS AT USING THEM

Emanuel Friedman, a pioneer of cervicometry represented by graphs on a partogram, was the first to measure the speed of labor and to create a mechanical cervicometer [34]. A similar instrument, consisting in the sophisticated use of a device that measures the progressive dilatation of the cervix, was developed by Krementsov [35]. Major drawbacks of these mechanical cervicometers were the impossibility to measure dilations in a continuous manner, and the distortion of the cervical dilation produced by the instrument.

The next step in the evolution of cervicometry was instruments that were comfortable and reliable, which were achieved by developing electromechanical devices. These tools were introduced by various scholars such as Smyth [36], Siener [37], Friedman and Von Micsky [38], and Richardson et al. [39]. Even these instruments, however, had significant problems, as they distorted the anatomy of the uterine cervix and were bulky. They also interfered with the vaginal exploration and blocked the birth canal at the time of birth.

Starting from this data, Kreiwall and Work subsequently developed an electromagnetic cervicometer based on changes of the magnetic field [40]. This instrument avoided some of the problems mentioned above, but the earth's magnetic field altered readings when dilations were greater than 6 cm.

Further innovations in the cervicometer occurred with the introduction of new ultrasonic instruments. This device was invented by both an American group, composed of Zador et al. [41], and a Dutch group, composed of Kok [42] and Eijskoot [43]. Ultrasonic transducers were placed on the patient's abdomen and the receivers were connected to the cervix. The real advantages of these devices were the smallness of the electrodes and the reliability of the reading compared to real obstetric data. Unfortunately, none of these cervicometers gained clinical consensus, and many of these were used on a relatively small number of patients (less than 100). In fact, only two journals collected this data and described the model and use of these instruments, due to lack of consensus among professionals.

It seems quite interesting that in the years between 1991 and 2000, besides the two aforementioned journals containing articles by Van Dessel [44] and Lucidi [45], not a single new publication about cervicometry was published. Letic published on mechanical cervicometry in 2005 [46]. Currently, to the state of our knowledge, there are only two other companies that look to ultrasound-based cervicometry. A research group has in fact presented its ideas on the possibility of creating an instrument based on ultrasound, but has not provided or published any data. The other group is that of Barnev, which instead has numerous publications [47–49] and has submitted its own data [50–54].

BARNEV CERVICOMETER FOR CONTINUOUS LABOR MONITORING (CLM)

The Barnev cervicometer is a tool based on ultrasounds [47] and uses transmitters placed on the abdomen of the patient to generate frequent waves. The receivers are placed on the head of the fetus and on the lateral margins of the external uterine orifice of the cervix. These measure the level of the presenting part of the fetus and monitor the fetal heart rate. In a manner that is similar to the monitoring of fetal cardiac activity, commercial scalp electrodes, modified for this purpose, are used to measure cervical dilatation (Figure 13.6). The time needed for the ultrasonic signal to travel from the abdominal transmitters to the neck or head electrodes is measured and used to calculate the distances between transmitters and receivers. By triangulating these distances with specific mathematical algorithms, it is possible to determine both the cervical dilation as well as the position of the fetal head.

The principles of the system are similar to the global standard of satellite positioning systems currently in vogue, i.e., the Global Positioning System (GPS). Data obtained by the cervicometer can be shown continuously on a small portable monitor (Figure 13.7) or sent to a monitor that shows the standard fetal heartbeat. Data can also be stored on an external storage unit along with other data, or it can be printed. The above-mentioned cervicometer produces real-time data on cervical dilatation and fetal head position.

Current applications of the Barnev cervicometer

The Barnev cervicometer has been used on more than three hundred patients in five centers and, to this day, has provided a continuous and accurate monitoring of cervical dilation, as reported in some trials. The application protocols of the cervicometer, however, require that it be positioned in the active phase of the first stage of labor. It also requires close monitoring of the position in the postpartum period. There may, in fact, be some small lacerations at the attachment point on the cervix. Until now only two minor abrasions have been recorded on more than 600 placements and only one patient required a small suture on the site of application of the internal electrode. No patient has complained about objective and symptomatic infections or bleeding.

The patients to which cervicometers were applied were given questionnaires on the acceptability of the system in general and in particular of the positioning of the internal electrodes. An analysis of the results has produced enthusiastic comments, and minimal discomfort during the

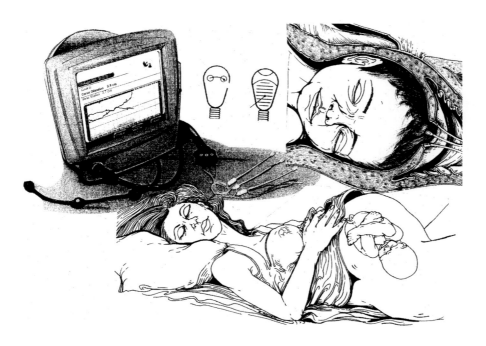

Figure 13.6 Application of electrodes on the fetal scalp and on the cervix, from the Barnev cervicometer, during the first stage of childbirth labor. (Modified from Malvasi A, Di Renzo GC. *Semeiotica Ostetrica*, Rome, Italy: CIC Edizioni Internazionali; 2012.)

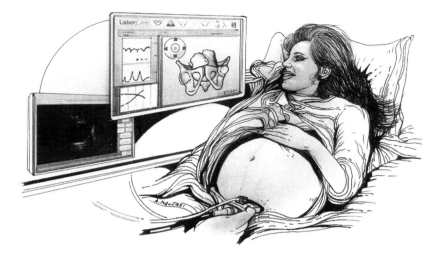

Figure 13.7 The LaborPro automatically computes data from the ultrasound image landmarks (biparietal diameter [BPD], head tip, orbits, etc.), providing precise measurement of fetal head station, head position, and head descent during contractions in relation to pelvic inlet plane and birth canal. (Modified from Malvasi A, Di Renzo GC. *Ecografia intraparto ed il parto*, Bari, Italy: Editori Laterza; 2012.)

application. It was an overall positive experience, particularly for some patients who could objectively assess their own labor.

In summary, the potential advantages of this system include

1. Generation of continuous and accurate data on two crucial parameters for the assessment of progression of labor: cervical dilatation and level of the fetal head.
2. Early detection of precipitous labor or arrest of labor.
3. Subjective and inaccurate assessment of cervical dilatation, as determined by vaginal examinations at intervals of 3–4 hours.
4. Reduction in the number of vaginal examinations, which may not be effective or may even be harmful for various reasons.
5. Generation of objective data and definite parameters on the progression of labor, which can be displayed on a computer in the room of the obstetrician-gynecologist on duty, thereby eliminating the need for multiple phone calls between medical and nursing staff.
6. Improvement of forensic documentation on the real evolution of labor.
7. Ability of the staff to make timely calls in case of imminent birth (obstetrician–gynecologist, obstetrician–anesthetist, obstetrician–neonatologist).

The disadvantages of the system can be broadly grouped into two categories. Cervicometer complications fall into the first category. Up to now in more than 300 cases analyzed, the risk of infection and bleeding is only theoretical, while the risk of cervical abrasion is very small (<0.5%). The second category involves the comfort and ergonomics of the instruments. An additional monitor would be used during labor, making delivery even less natural and more medicalized.

The benefits of this system, though, clearly outweigh these theoretical obstacles.

Possible future applications of cervicometry

The current applications of this system are considerable, yet in the near and imminent future these instruments might substantially change how labor is conducted.

In a preliminary study on the physiology of individual contractions [53], the Barnev cervicometer was used to evaluate the effect of individual contractions on dilation changes and the position of the presenting part. These preliminary data indicate a significant shift in the attitude by obstetricians regarding cervical dilations and the position of the head in response to uterine contractions. The data also suggest that this model can be very useful in identifying the exact moment in which the active phase begins and dilation is complete. Early detection of contractions not functional to dilation can be added to the cartographic parameters and can be concurrent with the diagnosis of slow dilation or poor descent of the fetal head. These data may lead to early obstetric interventions, thereby potentially reducing the need to resort to a cesarean delivery.

In light of the above, the authors suggest that analysis of rapid changes in cervical dilatation and/or engagement of the presenting part with a cervicometer could be an excellent diagnostic and therapeutic foundation. As mentioned, oxytocin, beta-agonist with a very short half-life, may be used based on the frequency and duration of contractions, both surrogate parameters in the evolution of childbirth labor. Cervical dilatation and descent of the head are, however, the two most reliable parameters for monitoring the progression of labor. It follows from the above that both can be evaluated with computerized cervicometry.

The authors of this chapter believe that, in a not-too-distant future, the dosage of oxytocin may be determined from short-term changes in cervical dilation and in the position of the head (both indicated by the cervicometer). This would eliminate the current long vaginal examination interval of 2–4 hours, in addition to reducing the number of vaginal examinations and resulting endometritis and chorioamnionitis.

A preliminary investigation of dystocic labor on an animal model has led to the conclusion that this instrument can potentially lead to an effective and timely obstetric intervention.

Short-term changes in dilation and in the position of the presenting part, in addition to the models provided by the instrument during the contractions, can provide good feedback for guiding the administration of oxytocin. As a result of its application there would be a reduction in vaginal visits, a lower rate of infection, a reduction in the rate of cesarean deliveries, and, probably, cesarean deliveries carried out early, with all the necessary indications [50–54].

CONCLUSIONS

Dystocia represents about 50% of the causes of operative deliveries and, in particular, of cesarean deliveries, while fetal distress represents 1%–2% of operative deliveries. However, while fetal distress can be measured with various instrumental techniques (cardiotocography, pulse oximetry, fetal electrocardiogram [ECG] or STAN), there have been no technological advancements in diagnosing dystocia, which to this day is done primarily by abdominal and vaginal examination.

An increase in legal disputes necessitates an objective assessment of maternal and fetal pathologies, and thus also of dystocia. Several studies have confirmed the diagnostic unreliability of vaginal examination, both in the first as well as in the second stage of labor. Therefore, the need in obstetrics for objective feedback has become more and more evident. The use of intrapartum ultrasound has been proposed to make up for the diagnostic inadequacy of the traditional obstetric examination, and this has significantly reduced the error in the diagnosis of fetal head position by 40%–70%. Nevertheless, a system that can objectively evaluate the different maternal and fetal delivery variables has not yet been validated.

Different instruments, named cervicometers, have been experimented with in the past, in the attempt to overcome this problem, but without significant clinical success. Researchers have achieved important results by using a ultrasound tool and placing transmitters on the abdomen of the patient, in order to produce waves that could be interpreted by special mathematical algorithms in a computer. The development of this instrument and the objective assessment of other parameters (currently not assessable) could represent a clinical application system that objectively determines dystocic birth, in the same manner as the cardiotocograph interprets fetal distress.

REFERENCES

1. Martin JA, Hamilton BE, Menacker F, Sutton PD, Mathews TJ. *Preliminary births for 2004: Infant and maternal health. Health E-stats.* Hyattsville, MD: National Center for Health Statistics. http://www.cdc.gov/nchs/products/pubs/pubd/hestats/prelimbirths04/prelimbirths04health.htm. Accessed November 15, 2005.
2. Martin JA, Hamilton BE, Sutton PD et al. Births: Final data for 2003. *National Vital Statistics Reports* 2005;54(2). Hyattsville, MD: National Center for Health Statistics. 2005. http://www.cdc.gov/nchs/data/nvsr/nvsr54/nvsr54_02.pdf. Accessed July 15, 2016.
3. Belizan JM et al. Rates and implications of caesarean sections in Latin America: Ecological study. *BMJ* 1999;319(7222):1397.
4. Wax JR, Cartin A, Pinette MG, Blackstone J. Patient choice cesarean: An evidence-based review. *Obstet Gynecol Survey* 2004;59(8):601–16.
5. Berger H, Revah G, AlSunnari S, Feig D, Chalmers B, Farine D. *Clinical Benefit Is Not a Factory Determining Acceptability of Screening for Gestational Diabetes.* SMFM, New Orleans, LA, 2004.
6. Paterson-Brown S. Should doctors perform an elective caesarean section on request? Yes, as long as the woman is fully informed. *BMJ* 1998;317(7156):462–3.
7. Turrentine MA Ramirez MM. Adverse perinatal events and subsequent cesarean rate. *Obstet Gynecol* 1999;94(2):185–8.
8. Ezra Y, McParland P, Farine D. High delivery intervention rates in nulliparous women over age 35. *Eur J Obstet Gynecol Reprod Biol* 1995;62(2):203–7.
9. American Congress of Obstetricians and Gynecologists (ACOG). ACOG Committee Opinion #319: The role of the obstetrician-gynecologist in the assessment and management of obesity. *Obstet Gynecol* 2005;106(4):895–899.
10. Feig DS, Palda VA. Type 2 diabetes in pregnancy: A growing concern. *Lancet* 2002;359(9318):1690–28.
11. Ananth CV, Wen SW. Trends in fetal growth among singleton gestations in the United States and Canada, 1985 through 1998. *Semin Perinatol* 2002;26(4):260–7.
12. Murphy K, Shah L, Cohen WR. Labor and delivery in nulliparous women who present with an unengaged fetal head. *J Perinatol* 1998;18(2):122–5.
13. Jafarey SN. Unengaged foetal head in Pakistani primigravida: Frequency and outcome. *Asia Oceania J Obstet Gynaecol* 1988;14(1):13–16.
14. Takahashi K, Suzuki K. Incidence and significance of the unengaged fetal head in nulliparas in early labor. *Int J Biol Res Pregnancy* 1982;3(1):8–9.
15. Zhang J, Troendle JF, Yancey MK. Reassessing the labor curve in nulliparous women. *Am J Obstet Gynecol* 2002;187(4):824–8.
16. Friedman EA. Primigravid labor: A graphicostatistical analysis. *Obstet Gynecol* 1955;6(6):567–89.
17. Hannah ME, Hannah WJ, Hewson SA, Hodnett ED, Saigal S, Willan AR. Planned caesarean section versus planned vaginal birth for breech

presentation at term: A randomised multicentre trial. Term Breech Trial Collaborative Group. *Lancet* 2000;356(9239):1375–83.
18. Blickstein I. Controversial issues in the management of multiple pregnancies. *Twin Research* 2001;4(3):165–7.
19. Robson M. Classification of cesarean sections. *Fetal Matern Med Rev* 2001;12(1):23–39.
20. Simpson KR, Atterbury J. Trends and issues in labor induction in the United States: Implications for clinical practice [see comment]. *J Obstet Gynecol Neonatal Nurs* 2003;32(6):767–79.
21. Sachs BP, Kobelin C, Castro MA, Frigoletto F. The risks of lowering the cesarean-delivery rate. *N Engl J Med* 1999;340(1):54–57.
22. Dupuis O, Silveira R, Zentner A, Dittmar A, Gaucherand P, Cucherat M, Redarce T, Rudigoz RC. Birth simulator: Reliability of transvaginal assessment of fetal head station as defined by the American College of Obstetricians and Gynecologists classification. *Am J Obstet Gynecol* 2005;192(3):868–74.
23. Carollo TC, Reuter JM, Galan HL, Jones RO. Defining fetal station. *Am J Obstet Gynecol* 2004;191:1793–6.
24. Sherer DM, Miodovnik M, Bradley KS, Langer O. Intrapartum fetal head position II: Comparison between transvaginal digital examination and transabdominal ultrasound assessment during the second stage of labor. *Ultrasound Obstet Gynecol* 2002;19(3):264–8.
25. Akmal S, Kametas N, Tsoi E, Hargreaves C, Nicolaides KH. Comparison of transvaginal digital examination with intrapartum sonography to determine fetal head position before instrumental delivery. *Ultrasound Obstet Gynecol* 2003;21(5):437–40.
26. Bergsjo P, Koss KS. Interindividual variation in vaginal examination findings during labor. *Acta Obstet Gynecol Scand* 1982;61(6):509–10.
27. Phelps JY, Higby K, Smyth MH, Ward JA, Arredondo F, Mayer AR. Accuracy and inter-observer variability of simulated cervical dilatation measurements. *Am J Obstet Gynecol* 1995;173(3 Pt 1):942–5.
28. Tuffnell DJ, Bryce F, Johnson N et al. Simulation of cervical changes in labour: Reproducibility of expert assessment. *Lancet* 1989;2:1089–90.
29. Seaward PGR, Hannah ME, Myhr TL et al. International multicenter term prelabor rupture of membranes study: Evaluation of predictors of clinical chorioamnionitis and postpartum fever in patients with prelabour rupture of membranes at term. *Am J Obstet Gynecol* 1997;177(5):1024–9.
30. Farine D, Jaffa A, Rosen B, Kreiser D, Schiff E, Kiss S, Shenhav M. The physiology of the cervix in labour: The effect of individual contractions. SMFM, Reno Nevada, February 2005. *Am J Obstet Gynecol* 2004;191(6 Suppl):S186.
31. Letic M. Inaccuracy in cervical dilatation assessment and the progress of labour monitoring. *Med Hypotheses* 2002;60(2):199–201.
32. Daniel-Spiegel E, Weiner Z, Ben-Shlomo I, Shalev E. For how long should oxytocin be continued during induction of labour? *BJOG* 2004;111:331–4.
33. Liston R, Crane J, Hughes O et al.; Fetal Health Surveillance Working Group. Fetal health surveillance in labour. *J Obstet Gynaecol Can* 2002;24(4):342–55.
34. Friedman EA. Cervimetry: An objective method for the study of cervical dilation in labour. *Am J Obstet Gynecol* 1956;71:1189–93.
35. Krementsov YG. Improved technique for measurement of cervical dilatation. *Biomed Eng* 1968;2:350.
36. Smyth CN. Measurement of the forces and strains of labour and the action of certain oxytocic drugs. *Proceedings of the International Congress of Gynaecology and Obstetrics*. Geneva, Switzerland; 1954:1030–39.
37. Siener H. First stage of labor recorded by cervical tocometry. *Am J Obstet Gynecol* 1963;86:303–9.
38. Friedman EA, Von Micsky LI. Electronic cervimeter: A research instrument for the study of cervical dilatation in labor. *Am J Obstet Gynecol* 1963;87:789–92.
39. Richardson JA, Sutherland IA, Allen DW. A cervimeter for continuous measurement of cervical dilatation in labour: Preliminary results. *BJOG* 1978;85:178–83.
40. Kriewall TJ, Work BA. Measuring cervical dilatation in human parturition using the Hall Effect. *Med Instrum* 1977;11:26–31.
41. Zador I, Neuman MR, Wolfson RN. Continuous monitoring of cervical dilatation during labor by ultrasonic transit time measurements. *Med Biol Eng* 1976;14:299–305.
42. Kok FT, Wallenburg HC, Wladimiroff JW. Ultrasonic measurement of cervical dilatation during labor. *Am J Obstet Gynecol* 1976;126:288–90.
43. Eijskoot F, Storm J, Kok FT et al. An ultrasonic device for continuous measurement of cervical dilatation during labor. *Ultrasonics* 1977;15:183–5.
44. van Dessel T et al. Assessment of cervical dilatation during labor: A review. *Eur J Obstet Gynecol Reprod Biol* 1991;41(3):165–71.
45. Lucidi RS, Blumenfeld LA, Chez RA. Cervimetry: A review of methods for measuring cervical dilatation during labor. *Obstet Gynecol Surv* 2000;55(5):312–20.
46. Letic M. Simple instrument for measuring cervical dilatation during labour. *Physiol Meas* 2005;26(1):N1–7.
47. Sharf Y, Farine D, Batzalel M, Megel Y, Shenhav M, Jaffa A, Barnea O. Continuous monitoring of cervical dilatation and fetal head station during labor. *Med Eng Phys* 2007;29(1):61–71.
48. Farine D, Shenhav M, Barnea O, Jaffa A, Fox H. The need for a new outlook on labor monitoring. *J Mat Fet Med Neonat Med* 2006;19(3):161–4.
49. Farine D, Hassan S Sorokin Y. Is cervicometry the future for labor movement? *Contemp Ob/Gyn* 2006;April:20–28.

50. Jaffa A, Shenhav M, Farine D. *Computerized Labor Management—A New Approach to Labor Management*. San Francisco, CA: Society for Maternal/Fetal Medicine;February 2003.
51. Shenhav M, Jaffa A, Kreiser D, Heifetz S, Schiff E, Farine D. *Computerized Real Time Labor Management*. New Orleans, LA: SMFM; February 2004.
52. Shenhav M, Kreiser D, Rosen B, Schiff E, Kiss S, Ariel J, Farine D. *Should Vaginal Examinations Be Performed Before, During or After Contractions?* Reno, NV: SMFM; February 2005.
53. Farine D, Jaffa A, Rosen B, Kreiser D, Schiff E, Kiss S, Shenhav M. *The Physiology of the Cervix in Labour: The Effect of Individual Contractions*. Reno, NV: SMFM; February 2005.
54. Jaffa A, Kreiser D, Schiff E, Farine D, Kiss S, Shenhav M. *Cervical Dilatation in Labour: Correlation Between Computerized Labor Monitoring (CLM) and Digital Examination (DE)*. Reno, NV: SMFM; February 2005.

FURTHER READING

Healthy People 2000 Review 1995–96, CDC, NCHS. *National Center for Health Statistics* 2000; (301):436–85.

Shoulder dystocia and cesarean delivery

ENRICO FERRAZZI

> … In spite of its low frequency, all physicians engaged in the delivery room should be prepared to handle the sudden and unpredictable onset of the dreaded complication that is shoulder dystocia [1].

INTRODUCTION

Understanding the mechanisms that lead to shoulder dystocia and, in particular, understanding which maneuvers need to be performed, requires a critical reassessment of the phases of the second stage of labor. For this purpose we start our analysis by taking a step back and looking at comparative anthropology.

The ratio between fetal head and birth canal in all anthropoid apes is such that the head of the fetus can progress into the birth canal once cervical dilatation occurs, without encountering any of the dimensional limits of the birth canal itself. The human species instead is the only one in which the head can move through the birth canal only through a complex internal rotation movement. This allows the head to engage and to overcome the mid-strait at its maximum diameter that is positioned differently than the maximum diameter of the superior strait (Figure 14.1).

This is the crucial difference compared to all other anthropoid species: the simple progression of a normally flexed head in the birth canal does not allow the delivery of full-term fetuses at normal weight (Figure 14.2). Such a limit, developed during the millions of years that have led to the upright position, has not allowed the brain weight to change (1.36 kg in an adult) [2,3].

Whatever mechanism has led to the development in our species of the brain/cranial cavity, it has been limited by the strong negative genetic pressure exerted by the fetal–pelvic disproportion, "any" fetus that has a larger brain dies at birth and, frequently, the mother also dies (Figure 14.3).

We could add to this paradigm another one: fetuses with higher percentiles of somatic development for our species encounter a second anthropomorphic limitation at childbirth. The bisacromial diameter, similarly, can move through the birth canal only to the extent that the diameter repeats the engagement mechanisms at the upper strait and the internal rotation at the mid-strait, concurrently with that of the head (Figure 14.4).

The second aspect that emerges from comparative anthropology is that delivery in all anthropoid apes is a "private" event. The female when giving birth distances herself from the group, so much so that even today there are very few images of childbirth in nature.

The selective advantage in hominids providing assistance to their females at childbirth increases the number of children in the group. This has likely resulted in childbirth being, in all human cultures, a social event in which women are assisted by third parties, both psychologically and physically.

Even today we can understand the dramatic impact of childbirth in the human species. Consider in fact the greater rate of maternal mortality and morbidity in those areas in which assistance during pregnancy and childbirth has remained unchanged for tens of thousands of years. In rural areas of Ghana the percentage of rectovaginal fistula for outcomes of arrest in the progression at mid-strait is 2% [4,5].

In 2000 the maternal mortality rate was 830 deaths per 100,000 women in Africa, in Asia 330 deaths/100,000 women (not including Japan and Korea), 240 deaths in Oceania (not including Australia and New Zealand), in Latin America 190 deaths, and in the industrialized countries 20 deaths per 100,000. The highest number of deaths in a single year was in India, with 136,000 expectant mothers who died. In 20 minutes, the time it takes to read this short text, in India alone 30 women will die during childbirth due to bleeding, infections, or obstructed labor.

In other countries, according to data from 2000, the number of maternal deaths per one hundred thousand childbirths is even higher than the previous figure: in Sierra Leone 2000 deaths per 100,000 births, in Afghanistan 1900 fatalities, in Malawi 1800, in Angola 1700, and in Niger 1600 (data from UNICEF/WHO/UNFPA: new report on maternal mortality from October 2003).

The efforts to understand and comprehend, as well as the classifications that have developed around the second stage of labor, start in the eighteenth century and continue in the Italian Porro in the second half of the nineteenth century, and in Clivio, a professor in Pavia in the 1940s. These efforts become more significant in light of all the dramatic struggles that reach far back into the history of mankind.

Since then nothing has obviously changed in human biology, with the possible exception of physical strength that, on average, is not as great as the strength we imagine our ancestors possessed. The second stage of labor therefore remains an event that is critically important in determining the quality of the childbirth for the mother–child dyad. On the other hand the general cultural context of human reproduction in the "Western" world has completely changed: society assists both pregnancy and childbirth, surgery, diagnostic techniques related to the well-being of the fetus (which we do not call mobile body

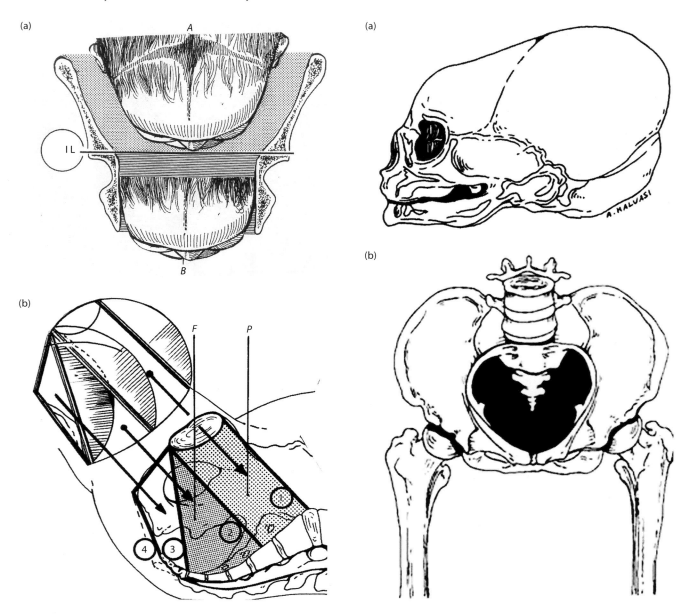

Figure 14.1 (a) Schematic frontal section of the basin (or bony pelvis). In the false (anatomical) pelvis (top image, A) the fetal head is not engaged in the pelvis. In the true (or obstetric) pelvis (bottom image, B) the fetal head is engaged. The line of separation passes through the superior strait and is called terminal line or ischiatic line (IL, in circle label). (b) Diameters of the mid-straits; Hodge's pelvic floor (P = Pigeaud's descending cylinder; F = Fouchier's disengagement triangle).

anymore), and image techniques used to objectively determine position and station [6].

THE SECOND STAGE OF LABOR
Critical points

First critical point

Traditional obstetrics divides the second stage of labor into six stages (Table 14.1). The first critical point is to define the beginning of the second stage of labor. If we

Figure 14.2 (a) Full-term human fetal skull. (b) A normal bony pelvis.

were to use Anglo-Saxon terminology, we would simply say that the second stage starts at full dilation, and that "it is characterized by the voluntary pushes of the patient" [7].

Apparently the simplification that the start of the second stage of labor = second-stage = full dilation is a descriptive advantage. Practically, however, it neglects two extraordinarily important events: the engagement of the head at the superior strait and the physiological mechanism that causes the somatic pain that induces the patient to "push out" the fetus.

According to authoritative texts the engagement of the fetal head in many nulliparae can occur before the onset of labor [8]. However, if what is meant by engagement is the widest cephalic circumference overcoming the superior

The second stage of labor 239

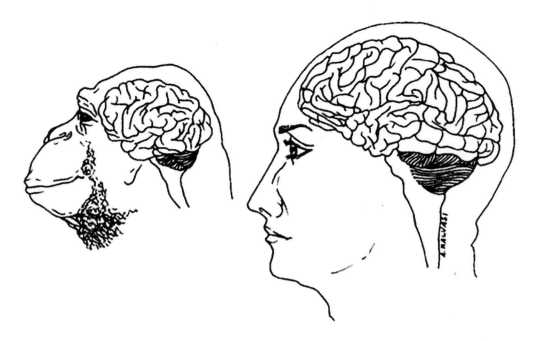

Figure 14.3 Comparison between the brain size of an adult gorilla (*left*) and the size of the human brain (*right*). (Modified from Malvasi A, Di Renzo GC. *Ecografia intraparto ed il parto*, Bari, Italy: Editori Laterza; 2012.)

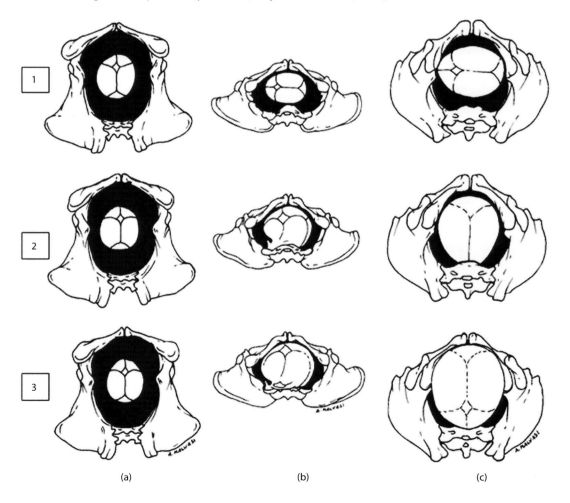

Figure 14.4 (a) The pelvis of an adult chimpanzee during childbirth: 1 = superior strait, 2 = mid-strait, 3 = inferior strait. (b) Australopithecus (A.L. 288–1) during childbirth. (c) *Homo sapiens* childbirth.

Table 14.1 Maternal-fetal childbirth stages

Active encounter	The presenting part encounters the oblique diameter of the superior strait
Reduction and engagement	The less favorable diameter of the fronto-occipital presenting part is replaced with a more favorable suboccipitobregmatic diameter, due to the force—contraction—and probably due to the combined effect of fetal posture and tone.
	Passage of the widest circumference of the presenting part in the superior strait, with suboccipitobregmatic diameter along one of the oblique diameters; generally, at this point the lowest part of the fetal head has reached the ischial spines.
Progression	The presenting part is forced to descend into the small pelvis maintaining the initial ratio of the suboccipitobregmatic diameter with an oblique diameter of the pelvis.
	The progression movement is completed when the most declivous part reaches the pelvic floor and when, concurrently, the only diameter that allows passage, or, the most favorable to passage, is the anterior–posterior. This movement corresponds to an initial spontaneous sense of contraction due to the pressure that the head exerts on the levator ani muscles.
Internal rotation engagement at the mid-strait	Rotation of the presenting part by one-eighth of a circle (45°), which moves the suboccipitobregmatic diameter along the more favorable anterior–posterior mid-strait diameter and brings the occiput up to the pubic symphysis: the occiput is thus secured under the symphysis and can start the deflection with leverage on the symphysis itself.
Disengagement of the presenting part	Overcoming the birth canal bend with extension of the head: squama occipitalis–atloido-occipital joint secured under the symphysis and uterine force applied initially to the frontal sinuses, then the nose, and finally the chin. The presenting part will move through the pelvic floor and the vulvar ring.
Restitution and external rotation concurrent with engagement of the shoulders and with internal shoulder rotation	Restitution: the head rotates from occiput anterior by 45° to the left or to the right, depending on the initial position, in the opposite direction to the internal rotation, thereby restoring the perpendicular orientation of its anterior–posterior diameter relative to the bisacromial diameter, that is now located at the superior strait, with anterior acromion on the right anterior oblique diameter.
	Rotation of the head by another 45°, clockwise, consensual with the rotation; rotation and engagement of the bisacromial diameter: from the superior strait—oblique diameter—to the mid-strait—anterior–posterior diameter. Subsequent securing of the anterior shoulder under the symphysis and progression of the posterior shoulder in the sacral concavity.
Total expulsion of the fetus	Engagement of the anterior shoulder under the symphysis, lateral flexion of the fetal trunk, disengagement of the posterior shoulder, and subsequent expulsion of chest, abdomen, and lower limbs.

strait, it occurs as a result of uterine contractions at the end of the dilation period [9].

The two concurrent events, complete dilation and engagement at the upper strait, mark the beginning of the second stage of labor. We know now that there may be a latency period, which can even be lengthy, between full dilation and engagement. In our experience in Milan, this latency, with a reassuring CTG, can last up to 3 hours, which then leads to a completely normal second stage of labor.

Ultrasound, combined with clinical obstetrics, teaches us that in about 20%–30% of labors at full dilation, the presentation is posterior [10,11]. Additionally we have learned that latency is determined by the amount of time needed by the fetus to bring the occiput to the front and therefore to engage in occiput anterior. Also, only a fraction of these fetuses begin the descent into the birth canal remaining in occiput posterior. This is the only knowledge that the masters of traditional obstetrics could not have had, thanks to modern-day ultrasound methods that are far more accurate than in the past. Well known, on the other hand, were the engagements in occiput posterior with progression and internal rotation at the mid-strait not of 45° (e.g., from left occiput anterior to anterior) but of 135° (i.e., from left occiput posterior to anterior).

This mechanism by which the fetal head adjusts to the best position for entrance to the superior strait is comparatively recently acquired knowledge. This justifies, if ever it were needed, the good obstetric practice of patiently waiting for full dilation and engagement, or rather, of waiting for full dilation, flexion, engagement, and progression of the head in the upper part of the birth canal. This until the appearance of the pushing sensation and of the desire on the part of the woman to perform spontaneous pushes due to the somatic pain from the pressure on the pelvic floor muscles.

When undue confusion is made between complete dilation and the beginning of the second stage of labor and hence, at complete dilation, the voluntary efforts of the parturient are being activated, maternal–fetal dystocias are likely to occur. The symptom, usually, is easily identifiable, but becomes difficult to evaluate in the presence of epidural analgesia, even when analgesia is adequately reduced at the end of the dilating period. In these cases, the obstetrician must be even more careful in determining when the patient shows objective symptomatological signs that indicate that the progression has occurred.

The active encounter mechanism—starting time for maternal–fetal events—would also justify (though this is more and more overlooked) the prompt rupture of the membranes to facilitate the movements of the fetus to adapt to the superior strait. Studies performed by Caldeyro-Barcia provide unequivocal scientific support to what normally occurs in nature: membranes rupture spontaneously in over 80% of cases, between 8 cm and complete dilation [12] (see Box 14.1).

Second critical point

The second critical point is well evidenced by the descriptive and semiological differences that exist between traditional Italian and Anglo-Saxon obstetrics. The differences are in how to describe that which we define the first three phases of the second stage of labor: I reduction and engagement, II spontaneous progression, and III internal rotation.

The objective diagnostics of the progression in the birth canal according to Anglo-Saxon criteria is based on identifying the station of the end of the presenting part, in relation to the level of the ischial spines, and expressed in the number of centimeters above (or below) the plane of the ischial spines (Figure 14.6).

A descriptive advantage of this semiotics is the parallel representation of the evolution of the dilation and the progression. The disadvantage of this semiotics is that less clinical diagnostic attention is paid to the movements of spontaneous progression and internal rotation, which would result in the head "engaging" the mid-strait from an optimal position. The same image that was used to "explain" the station of the presenting part in relation to the ischial spines makes you lose sight of the problem of internal rotation.

It is worth remembering, as a counterpoint, that humans are the only species that resort to this mechanism, in order for the cephalic extremity to advance in the birth canal. The birth canal therefore is not a tube with neutral landmarks as it would appear to be from the didactic representation used in Anglo-Saxon texts.

Box 14.1 Summary of first critical point

1. Add to the six traditional obstetrics movements the active encounter movement of the fetal head at the superior strait (Figure 14.5).
2. Define the beginning of the second stage of labor as the coexistence of complete dilation, occurred flexion, and engagement, associated with uncontrollable contractions on the part of the woman. It should be made clear that the second stage of labor can be considered started only in the presence of unrelenting contractions. This would avoid various iatrogenic situations caused by operators urging the woman to push in the absence of any spontaneous contraction.

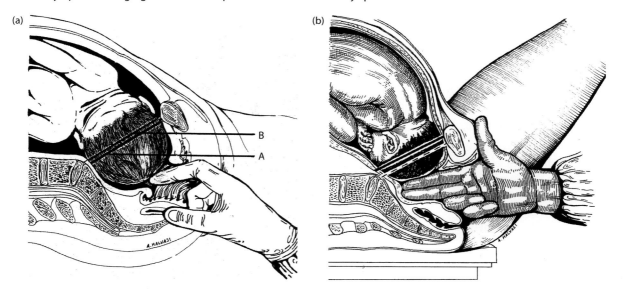

Figure 14.5 (a) Sagittal section of pelvis and of a fetal head that is encountering the superior strait in synclitism, while the operator palpates the left ischial spine (A = biparieta diameter, B =obstetric coniugate). (b) Sagittal section of the obstetric pelvis in the second stage of labor, in which the operator evaluates the encounter of the fetal head at the upper entrance (Farabeuf maneuver). ([b] Modified from Vincenzo T. *Semeiotica Ostetrica*, Bari, Italy: Editori Laterza; 1992.)

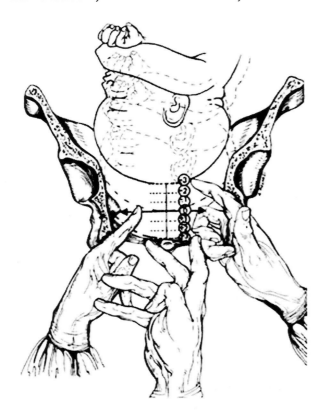

Figure 14.6 Stations of the fetal head in relation to the pelvis: the *plane* of the ischial spines is defined as station 0 (indicating the engagement). Above this plane the station is defined as −1, −2, and −3; as the fetal vertex descends the station is referred to as +1, +2, +3. The numbers refer to the distance (measured in centimeters), which separates the most prominent area of the fetal head from the area of the ischial spines.

Beck, in describing the third movement of the mechanical actions, i.e., internal rotation, uses the following definition: "… this movement is always associated with the descent of the presenting part and, usually, is not completed until the fetal head has reached the level of the ischial spines (+2) …" [7].

Semiotics of traditional Italian obstetrics, well highlighted by Pardi [9], proposed for recognizing and diagnosing these events is based, according to Clivio [13], not on the relation between cephalic extremity and spines, but rather on the relation between the fetal head and the pubic symphysis during progression in the upper part of the birth canal.

Here is the simple and elegant description provided by Clivio [13]:

> [I]t is said that the head is still mobile at the superior strait when fingers are able to push it back and run along the posterior surface of the pubic symphysis, up to its upper edge; that it is secured at the superior strait, when we are not able to push it back, and the upper edge of the pubic symphysis is no longer accessible [Figure 14.7]. We will say that the head is at the top part of the cavity when fingers are able to reach the lower two-thirds of the pubic symphysis; that it is in the mid or inferior part of the cavity when the lower half or third of the symphysis, respectively, are accessible. It will be said that the head is at the inferior strait when only the lower margin of the symphysis pubis [Figure 14.8], and the tip of the coccyx can be reached; in this case it will also be possible to see if the head has completed the rotation movement, by seeing if the sagittal suture is oriented according to the direction of the coccyx–pubic diameter.

The reproducibility of this semiotics, in its simplicity, is probably higher than that of the station in relation to the ischial spines. Mainly, however, it puts at the center of the first phase of the second stage of labor, the correct attainment of the mid-strait in occiput anterior.

It is important to reiterate the importance of the diagnosis of the position of the presenting part, as it influences the duration of the internal rotation and provides precise information on the fifth period of childbirth: moment of restitution and external rotation concurrent with engagement of the shoulders and with internal shoulder rotation. If those who are assisting the woman know the position of the fetal head at that moment, then they will know in which direction the head will make the restitution.

In 70% of cases the semiotics is simple, based on the identification of the longitudinal suture and the triangular fontanels. Unfortunately, this objective semiotics is most frequently uncertain when progression has slowed down or stopped. The therapeutic decision, in such cases, should be preceded by simple and reproducible ultrasound semiotics, as widely recommended in the literature and in the guidelines of the Canadian Society of Obstetrics.

The head overcomes the mid-strait (the longest segment in a eutocic birth) after it has engaged, when the occiput is balanced under the lower edge of the symphysis, to allow deflection and progression to the perineal level, which then stretches to allow disengagement of the head (fourth movement). The time from the engagement at the mid-strait to overcoming it can be very long, as the head, in spite of the rotation, may have to confront plastic changes in order to overcome this limit point.

In the past, that we can read about in historical texts on childbirth, or even today see in childbirth assistance in rural populations of the Third World, this time could last for hours or even days. This could result in the death of the fetus and in an acceleration of plastic phenomena, such as postmortem childbirth caused by muscle rigor of the dead mother, associated with postmortem phenomena of the fetal head.

Burial remains of women who died during childbirth have been found, in which a small fetal skeleton lies between the femurs of the woman. It was due to these postmortem childbirths that the first Christian-era emperors decided that doctors, who had assisted in childbirths that resulted in the death of the mother from "obstructed labor," had to perform a midline laparotomy

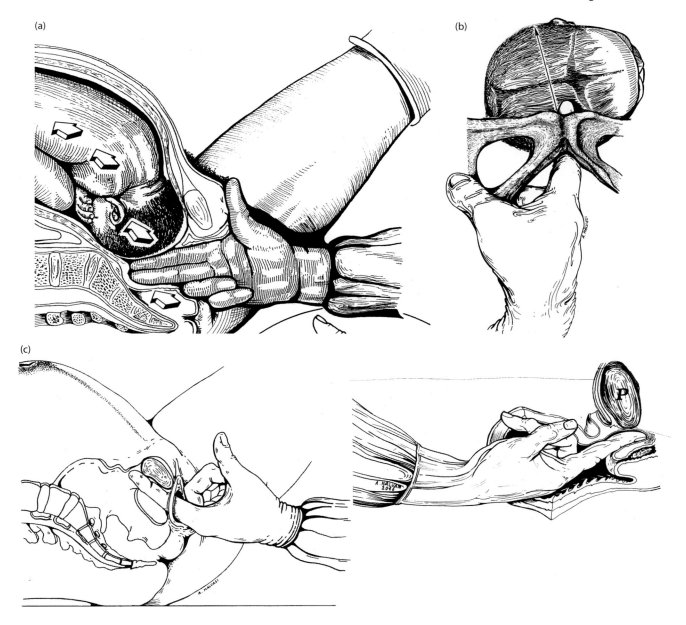

Figure 14.7 (a) Maneuver in which the disengaged fetal head is pushed back. (b) Exploring finger reaches the upper margin of the pubic symphysis, when the head is not engaged. (c) Palpation of the lower two-thirds of the pubic symphysis, when the fetal head is in the upper part of the pelvic cavity. ([a] Modified from Vincenzo T. *Semeiotica Ostetrica*, Bari, Italy: Editori Laterza; 1992.)

and a longitudinal cut on the uterus to remove the fetus. The fetus was laid next to the mother and buried, along with the mother, facing west. This was the so-called cesarean delivery—that is, required by law by the emperor Caesar. The law was to be strictly applied, to the point that Emperor Frederick II ordered the death of doctors who did not perform the postmortem cesarean delivery as per imperial (Cesarean) law (see Box 14.2).

Third critical point

The third critical point is represented by an inadequate focus, in the description of the restitution–external rotation of the head after disengagement, on the more important events that take place concurrently in the birth canal, related to the shoulder girdle and its bisacromial maximal diameter.

In fact the shoulder girdle in a normally developed full-term fetus performs the same movements as the head in passing through the birth canal. The only exception is that the oblique diameter at the superior strait in which the shoulders will engage is normally the anterior right in an OISA (anterior left iliac occiput) delivery. The diameter that encounters, engages, progresses, rotates at the medium cavity, and engages under the symphysis is the

244 Shoulder dystocia and cesarean delivery

> **Box 14.2 Summary of second critical point**
>
> 1. Reintroduce in partograms the six phases of the second stage of labor of traditional obstetrics, in addition to the definitions of station and position of the fetal head.
> 2. Jointly consider the two objective criteria: head symphysis relationship and head ischial spines relationship.
> 3. Consider internal semiotics alongside external suprapubic and abdominal semiotics, so as to be able to identify the fetal disposition, in order to improve diagnostic reproducibility as well as to learn to recognize the external findings that will be useful in those rare cases of shoulder dystocia.

bisacromial diameter. Any plastic modification is much easier to achieve through simple forward and/or downward flexion of the clavicles. Semiotics is simpler because in eutocic childbirths the head will indicate to us these movements, as long as it is observed without improperly interfering.

Once the disengagement of the head is completed we should observe (or feel with our hands, without performing any traction) the restitution–rotation of the head by 45°, from occiput anterior under the symphysis to left occiput anterior. This corresponds to the restitution of the head to a position that is orthogonal to the axis of the shoulders, which were engaged in the front

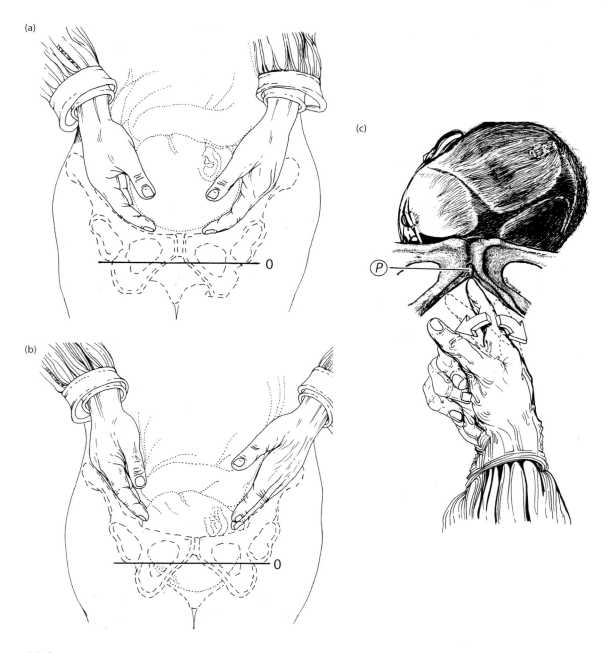

Figure 14.8 (a) Abdominal palpation (fourth Leopold maneuver) with disengaged fetal head; (b) engaged. The line shown on the pelvis represents level 0, the bisischial distance. (c) Palpation maneuver of only the lower margin of the pubic symphysis, with head engaged (*P* = pubis).

right anterior oblique diameter in the same direction as the disengagement of the head. The completion of the external rotation of the head by another 45° corresponds with the internal rotation of the shoulders at the mid-strait. This screwing movement allows the mid-strait to be overcome from the most favorable position—anterior–posterior—and brings the acromion under the symphysis (Figure 14.9).

Delivery assistance can provide a delicate rotating traction, only after observing the spontaneous restitution movement of the expelled head from left occiput anterior to left. This facilitates the progression of the front shoulder under the symphysis. When the acromion overcomes the lower margin of the symphysis, the disengagement of the rear shoulder can start. The mechanism is similar to that performed by the head (Figure 14.10).

Failure to comply with this critical point, the restitution of the head, and performing traction at this time, may cause iatrogenic shoulder pseudo-dystocias. These can be easily resolved if the fetus has a normal weight, but become complex and dramatic in macrocosmic fetuses.

In fact, traction performed before restitution can block the acromion at the symphysis (see Box 14.3).

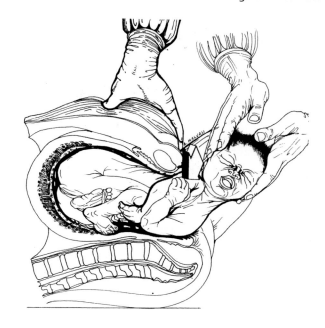

Figure 14.10 Disengagement maneuver of the rear shoulder. (Modified from Malvasi A, Di Renzo GC. *Semeiotica Ostetrica*, Rome, Italy: CIC Edizioni Internazionali; 2012.)

> **Box 14.3 Summary of third critical point**
>
> 1. Add to the terminology, as well as in conceptual terms, the movement of restitution with engagement of the shoulders and of external rotation of the head with internal rotation of the shoulders: shoulder engagement–restitution and external rotation–internal rotation of shoulders which defines the "consensual" rotation proposed by Pescetto.
> 2. Carefully define the main dystocias in the second stage of labor on the basis of the movements in a eutocic delivery, such as the lack of engagement at the superior strait, the lack of rotation and engagement at the mid-strait, the lack of engagement of the shoulders at the superior strait (Pescetto's type I), the lack of rotation and engagement of the shoulders at the mid-strait (Pescetto's type II).

Fourth critical point

The fourth critical point is the insufficient consideration given to the physiology of uterine contractions during labor and even more so in the second stage of labor.

According to studies [14], the lithotomy position increases the frequency of contractions but reduces the intensity. In fact measuring Montevideo units with internal pressure transducers, shows that the contractile force, developed in 10 minutes during the active dilating phase, is greater when the number of contractions are about three every 10 minutes (with sitting, squatting, or ambulatory patient), compared to the 4–5–6 contractions that we observe in the lithotomy position.

The possible cause of the increased activation of the uterine pacemakers may be the pressure generated on the presacral plexus by the gravid uterus. These observations

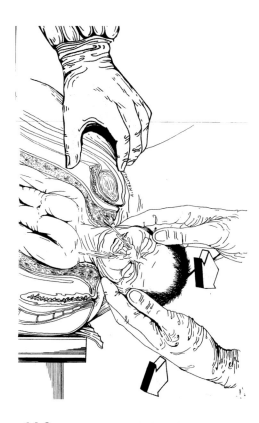

Figure 14.9 Front shoulder, below the mid-strait, in anterior–posterior position, with the acromion under the symphysis. (Modified from Malvasi A, Di Renzo GC. *Semeiotica Ostetrica*, Rome, Italy: CIC Edizioni Internazionali; 2012.)

> **Box 14.4 Summary of fourth critical point**
>
> Deal with our anxieties with more study and experience *and not* with maternal–fetal therapies.

could also explain why the contractions observed during the second stage of labor frequently slow down. It is possible that the less supine position of women in the second stage of labor reduces the neurogenic hyperstimulus of the uterine pacemakers. This does not mean that the overall force in the unit of time should be reduced, but may simply mean that the mechanical phenomena in the second stage of labor should be allowed to evolve.

Unfortunately, too many times in the delivery room we observe the bad habit of an oxytocic perfusion being applied, or increased, in the second stage of labor. The sole purpose, evidently, is to assuage the fear of the doctor, even though this damages the physiology of childbirth (see Box 14.4).

Fifth critical point

The fifth critical point is represented by the difficulty in correctly predicting the interaction between the two factors of childbirth that are crucial in achieving a eutocic outcome for both mother and child (ratio between birth canal and size of the fetus).

Basically, we know that the prediction of fetal weight by ultrasound measurement of standard fetal parameters—head, abdomen, legs—in 68% of cases is within 10% of the weight calculation determined by ultrasound calculation and in the remaining 32% can exceed this value. On the other hand, all the studies that have compared the ultrasound estimate with the objective estimation of the fetal weight have shown an even lower degree of accuracy.

Interesting prospects, in terms of accuracy, have emerged from the studies that associate ultrasound parameters to the biological data of mother and fetus (including its sex). Therefore, the error of 10% applies to over 80% of cases and, consequently, the average error for each single fetus is reduced [15–17].

In an integrated assessment of the risk of fetal pelvic disproportion, the ultrasound assessment of nontraditional parameters, such as fetal subcutaneous tissue, plays an important role [18,19].

> **Box 14.5 Summary of fifth critical point**
>
> 1. Acknowledge in an analytical way the risk factors specific to the individual case, of fetal–pelvic disproportion and making responsible medical decisions.
> 2. Share with the patient the extent and the potential risks related to the various possible methods for the delivery and to the child.
> 3. At the same time know that, in patients at risk of dystonias, the expulsive period should be assisted by the more experienced physicians and obstetricians on duty to avoid the treatment of emergencies by less-experienced physicians.

Semiotics, in the estimate of the normality of the pelvis, is based on traditional, inaccurate, and reproducible criteria. The evaluation of the physical maternal type—height, ethnicity—is probably an anamnestic–objective element, that is to be considered a risk factor in the clinical assessment of the individual case [10] (see Box 14.5).

SHOULDER DYSTOCIA

The cognitive "dissection" of the factors of childbirth—canal, fetus, contractions—and of childbirth phenomena, into maternal or dynamic, maternal–fetal or mechanical, fetal or plastic, is essential for focusing on each of the elements that contribute to the evolution of childbirth and, conversely, for properly diagnosing and treating dystocia. In terms of shoulder dystocia, the mechanisms by which the human fetus passes through the birth canal must be perfectly known. Indeed, therapeutic maneuvers aimed at preventing complications (even serious ones) (Table 14.2) should not be a mnemonic sequence of gestures or passed on through direct experience without any critical evaluation.

Therapies, in order to be successful, must be based on a correct diagnosis and must ensure that the bisacromial diameter, with the help of auxiliary forces, carries out the movements that it normally performs in the birth canal, and concurrent with the movements of the head. We also see that the purpose of the maneuver for extracting the rear shoulder is to allow engagement of the front shoulder at the superior strait, its progression and engagement under the symphysis. Shoulder dystocia or lack of shoulder engagement occurs at the superior strait (type I); lack of rotation and engagement of the shoulders occurs at the mid-strait (type II).

Definition of shoulder dystocia

The definition is implicit in the terminology itself. The use of this terminology would help the diagnosis and retrospective evaluation of cases and case studies.

Basically, it is a return to the general concept of the second stage of labor of the human fetus and to the presence of a pelvic limit in the descent into the birth canal. Therefore, there is a return to the mechanisms that enable–disable the engagement at the superior and mid-straits.

Table 14.2 Complications of shoulder dystocia

Maternal	Postpartum hemorrhage
	Recto-vaginal fistula
	Diastasis of the symphysis pubis, with or without transient femoral neuropathy
	Third- and fourth-degree lacerations
	Uterine rupture
Fetal	Brachial plexus palsy
	Fracture of the clavicle
	Fetal death
	Fetal hypoxia, with or without permanent neurological damage
	Fracture of the humerus

A third type, commonly referred to as iatrogenic dystocia of the shoulders, must be added to the first two types. It is usually a lack of engagement at the superior strait caused by traction on the head before restitution. This makes it impossible for the normally developed fetus to engage the bisacromial diameter on the oblique diameter of the superior strait.

Prevalence of shoulder dystocia

Objectively determining the prevalence of shoulder dystocia is not feasible, though it can help in understanding the risk factors.

The composition of the population—ethnicity, height, obesity, parity—and the prevalence of births by cesarean deliveries are essential determinants in the prevalence of this dystocia at childbirth. There is also uncertainty in the definition used in all recent works.

In countries with high prevalence of obese women and gestational diabetes, shoulder dystocia is a relatively common clinical event. In one review of 8000 nulliparous women in the urban area of Detroit [20], shoulder dystocia occurred in 0.8% of cases.

In urban areas of northern Italy, with a prevalence of cesarean deliveries of around 35% (10% above the North American level), shoulder dystocia can drop below 0.1%.

However, the definition proposed by Sokol [19] is the following: "impossibility of spontaneous disengagement of the shoulders caused by the impact of the front shoulder on the symphysis pubis."

Assistance at labor and delivery in the United States is carried out by doctors. In addition, typical obstetric practice is frequently characterized by traction on the head before restitution. As a result, part of the dystocias that were not assessed were likely of iatrogenic origin. On the other hand, shoulder dystocia occurrences due to the lack of internal rotation were not included.

This is the prevalence in "natural" populations at childbirth. Prevalence of shoulder dystocia instead was of 10% [21] in a Swiss multicenter series of 3356 fetuses weighing more than 4500 g.

Risk factors for dystocia

As can be seen from the analysis of the prevalence, all biological features linked to the development of macrosomic fetuses (previous macrosomia, in particular if it is caused by gestational diabetes and is therefore linked to truncal obesity, maternal obesity, and post-term pregnancy), as well as narrow pelvises (due to height, ethnicity, trauma) should be considered risk factors, as reported in Table 14.3.

It is interesting to note on the subject of risk factors, that Abramowicz et al. [19] reported a close association between the distribution of subcutaneous fat, typical of diabetic macrosoma (size of fetal cheeks) and dystocia in the second stage of labor.

In a second stage of labor in which the mid-strait is overcome through rotation, but is also due to accentuated plastic phenomena—events that can be diagnosed due to the amount of time that elapses starting from when the patient feels pain due to the pressure on the pelvic floor muscles;

Table 14.3 Risk factors for shoulder dystocia

Maternal	Gestational diabetes
	Pregnancy after term
	Previous shoulder dystocia
	Abnormal pelvic anatomy
	Short stature
Fetal	Suspected fetal macrosomia estimated weight > 4000 g
Related to labor	Operative vaginal delivery (vacuum extractor)
	Protracted active phase of the first stage
	Protracted second stage of labor due to slowdown of the third phase

this time should not exceed 2 hours, to avoid possible partial overlapping of the fissures of the cranial bones and/or caput succedaneum—vaginal operative delivery, subsequent difficult disengagement of the shoulders, as well as dystocia are all possible scenarios that must be dealt with by an experienced physician. The physician must be able to actively assist during an abnormal expulsive period.

Because the third period of the second stage of labor can have difficult dynamics, it is essential to have the most accurate information possible on the fetus (e.g., the estimated weight when more than 4000 g, the possible conformation determined by diabetic megalosomia, which accentuates the development of the trunk relative to the head). The same can be for the mother, so as to not deal with a vaginal operative delivery of the fetal head with a high subsequent risk of shoulder dystocia.

DIAGNOSIS OF DYSTOCIA

First type

The diagnosis of shoulder dystocia due to lack of engagement at the superior strait and to impact the anterior shoulder at the symphysis—shoulder dystocia of the first type—is typically characterized by the retraction of the head against the vulvar ostium after the expulsion (turtle sign). Restitution may be hinted at but is typically absent (Figure 14.11).

The objective impression that this type of dystocia immediately gives at its onset, is that of a single block between fetal body and birth canal. The diagnosis is completed by palpation (with flat hand) above the symphysis, in which normally the shoulder is perceived to be above the symphysis itself. In the clinical conditions in which the dystocia occurs, it is difficult if not impossible to be able to distinguish, at this stage, the shapes of the shoulders above the superior strait, from those in which the rear shoulder is beyond the superior strait, from which it may push the front shoulder even more above the symphysis.

Second type

Shoulder dystocia of the second type is characterized by normal disengagement of the head, absence of the "suction" effect of the head against the vulva, the restitution movement, as well as the absence of external rotation, which

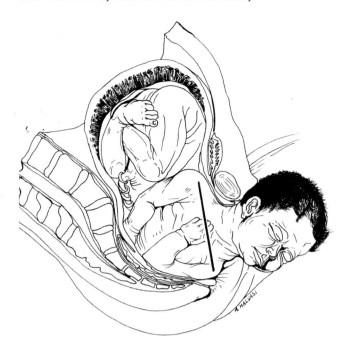

Figure 14.11 Type I shoulder dystocia, in which the anterior shoulder is blocked against the symphysis pubis.

should exactly correspond with the internal rotation and engagement of the shoulders at the mid-strait (Figure 14.12).

Prevention of dystocia

Even today, authoritative clinicians define shoulder dystocia as an obstetric emergency that is not predictable, which can be held to be generally true. However, knowing the risk factors of every individual case is essential in establishing a prudent and respectful approach to the mother–child dyad.

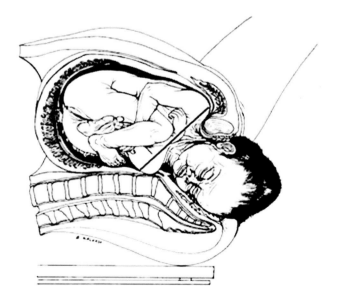

Figure 14.12 Type II shoulder dystocia, in which the anterior shoulder is blocked below the symphysis pubis, and the posterior is shoulder anchored behind the sacral promontory.

SHOULDER DYSTOCIA THERAPY

Shoulder dystocia due to lack of shoulder engagement

The idea behind the therapy is that it must lead to the extraction of the fetal body in no more than 4 minutes [22]. Four minutes is 240 seconds, a very long time for someone who knows what to do and what to tell others to do in the delivery room. This time estimate is indirectly inferred from the navel–head phase in breech delivery assistance. This is the amount of time between when the navel overcomes the rima vulvae (and essentially occludes) and the head disengages with the base deficit not exceeding −12 mmol/L.

We must however subtract from this time the effect of congestion of the cephalic extremity blood exposed to the atmospheric pressure, while the rest of the body continues to be subjected to a higher pressure.

Two hundred seconds are a very long time when one does not panic. After confirming the diagnosis and the type of shoulder dystocia, the assistants are to be gradually tasked with the therapeutic maneuvers, from the simplest to the most complex. For this to happen:

a. The entire obstetric medical team must have a detailed knowledge, even if only theoretical, of shoulder dystocia and of the diagnosis and therapy protocols adopted. This knowledge must be learned through specific annual discussions, held annually (at least) on the protocol adopted, as well as through individual study of each operator.

b. In cases at risk, the most expert doctor on duty must be present at the expulsive period. The same holds true for the obstetricians on duty. This will be possible if, during the evolution of the expulsive period, the risk elements that can lead to dystonia have been detected.

c. In cases in which the risk could not be predicted, there is an even greater need for the physician to know which maneuvers to carry out. Any maternal or fetal trauma that occurs, provided it is not on the brachial plexus, is the result of therapies that have the goal of preventing a greater evil: cerebral damage due to asphyxia.

The second premise concerns the knowledge of the following maneuvers: (a) "maternal" that affect the pelvic diameters and the soft parts, (b) maneuvers that can be performed on the fetal trunk, and (c) maneuvers that can be performed on the fetal head. The maneuvers are to be coordinated in order to obtain engagement of the shoulder and internal rotation, or disengagement of the posterior shoulder.

The third premise is that maneuvers passed on to us in the literature were born at a time when shoulder dystocia due to macrosomia could not be prevented with a cesarean delivery, even in the event of a clearly macrosomic fetus >4500–5000 g.

Their effectiveness, therefore, is not based on criteria that we would nowadays define as strictly "scientific," but on observations on their degree of effectiveness (and handed down clinically), or on epidemiological observations. This is what occurred, for example, with the maneuvers on the fetal trunk, introduced in the United States in the 1940s and which, in a decade, led to a marked reduction in the severe complications of shoulder dystocia [23]. Furthermore, the same definition frequently corresponds, in different traditions, to substantially different behaviors.

The first maneuver is the expansion of the mediolateral or paramedian episiotomy. The purpose is not to create more room behind the shoulders, which obviously cannot be achieved on the soft parts of the birth canal. Instead, this will facilitate any subsequent maneuver on the fetal trunk, as well as prevent third- and fourth-degree lacerations. The purpose of this act is often misunderstood.

Gurewitsch even compares a type of median episiorectotomy, unknown to us, with nonepisiotomy, thus coming to the conclusion that episiotomy does not prevent complications of the pelvic floor and rectal lacerations [24].

Without performing anything other than normal assistance, the obstetrician will attempt to counter-rotate the head, as if dealing with an iatrogenic dystocia. If this does not result in the rotation of the shoulders, the next step will be to perform the maneuvers related to the first type of dystocia (Figure 14.13).

The second maneuver is to move the pelvis of the patient to the edge of the bed, followed by the hyperflexion of the thighs toward the trunk by the obstetrician and a third assistant present in the room. The purpose of this maneuver, named the McRoberts' maneuver, is to increase the bony diameters (of the pelvic outlet) of the pelvis by moving back the promontory and bringing forward the symphysis (Figure 14.14).

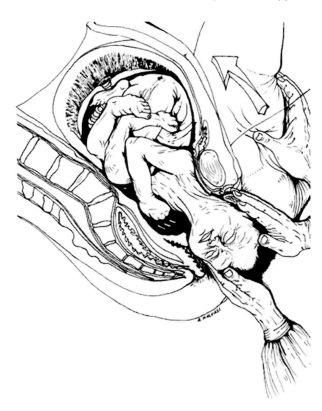

Figure 14.14 McRoberts' maneuver: the female pelvis is made to protrude from the delivery bed, while the staff assisting the delivery *hyperflexes* the thighs toward the trunk of the mother.

According to some protocols, before performing this maneuver the thighs must be extended and the legs brought down toward the floor. The purpose of this movement is to move it caudally, in order to widen the anterior–posterior diameter of the superior strait. This maneuver was named after Scipione Mercurio and Welcher (Figure 14.15), but its effectiveness is not confirmed in more recent assisted

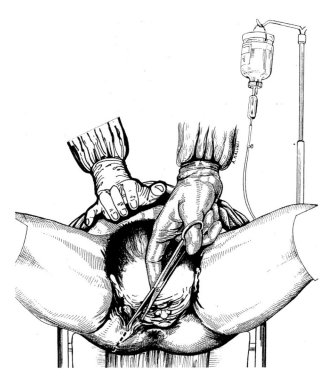

Figure 14.13 Extension of the episiotomy (typical "turtle" behavior of the head for the type 1 shoulder dystocia). (Modified from Malvasi A, Di Renzo GC. *Semeiotica Ostetrica*, Rome, Italy: CIC Edizioni Internazionali; 2012.)

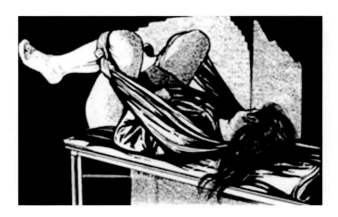

Figure 14.15 Depiction of McRoberts' maneuver, in home birth practice: the mother's thighs were hyperflexed with a cloth that also maintains her legs in this position. (Modified from Malvasi A, Di Renzo GC. *Ecografia intraparto ed il parto*, Bari, Italy: Editori Laterza; 2012.)

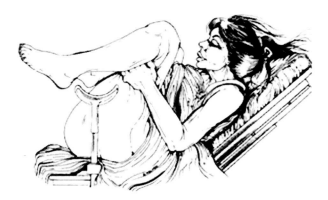

Figure 14.16 The patient on the delivery bed is able to perform the McRoberts' maneuver on her own.

deliveries. It may be appropriate, however, to hyperextend the woman's lower limbs and then to hyperflex the thighs. In emergency situations, when only the obstetrician is present in the delivery room, the hyperflexion of the patient's thighs can be performed by the patient herself (Figure 14.16).

The patient must be brought to the position with hyperflexed thighs (hyperextension of the lower limbs). One of the assistants alongside the woman (the obstetrician or the second doctor in the room) must feel the shoulder in front of the symphysis and exert pressure toward one of the oblique diameters of the superior strait, typically to the right (Figure 14.17). This will facilitate the engagement of the anterior shoulder. At the same time the mother's lower limbs are hyperflexed (legs on thighs and thighs on abdomen), increasing the mid-strait and inferior strait diameters, which, if the pressure is able to engage the anterior shoulder, will assist in the progression. For fans of nomenclatures with the author's name, we note that this maneuver is called Rubin's first maneuver.

The doctor must favor the engagement of the shoulder on the anterior–posterior diameter under the symphysis, with pulling and rotating movements of the head. This can occur only if there is a reasonable certainty of the engagement of the shoulder. The engagement of the anterior shoulder can be diagnosed by palpating over the symphysis and by the feeling of sliding of the shoulder into the superior strait, as well as by the corresponding improvement in the retraction of the head against the vulva.

According to Gherman, who in 1997 [25] reviewed a case study of 250 cases of shoulder dystocia in 44,000 consecutive deliveries, the sole McRoberts' position solved 40% of the dystocias. The cases resolved with the complete maneuver, without the use of other therapeutic procedures, were, however, of fetuses of less weight than the more complex cases. In reading these results there is real doubt on the actual dystocia of the cases treated.

Traction on the head, however, is critically important. The maneuver consists of three synergistic components: widening of the pelvis, pressure applied on the fetal trunk–shoulder from above the pubis, and traction on the head.

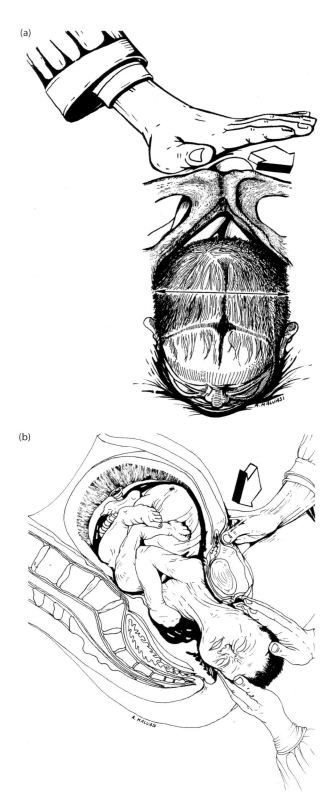

Figure 14.17 (a) Maneuver of suprapubic pressure to favor the positive engagement of the bisacromial diameter, in the case in which the anterior shoulder is anchored under the pubic symphysis; (b) completion maneuver, in which the anterior shoulder is released from the pubic symphysis, and it is possible to perform the traction of the head, without creating problems for the fetus.

In delivery rooms where the staff is familiar with the Kristeller maneuver, it must be performed immediately after pressure has been applied and the shoulder has overcome the symphysis, so as to not perform traction on the fetal head. Helping the engagement of the acromion under the symphysis with a downward pressure from the uterine fundus, reduces the need, even at a psychological level, of performing traction on the head.

The third maneuver regards the absolute necessity of not performing traction driven by panic and thus stressful on the head. The maneuver is guided by the need to not cause irreparable damage to the brachial plexus. At the same time it is important to know that a third maneuver of equal "simplicity" can be put in place and focuses, of the three components of the therapeutic action, on the fetal trunk. This reduces the pulling force to less than half of the force needed with pulling maneuvers for the same degree of dystocia [23].

This third maneuver, in some protocols, is the second. This maneuver (second maneuver of Rubin) consists of inserting two fingers of the right hand into the vagina on the posterior side of the shoulder blocked against the symphysis (Figure 14.18) and of trying to turn this shoulder toward the anterior oblique diameter, along with the effect of plastic reduction of the diameter in the displacement of the shoulder toward the thorax.

The push on the anterior shoulder may be carried out in combination with an equal and opposite thrust on the posterior shoulder, thus favoring the screwing of the shoulders. If in doing so the engagement takes place, then the maneuver is successful, at which point we will exert force in order to favor internal rotation and engagement under the symphysis—suprapubic pressure, lowering of the head without traction.

This maneuver, in which pressure is exerted on the fetal trunk, corresponds, in hindsight, to the counter-rotation and rotation movements usually carried out by obstetrics in the presence of mild or iatrogenic dystocia. Applying rotations and counter-rotations in the presence of severe dystocia would exert strong pressure to the fetal neck (with severe outcomes), whereas in this manner the pressure is applied to the fetal trunk (Figure 14.19).

The difficulty in comparing case studies in relation to diagnosis of admittance and to the treatment performed, is immediately apparent when comparing this sequence of maneuvers with those proposed on the American Congress of Obstetricians and Gynecologists (ACOG) website: the sequence is substantially identical. The only difference is that in the diagram the head is always shown in a complete external rotation position, which does not occur in severe shoulder dystocia of the first type, as we have seen.

The fourth maneuver (Jacquemier's maneuver) is the last maneuver described in this paragraph. It should be used when the previous maneuvers fail, which occurs after at least 2 minutes of time have passed. In this case, you should perform without delay the maneuver for extracting the posterior shoulder in order to reduce the diameter from bisacromial to acromion–subaxillary. The reason why, as a rule, this maneuver on the fetal body follows the others, is that it is likely to lead to the breaking of the clavicle or of the humerus, but without exerting traction on the fetal head.

This maneuver consists of placing the right hand of the doctor in the vagina in posterior–inferior position to the fetal back, and searching for the fetal arm, which at times is placed behind the back. The flat hand of the doctor is pushed up to the wrist and to the first third of the forearm, in the case where the posterior shoulder is placed over the superior strait. At this point the fetal elbow and forearm are flexed with a traction and rotation movement to the outside and downward. This maneuver may result in the breaking of the humerus or the fracture of the clavicle. Often the fetus at this point spontaneously rotates and the anterior shoulder engages below the symphysis and can be disengaged.

On a practical level it must be emphasized that when the doctor, who is attempting to rotate the trunk using internal pressure, realizes that the resistance to rotation cannot be overcome, the Jaquemier's maneuver must continue. Instead of inserting only two fingers proceed to immediately insert the entire hand and perform an energetic and continuous movement.

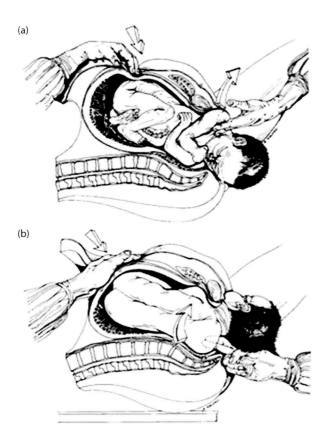

Figure 14.18 (a) Rubin's II maneuver: the operator, with his fingers on the posterior part of the shoulder blocked against the symphysis, rotates the shoulder until he disengages it below the symphysis. (b) Supplementary maneuver to Rubin II, in which the obstetrician provides an equal and opposite thrust on the posterior shoulder, thereby facilitating the screwing movement and a more favorable positioning of the bisacromial diameter.

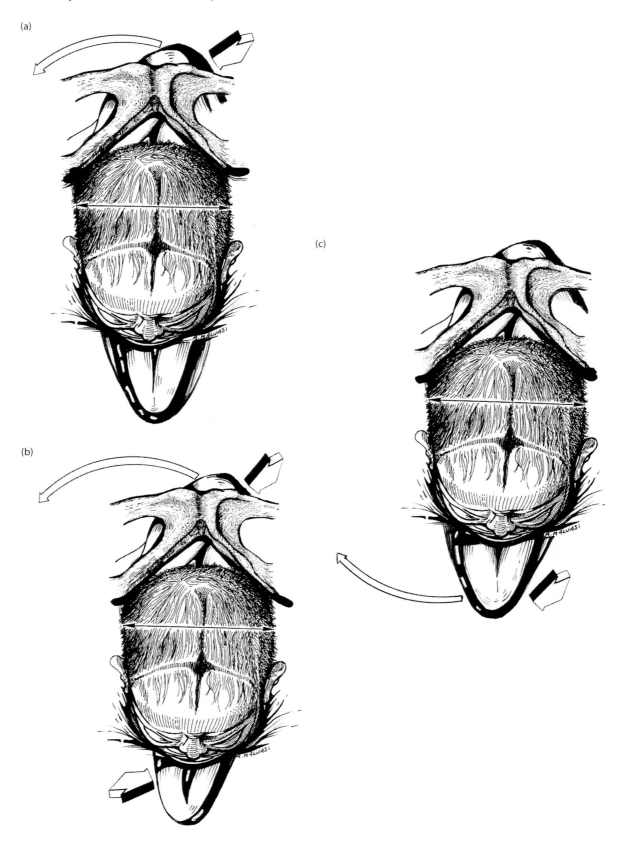

Figure 14.19 Diagram of the second Rubin maneuver: (a) place two fingers on the posterior side of the shoulder blocked against the symphysis and try to rotate the shoulder toward the oblique anterior diameter; (b) this push on the anterior shoulder may be done in combination with an equal and opposite thrust on the posterior shoulder, thus favoring the screwing of the shoulders; (c) if this maneuver is not successful, apply the force on the posterior surface of the posterior shoulder and try to rotate it 180° to below the symphysis.

When the situation is such that none of the maneuvers lead to the afterbirth of the shoulders, there are "heroic maneuvers" described in the literature. During these maneuvers the head is repositioned by flexion and pressure from the bottom upward in the birth canal. An emergency cesarean delivery is performed, preferably obtained with longitudinal incision of the abdominal wall and uterus to allow an extraction of, initially, the fetal body and then of the head (Figure 14.20).

Failure of internal rotation, dystocia (type II)

In type II shoulder dystocia, the bisacromial diameter of the fetus is engaged in the oblique diameter of the superior strait, but does not perform internal rotation to engage in the anterior–posterior diameter of the mid-strait, bringing the anterior shoulder under the symphysis pubis. The disengagement of the head is not followed by retraction toward the vulvar ring (turtle sign): the head moves away from the perineum and hints at the movement of restitution.

As in the first type of dystocia the premises previously mentioned are applicable and deserve to be pondered.

According to Pescetto, type I shoulder dystocias, resolved with one of the first three maneuvers of the protocol, can become a type II dystocia, with no subsequent internal rotation.

The first maneuver to perform, as in the type I dystocia, is the widening of the mediolateral or paramedian episiotomy so as to perform internal maneuvers on the body of the fetus.

The second maneuver is to perform ventral hyperflexion of the woman's thighs (McRoberts' maneuver, as described previously). This increases the anterior–posterior diameters and, at the same time, by placing flat hands on the fetal head, facilitates the internal rotation of the shoulders. This is followed by engagement at the mid-strait and subsequent progression into the inferior strait. Some authors propose to exert a prolonged pressure, in the caudal direction, with the fist in the suprapubic region, in order to avoid excessive traction on the fetal head. Kristeller's maneuver is recommended only when both the internal rotation and the engagement in the mid-strait have taken place.

The third maneuver is to be employed when the maneuvers described above fail. In this case perform a rotation, with internal maneuvers, along with a slow lowering of the fetal head to bring the anterior shoulder under the pubic symphysis (Figure 14.21).

The fourth maneuver is used if ultimately, no resolution is found: try to bring the fetal body back up into the birth canal in order to apply Jacquemier's maneuver.

Concluding remarks

The distinction in traditional Italian obstetrics of shoulder dystocia in the first and second types, ignored by Anglo-Saxon authors (2002 ACOG guidelines) is not an erudite nosological abstraction, but reflects easily distinguishable pathological events, without the need for sophisticated semiotics: the first type of shoulder dystocia presents an evident and dramatic adhesion of the head against the rima vulvae, as soon as the spontaneous birth takes place by Kristeller or vacuum extraction. The head does not tend to show any movement of restitution, let alone rotation (Figure 14.22).

In the second type of shoulder dystocia none of this happens: the presented head has a nearly normal restitution, but it does not perform the consensual external rotation. The second consideration concerns the general therapy principles based on the application of force to the mother, to the head of the fetus and to the trunk–limbs of the fetus.

Ideally, forces applied to the head must be no greater than those applied during assisted vaginal delivery. Therefore in carrying out the sequence of therapeutic

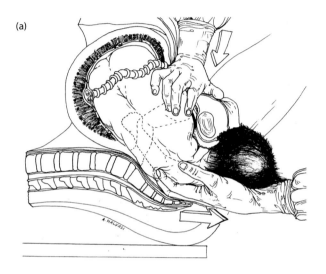

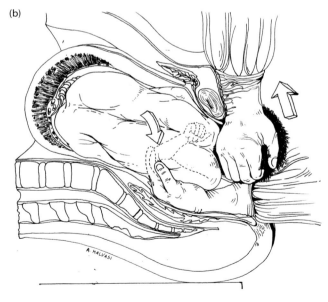

Figure 14.20 (a) The hand of the obstetrician reaches the wrist and the first third of the forearm, in case the shoulder is above the superior strait (type II dystocia). (b) The operator flexes the fetal elbow and forearm, with a traction and rotation movement to the outside and downward, while accompanying the rotation of the head.

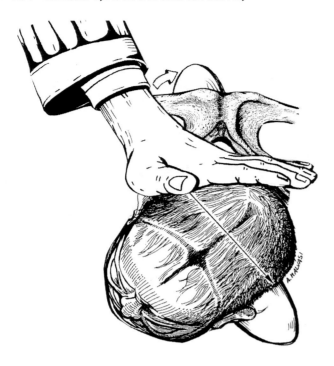

Figure 14.21 Third Rubin maneuver or reverse Rubin maneuver with downward pressure on the fetal head with flat hand.

movements it is recommended to initially apply maneuvers to the mother: hyperflexion of the thighs or external pressure on fetal shoulders (pressure applied above the symphysis) or internal maneuvers on the trunk–shoulders (rotational movements caused by the fingers). Traction on the head is to be banned and should simply serve to accompany the rotational movements of the shoulders.

Kristeller's maneuver, which we consider as a maneuver on the fetal trunk, should be performed only when the acromion rises to the symphysis, in order to be certain that the brachial plexus is not compressed against the symphysis itself.

The reduction of the bisacromial diameter to acromion axillary diameter (with its frequent bone trauma) must immediately follow the previous internal maneuvers, whenever these are not sufficient to carry out the necessary rotations to the fetal trunk.

In extreme cases, it may become necessary to fracture the clavicle to immediately reduce the bisacromial diameter and disengage the shoulders (Figure 14.23).

Zavanelli maneuvers

In certain dramatic cases the doctor may face a stop in the progression of the presenting part inside the female pelvis. In order to quickly resolve this delicate situation, it will be necessary to try to move the fetal head back up into the abdomen, in order to remove the fetus with an emergency cesarean delivery.

This type of movement can be performed through the Zavanelli maneuver [26]. It is an extreme and not frequently performed maneuver, in which the head may be outside the rima vulvae. It is performed for type II shoulder dystocia, that is when the fetus has been "expelled" and is beyond the rima vulvae with shoulders above the superior strait.

In this case the anterior shoulder is located below the symphysis pubis and the posterior shoulder is above the promontory. An emergency cesarean delivery is carried out to try to rapidly perform a vertex or breech extraction of the fetus, while the assistant tries to bring the head back

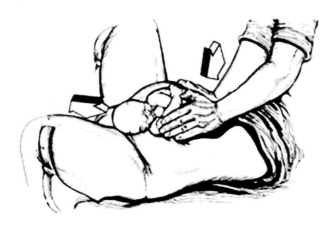

Figure 14.22 Kristeller's maneuver, in case of type II dystocia. The fetal head does not present restitution and rotation movements (*arrows*).

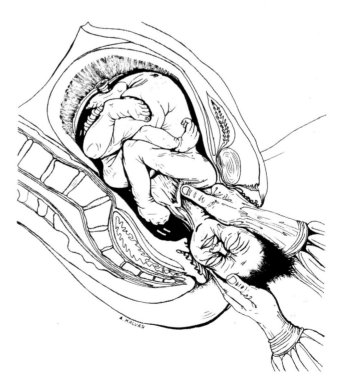

Figure 14.23 Clavicle fracture maneuver during shoulder dystocia.

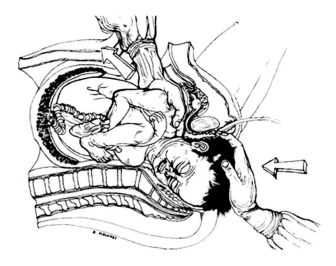

Figure 14.24 Zavanelli maneuver: the obstetrician grabs the anterior shoulder of the fetus, while the assistant pushes the presenting part back toward the abdomen.

into the pelvic cavity (Figure 14.24) and free it from the suffocating vulvovaginal grip [27].

The consequences of the Zavanelli maneuver on the newborn can be far more serious: some authors report injuries to the fetal column at a cervical level, or even the death of the fetus in the attempt to reposition the presenting part in the abdomen. Moreover, to reduce the extent of the Zavanelli maneuver, other authors have proposed to partially reposition the head in the vaginal canal. This is an attempt to rotate the shoulders with the McRoberts' maneuver, so that the fetus can then be extracted from the laparotomy wound [28].

The Zavanelli maneuver, however, is the last obstetric opportunity to resolve in a relatively short amount of time a compromised situation [29].

Brief emergency protocol for shoulder dystocia

If you are in the presence of a suspected shoulder dystocia, you need to call immediately for qualified help and proceed to the following initial steps: if the emergency provides for the time, call in the most experienced doctor on duty to the delivery room; otherwise proceed with the necessary interventions.

Check the clock of the delivery room, confirm the diagnosis, mentally review all the maneuvers that we may be called to perform. Do not let panic control your actions.

Let us summarize, point by point, the maneuvers to be implemented.

Episiotomy

Perform or complete a large paramedian episiotomy to allow internal therapeutic maneuvers.

Hyperflex the thighs on the abdomen (Mc Roberts' maneuver) with suprapubic pressure (if required)

Hyperflex the thighs on the trunk by the obstetrician and assistant present in the room, to increase the bony diameters of the pelvis by pulling back the promontory and bringing forward the symphysis. Exert direct pressure (with the fist) toward one of the oblique diameters of the superior strait and then direct caudally, while helping the anterior shoulder engage and progress. Concurrently perform a gentle traction and rotation of the fetal head toward the posterior perineum.

Internal maneuvers

Exert pressure on the shoulders with two fingers deep in the vagina, to facilitate the rotation of the anterior shoulder in an oblique diameter and below the symphysis.

Jacquemier's maneuver

Remove the rear arm from the birth canal and move the hand up the vagina, flex the fetal elbow and forearm with a traction and rotational movement directed externally and downward.

CONCLUSIONS

In the birth mechanism of the human species the birth of the head can be rightfully distinguished from the birth of the shoulders.

Comparative anthropology has shown that, much more so than in primates, dystocia (and of the shoulders in particular) is a frequent phenomenon in the human species. One of the main causes of dystocia in the human species is the volume of the fetal head, greater than that of other animal species. Another cause is the greater complexity of the female pelvis compared to those of other species.

Shoulder dystocia is not currently preventable, unless certain risk factors are taken into account (e.g., diabetes, obesity, fetal macrosomia, abnormal pelvis, maternal height).

It is important in diagnosing shoulder dystocia to distinguish the type. (Type II is the most severe.)

All obstetric teams should simulate this obstetric emergency which, although rare and unpredictable, is potentially dramatic. Shoulder dystocia "therapy" is based on several maneuvers, and requires perfect medical organization in the delivery room.

REFERENCES

1. Gherman RB, Chauhan S, Ouzounian JG, Lerner H, Gonik B, Goodwin TM. Shoulder dystocia: The unpreventable obstetric emergency with empiric management guidelines. *Am J Obstet Gynecol* 2006;195(3):657–72.
2. Rosenberg K, Trevathan W. Birth, obstetrics and human evolution. *BJOG* 2002;109(11):1199–206.
3. Rosenberg KR, Trevathan WR. The evolution of human birth. *Sci Am* 2001;285(5):72–77.
4. Baul MK, Manjusha. Maternal mortality—A ten-year study. *J Indian Med Assoc.* 2004;102(1):18–19, 25.
5. Danso KA, Martey JO, Wall LL, Elkins TE. The epidemiology of genitourinary fistulae in Kumasi, Ghana, 1977–1999. *Int Urogynecol J Pelvic Floor Dysfunct* 1996;7(3):117–20.

6. Akmal S, Tsoi E, Nicolaides KH. Intrapartum sonography to determine fetal occipital position: Interobserver agreement. *Ultrasound Obstet Gynecol* 2004;24(4):421–4.
7. Beck WW. *Ostetricia e ginecologia*. Chapter 4, Milan: Masson Edit; 1997:35.
8. Cunningham FG, Levono KJ, Bloom SL, Spong CY, Dashe JS et al., eds. *Williams Obstetrics*, 24th edition, McGraw-Hill; 2014.
9. Pardi G. In: Candiani GB, Danesino V, Gastaldi A, eds. *La clinica ostetrica e ginecologica*. Chapter 14, Milan: Masson Edit; 1996:706–707.
10. Akmal S, Tsoi E, Howard R, Osei E, Nicolaides KH. Investigation of occiput posterior delivery by intrapartum sonography. *Ultrasound Obstet Gynecol* 2004;24(4):425–8.
11. Barbera A, Giacomelli F. In: Arduini D, Gruppo di Studio SIGO, eds. *Trattato di Ecografia in Ostetricia e Ginecologia*. Milan: Poletto Edit; 1997:401–4.
12. Schwarcz RL, Belizan JM, Cifuentes JR, Cuadro JC, Marques MB. Caldeyro-Barcia R. Fetal and maternal monitoring in spontaneous labors and in elective inductions. A comparative study. *Am J Obstet Gynecol* 1974;120(3):356–62.
13. Clivio I et al. *Trattato di Ostetricia*, 4th ed. Milano, Italy: Vallardi; 1940.
14. Allman AC, Genevier ES, Johnson MR, Steer PJ. Head-to-cervix force: An important physiological variable in labour. Peak active force, peak active pressure and mode of delivery. *Br J Obstet Gynaecol* 1996;103(8):769–75.
15. Gardosi J. Customized fetal growth standards: Rationale and clinical application. *Semin Perinatol* 2004;28(1):33–40.
16. Sokol RJ, Chik L, Dombrowski MP, Zador IE. Correctly identifying the macrosomic fetus: Improving ultrasonography-based prediction. *Am J Obstet Gynecol* 2000;182(6):1489–95.
17. Ferrazzi E, Cortina Boria M, Fiore S. *Fetal weight estimation by standard ultrasound measurements and biological maternal and fetal data*. Rome, Italy: International Forum on Birth; 2005.
18. Padoan A, Rigano S, Ferrazzi E, Beaty BL, Battaglia FC, Galan HL. Differences in fat and lean mass proportions in normal and growth-restricted fetuses. *Am J Obstet Gynecol* 2004;191:1459e64.
19. Abramowicz JS, Rana S, Abramowicz S. Fetal cheek-to-cheek diameter in the prediction of mode of delivery. *Am J Obstet Gynecol* 2005;192:1205–13.
20. Mehta SH, Bujold E, Blackwell SC, Sorokin Y, Sokol RJ. Is abnormal labor associated with shoulder dystocia in nulliparous women. *Am J Obstet Gynecol* 2004;190(6):1604–7.
21. Raio L, Ghezzi F, Di Naro E, Buttarelli M, Franchi M, Durig P, Bruhwiler H. Perinatal outcome of fetuses with a birth weight greater than 4500 g: An analysis of 3356 cases. *Eur J Obstet Gynecol Reprod Biol* 2003;109(2):160–5.
22. Beer E, Folghera MG. Time for resolving shoulder dystocia. *Am J Obstet Gynecol* 1998;179(5):1376–7.
23. Gurewitsch ED, Kim EJ, Yang JH, Outland KE, McDonald MK, Allen RH. Comparing McRoberts' and Rubin's maneuvers for initial management of shoulder dystocia: An objective evaluation. *Am J Obstet Gynecol* 2005;192(1):153–60.
24. Gurewitsch ED, Donithan M, Stallings SP, Moore PL, Agarwal S, Allen LM, Allen RH. Episiotomy versus fetal manipulation in managing severe shoulder dystocia: A comparison of outcomes. *Am J Obstet Gynecol* 2004;191(3):911–6.
25. Gherman RB, Goodwin TM, Souter I, Neumann K, Ouzounian JG, Paul RH. The McRoberts' maneuver for the alleviation of shoulder dystocia: How successful is it? *Am J Obstet Gynecol* 1997;176(3):656–61.
26. Ross MG, Beall MH. Cervical neck dislocation associated with the Zavanelli maneuver. *Obstet Gynecol* 2006;108(3 Pt 2):737–8.
27. Zelig CM, Gherman RB. Modified Zavanelli maneuver for the alleviation of shoulder dystocia. *Obstet Gynecol* 2002;100(5 Pt 2):1112–4.
28. Kenaan J, Gonzalez-Quintero VH, Gilles J. The Zavanelli maneuver in two cases of shoulder distocia. *J Matern Fetal Neonatal Med* 2003;13(2):135–8.
29. Vollebergh JH, van Dongen PW. The Zavanelli manoeuvre in shoulder dystocia: Case report and review of published cases. *Eur J Obstet Gynecol Reprod Biol* 2000;89(1):81–84.

Multiple pregnancy and cesarean birth   15

GIAN CARLO DI RENZO, GIULIA BABUCCI, and ANTONIO MALVASI

...the more living beings are organised the fewer the descendants; therefore, in humans, who are highly developed, pregnancy and multiple births are relatively rare

(H. Marzius, *Trattato di Ostetricia*, 1953)

INTRODUCTION

Multiple pregnancies are an infrequent obstetric event. They represent 1% of all pregnancies, two-thirds of which are dizygotic, while one-third is monozygotic. The number of multiple pregnancies is on the rise due in part to an increase in the number of pharmacologically induced pregnancies, but also because of a more widespread use of assisted fertilization techniques.

From a physiological point of view, all dizygotic twins and a third of monozygotic twins are dichorionic, while slightly over 20% of all twin pregnancies are monochorionic [1].

Twin pregnancies are generally characterized by prematurity, an increase in the incidence of uterine hypokinesia (resulting from uterine overdistension), postpartum atony, and placental abruption.

Monochorionic twins usually have a worse prognosis than dichorionic twins, with perinatal morbidity and mortality that is three to five times higher. In these fetuses the prenatal diagnosis of chorionicity is essential (Figure 15.1) [2].

TWIN PREGNANCY: ETIOPATHOGENESIS

As mentioned, the number of twin pregnancies has been constantly increasing, which is reflected in a corresponding increase in cesarean deliveries related to twin pregnancies.

These increases can be tied to several factors. One such factor is assisted reproductive techniques (ARTs), which involve monozygotic as well as dizygotic pregnancies. Unlike dizygotic twins, in which two distinct ovocytes are fertilized by two different spermatozoids, monozygotic twins are the result of the fertilization of a single ovocyte with formation of a single zygote. In the first days after fertilization the ovule divides into two cellular entities that grow independently, each one generating a complete individual [3].

Therefore, the outcome for these types of twins depends on when the zygote division took place. In other words it depends on the amount of time between fertilization of the ovocyte and its division.

Contrary to what is widely believed, monozygotic twins occur sporadically, as no environmental factor is currently known to induce the duplication of the embryo. Duplication can, however, be achieved in the early stages of development through biological embryonic techniques, as is the case of multifetal pregnancies that originate from ARTs.

The incidence of multifetal pregnancies with the use of human menopausal gonadotropin (HMG) is approximately 8%, and the incidence with the use of clomifene is 1%. In case of in vitro fertilization (IVF) and gamete intrafallopian transfer (GIFT), it depends instead on how many gametes and embryos were transferred.

The overall incidence of multiple pregnancies is 3.5% for IVF (Figure 15.2) and 5% for GIFT. In the United States in recent years there has been a 33% increase in twin pregnancies and a 100% increase in triplet and multiple pregnancies. The incidence of triplet pregnancies in women over 35 years of age, who represent most patients who undergo IVF or GIFT programs, has increased by 179% [5].

From an embryogenetic point of view, monozygotic twin pregnancies are dichorionic diamniotic if the zygote divides within the fourth postconceptional day: in this case two separate placentas, which may be fused together, will form, as well as two chorionic sacs and two amniotic membranes, which wrap around the respective embryos.

If the division of the embryo occurs between the fourth and eighth days of development, the placentation will be diamniotic monochorionic: there will therefore be only one placenta, one chorionic sac, and two amniotic membranes. In case of a monochorionic monoamniotic twin pregnancy, the division of the embryo occurs after the eighth day of development. This type of pregnancy represents 5% of all monochorionic pregnancies and presents a single amniotic cavity and a single placenta from which originate two umbilical cords inserted very close to one another [6].

From an epidemiological point of view, dizygotic twins are always dichorionic and are more frequent in women over 35 years of age. This is due to the levels of gonadotropin (FSH and LH) present during this period of the woman's life. There is then the hereditary component in some families in which these gestations are likely to occur. Last, this can be due to the administration of drugs that induce ovulation.

In any case, whether it be monochorionic or dichorionic, twin pregnancies are always at greater risk than single fetus pregnancies due to the frequency of obstetric complications, and therefore need to be carefully monitored through clinical tests, ultrasound tests, and (at least monthly) flowmetry tests [7].

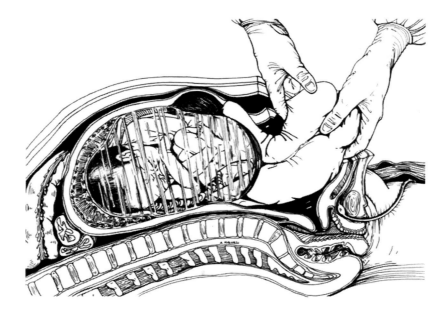

Figure 15.1 Monochorionic diamniotic twin pregnancy with rupture of the first amniotic sac and extraction of the first twin in breech presentation.

ULTRASOUND DIAGNOSIS OF PLACENTA IN TWIN PREGNANCY

The diagnosis of multiple gestation must be performed early, possibly during the first diagnostic ultrasound examination of pregnancy, and after the sixth or seventh week of amenorrhea. This diagnosis must take place even though the diagnosis of chorionicity, amnionicity, and zygosity is not always easy during the first ultrasound check.

Advances in ultrasound techniques and instruments have resulted in modern high-resolution ultrasound equipment capable of detecting well in advance the type of placentation in multiple pregnancies, with reliability around 95%.

The essential elements of an ultrasound examination are the number of placentas, the amniochorionic membranes, the thickness of the interamniotic septum, and the search for the "lambda" sign that corresponds to the duplication of the chorionic layers/membranes in the placental insertion point.

The additional identification of the discordant gender of the twins will help in the differential diagnosis of zygosity. The main difference in twin pregnancies is chorionicity and amnioticity, as monoamniotic twins are more likely to present a greater number of malformations than other pregnancies.

The main anatomical–clinical conditions are biovular, diamniotic, and dichorionic twins (Figure 15.3); biovular, diamniotic, and monochorionic twins (Figure 15.4); monochorionic, monovular, and diamniotic twins (Figure 15.5); and monochorionic, monoamniotic, and monovular twins (Figure 15.6).

The diagnosis of a monozygotic twin pregnancy can be determined with certainty only when the monochorionic pregnancy is indisputable. The diagnosis of a dizygotic pregnancy can be performed only in case of dichorionicity and different genders.

A diamniotic dichorionic pregnancy with concordant gender can be monozygotic: in these cases the patient will need accurate echocardiographs due to the high incidence of malformations that are typical of a monozygotic gestation [9].

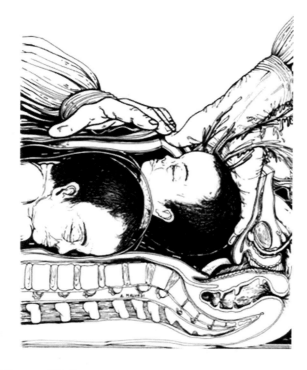

Figure 15.2 Dichorionic diamniotic twin pregnancy with fetuses in cephalic presentation during an elective cesarean delivery, in post-ART pregnancy.

Ultrasound diagnosis of placenta in twin pregnancy 259

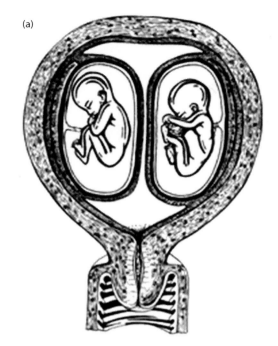

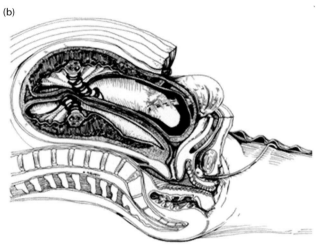

Figure 15.3 Biovular, dichorionic, diamniotic twin pregnancy: the fetuses have separate amniotic sacs, chorions, and deciduas. (a) Second trimester pregnancy. (b) Sagittal section of uterus during a cesarean delivery.

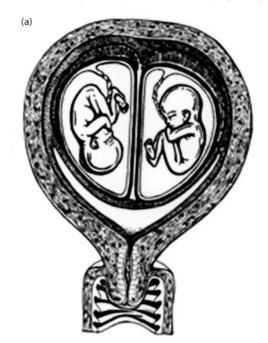

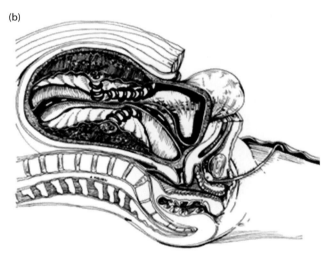

Figure 15.4 Biovular, monochorionic, diamniotic twin pregnancy: the "lambda" sign, corresponding to the duplication of chorionic layers in the placental insertion point, is visible (a), and for this reason the fetuses have separate amniotic sacs and chorions but shared decidua (b).

It is easy to differentiate a dichorionic from a monochorionic gestation in the first trimester, as the septum that differentiates the two sacs is clearly visible. It is rather difficult instead to differentiate monochorionic diamniotic gestation from monochorionic, monoamniotic gestation (Figure 15.7). This diagnosis can in fact be performed with a transvaginal probe and, in particular, by counting the number of vitelline sacs, the same as the number of amniotic sacs.

The amnionicity of a twin pregnancy, in a more advanced gestational stage and after the first trimester, can be identified using an ultrasound image of fused placentas with the help of the fetal gender: in the event of concordant gender the thickness of the amniotic septum must be evaluated, even if in a completely subjective manner.

If the membrane that separates the twins is not visualized in the second and third trimester, this should not lead to a hasty diagnosis of monoamnionicity, if it has not already been diagnosed in the first trimester. In fact in case of twin transfusion syndrome, the transfuser fetus may present significant oligohydramnios, to the point that the amniotic membranes appear crowded together and indistinguishable [10].

In order to safely establish a diagnosis of chorionicity, amnionicity, and zygosity, it is best to follow a diagnostic

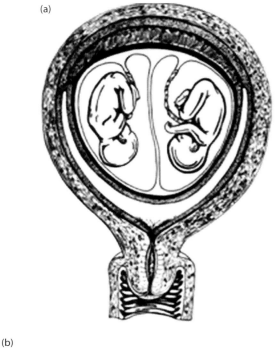

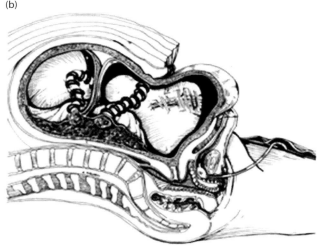

Figure 15.5 Monovular, monochorionic, diamniotic twin pregnancy (with shared chorion and decidua, but separate amniotic sacs): (a) second trimester pregnancy and (b) sagittal section of uterus during a cesarean delivery.

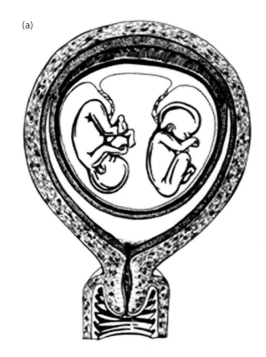

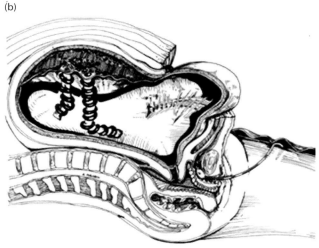

Figure 15.6 Monovular, monochorionic, monoamniotic twin pregnancy (with shared chorion, decidua, and amniotic sac). (a) Second trimester pregnancy. (b) Sagittal section of uterus during a cesarean delivery.

procedure that can in part change depending on the gestation period in which the ultrasound examination is performed.

DIAGNOSTIC PROBLEMS OF TWINS AND ANASTOMOTIC RISK

In case of a multiple pregnancy, in addition to the obstetric complications common in all twin pregnancies, the prognosis for monochorionic twins is worse than for dichorionic twins. This is due to malformations of one or both twins as well as vascular anastomosis in the placental areas, as all twin monochorionic pregnancies have vascular communications that connect the fetal circulations [11].

Venovenous and arterio-arterial anastomoses are superficial bidirectional communications located on the surface of the chorionic plate and constitute direct communications between the arteries and veins of the two fetal circulations.

They allow a flow in both directions and are found in 75% of monochorionic placentas, whereas venovenous anastomoses are found in only 20% of monochorionic placentas. Their role is not fully understood, though they seem capable of balancing any interfetal transfusions, albeit to a lesser degree than in venovenous anastomoses.

Venovenous anastomoses take place at the level of the placental cotyledons, which receive arterial blood from

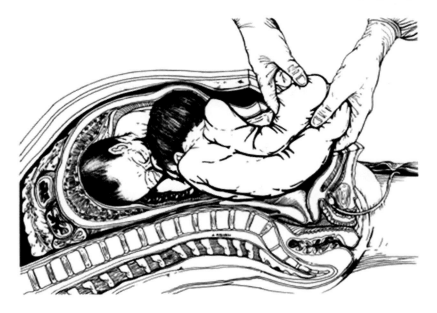

Figure 15.7 Monochorionic, monoamniotic twins with extraction of the first twin in breech presentation, buttocks variant.

one twin and provide blood to the other, creating a unidirectional flow with interfetal transfusion [12].

TWIN PREGNANCY WITH DEATH OF A TWIN

The intrauterine death of a twin occurs in 2%–5% of twin pregnancies and in 14%–17% of triplet pregnancies. This pathology affects monochorionic twins with a frequency three to four times greater than in dichorionic twins and is more common when one of the two fetuses has anatomical anomalies.

When the fetus dies in the late first trimester or in the early stages of the second trimester of gestation, the fetal remains appear as a small cystic shape that contains the "fetus papyraceus" (Figure 15.8) next to the placenta of the surviving fetus.

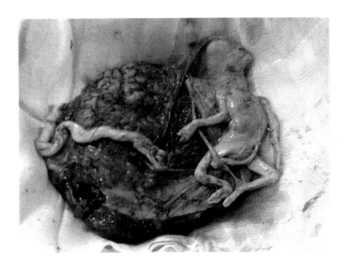

Figure 15.8 Fetus papyraceus at 37 weeks of gestation; after placental removal the fetus that had prematurely died appears.

The remaining or surviving fetus constitutes the main problem as the risk of morbidity and mortality ranges from 20% to 47% in various case studies and is tied to gestation chorionicity: more than 12% of monochorionic twins that survive the death of the second twin have various degrees of neurological and extraneurological damage [13].

The reason for this has never been determined, but the leading hypotheses all converge on the embolization of tissue products, similar to thromboplastin, by means of placental anastomosis with acute hypertension, deriving from massive blood transfusion from the surviving fetus to the deceased fetus, due to the existing pressure gradient.

From a physiopathological point of view the neurological damage consists of cerebellar necrosis, hydranencephaly, cerebral infarction, microcephaly, multicystic encephalomalacia, porencephaly, and spastic quadriplegia.

Extraneurological damage includes intestinal atresia, renal and pulmonary necrosis, and hepatic and splenic infarction [14].

The management of the twin's death varies in relation to the gestational age during which the fetal death occurred, the cause of death, and the chorionicity of the twins.

In the event of dichorionic twins, the absence of placental anastomosis improves the prognosis for the surviving twin, by allowing the continuation of the pregnancy until the pulmonary maturity of the fetus is achieved. If the gestational age at which the fetal death occurs is instead over 37 weeks, an urgent cesarean delivery is indicated.

In the event of monochorionic twins, the outcome for the surviving twin changes in relation to organ damage and preterm delivery damage. The choice of whether to continue the gestation or induce childbirth is tied to the gestational age at which the fetal death occurred and must be done in agreement with the wishes of the couple.

If a twin dies during the second trimester, the parents must be aware of the possible neurological and extraneurological damage to the surviving fetus, which may occur even weeks after the death of the second twin. Maternal risk is instead associated with the retention of abortive material and the onset of consumptive coagulopathy (for this reason it is recommended to constantly monitor the hemocoagulative profile of the pregnant woman) [15].

TWIN TRANSFUSION SYNDROME

As previously discussed, arteriovenous placental anastomoses result in a unidirectional blood flow with interfetal transfusion. In case of intraplacental reduction or the absence of bidirectional compensating vascular communications (of the superficial or deep, venovenous or arterio-arterial type), there is an imbalance of the interfetal blood flow, with hemodynamic instability and appearance of the twin transfusion syndrome (TTS) caused in part by discordant or asymmetrical development of the chorion [16]. This syndrome was defined for the first time in 1947 by Herlitz who observed anemia in one fetus and polycythemia in the other.

From a physiological point of view, the greater the placental anastomoses, the less likely it is that TTS will develop. TTS will establish itself only when the blood that passes through the arteriovenous shunt cannot return from the transfused fetus to the donor.

In the traditional TTS, the donor twin becomes progressively anemic, hypotensive, and hypovolemic, with oligohydramnios and intrauterine growth restriction (IUGR). At the same time, the recipient or acceptor twin becomes polycythemic, hypertensive, and hypervolemic with severe polyhydramnios.

Looking at it from an epidemiological point of view, more recent data show that TTS affects approximately 20% of monochorionic twin pregnancies. The onset period for TTS varies. It develops more frequently between the 16th and 25th weeks, and leads to the loss of both fetuses. It may also develop during the third trimester, with the only clinical condition being the discordant growth of the twins. In rare cases TTS may appear at the time of delivery, and its severity may vary, as neonates may have similar weight and length, but while one may be anemic and hypovolemic, the other may be polyglobulic and hypervolemic. This peripartum type rarely results in the simultaneous death of both fetuses [17].

There are acute and chronic forms of TTS. The "vanishing twin" syndrome is considered an acute form of TTS in the first trimester of pregnancy. If an acute form of TTS occurs in the second or third trimester of gestation, it may cause the death of one or both of the twins.

In the chronic form of TTS, the transfusion of blood from one fetus to the other occurs over a long period of time: the donor twin is hypovolemic and anemic, and displays growth delay and oligohydramnios. In the worst case, the donor twin can die in the uterus and appear at birth as a papyraceus fetus, while oligohydramnios pushes the donor twin to the uterine wall until it apparently adheres to it.

The transfused twin is hypervolemic, displays normal or increased biometrics, and can develop cardiac hypertrophy and congestive heart failure. Generally, the increase in urine production of the fetus results in polyhydramnios that rapidly worsens and is also responsible for the onset of preterm labor [18].

Characteristics of the TTS syndrome include diamniotic monochorionic twins, biometric disparity between twins (AC/AC > 20%), biometric disparity between amniotic sacs, biometric disparity (diameter) between umbilical cords, and hydrops, visceromegaly, and polyhydramnios of the recipient twin. The prognosis for early TTS syndrome is extremely grim, with perinatal mortality above 70%. Even in the case of intrauterine twin survival, cerebral lesions, which are more frequent in the event of endouterine fetal death, may occur.

The mechanism of cerebral, cardiac, and renal lesions of the surviving twin is apparently tied to the sudden hypotension that occurs at the time of death of the other twin. Hypotension is secondary to the fall in pressure in the circulatory system of the dead fetus and to the subsequent pressure imbalance, with sudden flow of blood from the live fetus to the dead fetus [19].

When this occurs the noninvasive therapeutic procedures (with very poor outcome), which vary depending on the gestational age during which the condition occurred, include the possibility of waiting or of providing medical treatment with indomethacin and digoxin. In case of invasive procedures, amnioreduction (evacuative paracentesis), selective feticide, or photocoagulation of placental vascular anastomosis can be performed.

Amnioreduction is a symptomatic treatment that extends pregnancies affected by TTS by diminishing uterine overdistension and the risk of preterm labor: polyhydramnios, which exerts a greater hydrostatic pressure than the fetal venous pressure, would worsen TTS and obliterate the superficial anastomoses among the placental circulations. Decompression with evacuative paracentesis would therefore help restore a new hemodynamic balance through new placental anastomoses.

Others have also attempted septostomy, which consists of creating a wide communication between the amniotic sacs. This improves amniotic fluid flow from the compartment of the recipient twin to that of the donor, as well as achieves a substantial balance of pressure, even though this method provides inadequate results due to the complications tied to artificially created monoamnionicity.

The percentage of fetal survival with selective feticide cannot be greater than 50%, unless the intervention is performed by clamping the umbilical cord. The risk of a retrograde hemorrhage toward the placenta of the dead fetus and the risk of neurological impairment of the surviving twin are both present.

Selective photocoagulation of placental anastomoses is performed with fetoscopy and involves both the anastomoses on the vascular equator as well as arteriovenous anastomoses. Unfortunately, in most cases the anastomoses in the placental area are deep and thus cannot be reached with a laser.

Little data on the outcome of fetuses that survive invasive treatment of TTS are available in the literature, as the main concern of prenatal treatment of TTS is that the extension of pregnancy might cause the survival of fetuses with severe neonatal and infantile complications [20].

MATERNAL RISK IN THE COURSE OF A CESAREAN DELIVERY

In addition to the above-mentioned fetal risks, twin pregnancies may present maternal complications with varying degrees of severity. In the first trimester of pregnancy there is an increase of nausea and vomiting, a greater risk of miscarriage and anemia, and significant increase of the plasma volume [21].

The risk of developing preeclampsia is five times greater in primigravid women with twins, while the risk for multigravida women is 10 times greater than for single pregnancies [21].

Furthermore, the risk of gestational hypertension seems to be higher for monozygotic twins. Postpartum hemorrhage is more frequent in twin pregnancies and seems to be caused by the larger placental insertion area and by uterine overdistension, with an increased tendency to atony in the early puerperium [22].

INTRAUTERINE GROWTH DELAY IN TWIN PREGNANCIES

Intrauterine growth restriction (IUGR) is very common in twin pregnancies with an incidence that varies from 25% to 33%: it is defined in terms of fetal biometrics (below the 10th percentile compared to the expected measurement of a single fetus for a given gestational age) and in terms of difference in the growth of the twins above 20%.

IUGR may involve one or both of the twins and is due to placental insufficiency and to other problems that are specifically related to twin pregnancies: a fetus can be small due to reduced blood flow, twin transfusion syndrome, or fetal malformation.

A fetus that is small due to reduced blood flow grows until 24–26 weeks at the same rate as a single fetus, but this is then followed by a reduced growth rate [23].

A biometric increase of 150 g a week is considered normal after the 26th week of gestation. For triplet pregnancies an increase of 100 g a week is considered acceptable (and so on in case of multiple pregnancies).

If the reduction in fetal growth occurs before the 24th week, one must consider the possibility of a malformed fetus, of the twin transfusion syndrome, or that a fetus in a twin pregnancy can at times display regular flowmetry while the other fetus is in distress [24].

MULTIFETAL PREGNANCY AND EMBRYONIC REDUCTION

The problem of multiple pregnancies and associated pathologies is extremely topical: in 85% of triplet pregnancies the birth is premature, with an average gestational age of 33 weeks. Neonates born before 32 completed weeks are obviously at greater risk of perinatal mortality and of serious long-term outcomes, while 25% of all triplet pregnancies end before 32 weeks of gestation are completed and 9% end before the 28th week [25].

The average gestational age at birth in quadruplet pregnancies is 29 weeks, whereas in pregnancies with a greater number of fetuses early fetal losses almost always occur. Although the percentage of preterm births varies in most case studies, there is a clear risk of extreme prematurity with severe long-term outcomes [26].

The limitation of multiple pregnancies is an extremely important and relevant problem that can be addressed in the preconceptional stage by regulating assisted fertilization techniques and in the postconceptional stage through multifetal pregnancy reduction (MFPR).

MFPR has been proposed in recent years as an attempt to decrease perinatal mortality and at the same time to improve the outcome of surviving fetuses, even though it does not represent the "ideal" solution to problems associated with multiple pregnancies. When performed by expert operators, MFPR poses a minimal risk of terminating surviving twin pregnancies and of maternal complications. It currently represents a reasonable alternative for those couples whose only choice in the past was to accept the risk of extreme neonatal prematurity or to terminate the pregnancy.

Although it is unanimously accepted that an unfavorable outcome is directly proportional to the number of fetuses, there is still disagreement on the indications for the reduction intervention, as well as on the number of fetuses to suppress. Some believe that the limit to look for should be pregnancies with four or more fetuses [27].

Currently MFPR is carried out transabdominally, as the transvaginal technique is subject to a high percentage of complications, in terms of fetal losses and infections, and therefore is only of historical interest.

There are greater technical problems before the ninth week of gestation due to the small size of the fetuses, the greater distance between fetuses and the maternal abdominal wall, and the limited resolution of transabdominal ultrasound in that stage. For these reasons the best period to perform MFPR is between the 9th and 12th weeks [28].

The choice of which fetuses to reduce is based on ease of access to the amniotic sac, crown–rump length (CRL) measurement, chorionicity, and contiguity to the uterine cervix. The need to avoid the suppression of the fetus closer to the cervix is tied to the risk of ascending infections. These infections are more likely to occur when the amniotic sac containing the nonviable fetus is contiguous to the cervical canal.

Reduction is achieved by reaching the fetal pericardial area with a spinal needle 20–22 G and injecting 0.2–0.4 mL of KCl; ultrasound monitoring is continuous, until asystole is reached, and then continues for three more minutes. Obviously, patients who undergo embryo reduction must

DIAGNOSIS OF FETAL LIE AND PRESENTATION IN TWIN PREGNANCIES

As mentioned, twin births are generally characterized by prematurity, an increase in the incidence of uterine hypokinesia (resulting from uterine overdistension), postpartum atony, and placental abruption. Uterine contractions (and therefore labor) in multiple pregnancies generally start before the presumed date of delivery. This increases the risk of premature delivery [29].

Because the fetuses have a reduced intrauterine size they are very mobile inside the uterine cavity and can be positioned in various ways, both in relation to each other and in relation to the uterus [30]. For this reason there are a high number of anomalous presentations in twin pregnancies, which can be summarized as follows:

- Longitudinal lie and cephalic presentation of both fetuses (50% of cases) (Figure 15.9)
- Longitudinal lie with one of the fetuses in breech presentation (approximately 30%–40% of cases) (Figure 15.10)
- Longitudinal lie with breech presentation of both fetuses (approximately 8%–10% of cases) (Figure 15.11)
- Transverse lie of one of the fetuses (Figure 15.12)
- Transverse lie of both fetuses (Figure 15.13)

CESAREAN BIRTH IN THE COURSE OF A TWIN PREGNANCY

Vaginal delivery in the event of a twin pregnancy with both twins in cephalic presentation (Figure 15.14) and a gestational age greater than 34 weeks is generally considered safe. Not all authors, however, agree on vaginal delivery for twin births in cephalic presentation, as the twins may lock during the expulsion phase.

Twin pregnancies have, therefore, become a more common relative indication for cesarean delivery, in part due to the fact that these pregnancies originate from an ART technique, which makes them even more valuable. In the case of other pathologies, such as fetal pelvic disproportion or fetal distress, a cesarean delivery is definitely preferable [29,30]. In addition to the aforementioned indications, there may be numerous other indications for performing a cesarean delivery in the case of twins in cephalic presentation. These include placenta previa, excessive fetal weight gain, placental abruption, maternal infections, cardiovascular pathologies, respiratory pathologies, renal pathologies, diabetes, etc. Other indications of a cesarean delivery in the course of a twin pregnancy are cephalic presentation of the first twin and breech presentation of the second twin (Figure 15.15), while few authors disagree with a cesarean delivery in case of breech presentation of both twins (Figure 15.16).

It is, however, always appropriate to evaluate the lie of the fetuses and the well-being of both fetuses and mother

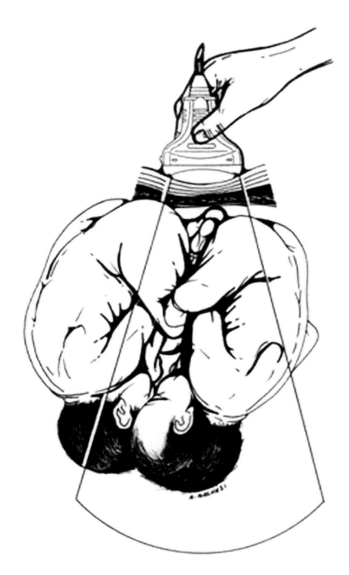

Figure 15.9 Twin pregnancy with longitudinal lie in cephalic presentation.

when deciding on the method of delivery. If the first twin is in breech presentation, this in itself is an indication for a cesarean delivery [31]. Nowadays, in the case of breech or transverse presentation of the second twin, with the first twin in cephalic presentation, a cesarean delivery is preferred. In fact, after vaginal birth of the first twin, complications can arise during the birth of the second twin in an anomalous presentation [32,33]. In any event many obstetricians, in order to avoid medical–legal complications, prefer to carry out the delivery of the twins with a cesarean delivery whenever both fetuses are not in cephalic presentation.

The use of a cesarean delivery is motivated by the need to prevent traumas to the fetuses (usually premature and hypodeveloped) and must be proposed whenever anomalous twin presentations occur [34]. When the first twin is in breech presentation a cesarean delivery is still preferred due to the possibility of a breech presentation that is incomplete or complicated, or in case

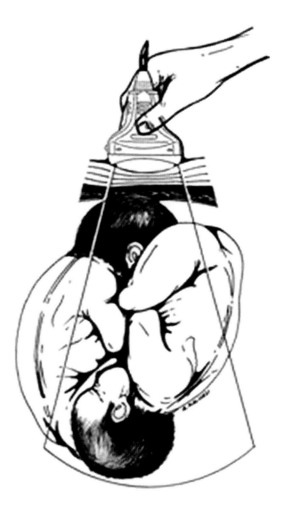

Figure 15.10 Twin pregnancy with longitudinal lie, in which the first twin is in cephalic presentation and the second twin is in breech presentation.

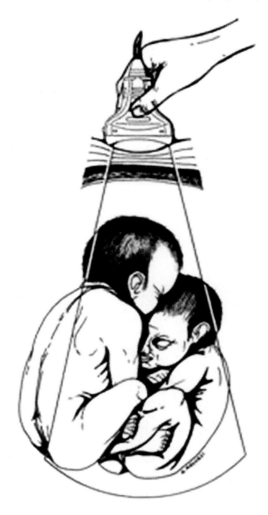

Figure 15.11 Twin pregnancy with longitudinal lie and bilateral breech presentation.

the limbs are blocked (Figures 15.17 and 15.18). In case of transverse lie of one of the twins, the operator must perform internal version (Figures 15.19 through 15.21). In case of a twin pregnancy with vaginal extraction of the fetuses, there may be a "locking" of the monoamniotic twins during the expulsion. When this occurs the head of the first breech twin is locked with the head of the second cephalic twin (Figure 15.22). Another less frequent complication that can arise in the cephalic presentation of both fetuses is interlocking at the exit or entry point of the birth canal (Figure 15.23). The locking of the fetuses during a breech presentation is a rare occurrence, as delivery is performed abdominally (Figure 15.24). The combination of a fetus in a transverse lie and a fetus in breech position is more likely to result in locking. It is an unusual condition that can originate when both fetuses at the beginning of labor are in a longitudinal lie and one of the two fetuses moves to the transverse position during advanced labor (Figure 15.25).

Another dystocic event that requires adequate preparation in the course of labor of twins in breech presentation is the "blocking" of upper limbs. When this occurs the blocked limb must be reduced before fetal extraction (Figures 15.26 and 15.27). The lower limbs may also be blocked, in which case they must be lowered before the fetus is extracted (Figure 15.28).

Before performing the cesarean delivery, the operator must also take amniochorionicity into account. In fact in diamniotic pregnancies it is easier to break the first sac, extract the first fetus and then determine the presentation of the second fetus, break the membranes, and extract the fetus. In monoamniotic twin pregnancies the operator instead must, through palpation, verify the easiest position for extraction of one of the two twins and then carry out the delivery.

After fetal extraction the placenta must be extracted in a similarly differentiated manner: generally, if the pregnancy is monochorionic, the single placenta is larger and can at times be succenturiata. In case of dichorionic pregnancy the two placentas may be separate or partially fused together.

In any case the operator must carefully palpate the cavity of the puerperal uterus to check whether any placenta residues were inadvertently left behind [29–34].

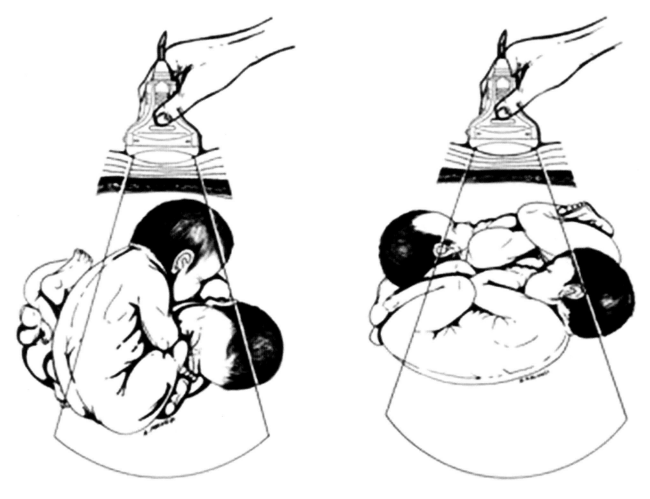

Figure 15.12 Twin pregnancy with bilateral transverse lie.

Figure 15.13 Twin pregnancy with transverse lie of a single fetus.

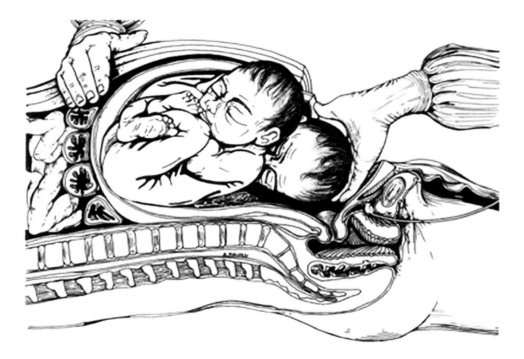

Figure 15.14 Twin pregnancy with fetuses in cephalic presentation in the course of a cesarean delivery.

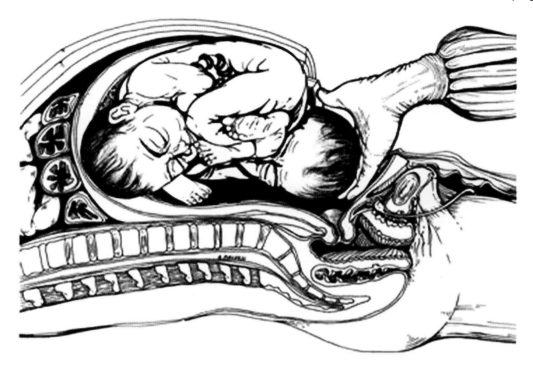

Figure 15.15 Monoamniotic, monochorionic twin pregnancy with the first fetus in cephalic presentation and the second fetus in breech presentation.

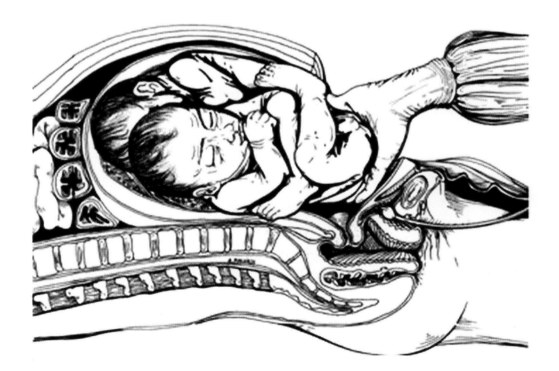

Figure 15.16 Monoamniotic, monochorionic twin pregnancy with both fetuses in breech presentation.

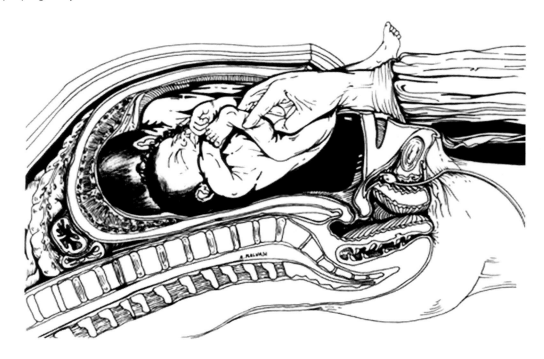

Figure 15.17 Monochorionic and monoamniotic twin pregnancy with the first fetus in breech presentation feet variant; the surgeon must search for the higher foot, grab, and lower it.

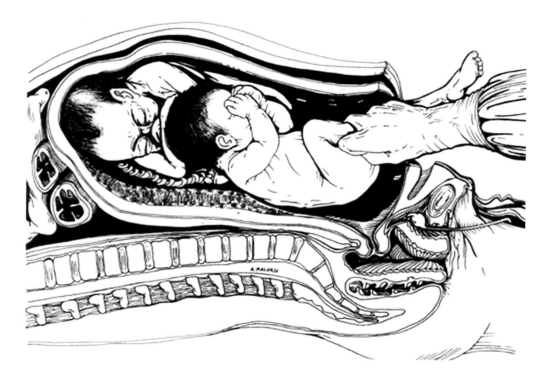

Figure 15.18 Monochorionic, monoamniotic twin pregnancy: the surgeon lowers the foot of the first twin to the uterine breech and then extracts the fetus with both feet lowered.

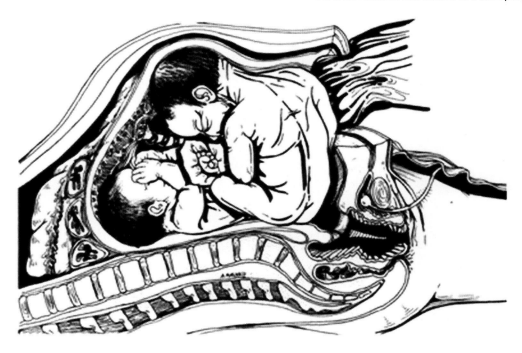

Figure 15.19 Monochorionic, monoamniotic twin pregnancy with the first fetus in transverse presentation, inferior dorsum position, and second fetus in breech presentation; the surgeon grabs the foot of the first twin.

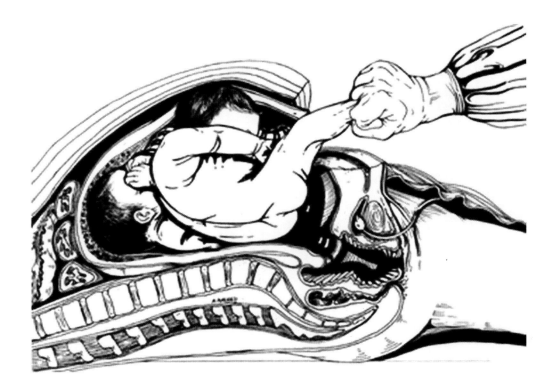

Figure 15.20 The surgeon rotates by 90° the fetus that is held by the lower limb (in this case the right limb).

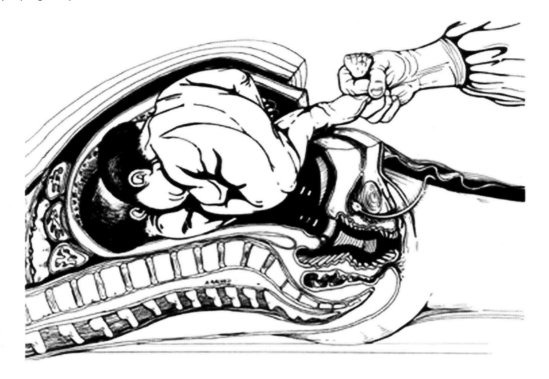

Figure 15.21 The surgeon brings the right foot toward the uterine breech and then moves the lower left limb in the same direction so that a breech presentation feet variant extraction can be performed.

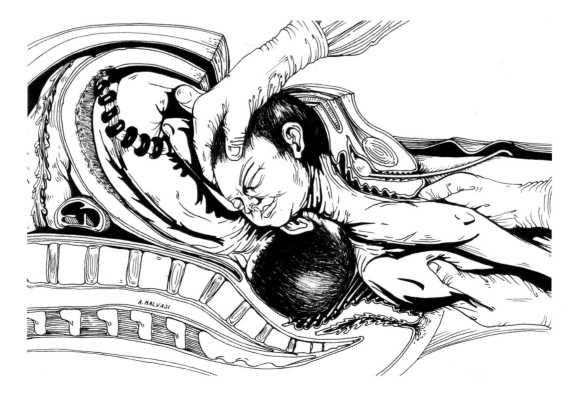

Figure 15.22 Locking or collision of twins during vaginal extraction with the first fetus in breech presentation and the second fetus in cephalic presentation. This results in an emergency cesarean delivery in which the operator attempts to unlock the two twins while an assistant at the lower end pushes the twin to facilitate the unlocking maneuver.

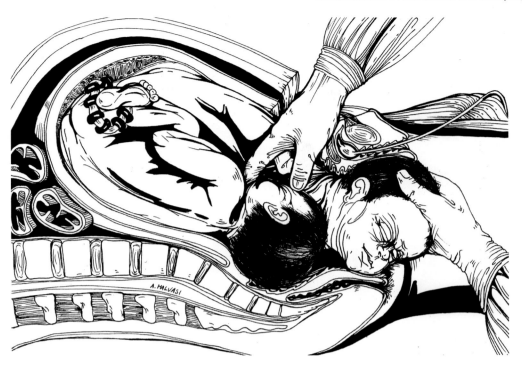

Figure 15.23 Locking or collision of twins in cephalic presentation: while the surgeon attempts to free the fetuses an assistant attempts to move back up the first wedged twin.

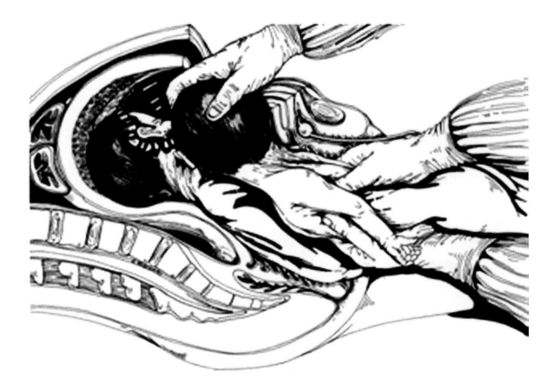

Figure 15.24 Locking or collision of twins in breech presentation: while the operator attempts to free the heads an assistant at the lower end facilitates the maneuver by pushing the first twin.

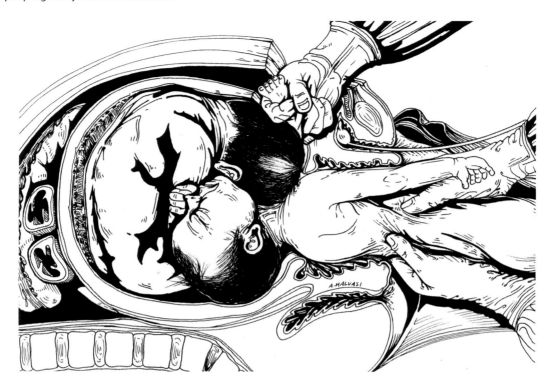

Figure 15.25 Locking of the twins with the second fetus in transverse lie, superior dorsum position, and the first twin in breech presentation. The operator must perform internal version in order to free the twins, while the assistant at the lower end pushes the breech fetus to facilitate these extreme maneuvers.

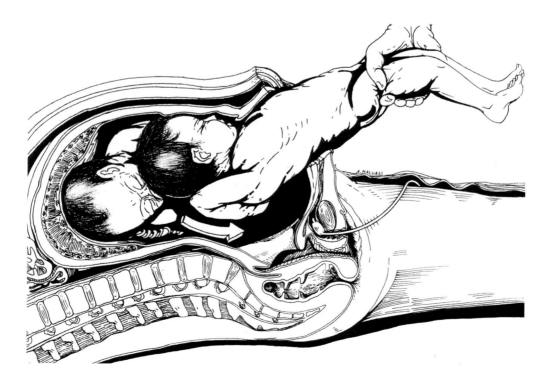

Figure 15.26 Blocked upper right limb of the first fetus in breech presentation (see arrow).

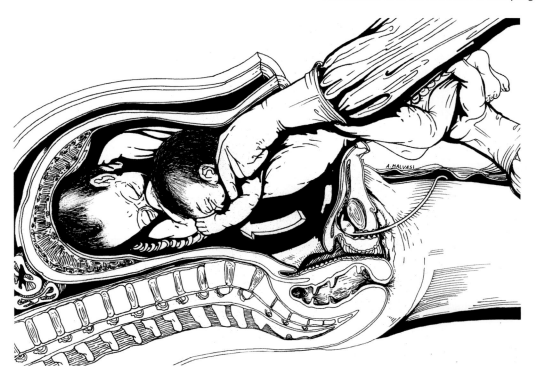

Figure 15.27 Lowering of the blocked limb after ventral rotation of the fetus.

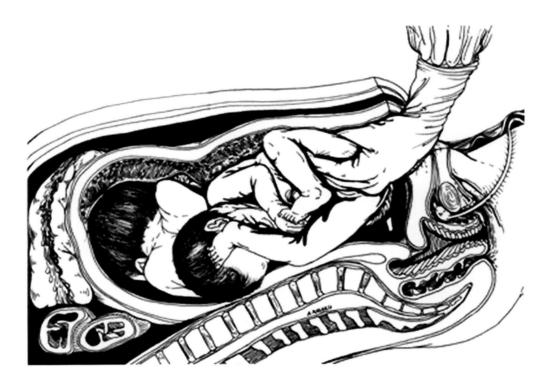

Figure 15.28 Lowering of the lower left limb of the first fetus in breech presentation in a monochorionic, monoamniotic, and monovular pregnancy, with a maneuver similar to the Pinard maneuver.

CONCLUSIONS

Twin pregnancies have become a relative indication for cesarean delivery, and their incidence has increased proportionally to the number of multiple pregnancies resulting from assisted reproductive techniques [35,36]. The diagnosis of a twin pregnancy is performed with obstetric ultrasound before and during the labor of birth [37].

Fetuses in cephalic presentation are, however, an indication for spontaneous delivery [38].

Cephalic presentation of the first fetus and breech presentation of the second fetus can lead to vaginal delivery, with special attention paid to the extraction of the second fetus [39].

Conversely, a breech presentation of the first fetus may result in the locking of the two fetuses, which may lead to a cesarean delivery for the second twin [40,41].

In twin pregnancies with both fetuses in breech and/or transverse presentation, cesarean deliveries are indicated and are done to avoid dangerous maternal–fetal complications [42].

REFERENCES

1. Horn J. Double trouble, twin triumph. *Pract Midwife* 2008;11(10):44–46.
2. Keith LG, Machin GA. *An Atlas of Multiple Pregnancy*. London, UK: Informa Healthcare; 1999.
3. Shebl O, Ebner T, Sommergruber M, Sir A, Tews G. Risk in twin pregnancies after the use of assisted reproductive techniques. *J Reprod Med* 2008;53(10): 798–802.
4. Badawy A, Elnashar A, Totongy M. Clomiphene citrate or aromatase inhibitors for superovulation in women with unexplained infertility undergoing intrauterine insemination: A prospective randomized trial [published online August 9, 2008]. *Fertil Steril* 2009;92(4):1355–9.
5. Blickstein I, Keith LG. *Multiple Pregnancy: Epidemiology, Gestation, and Perinatal Outcome*, 2nd ed. London, UK: Informa Healthcare; 2005.
6. Hack KE, van Gemert MJ, Lopriore E et al. Placental characteristics of monoamniotic twin pregnancies in relation to perinatal outcome [published online November 17, 2008]. *Placenta* 2009;30(1):62–65.
7. Monteagudo A, Timor-Trish IE. *Ultrasound and Multifetal Pregnancy*. Boca Raton, FL: Taylor & Francis; 1997.
8. Hack KE, Derks JB, Schaap AH et al. Perinatal outcome of monoamniotic twin pregnancies. *Obstet Gynecol* 2009;113(2 Pt 1):353–60.
9. Candiani GB, Danesino V, Gastaldi A. *La Clinica Ostetrica e Ginecologica*. Vol. 1. Milano, Italy: Masson; 1996.
10. Nicolaides KH, Snijders RJM, Sebire N. *The 11–14-Week Scan: The Diagnosis of Fetal Abnormalities*. New York, NY: Parthenon; 1999.
11. Wee LY, Muslim I. Perinatal complications of monochorionic placentation. *Curr Opin Obstet Gynecol* 2007;19(6):554–60.
12. Nakata M, Sumie M, Murata S, Miwa I, Matsubara M, Sugino N. Fetoscopic laser photocoagulation of placental communicating vessels for twin-reversed arterial perfusion sequence. *J Obstet Gynaecol Res* 2008;34(4 Pt 2):649–52.
13. Lee YM, Wylie BJ, Simpson LL, D'Alton ME. Twin chorionicity and the risk of stillbirth. *Obstet Gynecol* 2008;111(2 Pt 1):301–8.
14. Benirschke K, Kaufmann P. *Pathology of the Human Placenta*. 4th ed. New York, NY: Springer; 2000.
15. Winn HN, Hobbins JC. *Clinical Maternal-Fetal Medicine*. Boca Raton, FL: CRC Press/Taylor & Francis; 2000.
16. Habli M, Livingston J, Harmon J, Lim FY, Plozin W, Crombleholme T. The outcome of twin-twin transfusion syndrome complicated with placental insufficiency. *Am J Obstet Gynecol* 2008;199(4):424.e1–6.
17. Crombleholme TM, Shera D, Lee H et al. A prospective, randomized, multicenter trial of amnioreduction vs selective fetoscopic laser photocoagulation for the treatment of severe twin-twin transfusion syndrome. *Am J Obstet Gynecol* 2007;197(4):396.e1–9.
18. Quintero RA. *Twin-Twin Transfusion Syndrome*. London, UK: Informa Healthcare; 2007.
19. Said S, Flood K, Breathnach F, Fleming A, Kinsella CB, Geary M, Malone FD. Fetoscopic laser treatment of twin-to-twin transfusion syndrome (TTTS). *Ir Med J* 2008;101(6):191–3.
20. Habli M, Michelfelder E, Livingston J, Harmon J, Lim FY, Polzin W, Crombleholme T. Acute effects of selective fetoscopic laser photocoagulation on recipient cardiac function in twin-twin transfusion syndrome [published online August 22, 2008]. *Am J Obstet Gynecol* 2008;199(4):412.e1–6.
21. Luke B, Brown MB. Maternal morbidity and infant death in twin vs triplet and quadruplet pregnancies [published online February 21, 2008]. *Am J Obstet Gynecol* 2008;198(4):401.e1–10.
22. Keith LG, Machin GA. *An Atlas of Multiple Pregnancy*. London, UK: Informa Healthcare; 1999.
23. Morley R, Moore VM, Dwyer T, Owens JA, Umstad MP, Carlin JB. Maternal birthweight and outcome of twin pregnancy. *Paediatr Perinat Epidemiol* 2007;21(6):501–6.
24. Bowers N. *The Multiple Pregnancy Sourcebook: Pregnancy and the First Days with Twins, Triplets, and More*. New York, NY: McGraw-Hill; 2001.
25. Delbaere I, Verstraelen H, Goetgeluk S, Martens G, Derom C, De Bacquer D, De Backer G, Temmerman M. Perinatal outcome of twin pregnancies in women of advanced age [published online June 10, 2008]. *Hum Reprod* 2008;23(9):2145–50.
26. Gerris J. The near elimination of triplets in IVF. *Reprod Biomed Online*. 2007;15(Suppl 3):40–44.
27. Schmitz T, Carnavalet Cde C, Azria E, Lopez E, Cabrol D, Goffinet F. Neonatal outcomes of twin pregnancy according to the planned mode of delivery. *Obstet Gynecol* 2008;111(3):695–703.

28. Alexander JM, Leveno KJ, Rouse D et al. Cesarean delivery for the second twin. *Obstet Gynecol* 2008;112(4):748–52.
29. Vendittelli F, Rivière O, Pons JC, Lémery D, Berrebi A, Mamelle N; Obstétriciens du réseau sentinelle Audipog. Twin delivery: A survey of French obstetrical policies. *Gynecol Obstet Fertil* 2006;34(1):19–26.
30. Piekarski P, Czajkowski K, Maj K, Milewczyk P. Neonatal outcome depending on the mode of delivery and fetal presentation in twin gestation. *Ginekol Pol* 1997;68(4):187–92.
31. Kurzel RB, Claridad L, Lampley EC. Cesarean delivery for the second twin. *J Reprod Med* 1997;42(12):767–70.
32. Bider D, Korach J, Hourvitz A, Dulitzky M, Goldenberg M, Mashiach S. Combined vaginal-abdominal delivery of twins. *J Reprod Med* 1995;40(2):131–4.
33. Chauhan SP, Roberts WE, McLaren RA, Roach H, Morrison JC, Martin JN Jr. Delivery of the nonvertex second twin: Breech extraction versus external cephalic version. *Am J Obstet Gynecol* 1995;173(4):1015–20.
34. Chervenak FA, Johnson RE, Berkowitz RL, Hobbins JC. Intrapartum external version of the second twin. *Obstet Gynecol* 1983;62(2):160–5.
35. Sunderam S, Kissin DM, Flowers L, Anderson JE, Folger SG, Jamieson DJ, Barfield WD; Centers for Disease Control and Prevention (CDC). Assisted reproductive technology surveillance—United States, 2009. *MMWR Surveill Summ* 2012;61(7):1–23.
36. Ooki S. Concordance rates of birth defects after assisted reproductive technology among 17,258 Japanese twin pregnancies: A nationwide survey, 2004–2009. *J Epidemiol* 2013;23(1):63–69.
37. Lau TK, Jiang F, Chan MK, Zhang H, Lo PS, Wang W. Non-invasive prenatal screening of fetal Down syndrome by maternal plasma DNA sequencing in twin pregnancies. *J Matern Fetal Neonatal Med* 2013;26(4):434–7.
38. Breathnach FM, McAuliffe FM, Geary M et al.; Perinatal Ireland Research Consortium. Prediction of safe and successful vaginal twin birth. *Am J Obstet Gynecol* 2011;205(3):237.e1–7. doi:10.1016/j.ajog.2011.05.033.
39. Hoffmann E, Oldenburg A, Rode L, Tabor A, Rasmussen S, Skibsted L. Twin births: Cesarean delivery or vaginal delivery? *Acta Obstet Gynecol Scand* 2012;91(4):463–9.
40. Crowther CA. WITHDRAWN: Caesarean delivery for the second twin. *Cochrane Database Syst Rev* 20117;(12):CD000047. doi:10.1002/14651858.CD000047.pub2.
41. Steins Bisschop CN, Vogelvang TE, May AM, Schuitemaker NW. Mode of delivery in non-cephalic presenting twins: A systematic review. *Arch Gynecol Obstet* 2012;286(1):237–47.
42. Lee HC, Gould JB, Boscardin WJ, El-Sayed YY, Blumenfeld YJ. Trends in cesarean delivery for twin births in the United States: 1995–2008. *Obstet Gynecol* 2011118(5):1095–101.

Cesarean delivery for the preterm neonate

GABRIELE D'AMATO, SAVINO MASTROPASQUA, and ELENA PACELLA

INTRODUCTION

Premature births are one of the greatest challenges of perinatal care, and are an important risk factor for neurological impairment and disability. Premature birth constitutes the most frequent cause of perinatal mortality and morbidity. About 70% of deaths that occur during the perinatal period among neonates without obvious congenital anomalies can be attributed to preterm birth. It not only affects the infant and the family, that must remain in the hospital for several months, but it is also a significant health-care system cost.

An estimate from the United States, a country in which 500,000 preterm children are born each year, stated that $2 billion are spent each year for this problem. In addition, complications tied to prematurity, such as bronchopulmonary dysplasia, retinopathy, intraventricular hemorrhage, necrotizing enterocolitis, and infections that can create chronic disabilities, also add to the long-term costs [1,2].

THE PRETERM NEONATE
Definition

The criteria that define "prematurity," along with the scientific and diagnostic progress in neonatology, have gradually been defined over the course of the twentieth century. Even though the role of "maturity" in the neonate's survival and subsequent development was unanimously recognized in the first half of the 1900s, the criteria for its definition were neither clearly identified nor agreed upon.

In 1935 the American Academy of Pediatrics, followed in 1949 by the World Health Organization (WHO), assumed as the sole criterion for defining prematurity, a weight at birth of the neonate infant equal to or below 2500 g. This had the advantage of being a simple and economic criterion. Over the years, however, clinical practice showed a great degree of variability in the clinical conditions of neonates and in the relative therapeutic interventions needed for their survival. This constituted a barrier to the creation of guidelines for the treatment of the premature neonate, which could be applied to this entire category of patients. A more specific definition of prematurity was therefore needed, which had to include, at the least, a reference to the gestational age of the neonate.

In the early 1960s WHO redefined prematurity based on the following criteria:

- Weight at birth below 2500 g
- Gestational age below 37 weeks, corresponding to 259 days of gestation (National Health and Medical Research Council [NHMRC], 2000) [3].

Prematurity was therefore differentiated based on both weight at birth and gestational age.

Neonates can be classified on the basis of weight at birth as

- LBW (low birth weight) with a weight between 1500 and 2499 g
- VLBW (very low birth weight) with a weight between 1000 and 1499 g
- ELBW (extremely low birth weight) with a weight between 500 and 999 g

A preterm fetus is any fetus born before the 37th week of gestation, and can be classified as

- Preterm <37 weeks
- Very preterm <32 weeks
- Extremely preterm <28 weeks

The greater complexity of this new definition of prematurity is also reflected in the terminology. In fact, in 1969 WHO replaced the term "premature" with "preterm," underscoring that the definition was not based solely on the lack of maturation but also on the fact that the amount of time required to reach maturation was not achieved.

Advances in perinatal medicine allowed for an improved assessment of the gestational age of the fetus and facilitated the use of this new criterion (Table 16.1).

The gestational age determined from the early use of an ultrasound examination is more accurate than any other physical maturity point system attributed at birth.

A further step forward in defining prematurity, that would also be capable of categorizing the various categories of patients, was made at the end of the 1960s by Battaglia and Lubchenco [4]. They created a classification system with nine categories that combined the criteria of weight at birth with gestational age, and made use of the average prenatal growth curves.

This classification system has three general categories defined by gestational age:

- Term birth: >37 and <42 weeks
- Preterm birth: <37 weeks
- Post-term birth: >42 weeks

Each of these categories is subdivided into three subcategories based on appropriateness of weight at birth in relation to gestational age:

- Appropriate for gestational age (AGA)
- Small for gestational age (SGA)
- Large for gestational age (LGA)

Table 16.1 Criteria for determining the gestational age and weight of the fetus

- The gestational age calculation based solely on medical history (last menstrual cycle) can be from −6 to +14 days removed from the real age.
- The menstrual history, corroborated by the ultrasound examination result, provides the best estimate for gestational age. Complete antenatal annotations, including pelvic examination in the first trimester, previous ultrasound examinations, and symphysis fundal height measurement should also be assessed.
- If the gestational age is unknown, it can be adequately estimated from the ultrasound examination result. The ultrasound examination is reported to be accurate in terms of gestational age to within 8 days in the first trimester and 20 days in the second trimester.
- The estimate of the weight with ultrasound is within 10%–15% of the real weight and is a function of the amount of amniotic fluid, fetal position, and presentation, of the biometric data used to calculate the weight, and of operator experience. Utmost attention must be paid in the biometric examination in looking for congenital anomalies.
- Each maternal or fetal risk factor associated with the possible reduction in growth should be considered when interpreting the weight estimate.

Table 16.2 Definition of neonate according to the Società Italiana di Medicina Perinatale (SIMP) (Italian Perinatal Medicine Society)

Fetus with gestational age at birth between the beginning of the 23rd week (154th day or 22 complete weeks) and the end of the 36th week (258th day or 36 weeks and 6 days).

The neonate is defined "very preterm" if the gestational age is between 28 + 0 and 31 + 6 weeks and "extremely preterm" if between 22 + 0 and 27 + 6 weeks.

In relation to low weight at birth neonate infants are classified as
- LBW (low birth weight) weight between 1500 and 2499 g
- VLBW (very low birth weight) weight between 1000 and 1499 g
- ELBW (extremely low birth weight) weight between 500 and 999 g

Weight of neonate in relation to gestational age can be
- LGA (large for gestational age): high weight for gestational age (>90th percentile)
- AGA (appropriate for gestational age): appropriate weight for gestational age (between 90th and 10th percentile for gestational age)
- SGA (small for gestational age): low weight for gestational age (<10th percentile)

This differentiation is based on a statistical criterion: neonates with a weight below the 10th percentile of intrauterine growth curves are defined SGA, those with a weight above the 90th percentile are defined LGA, and those with a weight between the 10th and 90th percentile are considered AGA (Table 16.2).

In general, gestational age and weight at birth are inversely proportional to the increase in mortality and neonatal morbidity. In fact, most cases of mortality and morbidity are limited to "very preterm" neonates and in particular "extremely preterm" neonates.

Incidence

The overall incidence of preterm births in industrialized countries has not decreased in the last 30 years and represents approximately 9%–10% of live births. Some evidence shows a slight increase in these births, though the percentage of births with a gestational age less than 32 weeks has remained basically unchanged at around 1%–2% [5].

Numerous factors have contributed to the overall increase in the incidence of prematurity, including the increase in multiple births, the increased use of assisted reproduction, and a greater number of obstetric procedures. The apparent increase in preterm births can in part be explained by changes in clinical practice. One example is the ever-increasing use of ultrasound examinations to determine the gestational age, which has replaced the date of the last menstrual cycle. This increase can also be a result of the different classification systems used. This variability is dependent on whether a certain country considers a live birth any child born with a very short gestational age (<24 weeks). Moreover, although the law requires that live births should be registered, there is subjectivity in distinguishing between a live birth and a fetal loss, especially when the infant dies immediately after birth.

In the past some of these fragile neonates were regarded as spontaneous abortions and thus were not registered as live births. In fact in the United Kingdom, since October 1992, the reduction of the minimal gestational age required for fetal deaths to be considered stillborn, may have resulted in a greater percentage of extremely preterm pregnancies being registered as live births. The limit for infants to be declared and registered as a preterm live birth has been reduced from 28 complete weeks to 24 complete gestational weeks. At an international level, the limit varies from 22 gestational weeks in Japan, to 24 weeks in the United Kingdom, up to 28 weeks in many other European countries. In the United States, each state has its own registration system, with a majority of states adopting a gestational age of 20 weeks as the criterion for establishing a fetal death [6,7].

In light of this some estimates can be unreliable in epidemiological terms, which can explain the differences in survival percentages and the long-term neonatal outcomes described in the literature [5].

PERINATAL EPIDEMIOLOGY

The hospital discharge form (HDF) was created in 1994 and is now an established data collection tool used in hospitalization centers. Almost 100% of public and private structures make use of the form through which hospitalization stays can be precisely analyzed. Since 1997 the HDF must also be compiled for healthy neonates in nurseries.

Since 1998 there has been a significant increase in neonate registrations, which allow for specific analyses in the neonatal area. Since 2001 the data collected for babies discharged from the hospital have included information on the weight at birth. The coverage and quality of this information, however, does not allow complete prematurity analyses. Moreover, it will soon be possible to use the information contained in the CeDAP (delivery assistance certificates), which will significantly improve overall perinatal assistance.

Neonatal hospitalization

Neonatal hospitalization data of neonates with pathologies have been gathered by the Ministry of Health since 1994. Since 1997 the same information has been gathered for all neonates in hospital nurseries, including "healthy" infants, as defined by law DRG 391. Neonates in the DRG classification system are mostly grouped in MDC 15, neonatal disorders and illnesses, which includes seven DRGs (from 385 to 391). DRG 391 does not uniquely identify a healthy neonate, in that it includes cases of minor pathological conditions which do not absorb significant resources.

The number of neonates in the HDFs since 1998 has increased due to improved reporting and correct codification. This has increased the number of reported cases from 330,500 in 1998 to 541,306 in 2001 [8].

Besides the epidemiological aspect, the percentage of pathological neonates is an indicator of data quality and correct codification. Some concern is raised by the regional variability of neonates considered "not healthy" in the HDF. One neonate out of two is not considered healthy in Molise and Basilicata, while this drops to one out of four in the Autonomous Province of Trento, Veneto, Emilia Romagna, and Valle D'Aosta (Figure 16.1). To this end, in order to assess the causes of neonate hospitalization in the first 28 days of life, let us examine the list of the top 10 DRGs in terms of frequency (Table 16.3).

Since 2001 the weight of neonates hospitalized at birth has been a determining factor in the HDF record. The percentage of neonates with a low weight at birth is an important indicator of the health of the neonatal population. This percentage is a general indicator of reproductive health (in this sense, it is an outcome indicator), but it also represents a risk factor (especially for neonates with a weight <1500 g) and is an indicator of the needs of this same category of subjects. It is also one of the parameters considered by WHO that has set a goal of 3.8% for the year 2020 for this category of individuals.

The data from this indicator, as shown in the diagram, are incomplete. No data are available from three regions. A more precise analysis can be made when the CeDAP delivery assistance certificates are available (Figure 16.2).

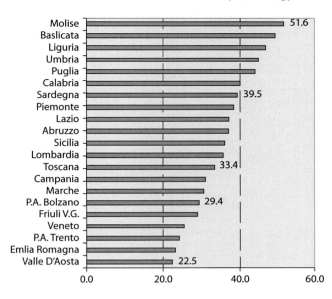

Figure 16.1 Percentage of pathological neonates 0–28 days. (Data from Eurostat 2003; graph from Fortino A, Lispi L. Ospedalizzazione pediatrica in Italia, 2001, in http://www.salute.gov.it/imgs/C_17_pubblicazioni_999_allegato.pdf. With permission.)

Table 16.3 Top 10 DRGs in neonates with 0–28 days of ordinary hospitalization

DRG	Description	Discharged n.	%
391	Healthy neonate	352,993	65.2
389	Full-term neonates with significant affections	57,039	10.5
390	Neonates with other significant affections	47,925	8.9
467	Other factors that affect health conditions	17,009	3.1
387	Prematurity with significant affections	12,465	2.3
388	Prematurity with significant affections	11,640	2.2
385	Neonates that are dead or transferred to acute care	7245	1.3
386	Neonates that are extremely immature or with respiratory distress syndrome	6070	1.1
137	Congenital cardiac and valvular diseases, age <18 years	4213	0.8
256	Other musculoskeletal system and connective tissue diagnoses	2391	0.4

Source: Fortino A, Lispi L, Ospedalizzazione pediatrica in Italia, 2001, in http://www.salute.gov.it/imgs/C_17_pubblicazioni_999_allegato.pdf. With permission.

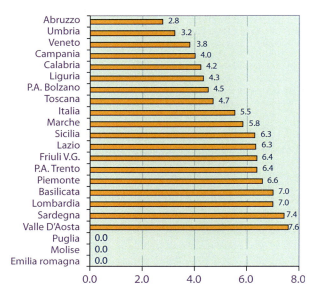

Figure 16.2 Percentage of neonates with weight at birth <2500 g in 2001. (From Fortino A, Lispi L. Ospedalizzazione pediatrica in Italia, 2001, in http://www.salute.gov.it/imgs/C_17_pubblicazioni_999_allegato.pdf. With permission.)

Neonatal mortality

Perinatal mortality, both in the fetal as well as in the neonatal component, is in constant decline, though it still remains high in many industrialized countries, including in Italy [9]. In particular, following the drastic reduction in postnatal mortality (from 1 month to 1 year of life), currently around 75% of infant-age (first year of life) deaths occur in the neonatal period (1 month) [10]. In addition, 50% of deaths that occur between 1 month and 1 year of life can be attributed to the same causes that lead to death in the neonatal period.

This explains the increasing attention paid to maternal–infant care in the perinatal period, so that interventions can be implemented that reduce both morbidity and mortality.

Infant mortality in Europe and Italy

Figure 16.3 shows the 2002 infant mortality rates from 15 European countries. Infant mortality rate was used instead of neonatal mortality, as this parameter is less susceptible to variations in the definitions used in various countries. In consideration of the fact that 75% of infantile age deaths occur within 28 days of life, and that a significant portion of deaths that occur between 1 month and 1 year is due to a pathology that came about in the perinatal period, there is a tendency to identify this rate with the neonatal rate. Figure 16.3 shows how much infant mortality in those 15 countries can vary, from 2.8‰ in Sweden, to 5.9‰ in Greece, with Italy having an intermediate value. Infant mortality has dropped 80% in Italy in the last 25 years, from 20.5‰ in 1975 to 4.7‰ in 2002 according to Eurostat data.

Considering only neonatal mortality, which constitutes the most significant portion of infant mortality, we can see that several regions in Northern and Central Italy have very low values (Friuli-Venezia Giulia and Autonomous Province of Bolzano 1.5‰ of live births, Veneto 2‰, Autonomous Province of Trento 2.1‰, Tuscany and Marche 2.3‰), with four Italian regions, prevalently from the South, that have values that are double: Sicily 4.8‰ of live births, Molise and Calabria 4.6‰, and Puglia with 4.1‰ [8,9] (Figure 16.4).

A main factor in the reduction of infant mortality is a significant reduction in postnatal mortality (between the 2nd and 12th months of life) and, albeit to a lower extent, of late neonatal mortality (between 7 and 30 days of life).

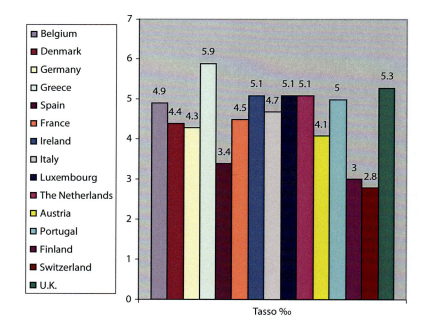

Figure 16.3 Infant mortality rates in Europe in 2003. (Data from Eurostat 2003.)

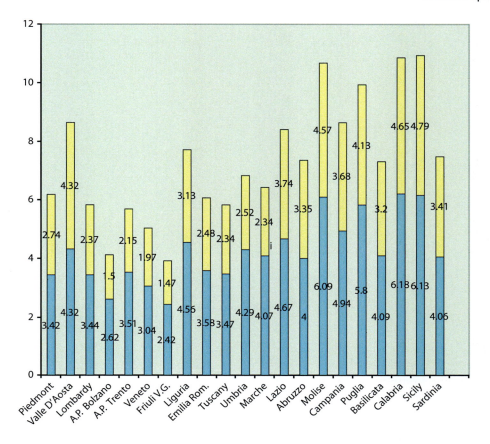

Figure 16.4 Infant and neonatal mortality rate per 1000 live births in Italian regions. (Data from ISTAT.)

In any event, neonatal mortality represents approximately 80% of infant mortality and the reduction of the incidence rates can be tied to several factors, for example, the increased use, starting in the 1970s, in Italy of Neonatal Intensive Therapies, distributed throughout the various regions, starting from the 1990s, according to specific criteria that are now widely accepted [11].

Neonatal mortality and the role of intensive care

Many works have been published in the last 20 years that show an improvement in the prognosis of VLBW neonates [12]. The collection of data regarding the survival of preterm neonates is important for several reasons. First, it can help inform the pregnant woman of the fetus' survival potential. Moreover, neonatal and perinatal mortality rates are frequently used to measure outcomes in studies that evaluate the effectiveness of therapeutic interventions.

There is an increased tendency to compare survival estimates among institutions as a way to verify obstetric and neonatal care. A large number of publications present estimates on preterm neonate survival rates in relation to each week of gestation. However, these curves show large differences among the percentages, especially in the group between 23 and 27 weeks of gestation. There are several potential explanations for this variability.

First, differences between studies may simply reflect differences in the populations studied (clinical variability), including sociodemographic factors. These variations may also depend on the time period examined or the use of interventions known to improve survival rates, such as, for example, antenatal steroids, or postnatal surfactant therapy. It is also possible that systematic errors are one of the causes of the variations in survival numbers. There may in part be a potential selection bias in those studies that only show the survival of neonates allowed in intensive care units and, to a lesser degree, in those studies that include live births but that do not include the stillborn [13].

The types of neonates that undergo intensive neonatal care are primarily preterm neonates with a weight <1500 g and/or gestational age <32 weeks. Most studies show that this category is less than 1% of total live births, but contributes to more than 40% of all neonatal deaths. Therefore, using data originating from single hospitals (center based), for this type of statistical analysis aimed at studying neonatal survival and outcomes, may be misleading due to spurious variations tied to the population of each center. To this end, it would be best to use data collected from a population from a more extended geographical area, such as a nation, region, or province (area based) [14].

Italy currently is without this type of data, though the data are available in single regions such as Friuli-Venezia Giulia, the Autonomous Provinces of Trento and Sassari and Lazio; one report contains a 2002 mortality estimate of VLBW neonates divided by three geographical areas in Italy (north, center, south) (Figure 16.5) [15].

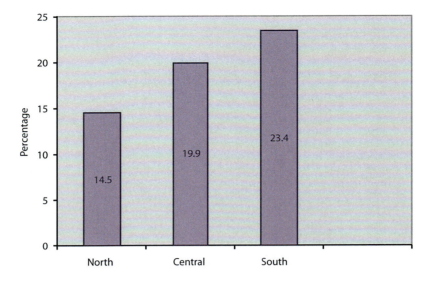

Figure 16.5 Mortality estimate of VLBW neonates. (From Corchia C. Epidemiologia dei VLBW in Italia, Acta IX National Congress SIN 2003. With permission.)

At an international level the Vermont Oxford Network, which gathers information from around 30,000 neonates that underwent a wide range of neonatal intensive care units in North America, shows survival rates stratified for each gestational age [16].

Another population study carried out in the United Kingdom and in the Republic of Ireland (EPICure) describes the survival and long-term outcome of live birth neonates below 26 complete weeks of gestational age (Figure 16.6) [17]. Overall, it can be said that the survival rate increases by 2%–4% for each intrauterine day from 23 to 26 weeks. Therefore, since 1990 intensive therapies have had a virtual survival rate ≥90% for neonates with weight at birth >1000 g. On the other hand, survival below 500 g can be considered a rare event. Thus, the entire ethical debate on intensive care is around a weight of approximately 500 g: to be precise in a weight range at birth of 500–1000 g.

A lot has changed in neonatal intensive care units (NICUs) in the last 15 years. Prenatal steroids are more widely used, ventilation techniques have improved, and surfactant is used. These measures have modified the epidemiology and the ethical considerations regarding the life and death of ELBW neonates in NICUs [18,19]. A study by Meadow from 2004 [20] analyzed this problem in 1142 ELBW neonates from 1991 to 2001 with a weight at birth <1000 g, with the following results:

1. There were substantially improved survival rates in those patients with a greater weight at birth and in those born in the last years of the past decade. However, since survival rates of the larger ELBW neonates have reached approximately 90% during the course of the entire decade, large-scale improvements for these patients are unlikely.
2. The greatest gains for smaller ELBW patients occurred at the beginning of the decade. From 1991 to 1997 survival rates improved by about 4% a year. However, starting in 1997 and continuing to 2001, no further improvements were observed.
3. The average hospital stay for deceased neonates increased from 2 to 10 days during this observation period, and consequently, the percentage of neonates with an "undeclared" outcome at 4 days of life increased from 10% to 20% for all ELBW patients and by 33% for those with a weight at birth between 450 and 700 g.
4. However, the percentage from 1991 to 2001 of hospital beds containing nonsurvivors remained low (7%).

This study concluded that very few of the ELBW neonate subgroups do not survive compared to the previous decade, with improvements especially in the 450–700 g weight range, which had and continues to have the highest mortality rate. In addition, this progress seems to have slowed down or come to a halt starting from the last years of the previous decade up to now. Although the majority of deaths in the ELBW subgroup with the lowest weight happen early, the life or death uncertainty persists for a longer period of time, although it remains acceptably short.

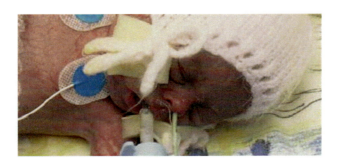

Figure 16.6 ELBW at 26 weeks of gestational age.

FACTORS ASSOCIATED WITH IMPROVEMENT OF SURVIVAL RATES

Antenatal steroids

Predicting and preventing preterm birth and choosing the best method of delivery, in order to reduce the number of preterm births and improve the outcomes for both mother and child, are today's challenges.

A large portion of preterm births result from unexplained labor or from rupture of the amniotic membranes. Up to 50% of births before 37 weeks are a result of idiopathic preterm labor, while another 30% is caused by preterm prelabor rupture of the amniotic membranes (PPROM) [21].

A great deal of work has been carried out to find diagnostic tests capable of accurately predicting whether women at risk will experience preterm labor, but with limited success. This would allow for an early and more efficient use of appropriate prenatal interventions.

Since "prevention of prematurity" cannot be effectively implemented, steroids have become an indispensable intervention in the event of a probable premature birth. More than 30 years have passed since Liggins studied the biochemical nature of delivery in animals and observed, after treatment with corticosteroids, an increase in the survival rate at earlier gestational periods and the histological maturation of the lung parenchyma. This was later applied to humans by administering betamethasone, which resulted in a reduction from 15.6% to 10% in the incidence of respiratory syndrome [22].

In 2000 these results were confirmed by a new recommendation from the National Institute of Health that confirmed the safety and effectiveness of this treatment and recommended its use in all pregnancies between the 24th and 34th weeks of gestation and at risk of delivery within 7 days (Table 16.4). Steroids achieve maximum effect 24 hours after administration and are associated with a significant reduction in respiratory distress syndrome (RDS) (from 23.7% to 8.8%) in children born 24 hours to 7 days after the treatment [23].

Neonatal mortality in the treated group is also reduced from 11.6% to 6%, as is the rate of intraventricular cerebral hemorrhages.

Steroids administered to the mother pass through the placenta and stimulate pulmonary maturation with surfactant produced by type II pneumocytes. They also stimulate the synthesis of proteins associated with surfactant and promote the structural maturation of the lung.

Surfactant therapy

A meta-analysis of several controlled and randomized clinical studies has shown the validity of surfactant therapy in reducing the severity of RDS and its complications. A certain number of reports show a reduction in the mortality of neonates <26 weeks of gestational age, which suggest that this was due to the routine clinical use of surfactant [24,25]. There is also, however, some direct evidence to support this claim as many clinical trials performed on individuals belonging to this category include too few neonates of this gestational age.

A combined study of antenatal steroids and surfactant therapy in pregnancies stratified by gestational age highlights the positive interaction of the two treatments at all gestational ages between 24 and 32 weeks. It can probably be assumed from this evidence that neonates with a low gestational age (survival threshold) benefit from these therapies. However, in certain cases, the effect of the therapy may not be as evident, due to intrinsic aspects of pulmonary immaturity.

Cesarean delivery

A survey of American gynecologists who were asked whether they would perform a cesarean delivery in an extremely preterm pregnancy due to fetal distress showed that 4% would perform this procedure at 23 weeks, 37% at 24 weeks, and 72% at 25 weeks. It is still debatable whether

Table 16.4 Recommendations on the use of antenatal corticosteroids

1. Prophylaxis with corticosteroids is recommended for all pregnant women between the 24th and 34th complete weeks of pregnancy at risk of preterm delivery, as the benefits (reduction in RDS [respiratory distress syndrome], ICH [intracranial hemorrhage], ROP [retinopathy of prematurity], NEC [necrotizing enterocolitis], and neonatal mortality) substantially outweigh the potential risks.
2. The therapy consists of two intramuscular injections, 12 mg each, of betamethasone, 24 hours apart.
3. The optimal effect is 24 hours from the initial administration and lasts for at least 7 days.
4. Reductions in fetal movements and heart rate may occur during the therapy, which however do not require therapeutic measures.
5. Therapy lasting less than 24 hours is effective even though to a lesser degree.
6. A concurrent tocolytic therapy can delay the delivery by at least 24–48 hours, which increases the effectiveness of the corticosteroid therapy.
7. Corticosteroid effectiveness is reduced after 7 days; the cycle should be repeated, though it is not mandatory.
8. In case of preterm prelabor rupture of the amniotic membranes (PPROM), corticosteroids are recommended for periods below 30–32 weeks and in the absence of clinical signs of chorioamnionitis. The prevalence of respiratory distress syndrome (RDS) and intraventricular hemorrhage (IVH) is significantly reduced, while that of maternal and neonatal infections may increase, though not substantially (antibiotic coverage should therefore not be omitted).
9. In case of hypertension; hemolysis, elevated liver enzymes, low platelet count (HELLP) syndrome; intrauterine growth restriction (IUGR); diabetes; and twins, corticosteroid therapy is advisable as no side effects are reported for the mother or infant.

this intervention can be justified in the presence of fetal distress.

Some argue that an extremely premature neonate is highly vulnerable to the normal labor process and that a cesarean delivery may be the best option [26]. Others suggest that the factors that originate unfavorable outcomes are already present at the start of labor, or at least when the decision to operate is taken.

Presumably, since the decision to perform a cesarean delivery is most likely made for those pregnancies with a better chance of survival or of a favorable outcome, epidemiological studies, similarly, show a positive association between cesarean deliveries and an increased survival rate. However, studies that used multivariate statistical analyses and logistic regressions do not show any benefit when certain variables such as, for example, gestational age, preeclampsia, or elective cesarean delivery are used.

Kitchen, in observing outcomes at 2 years, in 577 neonates with a weight at birth between 500 and 999 g, used a statistical analysis with logistic regression to show that the method of delivery did not affect the incidence of cerebral palsy. Similarly, other variables such as the Apgar score, rectal temperature, first arterial pH value, and assisted ventilation duration were not associated with the type of delivery [27].

In a review of all prospective studies on this subject, Grant used a meta-analysis to compare results of the elective cesarean delivery policy with those of the selective cesarean delivery. The small sample size was not enough to show significant data on the neonatal benefits of a cesarean delivery, but demonstrated that neonatal complications are more associated with breech presentation and that cesarean delivery is the main cause of maternal morbidity [28,29].

In conclusion, the effect of the method of delivery in preterm pregnancies on neonatal outcomes remains unclear. In addition, the current recommendations from the National Collaborating Centre for Women's and Children's Health on cesarean deliveries, published in April 2004 by the Royal College of Obstetrics and Gynaecologists (RCOG), show that this surgical procedure should not be routinely provided outside of research.

Regionalization of perinatal care

The improvement in the reduction of neonatal mortality is, in part, tied to the improvement in perinatal assistance under regional planning. The regionalization of perinatal care consists of implementing a coordinated and cooperating assistance system that defines the type of care that each hospital can provide to the mother and neonate.

This type of planning must take into account users, existing structures, and assistance capabilities. Therefore, to calculate the number of necessary beds it is essential to have data on neonatal birth rates and morbidity, as well as data on transfers, so as to define the neonatal transfer rates (transferred neonates/live neonates × 100).

The main goal of regionalization is to provide to the mother and neonate proper care in the nearest available structure, by planning a system that meets the patients' needs and improves the efficiency of intensive care units. Pregnancies at risk can thus be concentrated, and intensive care staff and equipment can be optimized. The structures throughout the territory are differentiated based on the level of care that they are able to provide [30,31].

NEONATAL OUTCOMES

The greatest increase in survival percentages, especially for ELBW preterm neonates, has occurred in the last 10 years. The survival limit is largely determined by pulmonary maturity, while subsequent morbidity in survivors is determined by the complications of the treatments for the underlying pulmonary disease. This increased success has coincided with the progress in perinatal medicine, neonatal surgery, anesthesia, and, in particular, intensive neonatal care.

Numerous strategies have been adopted to improve respiratory function (prenatal corticosteroids, surfactant, postnatal corticosteroids for chronic respiratory disease and more sophisticated means of assisted ventilation) and prevent serious illnesses such as intraventricular hemorrhage, patent ductus arteriosus, retinopathy of prematurity, necrotizing enterocolitis (NEC). Nutrition has also been improved through a more widespread use of human milk banks [32,33].

However, after a reduction in neonatal mortality and an increased survival rate (in particular of ELBW <1000 g), there has been an overall increase of neonatal outcomes.

Chronic respiratory disease: Bronchopulmonary dysplasia

The increased use of prenatal steroids and improved monitoring of pregnancy and fetal conditions has brought about a reduction in the incidence and severity of RDS in preterm babies. This is accompanied by the early and liberal use of exogenous surfactant, along with less traumatic and/or invasive mechanical ventilation (synchronized ventilation with trigger, pressure support ventilation, proportional assist ventilation, high-frequency oscillatory ventilation, continuous positive airway pressure with nasal cannulas, etc.), which have greatly improved the prognosis of RDS in affected neonates and simultaneously reduced the incidence of serious pulmonary illnesses such as bronchopulmonary dysplasia (Table 16.5) [34].

It is now widely accepted that administering exogenous surfactant to neonates with RDS decreases the severity of acute respiratory disease and allows for a less aggressive ventilation, thereby minimizing pressure and volumetric

Table 16.5 Main assisted ventilation techniques

Trigger ventilation (TV)
Pressure support ventilation (PSV)
Proportional assisted ventilation (PAV)
High-frequency oscillatory ventilation
Nasal continuous positive airway pressure (nCPAP)

trauma of the respiratory system and damage deriving from high inhaled O_2 concentrations (FIO_2).

The positive effect of surfactant may also be tied to the antimicrobial properties of SP-A and SP-D proteins that stimulate the phagocytosis of the neutrophils and of the pulmonary macrophages [35,36].

Despite this, there has been an increase in the less severe forms of chronic lung damage due to the increased overall survival rate. Many authors have a general name for this type of damage, chronic lung disease (CLD), and save the bronchopulmonary disease (BPD) name for cases of severe pulmonary damage [37].

Definition

BPD was described for the first time more than 35 years ago by Northway in neonates treated for hyaline membrane disease with ventilation therapy at high inspiratory pressure and high FIO_2 [38]. The original description contained four successive radiological and anatomopathological stages of the disease. However, not all radiological stages of BPD described by Northway can be observed among neonates with respiratory conditions similar to BPD, and so many other definitions, including several clinical conditions have been introduced over time. In most of these definitions the main diagnostic criterion was the need for supplemental oxygen, with or without ventilation support, and the presence of certain radiological conditions of the thorax.

Bancalari in 1979 [39] listed the following criteria to define BPD:

1. Need for intermittent positive pressure ventilation during the first week of life and for at least 3 days
2. Clinical signs of chronic respiratory disease (tachypnea, intercostal and diaphragmatic retractions, auscultatory sounds lasting for more than 28 days)
3. Need for supplemental O_2 for more than 28 days to maintain arterial PaO_2 at 50 mm Hg
4. Radiography of thorax with striations of persistent density in both lungs, alternated with areas of normal or increased transparency

The chronological duration of 28–30 days was the most widely used temporal diagnostic criterion.

Very premature neonates may, however, require supplemental oxygen at the postnatal age of 1 month due to the degree of immaturity and not necessarily because of a chronic pulmonary problem. Therefore, the need for supplemental O_2 at 36 weeks of corrected gestational age was suggested as a predictive criterion for abnormal pulmonary outcome. This became the most widely used definition in the literature, even though the predictive value of the BPD definition, based solely on duration of O_2 therapy, has been revised so that greater attention is paid to the radiological conditions in predicting future respiratory outcomes.

A U.S. workshop defined BPD using different criteria for neonates below or above 32 weeks of gestational age. It also has three categories of severity for the disease [40]. Radiological conditions are not present in this new definition, and the workshop recommends the use of the old "BPD" term for this type of respiratory illness in preterm neonates, while reserving the use of chronic lung disease (CLD) for a series of chronic respiratory illnesses related to subsequent ages.

Clinical presentation of the "new" BPD

With rare exceptions, BPD is preceded by the early use in the first days of life of mechanical ventilation, as a result of respiratory insufficiency due to hyaline membrane disease and/or pneumonia or insufficient breathing strength.

The "new BPD," as defined, is the most common and mildest clinical form, usually found in those small preterm neonates with weight <1000 g who survive prolonged mechanical ventilation. Generally, it has replaced the traditional BPD described by Northway, which has now become much less frequently used. The majority of these neonates have an initial RDS that responds favorably to the administration of surfactant. In addition, ventilation and oxygen support for these neonates is significantly reduced after a few days.

Despite this, after an initial period in which oxygen support is minimal or completely absent, pulmonary function deteriorates, and there are signs of progressive respiratory insufficiency (chest retractions, need for supplemental oxygen and mechanical ventilation), frequently caused by bacterial infections or by the ductus arteriosus that did not close [41].

Radiological manifestations usually do not appear (but may appear late) and include hyperinflation and nonhomogeneous lung tissue, with small or large dense areas that, in the more severe forms of BPD, tend to spread to the periphery. Radiological changes are less evident in the milder forms and primarily show a widespread opacification of the lung fields. When pulmonary damage is triggered, such neonates may need mechanical ventilation and an increased concentration of oxygen for a prolonged period of time (weeks or months).

Clinical progress of those who survive with BPD is slow but characterized by steady improvements in pulmonary functionality and radiological conditions, with a gradual weaning from oxygen and ventilation. Some neonates with the more severe forms of BPD may advance toward irreversible respiratory insufficiency and death, as a result of severe damage to the lungs and of pulmonary hypertension that evolves into cor pulmonale (Figure 16.7a and b).

Incidence of BPD

The incidence of BPD described in the literature varies widely, in part due to differences of susceptibility to the disease among the population. It is also a result of different therapeutic practices among institutions and of different criteria used to define BPD.

The incidence of BPD, defined as oxygen dependency at 36 weeks of postconceptional age, in neonates with a weight at birth between 500 and 1500 g varies between

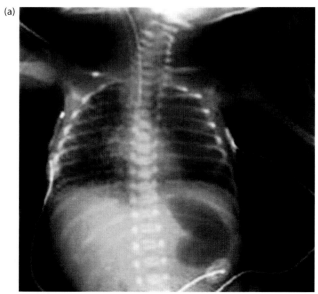

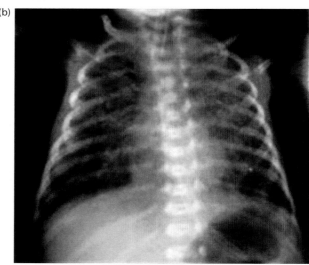

Figure 16.7 (a) BPD—Initial BPD in ELBW <26 weeks. (b) BPD—Severe BPD: anomalous dense areas and emphysema areas.

3% and 43% in various National Institute of Child Health and Human Development (NICHD) Neonatal Research Network centers [42].

Bancalari, in describing the data from his center, states that the incidence of BPD (defined as O_2 dependency of at least 28 days in the course of hospitalization) is inversely related to the gestational age and/or the weight at birth. These values vary from 67% in neonates between 500 and 750 g to less than 1% in neonates with a weight between 1251 and 1500 g [41].

Other incidence-related factors are tied to differences in the base populations used to calculate the incidence (e.g., a denominator that considers all preterm neonates or only survivors within a certain weight or category, etc.). They may also be tied to changes of the population at risk due to the introduction of prenatal steroids and surfactant.

Risk factors

Many single or combined factors have been involved in the pathogenesis of BPD. Because BPD is present almost exclusively in preterm neonates <1500 g who have undergone mechanical ventilation or oxygen therapy, prematurity, mechanical trauma, and O_2 toxicity have been considered crucial factors in the pathogenesis of the disease.

Other factors that appear to have an important role, include inflammation (by itself or associated with infection), pulmonary edema due to patent ductus arteriosus or to an excess of administered fluids, nutritional deficiencies, a predisposition to reactivity on the part of the respiratory system, and early adrenal insufficiency.

A study by Watterberg shows that the neonates with a lower level of plasma cortisol in the first week of life have an increased incidence of pulmonary inflammation and BPD. Early treatment instead with low doses of hydrocortisone increases the chances for survival without BPD [43].

There is a now a body of evidence that supports the role of infection and inflammation in the pathogenesis of BPD. This seems to be the case, especially for extremely small neonates without severe underlying pulmonary disorders who develop BPD after prolonged minimal ventilation support, used to support normal respiratory functions.

It has been demonstrated that a complex inflammatory reaction occurs in the interstitial space of immature lungs, followed by an accumulation of different cellular types (polymorphonuclear, macrophages, and chemical mediators (leukotrienes, interleukin 6 and 8, PAF, TNFα) [44,45]. The final result of this complex inflammatory process is an alteration of alveolar–capillary permeability, both during the acute phase of RDS and in its evolution to BPD, between the 10th and 14th days of life.

The stretching of lung tissue, secondary to an excessive volume (volutrauma) in the lungs of neonates ventilated with high tidal volumes, in particular in the absence of positive end-expiratory pressure, has been considered one of the factors that trigger these complex local inflammatory processes.

Another pathogenetic element of lung damage is the oxygen-free radicals produced when high fractions of oxygen are inhaled and/or when the preterm neonate does not have sufficient antioxidants (Figure 16.8) [46].

A greater role has been attributed to maternal infection, and specifically to chorioamnionitis, which apparently is associated with an increased risk of BPD. This correlation has been proven by a series of clinical and experimental observations that show a high presence of inflammatory cytokines in the fetal umbilical cord blood and in the amniotic fluid of mothers whose neonates subsequently develop a form of BPD [45].

Prognosis

The prognosis of these patients is conditioned by the degree of lung impairment. Although clinical conditions improve over time, most patients for several years continue to have increased airway resistance and bronchial

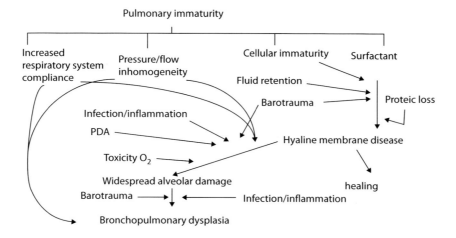

Figure 16.8 Pathogenesis of BPD.

hyperresponsiveness, reduced pulmonary compliance, as well as reduced ventilation/perfusion ratio (V/Q) and, from a radiological point of view, areas of atelectasis and/or emphysema. Rarely, chronic cor pulmonale may occur following chronic hypoxemia or pulmonary hypertension.

Prospective follow-up studies of all VLBW neonates show that the bronchial spasm rate is double in survivors with BPD. Lung function tests may still yield abnormal results with reduced tolerance for physical exercise up to the school age [47].

Pulmonary infections are common but tend to decrease over time and to disappear completely at 3 to 4 years of age.

Growth is generally insufficient due to a lack of nutrition and to the greater energy required for the increased respiratory functions. In the first 2 years of life, during which the respiratory situation of most infants with BPD may still be at risk, the length, weight, and cranial circumference values are significantly below average. For school-age children there are, however, no significant differences in somatic growth.

Neurological development can also be altered and is positively correlated with length of hospital stay and duration of oxygen dependency. Cognitive, motor, sensory, and language tests all show performance levels at 12 to 18 months that are significantly lower than in neonates with only RDS. At 3 years of age 29% of neonates with bronchopulmonary dysplasia (Northway stage 4) have an IQ between 80 and 90, while 40% have greater disabilities in the following areas: cerebral palsy, mental retardation, deafness, and blindness.

Mortality before discharge is generally caused by intercurrent infections, cor pulmonale, and respiratory insufficiency. The percentage of mortality in stage 4 of BPD, according to the Northway classification, is about 40%, with neonates dying approximately in the third month.

The survival percentage is correlated to hospitalization duration, with approximately 47% of neonates surviving when the hospital stay is less than 3 months. This percentage drops to 17% in those neonates who need hospitalization stays longer than 5 months.

Other predictive indicators include male gender and duration of ventilation support and supplemental oxygen therapy [48,49].

Central nervous system

The preterm neonate is at high risk of many insults to the central nervous system (CNS), usually represented by germinal matrix and intraventricular hemorrhage (GMH-IVH), intraparenchymal lesions (IPLs), posthemorrhagic hydrocephalus (PHVD), and cystic periventricular leukomalacia (PVL).

Germinal matrix and intraventricular hemorrhage

Intraventricular hemorrhage, or hemorrhage confined to the germinal matrix that surrounds the cerebral ventricles of the preterm neonate (GMH-IVH), is present in 35% to 50% of neonates with gestational age <32 weeks or with weight <1500 g at birth [50].

Since the 1990s there has been an overall decline in the incidence of IVH and IPL to around 20% of VLBW neonates (Table 16.6). The incidence and severity of these events is, however, inversely related to the gestational age, in part due to the extreme fragility of the capillary

Table 16.6 GMH-IVH classification

Grade	Hemorrhage extension
I	Germinal matrix hemorrhage with little or no intraventricular hemorrhage (<10% of the ventricular area in a parasagittal scan)
II	Intraventricular hemorrhage (10%–50% of the ventricular area in a parasagittal scan)
III	Intraventricular hemorrhage (>50% of the ventricular area in a parasagittal section); ventricles are usually relaxed
Other Notes	Periventricular echodensities (seat and extension)

Source: Reprinted from *Neurology of the Newborn*, 3rd ed. Volpe JJ, Saunders, Copyright 1995, with permission from Elsevier.

vascular bed of the germinal matrix that increases as age decreases [51].

Although GMH-IVH may occasionally occur in the uterus, most preterm neonates develop this complication after birth. Ultrasounds are able to accurately "time" these complications, which occur almost exclusively within 72 hours after birth (half within 24 hours). Only 10% of GMH-IVH appears after the first week.

The subependymal germinal matrix is a highly vascularized structure that contains glioblasts and neuroblasts, which take part in continuous mitotic activity and which subsequently migrate toward the cerebral cortex. This structure is prominent between 24 and 32 weeks of gestation but then regresses completely toward the end of the pregnancy.

The degree of prematurity and the presence of respiratory distress syndrome are reported as the main risk factors for the onset of GMH-IVH. This is due to changes in the cerebral blood flow and in the weak self-regulation mechanisms caused by insults such as hypoxia and acidosis, which occur more frequently in the course of a respiratory disease [52]. The loss of a self-regulating mechanism makes cerebral circulation dependent on arterial pressure, which therefore exposes the brain of the preterm neonate, which cannot protect itself from pressure changes, to a series of potential dangers. These arterial pressure changes have been noticed during the course of pneumothorax, endotracheal suctioning and manipulations, CO_2 retention, hypoxia, anemia, hypoglycemia, and mechanical ventilation.

Over time the cerebral ventricles in around 30% of preterm infants with GMH-IVH will dilate. The greater the degree of intraventricular hemorrhage (second–third degree), the higher is the risk of posthemorrhagic ventricular dilatation (PHVD).

This condition is subsequent to a process of adhesive arachnoiditis of the skull base and vault in which the arachnoid villi, damaged by phlogosis from blood in the subarachnoid space, stop reabsorbing the cerebrospinal fluid causing a type of communicating hydrocephalus.

A less common occurrence that follows intraventricular bleeding is the blockage of the aqueduct of Sylvius, which leads to the forming of a noncommunicating hydrocephalus [53].

PHVD develops in about half of those affected with third-degree GMH-IVH and poses a high risk of unfavorable neurobehavioral outcome (around 50%), which increases (75%) if a neurosurgical ventriculoperitoneal shunt procedure is used to control the progressive ventricular dilation [53].

Periventricular leukomalacia

Damage to the white matter of the semi-oval centers is the main cause of spastic diplegia, which is the most common form of unfavorable neurologic sequela of prematurity.

The difference in periventricular leukomalacia (PVL) incidence described in the literature is caused by the different classification systems used. Most studies, however, report a value between 3% and 10% for bilateral cystic PVL, which is the most severe form of damage to the periventricular white matter [54]. The timing of the appearance of this particular type of lesion is much more variable than GMH-IVH.

Occasionally, the reported damage is of prenatal origin, such as in the case of a twin dying, chorioamnionitis, prolonged premature rupture of membranes, or in the case of antepartum hemorrhages. In these situations periventricular cysts, visible via ultrasound a few days after birth, indicate that the pathogenetic causal event started during intrauterine life. The normal amount of time between the ultrasound showing a periventricular echodensity and the formation of cysts is about 2–3 weeks.

Pathogenesis of PVL is multifactorial and is, in any case, understood even less than events tied to hemorrhages. Currently, a lot of attention is paid to the hypoxic-ischemic and/or toxic damage to the intense metabolic activity of oligodendrocytes. These cells appear to be particularly vulnerable to the toxic damage of glutamate and cytokines (TNF) which can be released in response to bacterial endotoxins or vascular events of ischemic nature [55].

Many studies have long since identified arterial hypotension as a risk factor that is independent of PVL development. The deprivation of cerebral blood, that occurs during a large patent ductus arteriosus, modifies the diastolic phase of the cerebral blood flow (reverse flow), thus making several areas of the cerebral white matter that border different supply systems particularly susceptible to ischemic damage. This particular Doppler flowmetry pattern has been associated numerous times with the onset of PVL. The marked reduction of CO_2 in arterial blood (hypocapnia) also reduces cerebral blood flow and represents a risk factor associated with PVL.

There is no doubt that among all lesions diagnosed with ultrasound, cystic periventricular leukomalacia is the one that is closest to 100% in terms of predicting neonatal outcomes [56]. In numerous follow-up studies of VLBW neonates, any cases associated with the presence of cerebral palsy are almost always uniquely identified with an ultrasound diagnosis that shows a form of bilateral cystic periventricular leukomalacia. Single cysts and/or cysts confined to the frontal region seem to have a more favorable long-term neurological outcome [57].

The increased survival rate is a source of pride for the medical community, although long-term follow-up studies for this category of patients have brought to light many unresolved problems. Furthermore, it is well documented that VLBW neonates' neurological morbidity is a major part of the overall morbidity.

A meta-analysis done by Escobar in 1991 estimated the average incidence of neurological disabilities, after discharge, at approximately 25% for all VLBW neonates. The incidence of serious sensorimotor deficits, such as visual or hearing impairment and cerebral palsy, seems to be even higher in ELBW neonates [58].

Wood reports a 49% incidence of neurological disabilities in neonates <25 weeks of gestation. There also appears to be evidence that shows that even children apparently without significant neurological dysfunctions have "hidden" areas of impairment [59].

Multiple observational studies, with follow-ups that continue up to the school age, show lower cognitive test scores and an increased number of behavioral problems. A large collaborative study in the United States involved 1151 neonates with a weight between 401 and 1000 g that came from 12 National Institute of Child Health and Human Development (NICHD) Neonatal Research Network centers [60]. The study examined the neurosensorial, functional, and cognitive outcomes at 18 and 22 months of corrected age; in it, 25% of children presented an abnormal neurological examination, 37% had a mental development index (MDI) (Bayley Scales of Infant Development-II) <70, 29% had a psychomotor development index <70, 9% had visual impairment, and 11% had hearing impairment.

Neurological, cognitive, neurosensorial, and functional morbidities increased as the weight at birth decreased. Indeed 25% of infants between 901 and 1000 g had neurological anomalies, while this percentage rose to 43% for neonates between 401 and 500 g. Cerebral palsy in particular was diagnosed for 17% of neonates, with a range of values from 15% for 801–1000 g to 29% for 401–500 g.

The incidence of significant visual (3% blindness) and hearing impairments (3%) requiring assistance is similar to that of other studies.

Everyday functional abilities such as walking and using upper limbs for feeding or grabbing objects are achieved in 70%–80% of ELBW infants. However, only 57% of the group of patients <500 g is able to walk efficiently, 64% is capable of grasping, and 67% can eat on their own.

Significant factors associated with increased morbidity during neurological development are chronic respiratory disease (BPD), grade 3 intraventricular hemorrhages (IVH III), and parenchymal hemorrhage stroke (IPL), periventricular leukomalacia, necrotizing enterocolitis (NEC), and the use of steroids in the treatment of BPD in males.

A study by Kilbridge compared preschool outcomes of infants with weight at birth <800 g to those of full-term infants. At the time of the evaluation the average cognitive test scores were, on average, 10 points lower. In addition, scholastic abilities, in particular motor skills and linguistic capacities, were not as well developed [61]. This study therefore suggests that even though the environment is the same, biological events in the perinatal period will produce the aforementioned long-lasting effects.

Nuclear magnetic resonance (NMR) and other techniques have enormously increased the ability to understand the structure and function of the neonatal brain in normal conditions and after an insult. Currently, it is known that preterm neonates apparently without neurological deficits after birth do nonetheless show a reduction in volume of the cerebral cortex and of white matter, correlated with a reduction in cognitive test scores and behavioral alterations [62].

Besides these structural anomalies, there is evidence that shows there are long-term anomalies in brain function. Petersen compared, in studies of functional magnetic resonance imaging (fMRI), the cerebral activity of preterm neonates with that of full-term neonates, in relation to phonological and semantic processing mechanisms. He showed that preterm neonates with reduced linguistic abilities have an altered semantic capability in the phonological comprehension of sounds. This can explain the low verbal IQ and the language difficulties commonly noticed in school-age children.

Preterm infants therefore present an increased rate of neuronal death and an altered cerebral development. The mechanism associated with these changes in the structure of the brain is of great interest, and many studies performed on humans and animals suggest that these changes occur for the following reasons:

1. Immature neurons are vulnerable to degenerative processes.
2. Harmful environmental stimuli and clinical conditions have a significant impact on the growth and survival of neurons.

The second half of human gestation is characterized by rapid brain development. During this phase the number of neurons reaches a maximum level at 28 weeks which gradually decreases by about 70% reaching a stable level at birth. This critical period is also characterized by a marked synaptogenesis and by the development of populations of specific central nervous system receptors. Among these growing populations glutamate receptors (NMDA, AMPA) play a key role in cellular proliferation and in the migration, synaptogenesis, and plasticity of synapses in the developing brain. This is achieved by modulating the input of calcium and the activation of secondary messengers that alter gene regulation. Therefore, significant changes in glutamate or in excitotoxic neurotransmitters, which increase calcium input, render immature neurons vulnerable to stressful stimuli, such as background noise or high luminosity that normally are harmless.

Normal apoptosis and cellular death processes, which involve different cerebral regions in relation to the development phase, can be affected by stressful clinical and physiological events. This may lead to an alteration in development and in cerebral function [63]. This vulnerability is not limited only to neurons, but also involves oligodendroglia cells that are extremely sensitive to damage from free radicals. This susceptibility to damage also depends on the level of maturity, in that the differentiated stage of the oligodendroglial cell can tolerate stress due to free radicals better than its predecessor. This difference explains the particular susceptibility to damage of the periventricular white matter. This damage occurs during specific gestational ages (28–30 weeks) during which pre-oligodendrocytes are particularly active (periventricular leukomalacia) [64].

Preterm neonates usually have long hospital stays needed to stabilize and therapeutically support the functions of various organs by means of mechanical ventilation, positioning of catheters, etc. The combination of organ immaturity and the need for aggressive interventions places these neonates at risk of developing hemodynamic instability, infections, malnutrition, etc., which contribute in altering the structural and functional development of the brain. BPD and treatment with corticosteroids are independent factors associated with an unfavorable neurological outcome. Studies on animals have confirmed that recurrent hypoxic episodes can damage the CNS. In addition, corticosteroids induce neuronal death by means of oxidative stress or glutamate being released into the CNS, such as, for example infections, and hyperbilirubinemia.

Similarly, repeated or prolonged painful stimuli can alter the long-term behavior as documented in animal models.

Luminous intensity and noise from neonatal intensive therapies are also considered harmful for the development of the nervous system, which underscores the susceptibility of the preterm infant to environmental stresses [65]. The logical consequence of the above is to ask whether clinical interventions can be used to minimize neurocognitive and behavioral outcomes of VLBW neonates. Similarly, as the etiology of these deficits is multidimensional, so are the possible available interventions. For example, it is well established that breastfeeding is associated with improved neurocognitive and scholastic outcomes and that the longer breastfeeding lasts, the greater is the improvement.

Other beneficial maneuvers are analgesia techniques performed before painful procedures, as shown by the use of infusions with low doses of morphine that reduce the incidence of grade 3 IVH. Similarly, kangaroo care (skin-to-skin contact between mother and neonate) has a positive effect on neonatal morbidity, though the long-term effects remain unclear [66]. The effectiveness of avoiding environmental stresses, such as background noise or light, on cerebral development has yet to be determined.

After being discharged from intensive therapies other environmental factors such as family education, socioeconomic status, and maternal attitude play an important modifying role in the development of these children, at least up to 3 years of age, as documented in the Infant Health and Development Program (IHDP) [67].

Retinopathy of prematurity (ROP)

Retinopathy of prematurity (ROP) is a vascular proliferative ocular disorder that, in its most severe form leads to eyesight deterioration and blindness. It represents a high financial cost for the community, as well as a high individual cost for the child, with repercussions on language, motor, and cognitive development [68].

The "Vision 2020" program of the World Health Organization has identified ROP as one of the major causes of blindness in mid- to high-income nations. In the United States, ROP is the second most common cause of infant blindness [69].

Although there is a high prevalence of infant blindness in countries such as sub-Saharan Africa, with an infant mortality rate above 60 per 1000 live births, ROP is seldom reported in these nations due to the lack of intensive care for preterm neonates and their low survival rate.

In industrialized countries with infant mortality rates below 10 per 1000 live births, ROP is the reported cause of infant blindness in 6%–20% of cases [69,70]. Variations in incidence may also occur within a nation due to different levels of neonatal care.

There have been two epidemics of ROP in developed countries in the last 60 years. The severe form of ROP (initially named retrolental fibroplasia) was first described during an epidemic that took place in the 1940s [71]. In 1951, Campbell noted that providing supplemental uncontrolled oxygen to neonates was the main cause of the epidemic form of the illness. It was recommended to extend the pregnancy period, if possible, to 33 complete weeks of gestation and to proscribe the use of prophylactic oxygen in the treatment of cyanosis [72].

Later studies in the same decade confirmed that high O_2 concentrations resulted in the obliteration of neonatal retinal vessels. This epidemic was later brought to an end with the controlled use of O_2. Only in the United States the percentage of blindness due to retrolental fibroplasia dropped from 50% in 1950 to 4% in 1965 [73].

During the latter part of the 1970s and in the 1980s, despite careful monitoring of O_2 use in neonates, which had started in the 1950s, several studies described a second epidemic of ROP of similar proportions [74]. It was concluded that the event was due to the increased survival rate of VLBW neonates in the 750–999 g range and not to new iatrogenic factors.

Survival curves for preterm neonates <27 weeks continued to improve in the 1990s. Several studies reported a higher number of severe forms of ROP, but some evidence instead shows a decline in the incidence, severity, and progression of the threshold forms of the illness in developed countries [75]. ROP, however, remains prevalent among VLBW neonates, with 12.5% of neonates between 23 and 26 weeks of gestation requiring treatment of the "threshold" illness [76].

The International ROP Classification describes the seat of the lesion in relation to the optic nerve, the amount of vascularization, and the progressive stages of the illness. Stage 1 is the least severe, while stages 4 and 5 are associated with, respectively, the partial and total detachment of the retina. The term "plus" disease indicates signs of active progression of ROP that can accompany any stage. The term "threshold" indicates 5 consecutive hours, or 8 cumulative hours, of the optic disc of stage 3 in zones I or II and in the presence of "plus" disease, which indicates an increased likelihood that the disease will lead to retinal detachment [77] (Table 16.7).

Predisposing factors

Although many causal factors have been investigated in the development of ROP, only low birth weight, low gestational age, and supplemental oxygen therapy have been consistently associated with the disease.

Table 16.7 Classification in stages of retinopathy of prematurity

Stage 1: Demarcation line: thin flat white line that visibly separates the anterior avascular retina (toward the retinal edges) from the posterior vascularized retina.
Stage 2: Linear demarcation ridge: flat line of stage 1 grows in height, width, and volume and is white pinkish.
Stage 3: Demarcation ridge with extraretinal vascular proliferation.
Stage 4: Subtotal retinal detachment: In stage 4A the disease does not affect the macula and has a relatively favorable vision prognosis; in stage 4B the disease affects the fovea and has a usually unfavorable vision prognosis.
Stage 5: Total retinal detachment: detached funnel-shaped retina.
"Plus"disease: The "+" is placed after the disease stage when there are dilations of the posterior veins, tortuosity of retinal arteries, vitreous opacities, or pupil rigidity. If the "plus" disease is observed in the back part of the retina, the patient must be strictly monitored due to the high risk of ROP progressing to stage V within a few days.

An American multicentric study done between 1986 and 1987 showed that 81.6% of neonates weighing under 1000 g develop a form of ROP, while only 46.9% of those who weigh between 1000 and 1250 g develop the same type of disease. The severe forms are reported mainly in neonates <26 weeks, and the severity increases as the gestational age decreases [78].

Since the correlation between supplemental oxygen and ROP has been proven, much research has been done to identify the pathogenetic role of O_2. ROP starts to become evident between 32 and 34 weeks of postconceptional age relative to gestational age at birth, and has two separate phases.

During the first acute phase, normal retinal vasculogenesis is altered due to the relative hyperoxia of the extrauterine environment. This results in vessel obliteration and insufficient vascularization of certain areas of the anterior retina. The resultant hyperoxia causes a second chronic phase characterized by a proliferation of vascular and glial cells and formation of arteriovenous shunts that occasionally lead to involution or permanent cicatricial changes and visual impairment [79,80].

There is controversy on whether the duration of supplemental O_2 causes an increase in the incidence or severity of the disease. Some evidence shows that providing supplemental oxygen to neonates with moderate ROP does not reduce the incidence of progression toward the "threshold" stage. It seems instead that wide fluctuations in oxygen saturation condition the development of ROP and its progression [81].

Both hypoxia and unstable levels of O_2 in the rat animal model cause ischemic retinopathy. The significance of the oxygen levels lies in the nature of the choroidal circulation, which is unique, as it is without a self-regulation mechanism needed to respond to altered O_2 tension.

In conditions of hyperoxia, there is no choroidal vessel constriction, even though the retinal veins are capable of it. Consequently, the excess oxygen moves from the choroidal to the retinal circulation resulting in the obliteration of the retinal veins [82]. According to an alternative theory, the retinal vascular alterations can be attributed to the damage caused by reactive O_2 species (free radicals) capable of overcoming the defensive mechanisms put in place by the antioxidant enzymes, such as superoxide dismutase (SOD) and/or protective agents such as α-tocopherol [83].

Experimental studies on animal models and cell cultures have underscored the key role played by the VEGF-A cytokine (vascular endothelial growth factor A) in the abnormal development of retinal vasculature. High levels of VGEF-A have been found in human vitreous humor with ROP and in the subretinal fluid of eyes in the acute phase of stage 4, but not in stage 5. However, the absence of the RNA messenger of VEGF-A in the fetal retina (up to 20 weeks) and the finding that the insulin-like growth factor (IGF-1) contributes to optimizing VEGF-A activity of normal retina vascularization, underscore how other factors, besides hypoxia, regulate the gene expression of VEGF-A [84].

On the other hand, ROP can develop in preterm neonates who have received minimal or no supplemental O_2, and the causes that lead to retinal detachment in each neonate are unknown.

The hypothesis brought forward in the 1990s, in which genetic factors are capable of contributing to the development of ROP, is corroborated by variations seen in various ethnic groups. For example, some evidence suggests that African Americans are less inclined to develop the disease compared to whites. In addition, Alaska natives develop the "threshold" stage of ROP earlier than nonnatives, which confirms how genetic factors, along with socioeconomic and dietary factors, can play a role [85].

The clinical ocular characteristics of acute ROP, such as retinal folds, vitreoretinal traction, and detachment, show many similarities with a rare familial disorder, the Norrie disease, and with familial exudative vitreoretinopathy (FEVR). Due to similar ocular manifestations the putative genes of these two diseases were obvious candidates for describing ROP development. However, studies that attempted to quantify the contribution of the genes to the development and progression of the disease have proven inconclusive [86].

Many other risk factors have been associated with the onset of ROP, but it is not clear if these are actual independent risk factors or simply indicators of the degree of neonatal impairment. These factors include bronchopulmonary dysplasia, number of blood transfusions, parenteral nutrition, hypocapnia/hypercapnia, hypotension, patent ductus arteriosus, necrotizing enterocolitis (NEC), intraventricular hemorrhage (IVH), insufficient weight recovery after birth, and *Candida* sepsis [87].

Prognosis

Prognosis for most neonates who develop acute ROP is excellent. A great majority of stage 1 and 2 of the disease regresses without cicatrices.

Neonates with stage 3 limited to zone 3 have a similarly positive prognosis. Neonates instead with stage 3 "threshold" disease, which remains untreated, have a 50% risk of progressing toward total retinal detachment or severe cicatricial retractions.

Upon reaching the "threshold" disease, immediate treatment halves the risk of developing this outcome. However, approximately 20% of eyes in this condition progress toward retinal detachment or severe cicatricial retractions, even with optimal treatment. The prognosis with or without treatment, however, is worse when the disease affects zone 1 [49].

COMMUNICATION AND THE ELBW NEONATE

The advancement of medical technology has drastically improved the chances for survival for preterm neonates. However, the result of these intensive treatments can, at times, be of only delaying death or the neonate surviving with significant neurological disabilities. The effort undertaken to provide for neonatal care frequently is multidisciplinary, costly, and, at times, continues for the entire life of the patient.

The emotional and financial fallout on the family from the birth of an extremely premature child is the reason why it is important to inform the future parents on the impact of therapeutic options on life expectancy and outcomes. A reasonably acceptable approach to this dilemma is the "personalized" prognostic strategy. In this context neonatal care is provided at the appropriate level based on the expected outcome at the moment in which the therapies are performed. With this strategy, the neonate is continuously reevaluated, and the prognosis is reformulated according to the best available information and in conjunction with the best medical opinion. In this approach, the clinicians and medical team that care for the patient must bear significant responsibility due to the need for continuous and accurate assessments of neonatal conditions.

The family must be informed on the current situation and prognosis and must be involved in all major decisions that can alter the final outcome.

A possible compromise between extreme ethical positions (each human life must be defended and "do no harm") could be, on the one hand, to weigh on a case-by-case basis the probable benefits that can be achieved with the medical treatment and, on the other, the pain inflicted to the patient during the therapy (following the proportionality of treatment principle).

In any case, the reason that leads us to not start a treatment or to interrupt a treatment that is underway should be to prevent the neonate from suffering pain that is disproportionate to the benefits, and not to prevent survival with a possible disability.

For this method to be successful, both a medical staff spokesperson and a nursing staff spokesperson should be assigned with the task of discussing the various options with the family. The medical spokesperson must understand the worries and wishes of the parents, which many times are based on a complex combination of values and cultural influences, religious convictions, and education.

The parents must be encouraged to take an active part in the decisions and their rights must be respected. In case of disagreement or conflict between the medical recommendations and the parents' will, an option might be to involve the hospital bioethics committee. The clinician has the responsibility to explore and possibly try to change the decision reached by the parents, should the decision be contrary to the best interests of the neonate. If the clinician involved in the neonatal care is uneasy with the decision reached by the parents, even though this decision is a standard medical practice, the clinician may ask to be replaced.

Communication relative to potential neonatal outcomes

Most parents are not familiar with the complexity of the therapies required for an extremely premature neonate in an intensive care unit or after hospital discharge.

Many times the information must be provided in small fragments and at frequent intervals to help the parents understand the single problems that arise. The parents need clear and consistent explanations on the various support procedures necessary in the first days of life, along with information on the possible complications of extreme prematurity and intensive care. It is also necessary to provide information on the survival percentages for the specific gestational age and on the long-term outcomes. When providing this information both the current literature and local percentages must be considered [88].

Survival at 22 weeks and <500 g occurs sporadically, though survival without complications is basically nonexistent. According to data from a document by the "California Perinatal Quality Care Collaborative" (CPQCC), which collected information from NICUs in California, the mortality rate at 22 weeks is 100%. This percentage decreases to 71% at 23 weeks, and drops to 40% at 24 weeks. Survival is expected for most neonates over 24 weeks, with a survival rate of 68% at 25 weeks and 88% at 26 weeks. These data are similar to that obtained by the Vermont Oxford Network [89].

The incidence of handicaps usually defined by the presence of cerebral palsy, low intelligence test scores, blindness, or deafness is high and close to 70% in survivors at 23 weeks. This value decreases to 40% at 24 weeks and does not change for neonates up to 26 weeks of gestation [90].

In light of the mortality and morbidity of these fragile patients, planning with the parents is complex and requires profound and meditated discussions, preferably both before the birth and immediately after the birth, when an evaluation of the gestational age, weight, and actual neonate conditions are more accurate.

Recommendations

1. Parents are responsible for deciding which medical interventions are to be performed on their children that are at the viability threshold, and should be treated with respect and compassion.
2. All information needed for making informed decisions must be provided to the parents, who decide on the treatment their child will receive. In explaining the options it

is important to not guide the parents toward solutions, even though they may frequently have this need and appreciate these recommendations. Ideally, a close support relationship should be established with the parents.

3. If possible the gynecologist, neonatologist, and parents should all meet before the birth to discuss the possible outcomes and the treatment options.
4. Ideally, the initial conversation should take place as soon as the condition has been identified. The discussion should center on the specific problems present (prenatal steroids, PPROM, presence of IUGR, presence of congenital anomalies, or other factors that have repercussions on mortality and morbidity).
5. The neonatologist must emphasize that expectations for the neonate might change after birth, when the info on the estimate of gestational age, the real conditions at birth, as well as the response to reanimation and stabilization maneuvers can be based on more accurate criteria.
6. After birth, the parents must be informed of the expected outcome in the delivery room or in the neonatal intensive care unit.
7. If the initial evaluation differs from the expected one (different maturity, dimensions, conditions, anomalies) it must be communicated to the parents so they can act accordingly.
8. In situations in which
    a. There is ambivalence in the parents' decision
    b. The doctor is uncertain about the gestational age
    c. There is not enough time before birth to carry out a discussion

    It is best to resuscitate and then stop support, if deemed appropriate, rather than not intervening initially but only afterward. Decisions should always be based on frequently evolving evaluations of the clinical conditions and prognosis. The decision to provide complete neonatal support at birth is not irrevocable. Parents should be assisted in their decision on whether to suspend or continue life support interventions on the basis of the same continuously changing evaluations of the clinical conditions, prognosis, and best interest of the neonate.
9. Compassionate care must be provided to those neonates for whom it has been decided to not provide medical interventions after birth, and with gestational age and/or clinical conditions that have not changed from those established with the parents before birth. This includes maintaining a neutral environmental temperature, cleanliness, complete care management, human contact, and the use of analgesics when appropriate. The parents should be encouraged to touch and hold the child, if they so desire, both before and after the death.
10. Mortality and statistics on long-term outcomes constantly change with changes in perinatal care. Furthermore, due to the considerable variation among the various centers, it is also recommended that each hospital develop and update, at least annually, its own numbers on survival and outcomes. In addition, the approach in regard to perinatal outcomes should be based on the best local information available.

Communication before birth

- Proper communication between the parents and all the professionals involved in the treatment is of primary importance.
- The clinicians with the most experience chosen from the gynecologist, neonatologist, and obstetrician, should agree on a provisional treatment plan based on clinical information and on updated outcome data. If possible, time should be allocated so that all the interested parties can consider the various options and assimilate the information.
- The treatment plan should be clearly recorded and accessible to the entire medical staff.
- The parents should be encouraged to seek support from other family members and religious counselors.
- Clinicians should know the current statistics on survival and neonatal morbidity for their own operating unit and the major regional centers.

Recommendations for treatment

1. Neonates with gestational age of 22 complete weeks (from 154 to 160 days)
    a. Anecdotal evidence on the survival of these neonates indicates that it is dependent on individual physiological variation. There are no real evaluations on outcomes.
    b. The decision on which treatment to implement is primarily based on maternal health, and no cesarean delivery should be performed without taking into account the woman's health. Maternal request for cesarean delivery should be dissuaded.
    c. The neonatologist must be present at birth, if previously agreed, with the objective of supporting the parents and the medical team and for confirming the maturity.
    d. Only compassionate palliative care must be provided to the neonate. Active treatments must be implemented only upon request of the fully informed parents or if the gestational age at birth is underestimated.
2. Neonates with gestational age between 23 and 24 complete weeks (from 160 to 174 days)
    a. In these cases a cesarean delivery in the presence of fetal distress is not appropriate and is rarely performed due to the high percentage of mortality and the risk of negative outcomes for future pregnancies tied to the type of uterine incision performed (chances for survival are below 50% and the percentage of developing moderate to severe handicaps in survivors is even greater).
    b. An exception is a neonate close to 25 weeks.
    c. The will of the fully informed parents can override the opinion of the gynecologist in terms of inappropriateness of the cesarean delivery. In this case a second consultation is required and maternal care is transferred to another colleague.
    d. The initial treatment of the neonate at this age should be in agreement with the will of the parents.

However, there must be a discussion with the parents on the importance of being flexible in their decisions on how to start and suspend reanimation based on the conditions of the neonate.

e. Monitoring the fetal heart rate during natural birth can help the neonatologist decide whether reanimation or provisional intensive care is appropriate.

f. External cardiac massage and the use of adrenaline do not show any improvement in survival rates and are rarely appropriate <25 weeks.

g. Factors that must be considered in reanimation are
Evidence of perinatal asphyxia
Widespread ecchymosis
Low or no heart rate at the moment of birth

h. The fetal response to active reanimation is critical in deciding whether to implement provisional intensive care. If the heart rate rises rapidly and the color improves, it is recommended to transfer the neonate to the NICU for evaluation. Further treatment will depend on the response of the neonate to the treatment.

3. Neonates with gestational age between 25 and 26 complete weeks (from 175 to 188 days)

    a. Decisions regarding the "method of delivery" should be based on the best interest of the mother and neonate.
    b. In considering the increased survival rate at these gestational ages (50%–80% in worldwide literature), priority must be given to neonatal survival.
    c. Although there is a lack of evidence regarding the best way to perform a delivery, vaginal birth must be preferred in the case of rapid cervix dilation, with the fetus in the cephalic presentation.
    d. In the case of fetal impairment during labor, or in its absence with closed cervix, the cesarean delivery is the widely accepted method.
    e. In the case of breech presentation or of multiple births, there is general agreement on implementing an elective cesarean delivery.
    f. If the parents initially refuse a cesarean delivery, make sure that they fully understand the implications and the possible outcomes of their decision.
    g. The neonatologist actively reanimates the neonate in compliance with the previous criteria based on conditions at birth.
    h. If possible, a decision (commonly agreed to by the parents and the neonatal care team) should be taken after birth on whether to maintain or suspend the treatments, and these decisions must be clearly recorded on file.

REFERENCES

1. Guyer B, Martin JA, MacDorman MF et al. Annual summary of vital statistics 1996. *Pediatrics* 1997;100:905–18.
2. National Institutes of Health, Consensus Development Conference Statement. The effect of corticosteroids for fetal maturation on perinatal outcomes. *NIH Consensus Statement* 1994;12:1–24.
3. National Health and Medical Research Council (NHMRC). *Clinical Practice Guidelines. Care around Preterm Birth*; 2000. Canberra, Australia: NHMRC.
4. Battaglia FC, Lubchenco LO. A practical classification of newborn infants by weight and gestational age. *J Pediatr* 1967;71:159–63.
5. Tucker J, McGuire W. Epidemiology of preterm birth. *BMJ* 2004;329:675–8.
6. Gourbin C, Masuy-Stroobant G. Registration of vital data: Are live births and still births comparable all over Europe? *Bull World Health Organ* 1995;73:449–60.
7. Hartford RB. Definitions, standards, data quality and comparability. *International Symposium on Perinatal and Infant Mortality*, Bethesda, MD. April 30–May 2, 1990.
8. Fortino A, Lispi L. La rilevazione dei neonati attraverso la SDO. www.ministerosalute, luglio 2001.
9. Corchia C, Guercia A, Orzalesi M. La mortalità perinatale in Italia. *Prospettive in Pediatria* 1979;9(33):5.
10. Nordio S, De Vonderweit U. La valutazione delle terapie intensive neonatali. *Minerva Pediatrica* 1984;36:1.
11. Orzalesi M. Certezze e dubbi in medicina neonatale. *Quaderni ACP* 2004;11(3):122–7.
12. Parry GJ, Gould CR, McCabe CJ et al. Annual league tables of mortality in neonatal intensive care units: A longitudinal study. *BMJ* 1998;316:1931–5.
13. Evans DJ, Levene MI. Evidence of selection bias in preterm survival studies: A systematic review. *Arch Dis Child Fetal Neonatal Ed* 2001;84:F79–84.
14. Yu VYH, Doyle LW. Survival and disability in babies less than 26 weeks gestation. *Semin Neonatol* 1996;1:257–65.
15. Corchia C, Gualtieri R. Epidemiologia dei VLBW in Italia: Analisi territoriale dei centri di assistenza e della mortalità. *Atti IX Congresso Nazionale SIN*, Napoli, Italy; 2003.
16. Blanco F, Suresh G, Howard D, Soll RF. Ensuring accurate knowledge of prematurity outcomes for prenatal counseling. *Pediatrics* 2005;115:478–87.
17. Costeloe K, Hennessy E, Gibson AT et al. The EPICure study: Outcomes to discharge from hospital for infants born at the threshold of viability. *Pediatrics* 2000;106:659–71.
18. O'Shea TM, Klinepeter KL, Goldstein DJ et al. Survival and developmental disability in infants with birth weights of 500 to 800 g born between 1979 and 1994. *Pediatrics* 1997;100:982–6.
19. Meadow W, Reimshisel T, Lantos J. Birth weight specific mortality for extremely low birth weight infants vanishes by four days of life: Epidemiology and ethics in the neonatal intensive care unit. *Pediatrics* 1996;97:636–43.
20. Meadow W, Lee G, Lin K, Lantos J. Changes in mortality for extremely low birth weight infants in the 1990s: Implications for treatment decisions and resource use. *Pediatrics* 2004;113:1223–9.

21. Murphy DJ, Fowlie PW, McGuire W. Obstetric issues in preterm birth. *BMJ* 2004;329:783–6.
22. Liggins GC, Howie RN. A controlled trial of antepartum glucocorticoid treatment for prevention of the respiratory distress syndrome in premature infants. *Pediatrics* 1972;50:515–25.
23. National Institutes of Health (NIH), Consensus Development Conference Statement. *Antenatal Corticosteroids Revisited: Repeat Courses.* 2000;17(2):1–10.
24. Philip AGS. Neonatal mortality rate: Is further improvement possible? *J Pediatr* 1995;126:427–33.
25. Cooke RWI. Factors affecting survival and development in extremely tiny babies. *Semin Neonatol* 1996;1:267–76.
26. Holtrop PC, Ertzbischoff LM, Roberts CL et al. Survival and short-term outcome in newborns of 23 to 25 weeks gestation. *Am J Obstet Gynecol* 1994;170:1266–70.
27. Kitchen W, Ford GW, Doyle LW et al. Cesarean delivery or vaginal delivery at 24 to 28 weeks' gestation: Comparison of survival and neonatal and two-year morbidity. *Obstet Gynecol* 1985;66:149–57.
28. Grant A, Glazener CM. Elective or selective caesarean delivery of the small baby? A systematic review of the controlled trials. *Br J Obstet Gynecol* 1996;203:1197–200.
29. National Collaborating Centre for Women's and Children's Health. *Cesarean Delivery Clinical Guidelines April 2004.* London, UK: Royal College of Obstetricians and Gynecologists Press.
30. Yu VYH, Dunn P. Development of regionalized perinatal care. *Semin Neonatol* 2004;9:89–97.
31. Zeitlin J, Papiernik E, Bréart G, EUROPET Group. Regionalization of perinatal care in Europe. *Semin Neonatol* 2004;9:99–110.
32. Crowley P, Chalmers I, Keirse MJ. The effects of corticosteroid administration before preterm delivery, an overview of the evidence from controlled trials. *Br J Obstet Gynecol* 1990;97:11–25.
33. Schwartz RM, Luby AM, Scanlon JW et al. Effects of surfactant on morbility, mortality and resource use in newborn infants weighing 500–1500 g. *N Engl J Med* 1994;330:1476–80.
34. Donne S, Sinha S. Can mechanical ventilation strategies reduce chronic lung disease? *Semin Neonatol* 2003;8:441–8.
35. Wright JR. Immunomodulatory functions of surfactant. *Physiol Rev* 1997;77:931–6.
36. Jobe HA. Hot topics in and new strategies for surfactant research. *Biol Neonate* 1998;74(suppl):13–18.
37. Rojas MA, Gonzalez A, Bancalari E et al. Changing trends in the epidemiology and pathogenesis of neonatal chronic lung disease. *J Pediatr* 1995;126:605–10.
38. Northway WH Jr, Rosan RC, Porter DY. Pulmonary disease following respiratory therapy of hyaline membrane disease: Bronchopulmonary dysplasia. *N Engl J Med* 1967;276:357–68.
39. Bancalari E, Abdenour GE, Feller R et al. Bronchopulmonary dysplasia: Clinical presentation. *J Pediatr* 1979;95:819–23.
40. Jobe HA, Bancalari E. Bronchopulmonary dysplasia. *Am J Respir Crit Care Med* 2001;163:1723–9.
41. Bancalari E, Claure N, Sosenko IR. Bronchopulmonary dysplasia: Changes in pathogenesis, epidemiology and definition. *Semin Neonatol* 2003;8:63–71.
42. Lemons JA, Bauer CR, Oh W et al. Very low birth weight outcomes of the National Institute of Child Health and Human Development Neonatal Research Network, Jan 95–Dec 96. *Pediatrics* 2001;107:1–8.
43. Watterberg KL, Scott SM. Evidence of early adrenal insufficiency in babies who develop bronchopulmonary dysplasia. *Pediatrics* 1995;95:120–5.
44. Speer CP. Inflammation and bronchopulmonary dysplasia. *Semin Neonatol* 2003;8:29–38.
45. Yoon BH, Romero R, Jun J et al. Amniotic fluid cytokines (IL6, TNFα, IL1β, IL8) and the risk for the development of bronchopulmonary dysplasia. *Am J Obstet Gynecol* 1997;177:825–30.
46. Saugstaad OD. Bronchopulmonary dysplasia-oxidative stress and antioxidant. *Semin Neonatol* 2003;8:39–49.
47. Palta M, Gabbert D, Weinstein MR. Multivariate assessment of traditional risk factors for CLD in very low birth weight neonates. *J Pediatr* 1991;119:285–92.
48. Parat S, Moriette G, Delaperche MF et al. Long term of pulmonary functional outcome of BPD and premature birth. *Pediatr Pulmonol* 1995;20:289–96.
49. Rennie JM, Roberton NRC. *Textbook of neonatology.* 3rd ed. London, UK: Churchill-Livingstone; 2000:620–2.
50. Dolfin T, Skidmore MB, Fong KW et al. Incidence, severity and timing of subependymal and intraventricular hemorrhages in preterm infants born in a perinatal unit as detected by serial real-time ultrasound. *Pediatrics* 1983;71:541–6.
51. Van de Bor M, Verloove-Vanhorick SP, Brand R et al. Incidence and prediction of periventricular-intraventricular hemorrhage in very preterm infants. *J Perinat Med* 1987;15:333–9.
52. Perlman JM, McMenamin JB, Volpe JJ. Fluctuating cerebral blood flow velocity in RDS: Relation to the development of IVH. *N J Med* 1983;309:204–9.
53. Volpe JJ. *Neurology of the newborn.* 3rd ed. Philadelphia, PA: Saunders; 1995.
54. de Vries LS, Eken P, Dubowitz LM. The spectrum of leukomalacia using cranial ultrasound. *Behav Brain Res* 1992;49:1–6.
55. Oka A, Belliveau MJ, Rosenberg PA et al. Vulnerability of oligodendroglia to glutamate: Pharmacology, mechanism and prevention. *J Neurosci* 1993;13:1441–53.
56. de Vries LS, Eken P, Groenendaal F et al. Correlation between the degree of periventricular leukomalacia diagnosed using cranial ultrasound and RMI later in infancy in children with cerebral palsy. *Neuropediatrics* 1993;24:263–8.

57. Rogers B, Msall M, Owens T et al. Cystic periventricular leukomalacia and type of cerebral palsy in preterm infants. *J Pediatr* 1994;125:S1–8.
58. Escobar GI, Littenberg B, Petitti DB. Outcome among surviving very low birthweight infants: A meta-analysis. *Arch Dis Child* 1991;66(2):204–11.
59. Wood NS, Marlow N, Costeloe K et al. Neurologic and developmental disability after extremely preterm birth. EPICure study group. *N Engl J Med* 2000;343:373–84.
60. Vohr BR, Wright LL, Dusick AM et al. Neurodevelopmental and functional outcomes of ELBW infants in the National Institute of Child Health and Human Development Neonatal Research Network, 1993–1994. *Pediatrics* 2000;105:1216–26.
61. Kilbride HW, Thorstad K, Daily DK. Preschool outcome of less than 801-g preterm infants compared with full-term siblings. *Pediatrics* 2004;113:742–7.
62. Peterson BS, Anderson AW, Ehrenkranz R et al. Regional brain volumes and their later neurodevelopmental correlates in term and preterm infants. *Pediatrics* 2003;11:939–48.
63. Bhutta AT, Anand KJ. Vulnerability of the developing brain. Neuronal mechanisms. *Clin Perinatol* 2002;29:357–72.
64. Volpe JJ. Neurobiology of periventricular leukomalacia in the premature infant. *Pediatr Res* 2001;50:553–62.
65. Murphy BP, Inder TE, Huppi PS et al. Impaired cerebral cortical gray matter growth after treatment with dexamethasone for neonatal chronic lung disease. *Pediatrics* 2001;107:217–21.
66. Perlman JM. Neurobehavioral deficits in premature graduates of intensive care: Potential medical and neonatal environmental risk factors. *Pediatrics* 2001;108:1339–48.
67. McCormick MC, Workman-Daniels K, Brooks-Gunn J. The behavioural and emotional well-being of school-age children with different birth weights. *Pediatrics* 1996;97:18–25.
68. Mets MB. Childhood blindness and visual loss: An assessment at two institutions including a "new cause." *Trans Am Ophthalmol Soc* 1999;97:653–96.
69. Steinkuller PG, Du L, Gilbert C et al. Childhood blindness. *J AAPOS* 1999;3:26–32.
70. Gilbert C, Rahi J, Eckstein M et al. Retinopathy of prematurity in middle-income countries. *Lancet* 1997;350:12–14.
71. Terry TL. Extreme prematurity and fibroplastic overgrowth of persistent vascular sheath behind each crystalline lens. *Am J Ophthalmol* 1942;25:203–4.
72. Campbell K. Intensive oxygen therapy as a possible cause of retrolental fibroplasia: A clinical approach. *Med J Aust* 1951;2:48–50.
73. Hatfield EM. Blindness in infants and young children. *Sight Sav Rev* 1972;42:69–89.
74. Gibson DL, Sheps SB, Schechter MT et al. Retinopathy of prematurity: A new epidemic? *Pediatrics* 1989;83:486–92.
75. Fledelius HC. Retinopathy of prematurity in a Danish county. Trends over a 12-year period 1982–93. *Acta Ophthalmol Scand* 1996;74:285–287.
76. Todd DA, Cassell C, Kennedy J et al. Retinopathy of prematurity in infants <32 weeks' gestation at birth in New South Wales in 1993 and 1994. *J Pediatr Child Health* 1999;35:355–7.
77. The International Committee for the Classification of the Late Stages of Retinopathy of Prematurity. An international classification of retinopathy of prematurity. II. The classification of retinal detachment. *Arch Ophthalmol* 1987;105:906–12.
78. Coats DK, Paysse EA, Steinkuller PG. Threshold retinopathy of prematurity in neonates less than 25 weeks' estimated gestational age. *J AAPOS* 2000;4:183–5.
79. Chan-Ling T, Tout S, Holländer H. Vascular changes and their mechanisms in the feline model of retinopathy of prematurity. *Invest Ophthalmol Vis Sci* 1992;33:2128–47.
80. McLeod DS, Brownstein R, Lutty GA. Vaso-obliteration in the canine model of oxygen induced retinopathy. *Invest Ophthalmol Vis Sci* 1996;37:300–11.
81. The STOP-ROP Multicenter Study Group. Supplemental therapeutic oxygen for prethreshold retinopathy of prematurity (STOP-ROP), a randomized controlled trial. I: Primary outcomes. *Pediatrics* 2000;105:295–310.
82. Chan-Ling T, Stone J. Retinopathy of prematurity: Origins in the architecture of the retina. *Prog Ret Res* 1993;12:155–78.
83. Katz ML, Robison WG Jr. Autoxidative damage to the retina: Potential role in retinopathy of prematurity. *Birth Defects Orig Artic Ser* 1988;24:237–48.
84. Smith LEH. Pathogenesis of retinopathy of prematurity. *Semin Neonatol* 2003;8:469–73.
85. Flynn JT. The premature retina: A model for in vivo study of molecular genetics? *Eye* 1992;6:161–5.
86. Shastry BS, Pendergast SD, Hartzer MK et al. Identification of missense mutations in the Norrie disease gene associated with advanced retinopathy of prematurity. *Arch Ophthalmol* 1997;115:651–5.
87. Seiberth V, Linderkamp O. Risk factors in retinopathy of prematurity. A multivariate statistical analysis. *Ophthalmologica* 2000;214:131–5.
88. American Academy of Pediatrics, Committee on Fetus and Newborn, American College of Obstetricians and Gynecologists, Committee on Obstetrics Practice. Perinatal care at the threshold of viability. *Pediatrics* 1995;96:974–6.
89. Horbar JD, Badger GJ, Lewit EM et al. (Vermont Oxford Network) Hospital and patient characteristics associated with variation in 28-day mortality rates for VLBW infants. *Pediatrics* 1997;99:149–56.
90. Hack M, Friedman H, Fanaroff AA. Outcomes of extremely low birth weight infants. *Pediatrics* 1996;98:931–7.

The neonate from cesarean delivery

OLA DIDRIK SAUGSTAD

INTRODUCTION

Cesarean delivery (CD) in many cases contributes to a higher survival and better outcome for the newborn. In acute conditions it may prevent or limit perinatal adverse effects and reduce the risk of hypoxic ischemic encephalopathy (HIE). It seems, therefore, that a ratio that is too low is associated with an increased neonatal risk. On the other hand, a CD ratio above a certain level probably does not further reduce neonatal morbidity and mortality.

The challenge is therefore to find the right balance, because it may increase short- and long-term child morbidity. In a study from 19 countries from North and West Europe, North America, Australia, New Zealand, and Japan, Ye et al. [1] analyzed the relation between the ratio and neonatal and infant mortality. Once the delivery rate reached 10%, a further increase in the delivery rate had no impact on maternal, neonatal, and infant mortality rates (Figure 17.1).

Elective CD is increasing due to many factors including increased maternal age, assisted reproductive technology, fetal monitoring, breech delivery, and maternal request. The rise is predominantly attributed to the rise in rates of first-time CD, which may lead to repeat CD in 90% of cases. Maternal autonomy versus neonatal outcomes is therefore an important issue. Further, CD on demand will lead to more transfers to the neonatal intensive care unit (NICU) and the spending of more resources, with a financial and societal impact that should be considered.

It has been increasingly understood that there is increased risk even when uncomplicated deliveries occur 2–3 weeks before term. Studies have shown that increased morbidity in the newborn, especially respiratory morbidity. Already in 1995, Morrison et al. [2] published data from UK of term infants born between 1985 and 1993 comparing elective CD with vaginal delivery, showing that risk of respiratory morbidity was increased 7 fold, OR 6.8 (95% CI 5.2–8.9); however, CD infants had a gestational age of 37–39 weeks versus 40 weeks in the vaginal group. Kolås et al. [3] found, for instance, an almost doubled risk of transfer to the NICU after planned cesarean versus planned vaginal delivery (9.8% versus 5.2%); however, CD children had more than one week lower gestational age (mean 38.5 vs 39.7 weeks) than those delivered after planned vaginal birth. The recent years it has therefore been understood that there is increased neonatal morbidity even when uncomplicated deliveries occur only 2–3 weeks before term. Studies have shown that CD per se increases morbidity in the newborn, especially respiratory morbidity. Elective CD therefore leads to more transfers to the NICU and spending of more resources, with a financial and societal impact which should be considered [4]. This information has to be balanced against the risk of unexplained stillbirths which increases from 0.2/1000 deliveries at week 37 to 0.5/1000 deliveries week 38 [5]. Therefore, both British and American societies in obstetrics recommend elective CD to be scheduled after 39 completed weeks of gestation [6].

In this chapter short-term and potential long-term effects of CD on the child are discussed. It is not only a question of respiratory morbidity, but also whether immunology may be changed permanently after CD.

Delivery at term: Effect of gestational age

A number of studies have demonstrated increased neonatal morbidities even when the delivery was induced at 37 and 38 weeks' gestation. Typically, respiratory morbidities are about twofold increased at 37 weeks compared to 39 weeks. A large multicenter U.S. study by Tita et al. [7] on the effect of repeat elective CD of births between 1999 and 2002 concluded that elective repeat CD at 37 and 38 weeks compared with 39 weeks' gestation is associated with respiratory and other adverse neonatal outcomes. The composite outcome was neonatal death and adverse events such as respiratory complications, treated hypoglycemia, newborn sepsis, and admission to the NICU. The odds ratio (OR) for this adverse outcome was 2.1 (95% CI 1.7–2.5) for 37 weeks versus 39 weeks. For 38 versus 39 weeks OR was 1.5 (95% CI 1.3–1.7). RDS + TTN decreased from 8.2% to 3.4% from 37 to 39 weeks, need of ventilation decreased from 9.1% to 3.6%.

Wilmink et al. [8] in the Netherlands performed a retrospective cohort study including all elective CD of singleton pregnancies ($N = 20{,}973$) between 37 and 40 weeks' gestation. Of these 56% were performed < 39 + 0 weeks of gestation, 31.7% were performed at 39 + 0–6 weeks, and 11.7% ≥ 40 + 0 weeks. The composite neonatal outcome of death and neonatal morbidity (advanced resuscitation, sepsis, respiratory complications, need of ventilatory support, hypoglycemia, neurologic morbidity, admission to the NICU 5 days or more, and a 5 min Apgar score < 4).

The numbers of this outcome were 20.6% at 37 weeks, 12.5% at 38 weeks, and 9.5% for neonates at 39 weeks' gestation (ORs 2.4 [95% CI 2.1–2.8] and 1.4 [95% CI 1.2–1.5], respectively). Combined respiratory outcome was 6.8% at 37 weeks' gestational age, 3.5%, 2.1%, 2.0%, and 1.8% in 38, 39, 40, and 42 weeks, respectively. In babies 42 weeks and more there were only 0.8% having this outcome (Figure 17.2). Figure 17.2 shows the varying importance of outcome measures such as transferral to the NICU, transient tachypnea of the newborn (TTN), respiratory distress (RDS), use of continuous positive pressure ventilation (CPAP), and hypoglycemia from gestational week

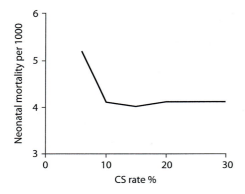

Figure 17.1 Cesarean delivery rate and neonatal mortality per 1000.

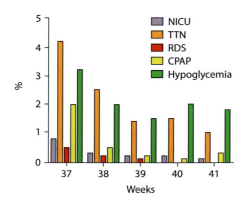

Figure 17.2 Outcome neonatal variables according to gestational age.

37 to week 41; weeks 37 and 38 have an increased morbidity compared to weeks 39, 40, and 41.

A similar study was carried out in Australia by Doan et al. [9] including 14,447 mother–baby pairs in the period of 1998–1999. CDs at 37 and 38 weeks were compared to 39–42 weeks' gestation. Serious neonatal morbidity (comprising all neonates admitted to the NICU and receiving assisted ventilation with mechanical ventilation and/or continuous positive airway pressure (CPAP) was more than doubled in the youngest group (1.16% versus 0.48%) with adjusted OR 2.74 (95% CI 1.79–4.21).

Nakashima et al. [10] from Japan compared elective CD at 37 weeks compared to 38 weeks between 2006 and 2012. At 37 compared to 38 weeks there was a significantly higher admission to NICU (8.2% versus 4.1%), number of respiratory complications (6.7% versus 2.4%), and number with hypoglycemia (7.7% versus 2.7%).

Hansen et al. [11] analyzed 34,458 deliveries in Denmark between 1998 and 2006, of which 2687 were elective vaginal deliveries between 37 and 41 weeks gestation. They showed that respiratory morbidities were higher in elective C-section versus planned vaginal delivery especially in gestational age weeks 37 and 38. Respiratory morbidity decreased from 10% at 37 weeks to 1.5% at 40 weeks. In a meta-analysis Hansen et al. [12] registering respiratory morbidity in term infants delivered at week 37, 38, and 39 it was found that elective CD increased the risk of various respiratory morbidities in the newborn, typically 2–3 times (however, data were not corrected for gestational age differences).

Planned vaginal versus elective CD

Effect of CD on respiratory morbidity

Even when gestational age for elective CD and planned vaginal delivery are matched a 2–3 fold increase of morbidities are found in the CD group when delivery occurs at week 37 and 38. When Morrison et al. [2] compared CD at 39 weeks with vaginal delivery at 40 weeks OR for respiratory morbidity was still high, 3.5 (95% CI 1.7–7.1).

In one study in newborn babies with gestational age >36 weeks, Kolas et al. [3] compared elective CD with uncomplicated vaginal delivery in a large cohort in Norway. When correcting for the difference in gestational age of 38.5 (SD 1.1) weeks in the elective CD group vs 39.7 (SD 1.3) weeks in the planned vaginal group, the difference in respiratory morbidity was only slightly reduced. However, for term infants ≥39 weeks there was no difference in the outcome between the groups. These results indicate that there were added morbidities when elective CD is carried out between 38 and 39 weeks, and that this increased morbidity exists at least up to 39 weeks of gestation.

Hansen et al. [11] compared respiratory morbidity in elective CD with planned vaginal delivery week by week between 37 and 41 weeks of gestation; there were higher rates in elective CD compared to planned vaginal delivery. At 37 weeks OR (95% CI) was 3.9 (95% CI 2.4–6.5) and 3.0 (95% CI 2.1–4.3) at 38 weeks. Even at 39 weeks these authors found an increased risk OR 1.9 (95% CI 1.2–3.0) for respiratory complications after elective CD. When analyzing low risk pregnancies alone more or less identical data were found. However, at 40 and 41 weeks there were no differences between elective CD and planned vaginal delivery. By excluding children with conditions that clearly add to child morbidity (such as meconium aspiration syndrome, sepsis, and pneumonia), the rates for OR (95% CI) for respiratory morbidity were 4.3 (2.6–7.2), 3.2 (2.2–4.6), 2.1 (1.3–3.4), and 1.2 (0.3–4.8) for weeks 37, 38, 39, and 40, respectively. This strongly indicates that increased child morbidity due to CD is present up to 40 weeks. Figure 17.3 shows the respiratory morbidity for elective CD and planned vaginal delivery in their study. Figure 17.4 shows the same pattern for serious respiratory morbidity.

An Italian study by Zanardo et al. [13] compared elective C-section and planned vaginal delivery between 37+0 and 41+6 weeks; in total 10,177 live births of women delivering between 1998–2000 were included. Gestational ages were 38.8 weeks in both groups. However, NICU admission was 1.3% versus 0.6% in the CD group and controlled vaginal delivery group, respectively. OR for neonatal respiratory

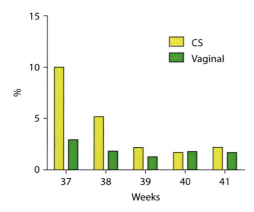

Figure 17.3 Rate of respiratory mortality between 37 and 41 weeks after cesarean delivery (CS) and vaginal birth (Vaginal).

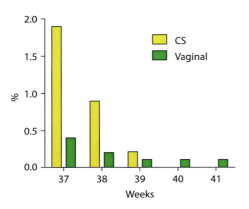

Figure 17.4 Serious respiratory morbidity between 37 and 41 weeks after cesarean delivery and vaginal delivery.

morbidity was 2.6 (95% CI 1.35–5.9). Respiratory problems (defined as respiratory distress and transitory tachypnea) were significantly higher in infants delivered by CD than in planned vaginal delivery at weeks 37 and 38; however, at weeks 39 and 40 there was no increased risk of respiratory adverse outcome between the groups.

A study by Stutchfield et al. [14] indicates that betamethasone may reduce respiratory morbidity after CD, even at term; from 37 to 39 weeks a risk reduction of 5.1% to 2.4% (RR 0.46 95% CI 0.23–0.93) after two doses of betamethasone was found. The European guidelines for respiratory distress syndrome therefore recommend betamethasone at elective CD <39 weeks [15] (Figure 17.5). The risk is of course an explosive use of antenatal betamethasone to fetuses near 40 weeks.

Effect on other morbidities

Neonatal infections are reduced by gestational age after planned CD compared to planned vaginal delivery. Wilmink et al. [8] found a reduction in neonatal sepsis from 0.8% at 37 weeks versus 0.4% 1 week later. Hypoglycemia

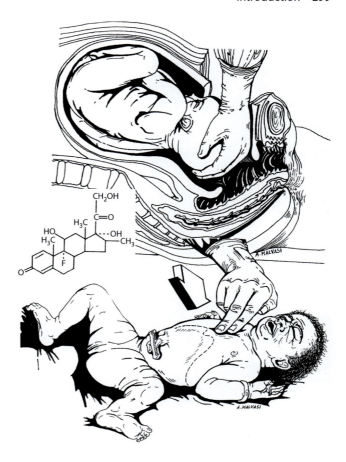

Figure 17.5 Cesarean delivery (top) and betamethasone (center left) use for neonatal respiratory morbidity reduction (bottom).

was not unexpectedly also higher in infants delivered at 37 weeks (3.2%) compared to 38 weeks (2.0%), 39 weeks (1.5%), and 40 weeks (2.0%); there was also more hyperbilirubinemia in the 37 week group (1.7%) versus 0.2% at 40 weeks (0.2%); there was no difference in convulsions [8]. Kolås et al. [3] found infections in 0.8% in the planned vaginal group vs 0.5% in the planned CD group; however, this difference was not significant (RR 0.63, 95% CI 0.23–1.60). CD can prevent a limited number of infections transmitted from the mother to the newborn: herpes simplex virus active in labor (Figure 17.6) and HIV (>1000 copies/mL) should be considered for possible CD (Figure 17.7). The NICE guidelines from the UK state that on grounds of HIV status CD should not be offered to a woman with a high active antiviral load of less than 400 copies/mL or a woman receiving any antiretroviral therapy with a viral load of less than 50 copies/mL [16].

Vaginal delivery is associated with a colonization of normal gut flora. Lack of this after CD may have long term consequences; data indicate that CD is associated with a 50% increased risk of severe asthma [17,18], as well as increased food allergy [19]. One study also indicated an increase in type 1 diabetes with childhood onset [20], OR 1.23 (95% CI 1.15–1.32).

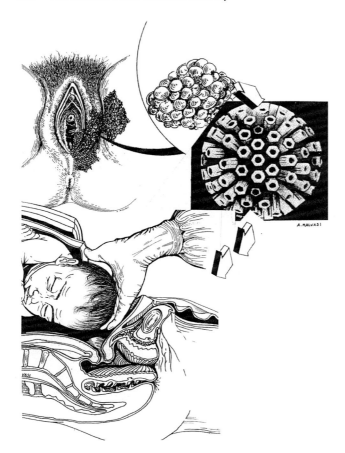

Figure 17.6 Genitalis infection of herpes simplex virus (HSV) (the microscopic HPS-2 three-dimensional model, top right) and elective cesarean delivery. (Modified from Malvasi A, Di Renzo GC. *Semeiotica Ostetrica*, Rome, Italy: CIC Edizioni Internazionali; 2012.)

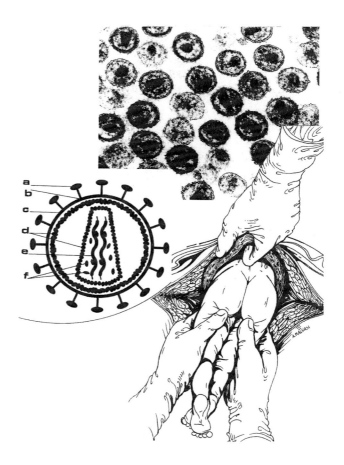

Figure 17.7 Cesarean delivery in patient with HIV infection (the electronic microscopic image of HIV and schematic virus ultrastructure, top and left). (Modified from Malvasi A, Di Renzo GC. *Semeiotica Ostetrica*, Rome, Italy: CIC Edizioni Internazionali; 2012.)

Fetal injury related to mode of delivery

Overall, fetal injury is greater in vaginal deliveries, particularly if instruments are used (Figures 17.8 and 17.9).

Such injuries are of course dependent on the size of the fetus. In the USA fetal macrosomia was reported in approximately 10% of all births from 1996–2002; birthweights above 4.5 kg were reported in approximately 1.5% of all births; the risk of shoulder dystocia increases with birthweight and is 5–10 times higher in children with birth weight >4.5 kg compared to 3.5–3.75 kg [21]. At 39 weeks shoulder dystocia was registered 0.047%–0.6% after vaginal and 0.0042 to 0.095% after CD at maternal request (Figure 17.10). It is estimated that 10000 CD are needed to prevent one permanent brachial plexus injury [21].

The fetal death rate increases toward term. Fretts et al. [22] reported a fetal death rate of 1.3 per 1000 live births at 37 weeks to 2.0 at 38 weeks, 2.9 at 39 weeks, 3.8 at 40 weeks, and 4.6 at 41 weeks. Both fetal death and hypoxic ischemic encephalopathy are significantly reduced by elective repeat CD compared to those who underwent trial of labor [23].

Although elective CD may be protective for the development of neonatal encephalopathy, to date it has not been proven to be protective on long-term neurological injuries.

Elective CD in week 39 versus expectant management showed that 1441 CDs were needed for preventing one death, and 2653 CDs to prevent one brachial/plexus injury.

Only a few congenital anomalies show a benefit for CD. These are hydrocephalus with macrocephaly (Figure 17.11), omphalocele with extracorporeal liver (Figure 17.12), anterior cystic hygroma (Figure 17.13), and hydrops fetalis. A vaginal delivery can be attempted in sacrococcygeal teratoma with a tumor less than 5 cm (Figure 17.14) [24].

CD IN PRETERM

A study from Germany by Bauer et al. [25] in extremely premature infants showed a more favorable outcome if they were born vaginally compared to CD; survival rates were 78% in infants born vaginally compared to 48% in the CD group. There were also fewer complications in the vaginal group compared to the CD group; intraventricular haemorrhage of grade III and IV was 18% versus 33% and periventricular leukomalacia 4% versus 14%; neonatal septicemia was also reduced (33% versus 52%).

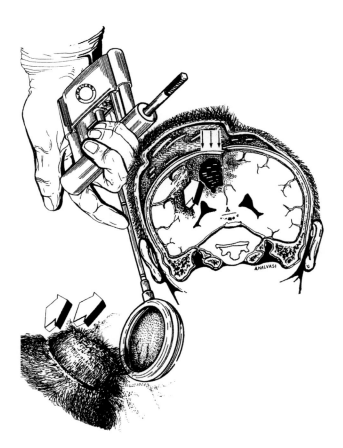

Figure 17.8 Vacuum extraction failure during vaginal delivery and neonatal brain hemorrhage.

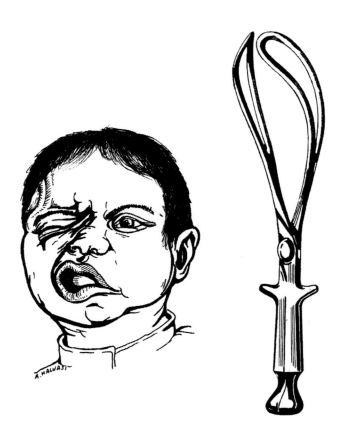

Figure 17.9 Left facial palsy in the baby, after forceps application in dystocic vaginal delivery and VIII cranial nerve injury.

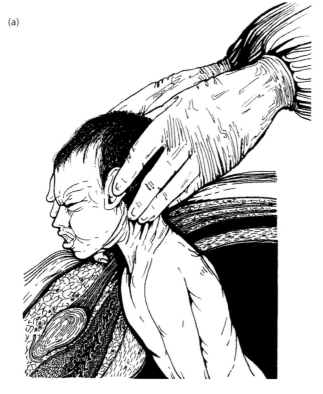

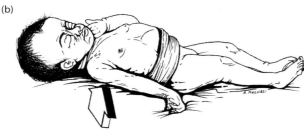

Figure 17.10 (a and b) Elective cesarean delivery for the shoulder dystocia and brachial plexus injury.

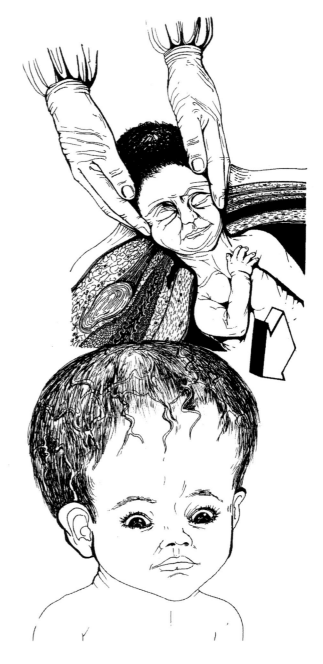

Figure 17.11 Elective cesarean delivery in case of fetus with hydrocephalus and macrocephaly.

However, vaginal breech delivery in low birth weight newborns in nulliparous women is associated with increased neonatal mortality [26]. In the birth weight group 500–100 gram OR(95% CI) for mortality was 11.7 (7.9–17.2) in vaginally versus SC delivery; for birth weights 1001–1500g and 1501–2000 g the risks were 17.0 (6.8–42.7) and 7.2 (2.4–21.4). Even for birth weights between 2001 and 2500 g OR for death was 6.6 (2.1–21.2) in vaginal versus CD children in breech position. Birth trauma was increased 4–5 fold in children with birth weight between 1500 to 2500 grams. A 3–4 fold increased risk of birth asphyxia in birth weights between 2000–2500 gram was also reported in breech if delivered vaginally compared to CD. Based on these data the vaginal route has an advantage compared to CD in immature infants; however, low birth weight infants in breech position should be delivered by CD (Figure 17.15).

CONCLUSIONS

CD is on the rise, and that is not always justified, especially not if the outcome for the child is taken into account. A CD rate of more than 10%–15% seems not to increase neonatal survival. Elective CD before 39 weeks carries unacceptable risks. In fact, elective CD in week 39 versus expectant management showed that 1441 CDs were needed for preventing one death, and 2653 CDs were needed to prevent one brachial/plexus injury.

For many societies, a high CD rate adds serious financial burdens that are not medically justified. Women

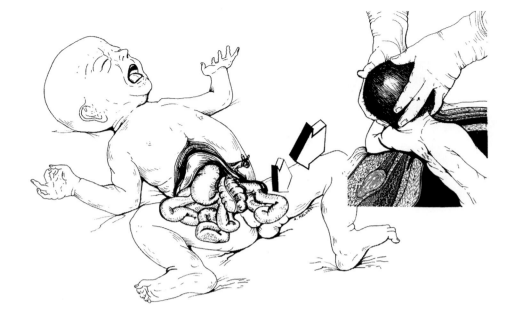

Figure 17.12 Omphalocele with extracorporeal liver (left arrow) require elective cesarean delivery (right).

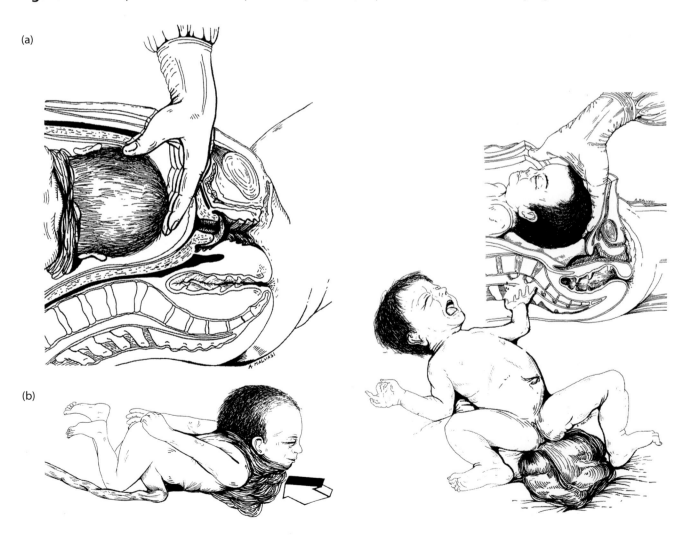

Figure 17.13 (a and b) Cesarean delivery in case of fetus with anterior cystic hygroma (arrow).

Figure 17.14 Cesarean delivery (top) in the fetus at gestational term with giant sacrococcygeal teratoma (bottom).

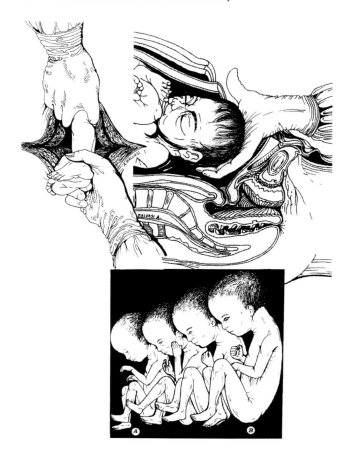

Figure 17.15 Cesarean delivery and preterm birth cephalic and breech presentation.

considering CD should be made aware of available data on potential risks and benefits for the fetus and the newborn. Due to the potential complications in the child, the ethics of accepting CD on demand, therefore, is debatable.

REFERENCES

1. Ye J, Betrán AP, Guerrero Vela M, Souza JP, Zhang J. Searching for the optimal rate of medically necessary cesarean delivery. *Birth* 2014;41(3):237–44.
2. Morrison JJ, Rennie JM, Milton PJ. Neonatal respiratory morbidity and mode of delivery at term: Influence of timing of elective caesarean section. *Br J Obstet Gynaecol* 1995;102(2):101–6.
3. Kolås T, Saugstad OD, Daltveit AK, Nilsen ST, Øian P. Planned cesarean versus planned vaginal delivery at term: Comparison of newborn infant outcomes. *Am J Obstet Gynecol* 2006;195(6):1538–43.
4. Zupanic JAF. The economics of elective cesarean section. *Clin Perinatol* 2008;35:591–599.
5. Wood SL, Chen S, Ross S, Sauve R. The risk of unexplained antepartum stillbirth in second pregnancies following caesarean section in the first pregnancy. *BJOG* 2008;115(6):726–31.
6. American College of Obstetricians and Gynecologists (ACOG). ACOG Committee Opinion No. 561: Nonmedically indicated early-term deliveries. *Obstet Gynecol* 2013;12:911–5.
7. Tita AT, Landon MB, Spong CY, Lai Y, Leveno KJ, Varner MW, Moawad AH et al. Eunice Kennedy Shriver NICHD Maternal-Fetal Medicine Units Network. Timing of elective repeat cesarean delivery at term and neonatal outcomes. *N Engl J Med* 2009;360(2):111–20.
8. Wilmink FA, Hukkelhoven CW, Lunshof S, Mol BW, van der Post JA, Papatsonis DN. Neonatal outcome following elective cesarean delivery beyond 37 weeks of gestation: A 7-year retrospective analysis of a national registry. *Am J Obstet Gynecol* 2010;202(3):250.e1–8.
9. Doan E, Gibbons K, Tudehope D. The timing of elective caesarean deliveries and early neonatal outcomes in singleton infants born 37–41 weeks' gestation. *Aust N Z J Obstet Gynaecol* 2014;54(4):340–7.
10. Nakashima J, Yamanouchi S, Sekiya S, Hirabayashi M, Mine K, Ohashi A, Tsuji S et al. Elective Cesarean delivery at 37 weeks is associated with the higher risk of neonatal complications. *Tohoku J Exp Med* 2014;233(4):243–8.
11. Hansen AK, Wisborg K, Uldbjerg N, Henriksen TB. Risk of respiratory morbidity in term infants delivered by elective caesarean section: Cohort study. *BMJ* 2008;336(7635):85–87.
12. Hansen AK, Wisborg K, Uldbjerg N, Henriksen TB. Elective caesarean section and respiratory morbidity in the term and near-term neonate. *Acta Obstet Gynecol Scand* 2007;86(4):389–94.
13. Zanardo V, Simbi AK, Franzoi M, Soldà G, Salvadori A, Trevisanuto D. Neonatal respiratory morbidity risk and mode of delivery at term: Influence of timing of elective caesarean delivery. *Acta Paediatr* 2004;93(5):643–7.
14. Stutchfield P, Whitaker R, Russell I; Antenatal Steroids for Term Elective Caesarean Section (ASTECS) Research Team. Antenatal betamethasone and incidence of neonatal respiratory distress after elective caesarean section: Pragmatic randomised trial. *BMJ* 2005;331(7518):662.
15. Sweet DG, Carnielli V, Greisen G, Hallman M, Ozek E, Plavka R, Saugstad OD et al.; European Association of Perinatal Medicine. European consensus guidelines on the management of neonatal respiratory distress syndrome in preterm infants—2013 update. *Neonatology* 2013;103(4):353–68.
16. Gholitabar, M, Roz Ullman R, James D, Griffiths M, on behalf of the Guideline Development Group Caesarean section. Summary of updated NICE guidance. *BMJ* 2011;343:d7108.
17. Huang L, Chen Q, Zhao Y, Wang W, Fang F, Bao Y. Is elective cesarean section associated with a higher risk of asthma? A meta-analysis. *J Asthma* 2015:52(1):16–25.

18. Tollånes MC, Moster D, Daltveit AK, Irgens LM. Cesarean delivery and risk of severe childhood asthma: A population-based cohort study. *J Pediatr* 2008;153(1):112–6.
19. Bager P, Wohlfahrt J, Westergaard T. Caesarean delivery and risk of atopy and allergic disease: Meta-analyses. *Clin Exp Allergy* 2008;38(4):634–42.
20. Cardwell CR, Stene LC, Joner G, Cinek O, Svensson J, Goldacre MJ, Parslow RC et al. Caesarean section is associated with an increased risk of childhood-onset type 1 diabetes mellitus: A meta-analysis of observational studies. *Diabetologia* 2008;51(5):726–35.
21. Hankins GD, Clark SM, Munn MB. Cesarean delivery on request at 39 weeks: Impact on shoulder dystocia, fetal trauma, neonatal encephalopathy, and intrauterine fetal demise. *Semin Perinatol* 2006;30(5):276–87.
22. Fretts RC, Elkin EB, Myers ER, Heffner LJ. Should older women have antepartum testing to prevent unexplained stillbirth? *Obstet Gynecol* 2004; 104:56–64.
23. Landon MB, Hauth JC, Leveno KJ, Spong CY, Leindecker S, Varner MW, Moawad AH et al.; National Institute of Child Health and Human Development Maternal-Fetal Medicine Units Network. Maternal and perinatal outcomes associated with a trial of labor after prior cesarean delivery. *N Engl J Med* 2004;35:2581–9.
24. Anteby EY, Yagel S. Route of delivery of fetuses with structural anomalies. *Eur J Obstet Gynecol Reprod Biol* 2003;106(1):5–9.
25. Bauer J, Hentschel R, Zahradnik H, Karck U, Linderkamp O. Vaginal delivery and neonatal outcome in extremely-low-birth-weight infants below 26 weeks of gestational age. *Am J Perinatol* 2003; 20(4):181–8.
26. Robilio PA, Boe NM, Danielsen B, Gilbert WM. Vaginal vs. cesarean delivery for preterm breech presentation of singleton infants in California: A population-based study. *J Reprod Med* 2007;52(6): 473–9.

General anesthesia for cesarean delivery
Indications and complications

KRZYSZTOF KUCZKOWSKI, YAYOI OHASHI, and TIBERIU EZRI

INTRODUCTION

Anesthesia for obstetrics is considered by many to be a high-risk subspecialty of anesthesiology, which is laden with clinical challenges and medicolegal liability [1]. Obstetric anesthesia-related complications are the sixth leading cause of pregnancy-related maternal mortality in the United States [2]. The vast majority of anesthesia-related maternal deaths occur under general anesthesia [1–13]. Most general anesthesia-related maternal deaths are attributed to failed intubation, failed ventilation/oxygenation, and/or pulmonary aspiration of gastric contents [1–13]. Predisposing factors include non-pregnancy-related maternal conditions (e.g., difficult airway and obesity), pregnancy-related maternal conditions (e.g., pregnancy-induced hypertension), and/or emergent circumstances requiring expeditious surgical delivery of the fetus (e.g., fetal distress) [12]. Ezri et al. created "the inverted traffic light"—a simple, difficult obstetric airway algorithm [3] (Figure 18.1).

ANESTHESIA-RELATED MATERNAL MORTALITY

Databases:

- Confidential Enquiry into Maternal and Child Health (CEMACH), United Kingdom
- Centers for Disease Control and Prevention (CDC), United States
- American Society of Anesthesiologists (ASA) closed claims reports

Obstetric anesthesia-related maternal mortality is decreasing [2,12]. One of the primary reasons behind this decrease in maternal mortality is the increased percentage of cesarean deliveries performed under regional versus general anesthesia. The primary causes of anesthesia-related mortality have also changed from airway problems and aspiration pneumonitis (in the 1980s) to high spinal block (complication of regional anesthesia), obesity, and airway problems (in the 1990s and 2000s) [14].

A report by Davies et al. comments on the results of the 1990–2003 closed claims analysis in obstetric anesthesia and compares them with the pre-1990 period in the United States [14]. While anesthesia-related maternal mortality was decreasing, there was still a significant (and very concerning) number of severe maternal and fetal complications and deaths. The causes of bad fetal outcome in some cases in this report were still linked to airway problems under general anesthesia [14].

The Confidential Enquiry into Maternal and Child Health (CEMACH) in the United Kingdom reported that in the analyzed period (2003–2005), six mothers died of direct anesthesia-related causes and 31 mothers died from indirect anesthesia-related causes. Maternal obesity was a leading predisposing cause of death [15]. Two parturients died due to lack of proper training and experience in difficult airway management by the anesthesia providers. Airway problems during extubation were often overlooked [15].

Rahman et al. reported that failed intubation in obstetrics occurred in 20 cases (1:238) during a 5-year period (1999–2003) in the United Kingdom [16]. The authors concluded that failed tracheal intubation is still managed badly (poor applications of algorithms and drills) in the United Kingdom.

The incidence of difficult and failed intubation and failed mask ventilation in obstetrics is uncertain, but it seems to be higher in pregnant compared to nonpregnant patients [3,12]. Difficult intubation occurs in 7.9% of the nonobese pregnant versus 1%–2% of the nonobese general surgical patients and in 35% in obese obstetric versus 12% in obese nonobstetric patients [17]. These findings are concerning as obesity among pregnant women in the United States and many other countries is on the increase [18]. The "ramped" position for intubation of obese parturients is recommended [3,12,19].

INDICATIONS FOR GENERAL ANESTHESIA IN CESAREAN DELIVERY

In the modern practice of obstetric anesthesia, regional anesthesia has become a "gold standard" for cesarean delivery, and it is used whenever possible. (Please see Chapter 19, "Local Anesthesia for Cesarean Delivery: Epidural, Spinal, and Combined Spinal-Epidural Anesthesia," for additional information.) General anesthesia is used only when it is absolutely necessary. As a result of increased popularity of neuraxial blocks in obstetrics, the use of general anesthesia has decreased over the last two decades (and continues to do so) [12,20,19].

However, general anesthesia is still indicated for emergent "stat" cesarean deliveries—when time of delivery is of essence [2,3,12]. In all urgent/emergent cases, the anesthesiologist, obstetrician, and neonatologist must weigh the severity of fetal distress against the risks of general anesthesia to the mother [21]. To complicate this matter further, most general anesthetics for urgent/emergent cesarean deliveries are administered to mothers with high

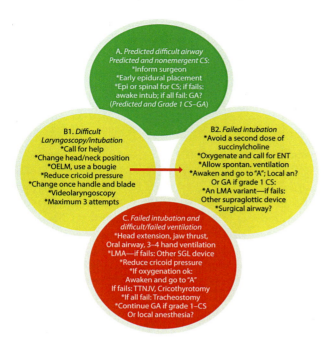

Figure 18.1 The "inverted traffic light" difficult obstetric airway management algorithm. (From Ezri T et al., *J Clin Monit Comput* 2012;26:491–492. With permission.)

incidence of coexisting disease (e.g., obesity) leading to higher incidence of adverse outcomes [18–21]. It is imperative to provide safe anesthesia for the mother without compromising the well-being of the fetus and newborn.

There are a few contraindications to general anesthesia for cesarean delivery, which include maternal conditions such as difficult airway, severe asthma, and history of malignant hyperthermia [2,3,12].

Given the decreased use of general anesthesia for cesarean delivery over the past two decades, concerns have been raised that anesthesia residents in training may not gain adequate experience in this technique, what has been described as the "vanishing art of general anesthesia in obstetrics" [22].

PREPARATION FOR ANESTHESIA

Irrespective of the type of anesthesia selected (general versus regional) for cesarean delivery, preparation for anesthesia is the same and includes several important steps, as outlined in Box 18.1. [3,6,8,9,12,13,17,19,20,23–30].

Box 18.1 Preparation for anesthesia

- Pre-anesthetic evaluation
- Pre-anesthetic medications
- Aspiration prophylaxis
- Intravenous fluids (crystalloid coloading or colloid loading)
- Maternal positioning
- Maternal monitoring

Pre-anesthetic evaluation

The Practice Advisory published by the American Society of Anesthesiologists (ASA) in 2012 requires a detailed review of the maternal medical, surgical, and anesthesia-related history; list of medications taken by the parturient; known drug allergies; results of pertinent laboratory tests; and basic maternal vital signs (e.g., blood pressure, heart, oxyhemoglobin saturation, and respiratory rate) prior to anesthesia (irrespective of the choice of anesthesia) [30]. In addition to preoperative assessment of the heart and lungs, physical examination of the pregnant women should include detailed evaluation of the airway. For regional anesthesia, close attention must be paid to maternal coagulation status and evaluation of the back area, with particular emphasis on the needle insertion site [31,32]. (Please see Chapter 19 entitled "Local Anesthesia for Cesarean Delivery: Epidural, Spinal, and Combined Spinal-Epidural Anesthesia," for details.)

Maternal coagulopathy (e.g., associated with hemolysis, elevated liver enzymes, low platelet count [HELLP] syndrome, placental abruption, and/or maternal sepsis), as well as maternal anatomical disorders (e.g., spina bifida and previous back surgery) or neoplasms at the site of needle insertion, may contraindicate regional anesthesia [19,20]. Maternal hypovolemia may constitute another contraindication to neuraxial anesthesia. In all these circumstances general anesthesia would be required.

Pre-anesthetic medications

Nonobstetric surgical patients often receive other (nonanesthetic) medications before anesthesia. Most pregnant women do not need sedative drugs before the administration of general anesthesia for cesarean delivery [12,17]. Sedative drugs should be avoided until after the delivery of the infant. Most pregnant patients want to enjoy and remember their childbirth experience as much as possible. If absolutely necessary, the anesthesia provider may administer a small intravenous dose of a benzodiazepine (e.g., midazolam 0.5–2 mg), and/or an opioid (e.g., fentanyl 25–50 mcg). Small doses of the above medications should have minimal effect on the fetus and neonate. A major disadvantage of the pre-anesthetic administration of benzodiazepines is their potential for amnesia (an effect clearly not desired in pregnant women) [12,17,19,20].

Aspiration prophylaxis

Prophylactic administration of nonparticulate antacids, H_2 receptor blockers, and/or metoclopramide should be considered prior to cesarean delivery under general anesthesia. [30,33–35]. Anticholinergic agents (e.g., atropine) decrease oral secretions and lessen the likelihood of maternal bradycardia during anesthesia. Atropine readily crosses the placenta; in contrast, glycopyrrolate does not readily cross the placenta, and it is the anticholinergic agent of choice in pregnant women. Glycopyrrolate may be given intravenously just before the administration of anesthesia (e.g., in urgent or emergent cesarean delivery) or intramuscularly 30–60 minutes before the induction of anesthesia (e.g., in elective cesarean delivery).

Metoclopramide is a procainamide derivative that is a dopamine receptor antagonist centrally and a cholinergic agonist peripherally. A small (e.g., 10 mg) intravenous dose of metoclopramide increases lower esophageal sphincter tone, has an antiemetic effect, and reduces gastric volume within 10–15 minutes by increasing gastric peristalsis [12,17].

Healthy parturients scheduled for elective cesarean delivery may be allowed to drink a modest amount of clear liquids until 2 hours before induction of anesthesia. Solid foods should be avoided for 6–8 hours prior to surgery [30].

Intravenous fluids: Crystalloid coloading or colloid loading

Pregnant women should receive an intravenous infusion of crystalloid solutions (e.g., 0.9% saline or Ringer's lactate) prior to anesthesia [12,17,20]. The intravenous crystalloid coloading is most effective if given within 20–30 minutes of induction of anesthesia. Alternatively, colloid solutions might be used for intravenous fluid therapy prior to anesthesia. The rationale behind this hydration strategy is to maintain adequate intravascular blood volume and prevent hypotension, which might develop after induction of regional (more likely) or general (less likely, however not uncommon) anesthesia. The incidence of hypotension is higher under neuraxial blocks, and subsequently, some practitioners believe that pregnant women undergoing cesarean delivery under regional anesthesia might require more volume for pre-anesthetic hydration than those whose surgery is conducted under general anesthesia [12,20]. However, this issue remains controversial.

Treatment of hypotension (in addition to intravenous crystalloid or colloid infusions/boluses) is either with ephedrine (intravenous boluses of 5–10 mg) or phenylephrine (which can be given by either boluses of 0.05–0.1 mg or infusion of 0.025–0.1 mg/min), will be discussed in detail in Chapter 19.

Maternal positioning

Maternal positioning for surgery and anesthesia should not be overlooked [12,20,30,36]:

- Pregnant women should not lie flat (be it in bed or on the operating table).
- In supine position, the gravid uterus compresses the aorta and the inferior vena cava against the bodies of the lumbar vertebrae leading to aorto-caval compression.
- Aorto-caval compression syndrome may develop.
- Aorto-caval compression should be avoided before and during cesarean delivery, regardless of the anesthetic technique used.
- It is necessary to maintain left uterine displacement before and during the performance of cesarean delivery.
- Special maternal head positioning (on the operating room table) for induction of general anesthesia in the "sniffing position" is required to facilitate airway instrumentation (e.g., laryngoscopy and intubation).
- The "ramped" position for intubation is indicated in obese parturients.

Maternal monitoring

Supplemental oxygen should be given to the mother during administration of either general or regional anesthesia (at least until delivery of the baby). Oxygenation should be monitored [37].

The American Society of Anesthesiologists (ASA) "Standards for Basic Anesthetic Monitoring" requires that, in addition to ECG, heart rate, and blood pressure measurement, "a quantitative method of assessing oxygenation such as pulse oximetry" be used during the administration of either regional or general anesthesia for surgery. It is especially important to monitor SpO_2 during the induction of general anesthesia [38].

The ASA also requires "continual monitoring for the presence of expired carbon dioxide" during the administration of general anesthesia. End-tidal carbon dioxide analysis allows rapid verification of correct placement of the endotracheal tube within the trachea. Failure to detect carbon dioxide should immediately signal the occurrence of esophageal intubation [38].

Monitoring must be initiated on admission to the labor and delivery room and/or operating room and continued until the end of anesthesia/recovery from anesthesia. Additional monitoring is individualized depending on institutional standards and the condition of the patient.

PREVENTION OF COMPLICATIONS

Prevention of anesthesia-related maternal complications should primarily focus on the anesthesia provider's ability to predict the likelihood of these complications (Box 18.2).

DENITROGENATION/PREOXYGENATION

After the pregnant patient is placed on the operating table, a folded blanket or a wedge is placed beneath the right hip (this is usually done by the obstetric nurse) to ensure proper left uterine displacement [12,20]. Appropriate monitors, including a nerve stimulator, are applied. The patient should then breathe 100% oxygen through a well-fitting facemask. Approximately 3–5 minutes represents the ideal interval to achieve denitrogenation (termed traditional or T method). When time is of the essence, the patient may take four vital-capacity breaths of 100% oxygen (termed

---

Box 18.2 Prevention of maternal complications under general anesthesia: Main focus

- Aspiration of gastric contents
- Difficult airway
- Hypotension

4DB/30 sec method) just before the induction of general anesthesia [12,19,20].

Induction of general anesthesia is performed after the gravid abdomen has been prepared and draped and the obstetrician is ready to begin cesarean delivery. A rapid sequence induction is used. This requires that a qualified assistant apply pressure to the cricoid cartilage to occlude the esophagus until an endotracheal tube has been inserted correctly, the cuff has been inflated, and ventilation of the lungs has been verified [20].

INDUCTION AGENTS

The goals of induction agents (Table 18.1) are to

- Ensure maternal hypnosis and amnesia
- Preserve maternal blood pressure, cardiac output, and uterine blood flow
- Minimize fetal and neonatal depression

Thiopental

The usual dose is 3–5 mg/kg. Thiopental provides prompt, reliable induction of anesthesia, it has few adverse effects on airway irritability, its pharmacokinetics are well understood, and it results in a smooth emergence from anesthesia [12,19,20,40]. The drug rapidly crosses the placenta, and it can be detected in umbilical venous blood within 30 seconds of administration. Several theories have been proposed to explain the scenario of an unconscious mother with an awake neonate. These include (1) preferential uptake of thiopental by the fetal liver, which is the first organ perfused by blood from the umbilical vein; (2) the higher relative water content of the fetal brain; (3) rapid redistribution of the drug into maternal tissues, which causes a rapid reduction in the maternal-to-fetal concentration gradient; (4) nonhomogeneity of blood flow in the intervillous space; and (5) progressive dilution by admixture with the various components of the fetal circulation [12,20]. Because of this rapid equilibration of thiopental and a lack of a significant concentration of thiopental in the fetal brain, there is no advantage in delaying delivery until thiopental concentrations decline. However there is no evidence of an adverse effect of thiopental on the fetus when the induction-to-delivery time is prolonged [12].

Table 18.1 General anesthesia in obstetrics: Induction agents for cesarean delivery

Agent	Dose	Maternal effect	UV/MV ratio	Neonatal effect
Thiopental	4.0 mg/kg	None	0.96	Low Apgar
Propofol	2.0 mg/kg	Pain (injection)	0.70	None
Ketamine	1–1.5 mg/kg	Dreams	Dose related	Hypertonus
Etomidate	0.2–0.3 mg/kg	Myoclonus	0.45	None

Propofol

The usual dose of propofol is 2–3 mg/kg. Propofol allows a rapid, smooth induction of anesthesia. Propofol attenuates the cardiovascular response to laryngoscopy and intubation much more effectively than thiopental [1,19,20,39–44]. Perhaps its major advantage is the rapid awakening that follows the discontinuation of an infusion of propofol. Moreover, intravenous infusion of propofol allows the anesthesiologist to give 100% oxygen. Some studies have noted that the administration of propofol results in a greater decrease in blood pressure than does thiopental. Decreased maternal blood pressure results in decreased uteroplacental perfusion and compromises fetal well-being. Other studies have not observed significant hypotension after the administration of propofol (2.0–2.8 mg/kg) before cesarean delivery [41–44].

Propofol is a lipophilic agent with a low molecular weight, and it rapidly crosses the placenta. Dailland et al. observed that the umbilical venous/maternal venous blood concentration ratio at delivery was 0.70 [43]. The authors also observed that propofol was rapidly cleared from the neonatal circulation, and they detected low concentrations of propofol in breast milk [12,20,42–44].

Propofol provides an excellent vehicle for the growth of bacteria, and for this reason, it should be used promptly after its withdrawal from the ampule. Propofol may be administered by continuous intravenous infusion for the maintenance of anesthesia [42,43]. Propofol does not offer significant advantages over thiopental during rapid sequence induction of general anesthesia in most obstetric patients. However, propofol blunts the hypertensive response to laryngoscopy and intubation more effectively than the other induction agents; thus it may be a good choice for the induction of general anesthesia in hypertensive patients (e.g., in women with preeclampsia) [12,20].

Most studies have noted that administration of propofol and thiopental results in similar Apgar scores.

Ketamine

The usual dose is 1 mg/kg. Ketamine is a very useful induction agent in obstetric patients [12,19,20]. Ketamine is also an excellent choice for the induction of general anesthesia for cesarean delivery. It has a rapid onset of action, it provides both analgesia and hypnosis, and it reliably provides amnesia [3]. In addition, its sympathomimetic properties are advantageous in patients with asthma or modest hypovolemia. Ketamine also is an excellent choice in cases of severe fetal distress; 100% oxygen can be administered until delivery, with a low risk of maternal awareness and recall [20].

When a dose of 1 mg/kg is used for induction, systolic blood pressure increases approximately 14% immediately after induction of anesthesia and approximately 30% after laryngoscopy and intubation. These hemodynamic changes result from ketamine's indirect sympathomimetic activity. Thus ketamine should be avoided in hypertensive patients.

Ketamine also results in direct myocardial depression and in decreased cardiac output and hypotension if the patient has severe hypovolemia [1,3]. Large doses of ketamine increase uterine tone.

Ketamine rapidly crosses the placenta, and it reaches a maximum concentration in the fetus approximately 1.5 to 2 minutes after administration [13].

After administration of ketamine, dreaming is common. Large doses of ketamine can cause dysphoria and hallucinations during emergence from anesthesia.

Etomidate

The usual dose is 0.2–0.3 mg/kg. Etomidate has been used in obstetric anesthesia practice since 1979. Etomidate produces a rapid onset of anesthesia in one arm-to-brain circulation time. It undergoes rapid hydrolysis, which results in a rapid recovery period [12,17,45]. Etomidate causes little cardiovascular depression; thus it is an excellent choice in patients with hemodynamic instability. Unfortunately, intravenous injection of etomidate may result in pain and myoclonus, which can be severe. Etomidate also may result in the suppression of neonatal serum cortisol concentrations, although it is unclear whether this level of suppression is clinically significant [12,46].

Muscle relaxants

Table 18.2 presents muscle relaxants used for cesarean delivery. In the United States the depolarizing agent succinylcholine 1.0–1.5 mg/kg remains the muscle relaxant of choice for most patients [12,20,46]. The nondepolarizing muscle relaxant rocuronium is a suitable alternative to succinylcholine when a nondepolarizing agent is preferred for rapid sequence induction of general anesthesia for cesarean delivery [46].

Regardless of the choice of muscle relaxant, laryngoscopy and intubation should not be attempted until adequate muscle relaxation has occurred.

Succinylcholine

The usual dose of succinylcholine is 1–1.5 mg/kg. Succinylcholine remains the muscle relaxant of choice for most pregnant women undergoing cesarean delivery under general anesthesia [13,19,20]. This dose provides complete muscle relaxation and optimal conditions for laryngoscopy and intubation within approximately 45 seconds of intravenous administration. Succinylcholine is highly ionized and water soluble, and only small amounts cross the placenta. Maternal administration of succinylcholine rarely affects neonatal neuromuscular function.

Succinylcholine is rapidly metabolized by plasma pseudocholinesterase. Pseudocholinesterase activity decreases 30% during pregnancy, but recovery from succinylcholine is not prolonged. The parturient's increased volume of distribution offsets the effect of the decreased pseudocholinesterase activity [20]. Administration of succinylcholine may result in neonatal apnea if the mother has homozygotic atypical pseudocholinesterase deficiency.

The anesthesiologist should confirm the return of neuromuscular function before giving additional doses of muscle relaxant [12,45].

Rocuronium

The usual dose of rocuronium is 0.6–1.2 mg/kg. Rocuronium is a suitable alternative to succinylcholine when a nondepolarizing agent is preferred for rapid sequence induction of general anesthesia for cesarean delivery [13]. Maximal effect is usually achieved within 90 seconds after administration of a dose of 0.6 mg/kg, and the neuromuscular blockade is satisfactorily reversed at the conclusion of cesarean delivery. Good conditions for laryngoscopy and intubation are accomplished within 70–80 seconds when 4–6 mg/kg of thiopental for the induction of anesthesia is used. A larger dose of rocuronium (e.g., 0.9 or 1.2 mg/kg) results in an onset of paralysis similar to that provided by succinylcholine, but the duration of action may be prolonged [45,46].

Vecuronium

The usual intubating dose is 0.1–0.2 mg/kg. Vecuronium may be administered when the use of succinylcholine is contraindicated; however, it has a significantly slower onset of action [45].

Atracurium

The usual intubating dose is 0.5–0.6 mg/kg. Atracurium is a less desirable agent for rapid sequence induction of anesthesia. The high dose required for a rapid onset of action may result in significant histamine release and hypotension.

The use of a nerve stimulator allows an objective assessment of the onset of paralysis and also guides the administration of additional doses of muscle relaxant [20,45]. Only very small amounts of the nondepolarizing muscle relaxants cross the placenta; thus the infant rarely is affected. Clinical studies have confirmed that maternal administration of a muscle relaxant does not affect Apgar or neurobehavioral scores.

Reversal agents

At the surgery conclusion and prior to emergence from anesthesia and extubation, muscle relaxation is reversed (Table 18.3) [20,45].

Table 18.2 General anesthesia in obstetrics: Muscle relaxants for cesarean delivery

Agent	Dose	Onset	Duration
Succinylcholine	1–1.5 mg/kg	45 seconds	13–14 minutes
Rocuronium	0.6–1.2 mg/kg	80 seconds	Variable/dose related
Vecuronium	0.2 mg/kg	175 seconds	115 minutes
Atracurium	0.3 mg/kg	>175 seconds	Variable/dose related

Table 18.3 General anesthesia in obstetrics: Reversal agents

Reversal agent	Dose	Onset
Neostigmine	0.05 mg/kg	9 minutes
Sugammadex	16 mg/kg	6 minutes

Endotracheal intubation

Equipment (basic):

1. Laryngoscope with two blade sizes
2. Endotracheal tube in two to three sizes plus guide
3. Suction tube
4. Nerve stimulator
5. Back-up equipment: oral and nasal airways, LMA, gum-elastic bougie

The anesthesia provider should not attempt ventilation before insertion of the endotracheal tube [13,20,45,46]. A short-handled laryngoscope is advantageous because it prevents contact with the enlarged maternal breasts. A 6- to 7-mm endotracheal tube is an ideal size for most pregnant women. After intubation, the presence of end-tidal carbon dioxide and bilateral breath sounds should be verified. At that time, the obstetric team may be given a "go-ahead" to start surgery [1].

Inhaled anesthetic agents

Inhaled anesthetic agents include nitrous oxide and various halogenated agents (sevoflurane, isoflurane, desflurane, and halothane) [20,46]. Characteristics of the ideal inhaled anesthetic agent include ample potency, low solubility (in both blood and tissues), resistance to metabolic degradation, and lack of injury to vital tissues [12,45]. The ideal anesthetic agent produces anesthesia while allowing the use of a high concentration of oxygen (ample potency) [46]. Solubility of an anesthetic agent in blood is quantified as the blood:gas partition coefficient. A low blood:gas partition coefficient reflects a low affinity of blood for the anesthetic, a desirable property in clinical practice. Similarly, the tissue:gas partition coefficient is the ratio of the concentration of an anesthetic in a tissue to the concentration of the anesthetic in the gas phase [45,46]. A low tissue:gas partition coefficient reflects low tissue solubility.

Differences in the solubility of inhaled anesthetic agents in blood and tissues have important clinical implications for the recovery from anesthesia. A lower solubility allows for a faster emergence from anesthesia. Desflurane tissue solubility is half that of sevoflurane, sevoflurane is half as soluble as isoflurane, and isoflurane is half as soluble as halothane.

To minimize waste of anesthetic agents and decrease cost, potent inhaled anesthetic agents are delivered in a circle absorption system (with absorbents that remove carbon dioxide and allow for the rebreathing to take place). Desflurane, halothane, and isoflurane all are metabolized to trifluoroacetate, which can cause hepatotoxicity. Seizures and agitation have been reported in patients (primary children upon emergence, and possibly in parturients) receiving sevoflurane [47,48]. Desflurane, halothane, isoflurane, and nitrous oxide are not associated with seizures.

Inhaled anesthetics differ in their pungency and tendency to irritate the human airways. Because of its low pungency and low risk of respiratory irritation, sevoflurane is currently the agent of choice for inhalation induction of anesthesia in the United States. This is less relevant to OB patients because parturients do not receive mask induction. Potent inhaled anesthetic agents differ minimally in their circulatory effects. Selecting the appropriate agent may at times be difficult. Although halothane has many ideal inhaled anesthetic agents (e.g., ample potency and lack of respiratory and circulatory stimulation), the high solubility and hepatotoxicity limit its clinical applications [45]. Choosing among sevoflurane, desflurane, and isoflurane involves weighing the advantages and disadvantages of each agent. Nitrous oxide is not metabolized.

MAINTENANCE OF ANESTHESIA

After the delivery of the fetus, the inspired concentration of nitrous oxide is increased. Some anesthesia providers choose to decrease or discontinue the administration of the volatile halogenated agent to allow for optimal uterine involution [45]. However, the uterus should contract adequately in response to oxytocin, despite the administration of a low concentration of a volatile halogenated agent.

The authors of this chapter discontinue the volatile halogenated agent only if there is evidence of uterine atony that is unresponsive to oxytocin. We then administer modest doses of opioid as needed to maintain adequate maternal anesthesia [12,20].

Muscle relaxation may be maintained with any of the nondepolarizing agents or with an infusion of succinylcholine. We prefer rocuronium for maintenance of muscle relaxation. At the end of surgery, residual nondepolarizing neuromuscular blockade is reversed.

The upper airway is suctioned and extubation is performed when the patient has regained her protective reflexes, can maintain her own airway, and responds appropriately to verbal commands [45]. It is noteworthy that in preeclamptic patients treated with magnesium, the effect of nondepolarizing relaxants may be prolonged, and neostigmine may be ineffective in the presence of a deep block caused by magnesium potentiation of the relaxants.

EFFECTS OF GENERAL ANESTHESIA ON THE FETUS AND NEONATE

The goal of anesthesia is to provide safe anesthetic to the mother without jeopardizing the condition of fetus and newborn. The placental transfer of drugs administered to the mother may directly affect the fetus [49–54]. These drugs may cause clinically apparent depression of the infant at delivery or subtle neurobehavioral changes during the first several hours after birth.

Maternal hypotension or the administration of uterine artery vasoconstrictive drugs results in decreased

> **Box 18.3 Prevention of fetal hypoxemia and acidosis**
>
> - Providing left uterine displacement to prevent aortocaval compression
> - Ensuring adequate maternal oxygenation
> - Avoiding maternal hyperventilation
> - Avoiding excessive doses of anesthetic agents
> - Treating hypotension promptly

uteroplacental blood flow, which may cause fetal hypoxia and acidosis (Box 18.3). Maternal hypoxemia also adversely affects the fetus [53].

One factor that may affect oxygenation and acid–base status at delivery is the uterine incision-to-delivery (U-D) interval. A U-D interval longer than 3 minutes is associated with an increased incidence of low umbilical cord blood pH measurements and low Apgar scores, regardless of the anesthetic technique. The obstetrician should minimize the U-D interval, regardless of the type of anesthesia that is used [45,50–54].

A prolonged I-D interval results in greater fetal exposure to nitrous oxide and the volatile halogenated agent. Thus, a prolonged I-D interval may result in a greater risk of neonatal depression at delivery, despite the presence of normal umbilical cord blood gas and acid–base measurements [53,54].

Nitrous oxide has been implicated as a cause of neonatal depression. Nitrous oxide rapidly crosses the placenta.

The next section of this chapter reviews complications of general anesthesia in obstetrics, which are included in Box 18.4.

Awareness during anesthesia

The risk of maternal awareness is the highest between induction of general anesthesia and delivery of the infant. Administration of 50% nitrous oxide in oxygen *without* another agent results in maternal awareness in 12%–26% of cases [12,45]. Awareness is inhumane for the mother and results in high maternal concentrations of catecholamines, which result in uterine artery vasoconstriction and reduced oxygen delivery to the fetus [55–64].

The Bispectral Index (BIS), a multivariable processed electroencephalographic monitor, is potentially a useful aid in titration of inhalational agents in parturients undergoing cesarean delivery under general anesthesia (to ensure adequate hypnosis without compromising the fetus) [63,64].

A common approach to prevent awareness is to administer 50% nitrous oxide in oxygen in combination with a low concentration of a volatile halogenated agent (e.g., isoflurane 0.6%, or sevoflurane 1.0%) [45,46]. This method is simple and reduces the incidence of maternal awareness to less than 1%. A low concentration of a volatile halogenated agent is adequate for most patients because pregnancy decreases anesthetic requirements by as much as 30%–40%. Predelivery administration of a low concentration of a volatile halogenated agent does not adversely affect neonatal condition, and it does not significantly increase maternal blood loss [56,63,64].

In most cases, we administer 30%–50% nitrous oxide in oxygen and a low concentration (0.5 MAC) of a volatile halogenated agent (e.g., isoflurane, sevoflurane, and desflurane) [45,46,57–63].

Intraoperative awareness can occur in emergent cesarean deliveries under general anesthesia in hemodynamically unstable patients unable to tolerate a sufficient depth of anesthesia. Czarko et al. and Paech et al reported that the incidence of intraoperative awareness might be as high as 1 in 88–382 (0.26%–1.1%) [56,57]. Intraoperative awareness under general anesthesia may cause severe postoperative psychological sequelae, including post-traumatic stress disorder, anxiety, neurosis, nightmares, fear of hospitals, and even death [58].

Factors predisposing to intraoperative awareness [57,58]

- High cardiac output = wider drug distribution = lower blood drug levels
- No premedication given
- Decreased concentrations of volatile anesthetic agents used
- Withholding of benzodiazepine and opioids until delivery to avoid fetal exposure and mother's anterograde amnesia

Preventative measures should be taken to avoid intraoperative awareness. Monitoring minimum alveolar concentration (MAC) can be one of the means of prevention of intraoperative awareness. The use of nitrous oxide should be considered. Nitrous oxide does not alter the bispectral index [60–62]. Although 50% oxygen concentration is commonly required before delivery, it has been shown that 33% of oxygen can be an acceptable alternative without fetal compromise [59].

Bispectal index (BIS) and Entropy module are widely used to monitor the depth of anesthesia. The B-Aware trial showed an 82% reduction in the incidence of awareness in patients at risk of perioperative awareness including cesarean delivery patients [63]. BIS < 60 is a commonly accepted index (state of unconsciousness). However, of note is the fact that low BIS score does not guarantee unconsciousness [64]. One study suggested that BIS needs to be lower than 27 in order to prevent 100% potential for intraoperative awareness in cesarean delivery patients [58].

> **Box 18.4 Complications**
>
> - Maternal awareness
> - Difficult airway (inability to maintain a patent airway)
> - Hypoxia
> - Aspiration pneumonitis (Mendelson syndrome)
> - Cerebrovascular stroke
> - Chronic postcesarean pain
> - Fetal and neonatal respiratory depression

The potential of intraoperative awareness should be discussed in advance with patients who undergo cesarean delivery under general anesthesia.

Difficult airway

It is a general consensus that intubation of a full-term pregnant women can be difficult for a number of reasons, including non-pregnancy-related (e.g., obesity) or pregnancy-specific (large breasts) predisposing factors [4,8,65,66]. McDonnel et al. conducted an observational study of airway management and complications associated with general anesthesia for caesarean section [4]. The authors reported the incidence of difficult intubation in pregnant women to be as high as 1 in 20–30 (3.3%–4.7%) [4]. In another study failed intubation in pregnant women was reported to be 1 in 100–1316 (0.08%–1%) [5]. One in 250 is a generally quoted ratio. Difficult and/or failed intubation in obstetric population is known to be 8–10 times higher than that in the nonobstetric surgical population [6].

Quinn et al. found that older age, high body mass index (BMI), and the Mallampati score were significant independent predictors for difficult intubation [7]. Of note is the fact that with every 1 kg/m² increase in BMI, there is a 7% increase in the risk of failed intubation [7]. Two studies have reported rapid and significant changes (increase) in the Mallampati score during pregnancy and in labor [8,9]. There was a 1.4- to 3.4-fold increase of Mallampati scores of 3 and 4 in parturients during labor or immediately after labor [8,9] (Figure 18.2). This tendency worsens in patients with preeclampsia or eclampsia. In obstetric population, Mallampati classes 3 and 4 are strongly associated with difficult laryngoscopy, with an increased relative risk of 7.6 and 11.3, respectively [10].

Ushiroda et al. reported a life-threatening airway obstruction due to upper airway edema and marked neck swelling after labor and delivery [11]. The neck swelling and pharyngolaryngeal edema appeared during labor. Kuczkowski and Benumof reported on the parturient with prepregnancy subglottic tracheal stenosis, which worsened during pregnancy, creating serious airway management dilemma [67].

The supraglottic airway devices have been used successfully in slim, fasted pregnant women for elective cesarean deliveries under general anesthesia [24,25], as well as rescue devices for emergent difficult airway management [7]. The LMA classic is easy to insert, the ProSeal and Supreme have a drainage tube, while the intubating LMA may serve as a conduit for fiberoptic intubation [3].

Definition of a "difficult" airway

- Difficult laryngoscopy
- Difficult intubation
- Difficult mask ventilation
- Combination of all the above factors

The airway difficulty can be assessed by an experienced anesthesiologist during a single attempt at laryngoscopy.

Factors predisposing to difficult airway in obstetrics

- Pregnancy-related airway changes
  - Airway edema (water retention)
- Other physiological changes of pregnancy
  - Large breast impairing laryngoscopy
- Tendency to rapid development of hypoxemia
  - Decreased functional residual capacity (FRC) in the lungs
  - Increased oxygen consumption (maternal and fetal needs)
- Maternal anatomical abnormalities
- Coexisting diseases
  - Obesity
- "Technical" issues
  - Emergency cesarean delivery
  - Lack of communication
  - Lack of organization
  - Lack of expertize (senior anesthesiologist's backup needed)
  - Lack of equipment

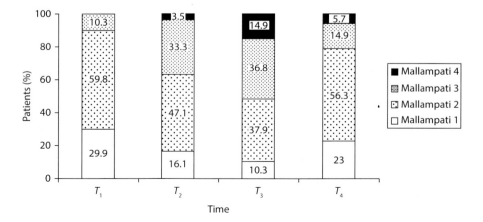

Figure 18.2 Mallampati classes at different time points: T1: 8 months of pregnancy, T2: during labor, T3: 20 minutes after delivery, T4: 48 hours after delivery. (From Boutonnet M et al., *Br J Anaesth* 2010;104:67–70. With permission.)

Assessment of the obstetric airway

- History: from—patient, family, chart
- Airway examination—look for predictors of difficult airway
  - The Mallampati classification (This is nonspecific, if used alone[!]; increases are made throughout labor due to water retention, straining, pushing efforts, and Trendelenburg position.)
  - The Wilson sum score (predicted difficulty with a score >4) (Table 18.4)

Management of the obstetric airway

- Personnel/skills/call for help!
- Equipment
- Protocols/drills/algorithms
- Communication/organization
- Continuing medical education (CME)
- Applying judgment/knowledge/common sense

Airway equipment

In the last 20 years, the development of the fiberoptic bronchoscope for intubation of patients with predicted difficult airway, and the laryngeal mask as a rescue ventilation device and conduit for intubation, have revolutionized airway management [3].

Classification of airway devices

- Devices used for ventilation—supraglottic airways
- Devices used for intubation
- Surgical airway devices
- Devices used for CO_2 detection

Supraglottic (extraglottic) devices

LMA devices include the following: Classic, ProSeal, Fastrach (intubating LMA), and Supreme.

With failed intubation and difficult mask ventilation, the ProSeal may be preferred as it has a drain tube for the regurgitant fluid. The Fastrach may be preferred if a definitive airway (i.e., endotracheal intubation) is required for prolonged surgeries (i.e., cesarean hysterectomy), and it enables intubation with the aid of a fiberoptic bronchoscope. The new LMA Supreme possesses both advantages,

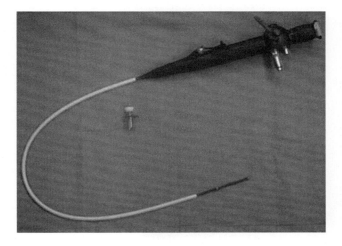

Figure 18.3 The Aintree intubation catheter.

thus allowing both drainage of regurgitant fluids and intubation. The LMA Classic enables fiberoptically aided intubation through it, although it is too long, which carries the risk of endotracheal tube dislodgement. The drawback can be solved by using the Aintree intubation catheter [3] (Figure 18.3).

It should be noted that no LMA prevents the aspiration of gastric contents. It is also important to have alternative supraglottic airway devices, as discussed subsequently, available in case ventilation with the LMA is not possible [3,12,19,20].

The Laryngeal suction tube (Figure 18.4)

- The EasyTube (Figure 18.5)
- The Cobra-PLA (Figure 18.6)
- The I-Gel (Figure 18.7)

Table 18.4 The Wilson sum score (predicted difficulty with a score >4)

	Parameter risk level
Weight	0–2 (>90 kg = 1; >110 kg = 2)
Head and neck movement	0–2
Jaw movement	0–2
Receding mandible	0–2
Buck teeth	0–2
	Total = Maximum 10 points

Source: From Wilson ME et al., Br J Anaesth 1998;61:211–6. With permission.

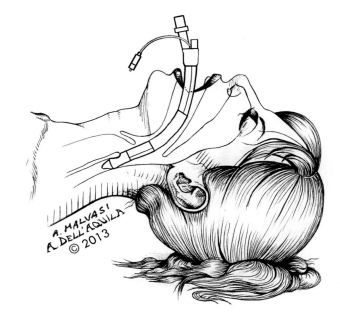

Figure 18.4 The laryngeal suction tube.

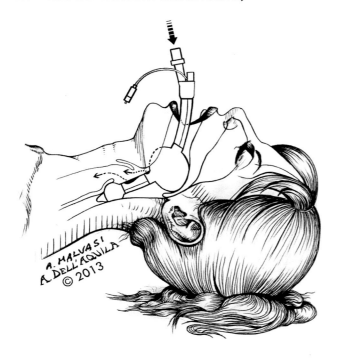

Figure 18.5 The EasyTube (a less traumatic variant of the Combitube).

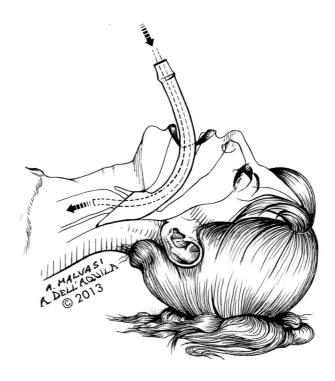

Figure 18.7 The I-Gel.

Difficult airway management: Selected scenarios

1. Alertness to parturients at risk for difficult airway. According to the American College of Obstetricians and Gynecologists (ACOG): "As primary physician, the obstetrician should be alert to the presence of risk factors that place patient at risk for complications ... and could alert the anesthesiologist of airway-related problems" [21]. "Early" epidural placement would be indicated.
2. The anesthesiologist (and the patient) should be prepared for general anesthesia in case of failed spinal anesthesia, total spinal, cardiac arrest, massive hemorrhage.
3. Anticipated difficult airway.
4. Unanticipated difficult airway.
5. Failed intubation, increasing hypoxemia, and difficult ventilation in the paralyzed, anesthetized patient—modified UK Guidelines.
    a. *Failed intubation and difficult ventilation* (other than laryngospasm)
        i. Face mask
        ii. Oxygenate and ventilate the patient
        iii. Maximum head extension
        iv. Maximum jaw thrust
        v. Assistance with mask seal
        vi. Oral ± 6-mm nasal airway
        vii. Reduce cricoid force, if necessary
    b. *Failed oxygenation with facemask* (e.g., $SpO_2 < 90\%$ with $FIO_2 = 1$)
        i. Call for help
        ii. LMA—Oxygenate and ventilate patient

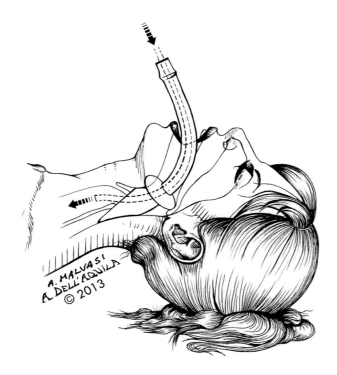

Figure 18.6 Cobra-PLA.

A new technological development that may help in cases of unexpected difficult intubation is videolaryngoscopy (i.e., Storz, Glidescope videolaryngoscopes). This technology also provides an excellent teaching tool (Figure 18.8).

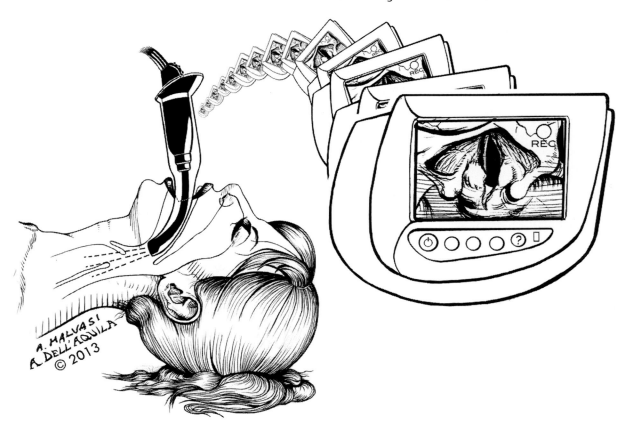

Figure 18.8 The Glidescope.

    iii. Maximum two attempts at insertion
    iv. Reduce any cricoid force during insertion
    v. If oxygenation satisfactory and stable, maintain oxygenation and start cesarean delivery—deliver baby
  c. "Can't intubate, can't ventilate" situation with increasing hypoxemia
    i. Trans-tracheal jet ventilation
    ii. Cannula cricothyroidotomy
    iii. Surgical cricothyroidotomy
    iv. Tracheostomy

Cannula cricothyroidotomy

Equipment: Kink-resistant cannula, for example, Patil (Cook) or Ravussin (VBM); high-pressure ventilation system, for example, Manujet III (VBM).

1. Insert cannula through cricothyroid membrane.
2. Maintain position of cannula—assistant's hand.
3. Confirm tracheal position by air aspiration—20-mL syringe.
4. Attach ventilation system to cannula.
5. Commence cautious ventilation.
6. Confirm ventilation and exhalation through upper airway.
7. If ventilation fails, or any other complication develops—convert immediately to surgical cricothyroidotomy.

Surgical cricothyroidotomy

Equipment: Scalpel—short and rounded—no. 20 or Minitrach scalpel; small (e.g., 6 or 7 mm) cuffed tracheal or tracheostomy tube.

Four-step technique:

1. Identify cricothyroid membrane.
2. Stab incision through skin and membrane, enlarge incision with blunt dissection (e.g., scalpel handle, forceps, or dilator).
3. Ensure caudal traction on cricoid cartilage with tracheal hook.
4. Insert tube and inflate cuff.
  a. Ventilate with low-pressure source.
  b. Verify tube position and pulmonary ventilation.

Difficult airway: Conclusions

- The obstetrician and anesthesiologist should be alert to the presence of problematic airway.
- Most emergency cesarean deliveries can be done under regional anesthesia.
- Preplanned strategy, airway devices, and expert anesthesiologists may lead to improved outcome.
- Induction of general anesthesia should be implemented only in cases of severe fetal bradycardia with contraindication to regional anesthesia or maternal hemorrhage.
- Prediction of difficult airway reduces the likelihood of adverse outcomes.

HYPOXIA

Failed intubation is associated with a higher incidence (71% versus control 2%) of hypoxemia ($SpO_2 < 90\%$). Reduced functional residual capacity (FRC) and an increased metabolic rate in pregnancy lead to a rapid progression to hypoxia after the apnea period during induction [7]. Hignett et al. demonstrated FRC was increased by a mean of 188 mL from the supine to the 30° head-up position [12]. Proper positioning for oxygenation and intubation is crucial in parturients with difficult airway.

Repeated attempts at intubation are contraindicated after ineffective external laryngeal manipulation and progressive hypoxia [65]. The airway needs to be secured with alternative methods (see the inverted traffic light algorithm), and oxygenation must be maintained. We must not allow the situation to worsen and progress to a "cannot intubate, cannot ventilate, and cannot oxygenate" situation.

How can we avoid hypoxia during induction of general anesthesia?

- Pre-oxygenation: eight deep breaths over 60 seconds
- Pre-oxygenation with 25° head-up
- Maximum of three attempts at laryngoscopy
- Use of the "ramped" position for intubation (useful for obese pregnant women)
- Extubation in semi-upright position

Folded blankets are added or removed (as needed) to

1. Keep the patient's head above her shoulders.
2. Keep the external auditory meatus and the sternal notch in the same horizontal plan.

This is better than the "sniff position" for alignment of the oral, pharyngeal, and laryngeal axes.

How should we deal with hypoxia during induction of general anesthesia?

- Ventilate–Call for help–Ventilate!
- Failed intubation should not lead to death or brain damage.

Aspiration pneumonitis (Mendelson syndrome)

Aspiration pneumonitis (Mendelson syndrome) and its mechanism under the settings of anesthesia for obstetric patients was first reported by an obstetrician—Dr Mendelson.

It is our opinion that all pregnant women should receive acid aspiration prophylaxis regardless of the NPO status or the planned anesthetic technique for cesarean delivery [12,19,20]. We administer metoclopramide routinely, and H2 blocker in selected cases, such as diabetes or morbid obesity, on top of the antacid sodium citrate.

Aspiration pneumonitis used to be one of the major causes of perioperative maternal death. A number of preventative measures have been introduced over time to prevent this lethal condition. Rapid sequence induction technique with cricoid pressure and use of sodium citrate and H2 blockers have decreased the incidence of aspiration of gastric contents [66].

The incidence of aspiration of gastric contents is widely quoted to range from 1 in 900 to 1 in 1547 (0.064%–0.11%) [4,33,34]. A prospective observational study from Australia and New Zealand showed that regurgitation of gastric contents during general anesthesia for cesarean delivery occurred in eight cases out of 1095 (0.7%), with four episodes at induction of anesthesia and five episodes at extubation (one at both intubation and extubation) [4]. It must be emphasized the importance of extubating the patients after caesarean delivery when they are fully awake [45].

Quinn et al. reported that failed intubation was related to the higher aspiration rate compared to the control group (8% versus control 1%) [7]. Pregnant woman should be considered as "full stomach" regardless of the fasting status. Older studies have showed that gastric emptying does not alter during pregnancy. However, of note is the fact that once labor starts, a delay in gastric emptying occurs [7].

Paranjothy et al. studied the effectiveness of various interventions at cesarean delivery for reducing the risk of aspiration pneumonitis [35]. The authors concluded that the effects of interventions such as administration of H2 receptor blockers and/or sodium citrate are less consistent than previously believed. However, the authors concluded that their use should still be strongly considered [35].

Cerebrovascular stroke

In addition to physiological changes during pregnancy, pregnancy-related disorders such as preeclampsia and/or eclampsia can contribute to the increased incidence of cerebrovascular and intracranial adverse events during pregnancy, labor, and postpartum. Feske and Singhal reported that the incidence of all types of strokes is four to seven cases in 100,000 pregnancies [68]. Lanska and Kryscio reported that cesarean delivery was associated with a 3- to 12-fold increased risk of peripartum and postpartum stroke [69]. Meticulous attention to the hemodynamic stability during general anesthesia, especially in preeclamptic or eclamptic patients during the induction of anesthesia and intubation is essential to avoid any intracranial adverse events.

Intracranial hemorrhagic stroke

Intracranial hemorrhage is the most common cause of maternal death from stroke in patients with preeclampsia or eclampsia [70]. The incidence of peripartum intracranial hemorrhage is quoted to be as high as 6.1–31.4 cases in 100,000 deliveries [71–72] The incidence of hemorrhagic stroke increases from 2.5-fold in the antenatal period to 23.8-fold in the postpartum period [70].

Takahashi et al. conducted a survey of neurosurgical institutes across Japan to determine the most common causes of cerebrovascular disease in pregnancy [73]. Arteriovenous malformations (AVMs) were the most frequent causes of intracranial hemorrhage, followed by cerebral aneurysms and moyamoya disease. Systemic obstetric complications including coagulopathies; preeclampsia and eclampsia were identified as the risk factors for intracranial hemorrhage [73].

Intracranial ischemic stroke

Foo et al. reported that the incidence of maternal death from ischemic stroke was 1.6 in 100,000 maternities, with a 13.9% (95% CI 12.6–15.3) mortality rate [70]. Cardioembolism, preeclampsia or eclampsia (11%–47% of stroke cases), and cerebral venous sinus thrombosis account for most pregnancy-related ischemic strokes [68].

Chronic postcesarean pain

The prevalence of postpartum pain at 2 months after vaginal delivery has been reported at 10% [74], while the prevalence of pain following cesarean delivery has been reported at 18% at 3 months and 12% at 10 months, respectively, after the surgery [75]. The potential implications of postpartum pain on daily function, mother–infant bonding, and postpartum depression should not be ignored.

Fetal and neonatal respiratory depression

In recent years, remifentanil has been used for the induction of general anesthesia for cesarean delivery. Remifentanil crosses the placenta easily, but is cleared rapidly from the neonatal plasma. One review of remifentanil use for cesarean delivery indicates that remifentanil is highly effective in blunting the sympathetic response (increase in blood pressure and heart rate) to laryngoscopy, intubation, and surgery. Furthermore, pH and base excess were higher in infants of remifentanil-treated mothers. There was no difference regarding the neonatal outcome parameters such as postdelivery mask ventilation, intubation, and Apgar score [49]. However, there were reported cases of neonatal depression when remifentanil was used as bolus followed by continuous infusion. Brief mask ventilation was required in six out of 13 neonates studied.

For many years thiopental has been the drug of choice for induction of general anesthesia for cesarean delivery. However, over the last 10 years production of thiopental was discontinued in several countries, and propofol has become an attractive alternative to thiopental. Propofol rapidly crosses the placenta but is rapidly cleared from the neonatal circulation [50,51]. Celleno et al. studied the neurobehavioral effects of propofol on the neonate following elective cesarean delivery [52]. The authors reported that in the propofol group the Apgar scores and neurobehavioral scores recorded 1 hour after delivery were lower than in the thiopental group [52]. Gin et al. studied plasma catecholamines and neonatal condition after induction of anesthesia with propofol or thiopentone at cesarean delivery [53]. The authors reported no adverse drug effects on maternal hemodynamics, umbilical cord blood gases, Apgar scores, and neurobehavioral scores [53]. Abboud et al. studied the neonatal effects of intravenous propofol versus thiamylal-isoflurane for cesarean delivery [54]. No adverse effects were reported.

REFERENCES

1. Kuczkowski KM. Medico-legal issues in obstetric anesthesia: What does an obstetrician need to know? *Arch Gynecol Obstet* 2008;278:503–5.
2. Hawkins JL, Koonin LM, Palmer SK, Gibbs CP. Anesthesia-related deaths during obstetric delivery in the United States, 1979–1990. *Anesthesiology* 1997;86:277–84.
3. Ezri T, Weisenberg M, Cohen Y, Evron S, Kuczkowski KM. The "inverted traffic light" obstetric difficult airway management algorithm. *J Clin Monit Comput* 2012;26:491–2.
4. McDonnell NJ, Paech MJ, Clavisi OM, Scott KL; ANZCA Trials Group. Difficult and failed intubation in obstetric anaesthesia: An observational study of airway management and complications associated with general anaesthesia for caesarean section. *Int J Obstet Anesth* 2008;17:292–7.
5. McKeen DM, George RB, O'Connell CM, Allen VM, Yazer M, Wilson M, Phu TC. Difficult and failed intubation: Incident rates and maternal, obstetrical, and anesthetic predictors. *Can J Anaesth* 2011;58:514–24.
6. Palanisamy A, Mitani AA, Tsen LC. General anesthesia for cesarean delivery at a tertiary care hospital from 2000 to 2005: A retrospective analysis and 10-year update. *Int J Obstet Anesth* 2011;20:10–16.
7. Quinn AC, Milne D, Columb M, Gorton H, Knight M. Failed tracheal intubation in obstetric anaesthesia: 2 yr national case–control study in the UK. *Br J Anaesth* 2013;110:74–80.
8. Kodali BS, Chandrasekhar S, Bulich LN, Topulos GP, Datta S. Airway changes during labor and delivery. *Anesthesiology* 2008;108:357–62.
9. Boutonnet M, Faitot V, Katz A, Salomon L, Keita H. Mallampati class changes during pregnancy, labour, and after delivery: Can these be predicted? *Br J Anaesth* 2010;104:67–70.
10. Rocke DA, Murray WB, Rout CC, Gouws E. Relative risk analysis of factors associated with difficult intubation in obstetric anesthesia. *Anesthesiology* 1992;77:67–73.
11. Ushiroda J, Inoue S, Egawa J, Kawano Y, Kawaguchi M, Furuya H. Life-threatening airway obstruction due to upper airway edema and marked neck swelling after labor and delivery. *Braz J Anesthesiol* 2013;63:508–10.
12. Kuczkowski KM, Reisner LS, Benumof JL. Airway problems and new solutions for the obstetric patient. *J Clin Anesth* 2003;15:552–563.
13. Kuczkowski KM. Trauma in pregnancy: Perioperative anesthetic considerations for the head-injured pregnant trauma victim. *Anaesthesist* 2004;53:180–2.
14. Davies JM, Posner KL, Lee LA, Cheney FW, Domino KB. Liability associated with obstetric anesthesia: A closed claims analysis. *Anesthesiology* 2009;110:131–9.

15. Cooper GM, McClure JH. Anaesthesia chapter from Saving Mothers' Lives: Reviewing maternal deaths to make pregnancy safer. *Br J Anaesth* 2008;100: 17–22.
16. Rahman K, Jenkins JG. Failed tracheal intubation in obstetrics: No more frequent but still managed badly. *Anaesthesia* 2000;60:168–71.
17. Soens MA, Birnbach DJ, Ranasinghe JS, van Zundert A. Obstetric anesthesia for the obese patient: An ounce of prevention is worth more than a pound of treatment. *Acta Anaesthesiol Scand* 2008;52:6–19.
18. Kuczkowski KM. Labor analgesia for the morbidly obese parturient: An old problem—New solution. *Arch Gynecol Obstet* 2005;271:302–3.
19. Kuczkowski KM, Reisner LS, Benumof LJ. The difficult airway: Risk, prophylaxis and management. In: Chestnut DH, ed. *Obstetric anesthesia: Principles and practice*, 3rd ed. Philadelphia, PA: Elsevier Mosby; 2004:535–61 (Chapter 31).
20. Ezri T, Szmuk P, Evron S, Geva D, Hagay Z, Katz J. Difficult airway in obstetric anesthesia: A review. *Obstet Gynecol Surv* 2001;56:631–41.
21. Gaiser RR, McGonigal ET, Litts P, Cheek TG, Gutsche BB. Obstetricians' ability to assess the airway. *Obstet Gynecol* 1999;93:648–52.
22. Tsen LC, Pitner R, Camann WR. General anesthesia for cesarean delivery at a tertiary care hospital 1990–1995: Indications and implications. *Int J Obstet Anesth* 1998;7:147–52.
23. Wilson ME, Spiegelhalter D, Robertson JA, Lesser P. Predicting difficult intubation. *Br J Anaesth* 1988;61:211–6.
24. Halaseh BK, Sukkar ZF, Hassan LH, Sia AT, Bushnaq WA, Adarbeh H. The use of ProSeal laryngeal mask airway in caesarean section—Experience in 3000 cases. *Anaesth Intensive Care* 2010;38:1023–8.
25. Han TH, Brimacombe J, Lee EJ, Yang HS. The laryngeal mask airway is effective (and probably safe) in selected healthy parturients for elective Cesarean delivery: A prospective study of 1067 cases. *Can J Anaesth* 2001;48:1117–21.
26. Kuczkowski KM, Benumof JL. Anaesthesia and hair fashion. *Anaesthesia* 2001;56:799–800.
27. Kuczkowski KM, Benumof JL. Tongue piercing and obstetric anesthesia: Is there cause for concern? *J Clin Anesth* 2002;14:447–48.
28. Kuczkowski KM, Benumof JL, Moeller-Bertram T, Kotzur A. An initially unnoticed piece of nasal jewelry in a parturient: Implications for intraoperative airway management. *J Clin Anesth* 2003;15:359–62.
29. Kuczkowski KM, Bui PK. Maxillary jewelry in a parturient: A new cause for concern. *Can J Anaesth* 2004;51:519.
30. Apfelbaum JL, Connis RT, Nickinovich DG et al. Practice advisory for preanesthesia evaluation: An updated report by the American Society of Anesthesiologists Task Force on Preanesthesia Evaluation. *Anesthesiology* 2012;116:522–38.
31. Horlocker TT, Wedel DJ, Rowlingson JC et al. Regional anesthesia in the patient receiving antithrombotic or thrombolytic therapy: American Society of Regional Anesthesia and Pain Medicine Evidence-Based Guidelines, 3rd ed. *Reg Anesth Pain Med* 2010;35:64–101.
32. Practice guidelines for obstetric anesthesia: An updated report by the American Society of Anesthesiologists Task Force on Obstetric Anesthesia. *Anesthesiology* 2007;106:843–63.
33. Dindelli M, La Rosa M, Rossi R, Di Nunno D, Piva L, Pagnoni B, Ferrari A. Incidence and complications of the aspiration of gastric contents syndrome during cesarean delivery in general anesthesia. *Ann Ostet Ginecol Med Perinat* 1991;112:376–84.
34. La Rosa M, Piva L, Ravanelli A, Dindelli M, Pagnoni B. Aspiration syndrome in cesarean delivery. Our experience from 1980 to 1990. *Minerva Anestesiol* 1992;58:1213–20.
35. Paranjothy S, Griffiths JD, Broughton HK, Gyte GM, Brown HC, Thomas J. Interventions at caesarean section for reducing the risk of aspiration pneumonitis. *Int J Obstet Anesth* 2011;20:142–8.
36. Hignett R, Fernando R, McGlennan A, McDonald S, Stewart A, Columb M, Adamou T, Dilworth P. A randomized crossover study to determine the effect of a 30° head-up versus a supine position on the functional residual capacity of term parturients. *Anesth Analg* 2011;113:1098–102.
37. Practice guidelines for obstetric anesthesia: An updated report by the American Society of Anesthesiologists Task Force on Obstetric Anesthesia and the Society for Obstetric Anesthesia and Perinatology. *Anesthesiology*. 2016;124(2):270–300.
38. American Society of Anesthesiologists. *Standards for Basic Intra-Operative Monitoring*. Park Ridge, IL: American Society of Anesthesiologists; October 21, 1998.
39. Gin T, Gregory MA, Oh TE. The hemodynamic effects of propofol and thiopentone for induction of caesarean section. *Anaesth Intensive Care* 1990;18: 175–9.
40. Moore J, Bill KM, Flynn RJ, McKeating KT, Howard PJ. A comparison between propofol and thiopentone as induction agents in obstetric anaesthesia. *Anaesthesia* 1989;44:753–7.
41. Gregory MA, Gin T, Yau G, Leung RK, Chan K, Oh TE. Propofol infusion anaesthesia for caesarean section. *Can J Anaesth* 1990;37:514–20.
42. Yau G, Gin T, Ewart MC, Kotur CF, Leung RK, Oh TE. Propofol for induction and maintenance of anaesthesia at caesarean section: A comparison with thiopentone/enflurane. *Anaesthesia* 1991;46:20–23.
43. Dailland P, Cockshott ID, Lirzin JD, Jacquist P, Jorrot JC, Devery J, Harmey JL, Conseiller C. Intravenous propofol during cesarean delivery: Placental transfer, concentrations in breast milk, and neonatal effects—A preliminary study. *Anesthesiology* 1989;71:827–34.

44. Alon E, Ball RH, Gille MH, Parer JF, Rosen MA, Shnider SM. Effects of propofol and thiopental on maternal and fetal cardiovascular and acid-base variables in the pregnant ewe. *Anesthesiology* 1993;78:562–76.
45. Kuczkowski KM, Reisner LS, Lin D. Anesthesia for Cesarean delivery. In: Chestnut DH, ed. *Obstetric Anesthesia: Principles and Practice,* 3rd ed. Philadelphia, PA: Elsevier Mosby; 2004:421–46 (Chapter 25).
46. Kuczkowski KM. Anesthetic considerations for complicated pregnancies. In: Creasy R, Iams JD, eds. *Maternal-Fetal Medicine,* 6th ed. Philadelphia, PA: Saunders Elsevier; 2009:1147–65 (Chapter 56).
47. Kuczkowski KM. Seizures on emergence from sevoflurane anaesthesia for Caesarean section in a healthy parturient. *Anaesthesia* 2002;57:1234–5.
48. Kuczkowski KM. Sevoflurane and seizures: Déjà vu. *Acta Anaesthesiol Scand* 2004;48:1216.
49. Heesen M, Klöhr S, Hofmann T, Rossaint R, Devroe S, Straube S, Van de Velde M. Maternal and foetal effects of remifentanil for general anaesthesia in parturients undergoing caesarean section: A systematic review and meta-analysis. *Acta Anaesthesiol Scand* 2013;57:29–36.
50. Devroe S, Van de Velde M, Rex S. General anesthesia for cesarean section. *Curr Opin Anaesthesiol* 2015;28(3):240–6.
51. Sánchez-Alcaraz A, Quintana MB, Laguarda M. Placental transfer and neonatal effects of propofol in caesarean section. *J Clin Pharm Ther* 1998;23:19–23.
52. Celleno D, Capogna G, Tomassetti M, Costantino P, Di Feo G, Nisini R. Neurobehavioural effects of propofol on the neonate following elective caesarean section. *Br J Anaesth* 1989;62:649–54.
53. Gin T, O'Meara ME, Kan AF, Leung RK, Tan P, Yau G. Plasma catecholamines and neonatal condition after induction of anaesthesia with propofol or thiopentone at caesarean section. *Br J Anaesth* 1993;70:311–6.
54. Abboud TK, Zhu J, Richardson M, Peres Da Silva E, Donovan M. Intravenous propofol vs thiamylal-isoflurane for caesarean section, comparative maternal and neonatal effects. *Acta Anaesthesiol Scand* 1995;39:205–9.
55. Kuczkowski KM. Cesarean hysterectomy in the parturient with abnormal placentation: An evidence based strategy. In: Kuczkowski KM, Drobnik L., eds. *International Textbook of Obstetric Anaesthesia and Perinatal Medicine: Principles and Practice.* Warsaw, Poland: MedMedia; 2009:95–101 (Chapter 12).
56. Czarko K, Kwiatosz-Muc M, Fijałkowska A, Kowalczyk M, Rutyna R. Intraoperative awareness—Comparison of its incidence in women undergoing general anaesthesia for caesarean section and for gynaecological procedures. *Anaesthesiol Intensive Ther* 2013;45:200–4.
57. Paech MJ, Scott KL, Clavisi O, Chua S, McDonnell N; ANZCA Trials Group. A prospective study of awareness and recall associated with general anaesthesia for caesarean section. *Int J Obstet Anesth* 2008;17:298–303.
58. Zand F, Hadavi SM, Chohedri A, Sabetian P. Survey on the adequacy of depth of anaesthesia with bispectral index and isolated forearm technique in elective Caesarean section under general anaesthesia with sevoflurane. *Br J Anaesth* 2014;112(5):871–8.
59. Lawes EG, Newman B, Campbell MJ, Irwin M, Dolenska S, Thomas TA. Maternal inspired oxygen concentration and neonatal status for caesarean section under general anaesthesia. Comparison of effects of 33% or 50% oxygen in nitrous oxide. *Br J Anaesth* 1988;61:250–4.
60. Barr G, Jakobsson JG, Owall A, Anderson RE. Nitrous oxide does not alter bispectral index: Study with nitrous oxide as sole agent and as an adjunct to i.v. anaesthesia. *Br J Anaesth* 1999;82:827–30.
61. Anderson RE, Jakobsson JG. Entropy of EEG during anaesthetic induction: A comparative study with propofol or nitrous oxide as sole agent. *Br J Anaesth* 2004;92:167–70.
62. Robins K, Lyons G. Intraoperative awareness during general anesthesia for cesarean delivery. *Anesth Analg* 2009;109:886–90.
63. Myles PS, Leslie K, McNeil J, Forbes A, Chan MT. Bispectral index monitoring to prevent awareness during anaesthesia: The B-Aware randomised controlled trial. *Lancet* 2004;363:1757–63.
64. Mychaskiw G, Horowitz M, Sachdev V, Heath BJ. Explicit intraoperative recall at a Bispectral Index of 47. *Anesth Analg* 2001;92:808–9.
65. Pilkington S, Carli F, Dakin MJ, Romney M, De Witt KA, Doré CJ, Cormack RS. Increase in Mallampati score during pregnancy. *Br J Anaesth* 1995;74:638–42.
66. Habib AS. Is it time to revisit tracheal intubation for Cesarean delivery? *Can J Anaesth* 2012;59:642–7.
67. Kuczkowski KM, Benumof JL. Subglottic tracheal stenosis in pregnancy: Anaesthetic implications. *Anaesth Intensive Care* 2003;31:576–7.
68. Feske SK, Singhal AB. Cerebrovascular disorders complicating pregnancy. *Continuum (Minneap Minn)* 2014;20:80–99.
69. Lanska DJ, Kryscio RJ. Risk factors for peripartum and postpartum stroke and intracranial venous thrombosis. *Stroke* 2000;31:1274–82.
70. Foo L, Bewley S, Rudd A. Maternal death from stroke: A thirty year national retrospective review. *Eur J Obstet Gynecol Reprod Biol* 2013;171:266–70.
71. Liang CC, Chang SD, Lai SL, Hsieh CC, Chueh HY, Lee TH. Stroke complicating pregnancy and the puerperium. *Eur J Neurol* 2006;13:1256–60.

72. Bateman BT, Schumacher HC, Bushnell CD, Pile-Spellman J, Simpson LL, Sacco RL, Berman MF. Intracerebral hemorrhage in pregnancy: Frequency, risk factors, and outcome. *Neurology* 2006;67:424–9.
73. Takahashi JC, Iihara K, Ishii A, Watanabe E, Ikeda T, Miyamoto S. Pregnancy-associated intracranial hemorrhage: Results of a survey of neurosurgical institutes across Japan. *J Stroke Cerebrovasc Dis* 2014;23:e65–71.
74. Eisenach JC, Pan P, Smiley RM, Lavand'homme P, Landau R, Houle TT. Resolution of pain after childbirth. *Anesthesiology* 2013;118:143–51.
75. Nikolajsen L, Sørensen HC, Jensen TS, Kehlet H. Chronic pain following Caesarean section. *Acta Anaesthesiol Scand* 2004;48:111–6.

Local anesthesia for cesarean delivery
Epidural, spinal, and combined spinal–epidural anesthesia

KRZYSZTOF KUCZKOWSKI, TOSHIYUKI OKUTOMI, and RIE KATO

INTRODUCTION

Obstetric anesthesia is responsible for 3%–12% of all maternal deaths [1,2]. The majority of maternal deaths occur during administration of general anesthesia and result from airway management-related complications (e.g., failed intubation, failed ventilation, and inadequate oxygenation) [1]. Subsequently, many obstetric anesthesiologists are recommending administration of regional anesthesia when possible, and that general anesthesia be given only when it is absolutely indicated [1–3]. Regional anesthesia is the technique of choice for cesarean delivery for the following reasons: (1) it is safer for the mother, (2) it has less depressant effects on the baby, (3) it allows mothers to be awake during the birth of their babies, and (4) the technique is simpler. Neuraxial techniques include three choices: spinal, epidural, and combined spinal–epidural (CSE) anesthesia. One of them is chosen based on its characteristics, maternal preference, maternal general health condition, and the indications (e.g., fetal distress) for cesarean delivery.

SINGLE-SHOT SPINAL AND *DE NOVO* EPIDURAL TECHNIQUE

Spinal anesthesia is an appropriate choice for most elective and urgent cesarean deliveries in parturients without preexisting epidural anesthesia because of its simplicity, speed, and reliability. In contrast, the popularity of *de novo* epidural anesthesia for elective cesarean delivery is decreasing (somewhat less reliable and currying higher risk of local anesthetic toxicity). In the past, epidural anesthesia was believed to be superior to spinal anesthesia for a parturient with preeclampsia because its slow onset guaranteed more hemodynamic stability. However, several studies have shown that the hemodynamic effects of spinal anesthesia are similar to those of epidural technique [4,5] (Table 19.1).

EXTENSION OF EPIDURAL LABOR ANALGESIA FOR NONELECTIVE CESAREAN DELIVERY

If the epidural catheter is already in situ and fully functional and tested for labor analgesia (and time permits), the indwelling epidural catheter is utilized for epidural anesthesia for nonelective cesarean delivery.

COMBINED SPINAL–EPIDURAL TECHNIQUE

Combined spinal–epidural (CSE) anesthesia has gained significant (and still increasing) popularity in contemporary obstetric anesthesia practice worldwide. CSE may be the technique of choice when the ability of rapid-onset, dense spinal block and the flexibility to prolong the duration of anesthesia in time (as needed) via an epidural catheter is desired [6]. CSE was first introduced as two interspace techniques (separate spinal and epidural needles inserted at different interspaces). However, the needle-through-needle technique with special CSE-specific needle design (via a single interspace) is now almost universally used [6].

The needle-through-needle CSE technique is advantageous for the obese parturient [7]. In the United States more than 30% of parturients presenting for obstetric anesthesia are overweight and/or obese. In the obese patients, the spinal needle may not be advanced straight and easily into the subarachnoid space, because the distance from skin to the subarachnoid space is much longer than in nonobese parturients. With a CSE technique, the epidural needle can be used as an "introducer" for the spinal needle. Once epidural space is identified with a loss of resistance technique, the spinal needle may be easily advanced through the epidural needle. CSE is also preferred in cases where anesthesia-related rapid hemodynamic changes should be avoided, such as for parturients with cardiac disease [8]. Prior to the initiation of epidural anesthesia, the degree of the residual spinal anesthetic effects should be considered.

SPINAL ANATOMY

In adults, the spinal cord typically extends to the lower border of L1 vertebrae or L1/2 interspace level [9]. Hence, spinal needle insertion must be performed at L2/3 or more caudal interspaces in order to avoid direct trauma to the spinal cord. The primary insertion level for cesarean delivery is the L3/4 or L4/5 interspace. Figure 19.1 depicts a transverse section image at the fourth lumbar vertebra. The main constituents in the subarachnoid space at this level are cerebral spinal fluid, cauda equina, and blood vessels. The target area for spinal anesthesia should be this space. The arachnoid and the dura matter constitute the outer layer of the subarachnoid space. Surrounding the dura matter is the epidural space, the dorsal part of which is used for epidural anesthesia. The ligamentum flavum, the key structure to identify the epidural space, is located immediately dorsal to it. An epidural catheter for cesarean delivery is usually placed through L3/4 or L4/5 so that T4–S5, the necessary block range for the surgery, is successfully blocked.

Table 19.1 Advantages and disadvantages: Spinal, epidural, combined spinal–epidural (CSE) anesthesia

	Spinal	Epidural	CSE
Technique	Simple	Moderate	Complex
Speed of induction	Fast	Slow	Moderate
Reliability	Reliable	Least reliable	Less reliable
Effect duration	Limited	Can be extended	Can be extended
Dose of local anesthetic	Low	High	Moderate
Hemodynamic changes	Rapid and large	Slow and small	Moderate
Local anesthetic toxicity	None	Can be caused	Can be caused

MEDICATIONS

Spinal anesthesia

The choice of any particular local anesthetic primarily depends on the availability of the agent, condition of the patient, obstetrical indications for delivery, and preference of the anesthesia provider. The use of lidocaine should be withheld because of concerns about neurotoxicity (e.g., transient neurologic syndrome) [10,11]. Whichever agent is chosen, a hyperbaric anesthetic is generally selected for cesarean delivery. An isobaric anesthetic is diffused in the subarachnoid space from the injection site, and a hyperbaric one is spread by gravity along the physiological spinal curvature (Figure 19.2). Hence, block to T4 dermatome is more rapidly achieved with hyperbaric solutions of local anesthetics.

Fentanyl or sufentanil (most popular opioids in obstetrics) are commonly added to the local anesthetic agent. These opioids are known to extend duration of anesthetic effects and also decrease intraoperative nausea and vomiting. However, they do not contribute to postoperative analgesia because of short duration of action. Therefore, morphine is often administered in addition to either of the short-acting opioids. Side effects of intrathecal morphine include postoperative nausea/vomiting, pruritus, and delayed respiratory depression. Respiratory depression is usually minimal but can be life threatening [12]. Therefore, respiratory rate and pulse oximetry should be monitored for at least 24 hours after administration of intrathecal (spinal) morphine.

It must be noted that nerve roots inside the subarachnoid space are highly vulnerable to chemical injury (e.g., adhesive arachnoiditis). A small amount of noxious agent can result in significant neurologic deficits. Although anesthetic agents with preservatives are commonly used for epidural anesthesia, preservatives should not be injected into the subarachnoid space. Caution should be exercised to avoid contamination of subarachnoid injectate with preservatives. See Table 19.2.

Epidural anesthesia

Local anesthetic used for epidural anesthesia is similar to that used for spinal anesthesia, but the epidural dose is much higher than the spinal dose. The drug choices for elective cesarean delivery or extension of epidural labor analgesia for nonurgent cesarean deliveries include 0.5% bupivacaine or levobupivacaine, 2%–3% chloroprocaine, and 0.5%–0.75% ropivacaine. Bupivacaine 0.75%, which had been used in the United States in the past for spinal anesthesia, is no longer approved for this purpose in the United States

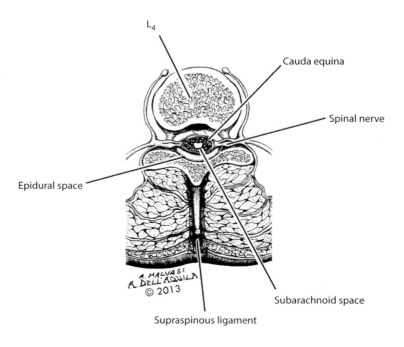

Figure 19.1 Cross section of spinal anatomy.

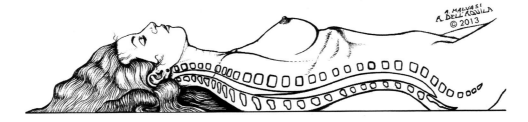

Figure 19.2 Physiological curvature of the spine: hyperbaric anesthetic solution injected at lower lumbar flow down to the thoracic and sacrum kyphosis.

Table 19.2 Local anesthetic agents and opioids used for spinal anesthesia

		Dose	Duration (hours)
Local anesthetics	Bupivacaine	10–15 mg	1–2
	Levobupivacaine	10–15 mg	1–2
	Ropivacaine	15–25 mg	1–2
	Lidocaine	60–80 mg	0.75–1.25
Opioids	Fentanyl	10–20 mcg	3–4 (for postoperative analgesia)
	Sufentanil	2.5–5 mcg	3–4 (for postoperative analgesia)
	Morphine	0.1–0.2 mg	6–12 (for postoperative analgesia)

Table 19.3 Local anesthetic agents and opioids used for epidural anesthesia

		Concentration/dose	Volume
Local anesthetics	Chloroprocaine	2%–3%	15–20 mL
	Lidocaine	2%	15–20 mL
	Bupivacaine	0.5%	15–20 mL
	Levobupivacaine	0.5%–0.75%	15–20 mL
	Ropivacaine	0.5%–0.75%	15–20 mL
Opioids	Fentanyl	100 mcg	—
	Sufentanil	5–10 mcg	—
	Morphine	2–3 mg	—

by the U.S. Food and Drug Administration (FDA). This is due to case reports of unintentional intravenous injections of 0.75% bupivacaine leading to maternal cardiac arrest. Levobupivacaine and ropivacaine are relatively new L- or S-isomer agents, resulting in less potential for cardiotoxicity.

For urgent cesarean deliveries, chloroprocaine or lidocaine is usually used. When the surgery is urgent, 2% lidocaine combined with 8.4% (1 mEq/mL) sodium bicarbonate is usually used. The ratio of 2% lidocaine:sodium bicarbonate is about 10–20:1 in volume. The alkalization of local anesthetic by sodium bicarbonate not only shortens the onset of blockade but also improves its quality, and prolongs the duration of the blockade. Alkalization increases the nonionized form of local anesthetic molecules, which pass more easily through the neuronal membrane than ionized molecules. When selecting an appropriate anesthetic agent it is important to remember that the duration of action of chloroprocaine and lidocaine is shorter than the duration of action of bupivacaine, levobupivacaine, and ropivacaine. Subsequently, top-up boluses may be necessary during surgery when either chloroprocaine or lidocaine is selected.

Neuraxial opioids are often combined with local anesthetic in order to shorten the onset of anesthesia, and improve and prolong the duration of surgical anesthesia.

One meta-analysis showed that 100 mcg fentanyl combined with 2% lidocaine, or 75 mcg fentanyl combined with levobupivacaine shortened (by 2 minutes) the onset of surgical anesthesia [13]. The study in question also demonstrated that a mixture of lidocaine and epinephrine, with or without fentanyl, shortened the onset of surgical anesthesia.

Short-acting opioids (e.g., fentanyl) are used for their intraoperative analgesic effects, and morphine (a long-acting opioid) is used for its postoperative analgesia. These neuraxial opioids have side effects, such as pruritus, nausea and vomiting, delayed gastric emptying, urinary retention, sedation, and respiratory depression. Morphine-induced respiratory depression is usually minimal, but might be life threatening. Therefore, the patient who received epidural morphine should be continuously monitored (with pulse oximetry) for at least 24 hours after morphine administration. See Table 19.3.

Combined spinal–epidural anesthesia

The CSE technique offers the possibility of combining rapid onset of subarachnoid anesthesia with the flexibility of continuous epidural anesthesia during cesarean delivery [14]. Selection of local anesthetics and opioids is identical to what has been outlined above for each technique when used alone.

PREPARATION FOR ANESTHESIA

Although the technique of neuraxial anesthesia is simpler than that of general anesthesia, preparation for both techniques is the same and includes pre-anesthetic evaluation, administration of pre-anesthetic medications and intravenous fluids, maternal positioning and monitoring of both the mother and the fetus [1,3,7,8].

Pre-anesthetic evaluation

As outlined in Practice Advisory published by the American Society of Anesthesiologists [15] a detailed maternal medical and anesthetic history, medications, allergies, laboratory data, and baseline blood pressure and heart rate must be obtained prior to anesthesia. Physical examination includes evaluation of airway (please see Chapter 18, "General Anesthesia for Cesarean Delivery: Indications and Complications"), heart, and lungs. For neuraxial anesthesia, close attention must be paid to maternal coagulation status and the needle insertion site (evaluation of the back area) [16,17].

Coagulopathy is one of the contraindications to neuraxial anesthesia, as it can result in epidural hematoma. When acquired coagulopathy is suspected (e.g., hemolysis, elevated liver enzymes, low platelet count [HELLP] syndrome, placental abruption, and/or maternal sepsis), coagulation studies (e.g., platelet counts, prothrombin time, and activated partial thromboplastin time) must be obtained prior to regional anesthesia. It needs to be emphasized that there are no universal criteria for laboratory parameters which would guarantee safe neuraxial anesthesia [18]. As for parturients on anticoagulant therapy, it is sensible to refer to the evidence-based practice guidelines [19,20].

Anatomical disorder, infection, and neoplasms at the site of needle insertion may be contraindications to neuraxial technique [21]. Maternal hypovolemia is another contraindication to neuraxial anesthesia. When sensory nerves are blocked by neuraxial anesthesia, sympathetic nerves are also blocked, resulting in vasodilation. This causes hypotension, which requires aggressive and prompt treatment to avoid maternal and fetal complications. Anesthesia-related hypotension is aggravated by pre-existing hypovolemia [1,7,8,14].

Aspiration prophylaxis

Laboring women can drink clear water as they desire, but solid foods should be avoided in labor [22,23]. Healthy parturients undergoing elective cesarean delivery may drink a modest amount of clear liquids (e.g., water, tea/coffee without milk/creamer) until 2 hours before induction of anesthesia, regardless of the anesthetic method used. Solid foods should be refrained from for 6–8 hours [22,23] prior to surgery.

Prophylactic administration of H_2 receptor blockers, nonparticle antacids, and/or metoclopramide should be considered for elective cesarean delivery [14,15].

Monitoring

Basic monitoring of maternal pulse, oximetry, ECG, and blood pressure, is mandatory in all cesarean delivery patients. Monitoring must be initiated on admission to the labor and delivery room and/or operating room and continued until the end of anesthesia/recovery from anesthesia. Additional monitoring is individualized depending on institutional standards and the condition of the patient.

TECHNICAL ISSUES OF OBSTETRIC ANESTHETIC CARE

Positioning

The "ideal" patient positioning for neuraxial needle insertion requires (1) straight spinal column, (2) wide interspinous spaces, and (3) easy identification of the spinal column by palpation. Patients are usually required to hunch in a sitting or lateral decubitus position (Figure 19.3). The sitting position is preferred by many anesthesia providers because it is easier to identify the midline axis. However, orthostatic hypotension is more likely to occur in the sitting position. It is important to make sure that parturients in the sitting position do not lean sideways. A footstool or a pillow on the lap may help them maintain a straight position. When performing neuraxial anesthesia in the lateral decubitus position, right lateral (rather than left lateral) position is usually chosen, because it enhances the speed of bilateral block with left uterine displacement [24]. In either sitting or lateral decubitus, "tight curl" position should be avoided in women with a gravid uterus at term as it may cause aorto-caval compression [25,26]. The authors recommend that the duration of the curl position be as short as possible.

Locating the needle insertion site

The anatomical landmark for the estimation of vertebral level is the intercristal line (Tuffier's line, Jacoby's line), which is known to most frequently cross L4 vertebral body level (Figure 19.4). The anesthetist must palpate the iliac crest and estimate vertebral levels before needle insertion.

However, this widely used palpation method is far from accurate. It is a common belief that palpation estimates in the sitting position are ≥1 vertebral higher than the anatomical position [27,28]. Estimate errors can also arise in the lateral decubitus position (Figure 19.5). Ultrasound-guided vertebral-level estimation may be a promising technique for more accurate estimation. Paramedian longitudinal views enable us to identify sacrum, lumbar vertebrae, and intervertebral spaces; it is also possible to estimate the depth of the epidural space in the transverse view [29].

Pre-anesthetic antiseptic preparations

Hand washing by the practitioner

Prior to any anesthetic procedure, the practitioner should consider proper hand preparation (e.g., washing). Basic soap and water simply move bacteria on the skin surface, instead of removing them, and therefore, these are not effective in killing microorganisms. Therefore, the use of alcohol-containing solutions or alcohol is recommended, especially by rubbing the practitioner's hands. This is superior to hand washing with nonalcoholic antiseptic solutions such as povidone iodine or chlorhexidine [30].

Technical issues of obstetric anesthetic care 327

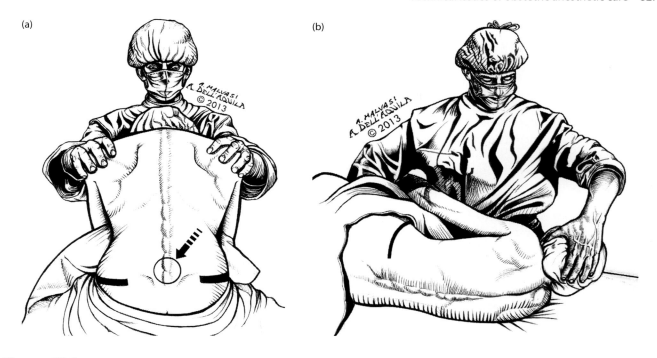

Figure 19.3 (a) Patient positioning for neuraxial anesthesia procedures, sitting position. (b) Patient positioning for neuraxial anesthesia procedures, lateral position.

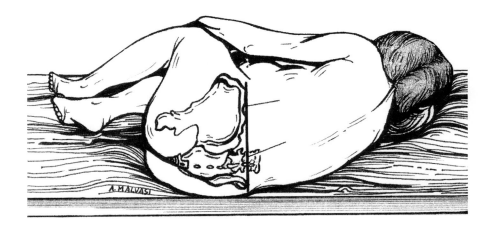

Figure 19.4 Intercristal line.

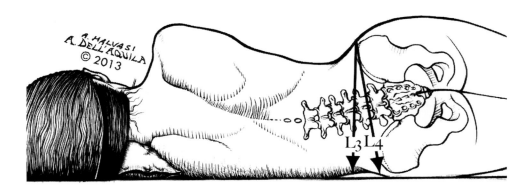

Figure 19.5 Possible interspace estimation error in the lateral position. The error may be more likely in pregnant women at term whose hips are greater in size.

Masks, gowns, and gloves

The clinical significance of wearing a surgical gown for neuraxial anesthesia is not supported by evidence, and remains controversial. Gown technique is common in the United Kingdom, but not in the United States, France, and Japan [31].

To the contrary, anesthetic providers should always wear a surgical mask during neuraxial procedures. The practice advisory of the American Society of Anesthesiologists recommends use of surgical masks during administration of all kinds of regional anesthesia [32]. In spite of these recommendations, five healthy women who underwent spinal anesthesia for labor developed bacterial meningitis, and one of them subsequently died [33]. Four of the cases were confirmed to be infections with *Streptococcus salivarius*, a bacterium of the normal human mouth flora.

It is routine practice to wear sterile gloves for neuraxial techniques. Latex or vinyl gloves are usually worn depending on institutional guidelines and/or provider's preference.

Skin preparation at the needle insertion site

The importance of aseptic skin preparation technique at the site of neuraxial needle insertion site cannot be overemphasized. The aseptic skin preparation should be performed after the proper patient positioning (for induction of regional anesthesia) is established [14].

Although the most commonly used disinfectants include povidone iodine- and chlorhexidine-based solutions, the ideal solution is still controversial. Chlorhexidine with or without alcohol (isopropyl alcohol or ethanol) is recommended for prevention of intravenous catheter-related infections. However, the evidence is not conclusive that chlorhexidine-based solutions reduce infectious complications associated with neuraxial anesthesia.

The American Society of Anesthesiologists Task Force published the recommendation to use the alcohol-based solutions in 2010 [32]. The superiority of alcohol-based solutions is based on the fact that they eliminate the *Staphylococcus* flora in the corneal layer of the skin better than non-alcohol-based skin prep solutions. Disadvantages of alcohol-based solutions include its flammability (fire hazard in the operating room) and irritant properties to skin and/or mucus membranes.

Needles, syringes, catheters

Spinal needles

Spinal needles fall into two categories: those with beveled tips and cutting edges and those with pencil-point tips. The pencil-point tip needles are recommended because they reduce the incidence of postdural puncture headache [14,34,35]. Pencil-point needles also provide better tactile feel as they pass through layers of tissues, especially the dura.

Smaller-gauge needles are less likely to cause postdural puncture headache [34] but more likely to deflect than larger-gauge needles. The most commonly used needle size for cesarean delivery is 25–27 gauge.

Epidural needles

The most common types of epidural needles used in obstetrics are the 17- to 18-gauge Tuohy (or Tuohy–Schliff) needles with a curved tip and a lateral facing orifice. This lateral orifice avoids the undesired insertion of the epidural catheter toward the dura mater and facilitates smooth catheter insertion.

CSE needles

It has been reported that combining spinal and epidural blocks may appear cumbersome and time consuming [14]. However, newer CSE trays have eliminated many equipment limitations, and thus reduced preparation time. In experienced hands the entire procedure should not take longer than approximately 4–5 minutes. An 18-guage Tuohy (or other type) epidural needle, placed in the lumbar epidural interspace, serves as an introducer to a long 27-gauge pencil-point spinal needle that punctures the dura and subarachnoid mater of the spinal cord allowing the initial injection of the subarachnoid dose for induction of labor analgesia [14]. There is even a special CSE needle set on the market, which allows the spinal needle to be "locked" on the epidural needle, so it is kept in fixed position during administration of spinal medications (Figure 19.6).

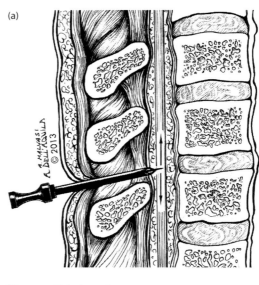

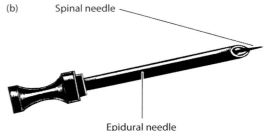

Figure 19.6 (a and b) Combined spinal and epidural needle; the spinal needle is inserted through the epidural needle.

Loss of resistance (LOR) syringes

In the LOR syringe the internal wall of the barrel is coated with silicon to reduce friction between the barrel and plunger. This helps the operator to feel the resistance change when an epidural needle tip enters the epidural space.

Catheters

The epidural catheter may either have a single orifice or multiple orifices. A multi-orifice catheter may result in a smaller incidence of patchy or unilateral blocks [36]. Some practitioners prefer wire-embedded catheters because of less likelihood of an unintentional intravenous catheter insertion [37]. However, the outcome with the use of either single-orifice or multi-orifice catheters is similar [38].

Words of wisdom—spinal anesthesia

Midline approach using non-cutting-edge needle (Figure 19.7):

1. Identify the interspinous space (L3/4 or L4/5*) in the midline (Figure 19.8a).
2. Make a skin wheel with local anesthetic over the selected injection site.
3. Insert the introducer† in the midline. (Figure 19.8a).
4. Hold the introducer with the nondominant hand (index finger and thumb) and insert the spinal needle through the introducer using the dominant hand (Figure 19.8b).
5. Advance the spinal needle in the midline slowly to sense the resistance of the needle.‡ There are two resistance changes until it enters the subarachnoid space. The first subtle "pop" is noted as the needle passes through the ligamentum flavum. This is followed by the second bigger "pop" as it goes through the dura.
6. Remove the stylet of the needle while grasping the needle hub with the nondominant index finger and thumb. The cerebrospinal fluid (CSF) should flow into the needle hub.
7. Keep the needle steady and connect a medication syringe (Figure 19.8c).
8. Confirm easy aspiration of the free-flowing CSF with the syringe, and then administer medications at a rate of approximately 0.2 mL/s.

---

* When interspaces were identified by palpation of the intercristal line, it is prudent not to choose L2/3 interspace for needle insertion in order to avoid traumatic injury to the spinal cord. Note that palpation estimates are often ≥1 vertebral higher than the anatomical position [28,39].

† It is recommended to insert a non-cutting-edge needle through an introducer in order to avoid needle deflection (Figure 19.8d) and contamination with skin flora.

‡ Great care should be taken to avoid displacement of the needle tip from the subarachnoid to the epidural space. It is recommended that the dorsum of the nondominant hand should be anchored against the patient's back while the fingers and thumb grasp the needle (Figure 19.8c).

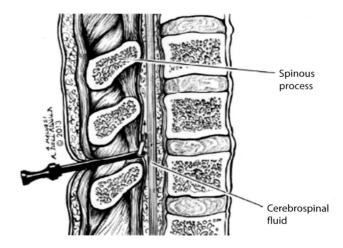

Figure 19.7 Needle placement—midline approach, sagittal image.

Troubleshooting:

- If the needle contacts a bone, redirect it to a slightly cephalad (or caudal) direction. If redirection does not help, withdraw the needle completely and move the insertion site slightly cephalad or caudal in the midline. Change the interspace if the needle still contacts a bone.
- If CSF does not appear in the needle hub after removing the stylet following the characteristic "pop," rotate the needle in 90° increments until CSF appears. If CSF still does not appear, advance the needle by 1 mm with caution.
- If CSF flow is minimal when aspirated, it can be either that the needle tip hole is not completely placed in the subarachnoid space (Figure 19.9), or cauda equina is plugging the needle hole. Advance the needle by 1 mm and check for free-flowing CFS again.

Words of wisdom—epidural anesthesia

Midline approach (Figure 19.10):

1. Identify the interspinous space (L3/4 or L4/5) in the midline.
2. Make a skin wheel with local anesthetic over the selected insertion site.
3. Advance the epidural needle in the midline through the supraspinous ligament and interspinous ligament to the ligamentum flavum (Figure 19.11a). The practitioner should be able to discriminate different ligaments by tactile sensation.
4. With the needle tip in the ligamentum flavum, remove the stylet and connect an LOR syringe (or other) filled with saline or air§ to the hub of the epidural needle.
5. Grasp the needle wing with the nondominant hand and push toward the epidural space, while applying constant pressure on the LOR (or other) syringe plunger with the dominant thumb (Figure 19.11b). When the needle tip

---

§ Saline is safer than air because air can cause pneumocephalus in case of unintentional dural puncture, resulting in severe headache [40]. Injection of air into the epidural space can also lead to patchy block.

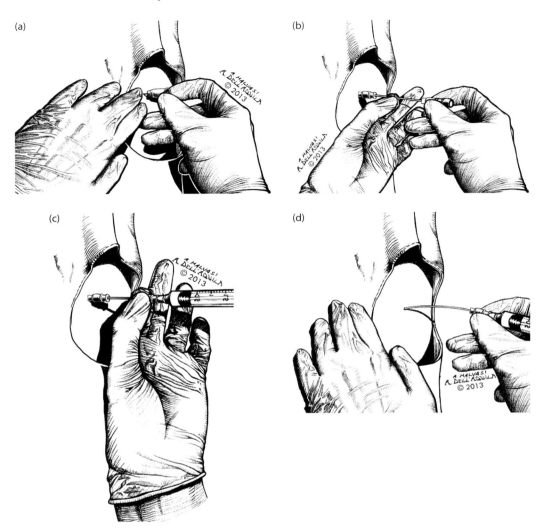

Figure 19.8 Procedures for spinal anesthesia: (a) insertion of an introducer, (b) spinal needle insertion through the introducer, (c) administration of medications to the subarachnoid space, and (d) deflection of spinal needle.

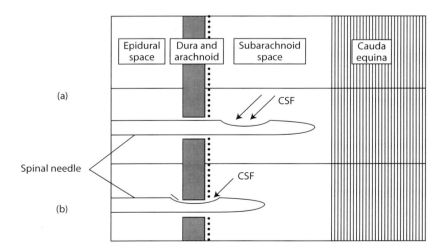

Figure 19.9 Spinal needle orifice position. (a) The needle is placed in an appropriate position. (b) Although the very tip of the needle is in the subarachnoid space, the orifice is not completely placed inside the subarachnoid space.

Technical issues of obstetric anesthetic care 331

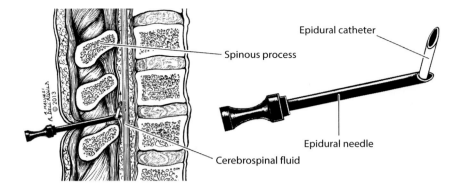

Figure 19.10 Epidural catheter placement.

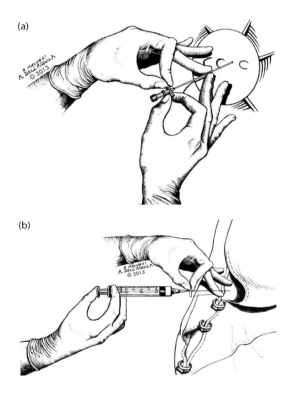

Figure 19.11 Procedures for epidural anesthesia: (a) epidural needle insertion to the ligamentum flavum, (b) loss of resistance technique.

enters the epidural space, the nondominant hand feels reduction in resistance and the syringe plunger allows the saline or air to flow without resistance into the epidural space.
6. Thread an epidural catheter slowly through the epidural needle 4–5 cm into the epidural space.*
7. Remove the epidural needle slowly, while the catheter is kept in place.
8. Once the epidural catheter is placed in the desired position, secure it with a transparent adhesive dressing.

---

* The shorter the length of the catheter in the epidural space, the higher is the incidence of catheter displacement. To the contrary, the risk of unilateral blockade is higher when the catheter length in the epidural space is longer.

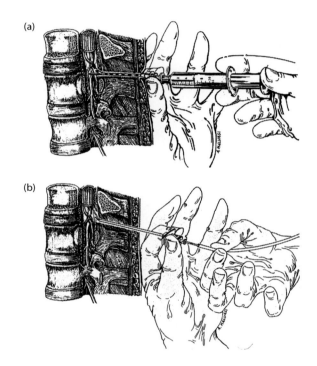

Figure 19.12 (a and b) Combined spinal and epidural anesthesia.

Words of wisdom—CSE anesthesia, needle-through-needle technique (Figure 19.12)

Midline approach:

1. Please see items 1–5 of "Technical aspects for epidural anesthesia" described above.
2. Once the epidural space is identified, remove the stylet of the epidural needle, and insert the spinal needle through the epidural needle while holding the epidural needle.
3. When a "pop" or "click" sensation is felt, remove the stylet of the spinal needle while grasping the spinal needle hub with the nondominant hand.
4. With confirmation of CSF flow into the spinal needle hub, connect a medication syringe, then administer medication (same way as with spinal anesthesia).

5. Remove the spinal needle with an empty medication syringe.
6. Thread an epidural catheter slowly (same way as with epidural anesthesia).

Confirming anesthetic block effects

A dermatome is an area of skin supplied by a single spinal nerve root (Figure 19.13). Knowledge of dermatomes is crucial when evaluating the extent (height) of neuraxial blockade. Some landmark dermatomes are shown in Table 19.4.

Bilateral block height from S5 to T4 is needed for cesarean surgery. It is sometimes misunderstood that only T10–12 blockade is necessary (as surgical site is the lower abdomen and pelvis). Although skin incision is made on the skin innervated by T10–12, sensory nerves to the uterus and surrounding organs must also be blocked to provide comfortable surgery to the parturient.

Block height is determined by lack or deficit of pain or cold sensation of the skin. The sense of pain is assessed by pin-prick, ice, or alcohol swab. Contrary to the sense of pain and cold, the sense of touch and position are usually preserved after introduction of spinal/epidural/CSE anesthesia. Patients should be informed and prepared to expect touch sensation, pressure, and traction during surgery.

With spinal anesthesia a blockade to T4 level is usually achieved within 10 minutes. The onset of de novo epidural anesthesia develops much slower (e.g., 20 minutes for bupivacaine, levobupivacaine. or ropivacaine without fentanyl or sodium bicarbonate and approximately 10 minutes for lidocaine combined with fentanyl and sodium bicarbonate).

Inadequate spinal/epidural block

Causes of insufficient spinal block after seemingly successful spinal injection include misplaced injection, abnormal

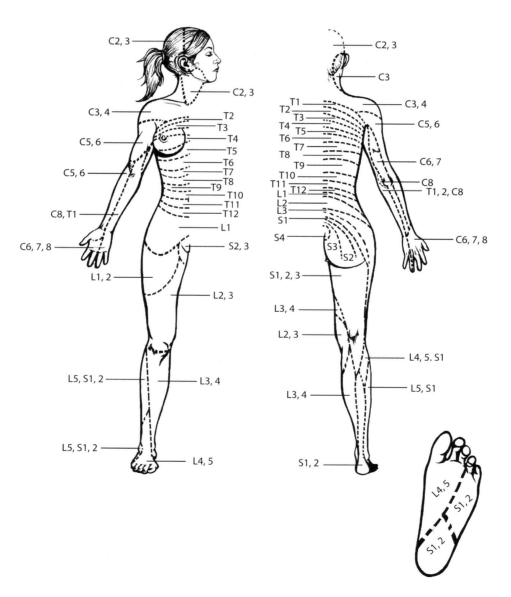

Figure 19.13 Dermatomes.

Table 19.4 Landmark dermatomes

Area of skin	Dermatome
Nipple	T4
Tip of xiphoid process	T6
Umbilicus	T10
Perineum	S2–4

anatomy, and medication errors [41]. Figure 19.13 shows an example of misplaced injection. Some injectate is lost to the epidural space, hence an insufficient blockade. Rarely, cauda equina or ligaments, which support the spinal cord within the subarachnoid space, can behave as a barrier preventing anesthetics from spreading.

Performing a second spinal injection in case of insufficient spinal block is controversial. As the second full dose might result in high spinal block, it is reasonable to reduce the second dose.

The success rate of epidural anesthesia is lower than that of spinal anesthesia. Asymmetric block is not uncommon. One of the causes of this phenomenon is an epidural catheter migration to the paravertebral space. Patchy block occurs when a catheter is unintentionally placed in the subdural space.

SIDE EFFECTS AND COMPLICATIONS
Hypotension

Hypotension is a side effect quite commonly observed after induction of spinal, epidural, and CSE anesthesia. Hypotension is especially noticeable with spinal anesthesia where the incidence can be as high as 80%. Hypotension is less common in epidural anesthesia because the incidence and severity of hypotension are partly determined by the speed of onset of epidural block. Neuraxial anesthesia-related hypotension is caused by blockade of sympathetic vasomotor activity that is innervated through spinal nerves. When the parturient is turned to the supine position, gravid uterus compresses the descending aorta and inferior vena cava (aorto-caval compression syndrome) and can further lower the maternal blood pressure.

Hypotension can result in maternal nausea/vomiting, unconsciousness, and cardiac arrest. However, uteroplacental perfusion and fetal compromise might be more vulnerable to its effects. Hypotension must be prevented and treated aggressively when it occurs (Box 19.1). Parturients of 20 or more weeks' gestation should have a left tilt when positioned in the supine position. Intravenous fluid

Box 19.1 Prophylaxis and management of hypotension

- Crystalloid coloading or colloid loading
- Left uterine displacement
- Ephedrine/phenylephrine

preloading with 500–1000 mL of crystalloid solution is a classical prophylactic method against hypotension. However, it has been reported that intravascular colloid infusions might be more effective [42].

Left uterine displacement and/or intravascular fluid infusions do not completely prevent hypotension after neuraxial anesthesia. Hence, vasopressors must be ready at hand. For decades, ephedrine (an adrenalin α, β-agonist) was believed to be the vasopressor of choice for treatment of hypotension during neuraxial anesthesia for cesarean delivery. However, some studies have demonstrated that phenylephrine (an α-agonist) is equally effective and safe to prevent and treat hypotension induced by spinal anesthesia [43]. It seems reasonable to choose either vasopressor depending on maternal heart rate; when the parturient is bradycardic ephedrine would be the first line, and when tachycardic, phenylephrine should be used. Ephedrine is usually administered by intravenous boluses of 5–10 mg. Phenylephrine can be given by either boluses of 0.05–0.1 mg or infusion of 0.025–0.1 mg/min.

Postdural puncture headache (PDPH)

Postdural puncture headache (PDPH) also known as spinal (or postspinal) headache remains a disabling complication of needle insertion into the subarachnoid space. Parturients are at increased risk of dural puncture, and the subsequent headache, because of sex, young age, and the widespread use of regional anesthesia in obstetrics [7,14,35,40].

The incidence of this complication depends on the type and size of needle used. However, several articles reported that the frequency of PDPH did not increase with CSE technique when compared with spinal [44] or epidural anesthesia [45,46]. Typically the headache is pulsatile, frontal to parietal, and occasionally occipital in location. It is positional, exacerbated by sitting or standing, but gradually relieved in the supine position. Neck pain, nausea and vomiting, tinnitus, and diplopia may accompany the often severe cephalgia. Symptoms usually develop within 2–3 days following dural puncture with a needle. Most cases of PDPH resolve within a few weeks. However, some headaches might last for several months or over a year. The differential diagnosis includes severe preeclampsia or eclampsia, posterior reversible encephalopathy syndrome, subdural hemorrhage [47], venous sinus thrombosis/cortical vein thrombosis, pneumocephalus, and meningitis. Etiology may be due to the decrease in the CSF volume or pressure, or both, leading to traction on pain-sensitive brain structures. Cerebral vasodilation via adenosine receptor activation may be a contributing factor.

Pre-anesthetic preventive strategies:

- *Pencil-point spinal needles for spinal anesthesia*: Pencil-point needles are recommended in obstetric anesthesia practice [34]. This non-cutting-edge type of needle design is believed to separate the dural fibers instead of cutting them, so the CSF leakage is less significant when the needle is removed. Microscopic studies clearly show that the CSF leakage is less in non-cutting-edge needle than in cutting-edge needle [48]. One study showed that non-cutting needle produced a traumatic opening with tearing and severe crush of the collagen fibers while cutting needle created a sharp-cut opening of the fibers. It is believed that non-cutting needles exacerbate the inflammation reaction of the dural hole, subsequently facilitating fibroblastic proliferation of the tissues and repair of the dural hole [49]. In order to reduce the incidence of PDPH, direction of the cutting bevel should be inserted parallel to the longitudinal dural fibers [50].

- *Needle size for spinal anesthesia*: Spinal needle size is important, affecting the incidence of PDPH. However, very slow CSF flow from very small needles might require several attempts, lead to multiple dural punctures, greater failure rate, and subsequently not reduce the incidence of PDPH. It is believed that 27–25 gauge is an optimal needle size for spinal anesthesia.

Other techniques for preventing PDPH:

- Ultrasound-guided neuraxial approach may help identify the correct needle insertion site, and guide the depth and angle of the needle insertion. This may reduce unnecessary dural punctures [51,52].
- Some authors have recommend insertion of the Tuohy (or other) needle with the bevel parallel to the long axis of spine if midline approach is used [53,54], or use of paramedian approach instead [55,56]. However, this is still controversial.

Psychological support

Since PDPH is an iatrogenic complication, patients are often depressed, anxious, restless, and even angry. Therefore, it is essential that the practitioner visits the patient at least once daily to explain symptoms and prognosis with and without treatment. Psychological support and other therapeutic options in some cases might be necessary. After discharge, follow-up telephone conversation may be indicated.

Prevention of PDPH after accidental dural puncture

Although a few measures have been proposed to prevent PDPH (subarachnoid injection of normal saline, insertion of the epidural catheter into the subarachnoid space through the dural hole, etc.), none have been shown to work with certainty to date [57–63].

Kuczkowski and Benumof [64] reported that following accidental dural puncture with an 18-gauge epidural needle in pregnant women, sequential (Table 19.5) (1) injection of the CSF in the glass syringe back into the subarachnoid space through the epidural needle, (2) insertion of an epidural catheter into the subarachnoid space, (3) injection of a small amount of preservative-free saline (3–5 mL) into the subarachnoid space through the subarachnoid catheter, (4) administration of bolus and then continuous intrathecal labor analgesia, and (5) leaving the catheter in situ in the subarachnoid space for a total

Table 19.5 Prevention of PDPH in pregnant women: Maintaining CSF volume

1. Injecting the CSF in the glass syringe back into the subarachnoid space through the epidural needle
2. Passing the epidural catheter through the dural hole into the subarachnoid space
3. Injecting 3–5 mL of preservative-free saline into the subarachnoid space through the subarachnoid catheter
4. Administering bolus and then continuous intrathecal labor analgesia through the subarachnoid catheter
5. Leaving the subarachnoid catheter in situ for a total of 12–20 hours

Source: Adapted from Kuczkowski KM, Benumof JL. *Acta Anaesthesiol Scand* 2003;47:98–100.

of 12–20 hours decreased the incidence of PDPH from 76%–85% to 14% [64].

Since their original report the authors encountered eight more pregnant women in whom the performance of epidural analgesia was complicated by an accidental dural puncture with an 18-gauge epidural needle. In all eight additional cases, the accidental dural puncture was followed by the same five maneuvers and no PDPH was reported in any of these patients. These additional eight cases combined with the original seven patients ($N = 15$) suggest that following an accidental dural puncture with an 18-gauge epidural needle in parturients, sequential performance of these five maneuvers decreased the incidence of PDPH from 76%–85% (13) to 6.6%. (PDPH occurred only in one out of our total number of 15 pregnant patients.) All of these five components were aimed at maintaining CSF volume [64].

Pharmacological therapy

The first-line (conservative) therapy with medications for PDPH includes acetaminophen/paracetamol, ibuprofen, naproxen, and other nonsteroidal anti-inflammatory drugs (NSAIDs). These agents should be administered as scheduled dosing for 1–2 days instead of "as needed" dosing. For severe headache, oral or intravenous opioids may also help relieve it.

In the past years, several agents such as caffeine, sumatriptan, gabapentin, theophylline, hydrocortisone, or adrenocorticotropin (ACTH) have been investigated as treatment for PDPH. A Cochrane review in 2011 showed that each drug was effective to reduce PDPH when compared to placebo [65]. Caffeine is the most popular agent for treatment of PDPH. However, it lasts for a limited period of time. The optimal dose of caffeine is also still controversial.

Therapeutic epidural blood patch

This therapy has been clinically accepted as the "gold standard" of treatment of severe PDPH [66]. Speculative mechanisms of headache relief by epidural blood patch include (1) increase in intracranial blood pressure via compressing the thecal sac by epidural blood, resulting in restoration of tractional brain structure, (2) deactivation of adenosine receptor and reversal of cerebral vasodilation by increase in intrathecal pressure, (3) fibrin clot formation, and sealing of the dural hole with injected epidural blood.

Optimal blood volume for the epidural blood patch is controversial. Some researchers suggest that 12–15 mL blood be used for epidural blood patch [67,68], while others conclude that 7.5–10 mL is enough [69,70]. One study showed 20 mL blood relieved headache more frequently than 15 mL blood [71]. In this study, all of the subjects received their epidural blood patch more than 24 hours after the dural puncture.

If the practitioner decides to perform epidural blood patch, the procedure should be done under sterile conditions. Most practitioners let their patients remain supine for 30 minutes to 2 hours after epidural blood patch. If the treatment is effective, headache will cease within 48 hours. The overall success rate of the epidural blood patch is about 70% [72,73]. If an epidural blood patch is ineffective in relieving the headache, repeated blood patch has a similar success rate. In case of the second patch failure, repeating the patch for a third time may be considered. However, first alternative causes should be considered for persistent severe headache. The timing of the epidural blood patch is also controversial. One study shows that an epidural blood patch prior to 48 hours after dural puncture has no advantages [73]. A possible blood patch complication is a backache at the site of injection. If a patient has a fever, infection at the puncture site, or any coagulation abnormalities, treatment with blood patch is contraindicated.

Local anesthetic systemic toxicity

Local anesthetic toxicity occurs when plasma concentration of a local anesthetic increases to toxic levels. This usually happens when the epidural dose of a local anesthetic is unintentionally administered into the vessel in the epidural space. The epidural vessels are known to be engorged during pregnancy. Toxicity can also occur when a relatively large (too large) dose of local anesthetic is administered to the epidural space and slowly absorbed into the circulation. Symptoms of local anesthetic toxicity vary depending on the plasma concentration of the local anesthetic (Table 19.6). They are caused by blockade of voltage-gated Na channels in the central nervous system (CNS) and cardiovascular system (CVS).

The CNS toxicity (e.g., seizures) is due to drug potency. Equipotent doses of different local anesthetics can cause similar symptoms of toxicity. However, L- or S-isomers have less propensity to cause seizure than racemic forms of local anesthetics. Therefore, levobupivacaine and ropivacaine (L- or S-isomer) are safer than bupivacaine regarding CNS toxicity. In contrast, CVS toxicity varies among different concentrations of each drug. For example, lidocaine has a greater margin of safety than bupivacaine. Bupivacaine (7–12 mcg/mL) can produce CVS toxicity at much lower drug blood concentrations. Furthermore, a lipophilic drug such as bupivacaine is more likely to cause irreversible heart conduction blocks. Among lipophilic drugs, levobupivacaine (L- or S-isomer bupivacaine), or ropivacaine are less likely to lead to CVS compared to bupivacaine. Bupivacaine, a low-cost local anesthetic, remains popular and safe in obstetric patients, if used in low (diluted) concentrations.

Prevention of local anesthetic toxicity far outweighs treatment [74]. Aspiration of epidural catheter prior to injection and a test dosing are essential. Although epinephrine 10–20 mcg combined with a local anesthetic as a test dose may increase maternal heart rate around 10 bpm systolic blood pressure 10–20 mm Hg, it might be less sensitive and less specific in laboring women. Another preventive strategy includes slow incremental administration of local anesthetics.

When severe systemic local anesthetic toxicity occurs, airway management is essential, because hypoxemia and acidosis decrease the seizure threshold and enhance myocardial depression with increase of arrhythmogenic effect. Although benzodiazepines (e.g., diazepam and midazolam) and propofol may suppress the seizure activities, they have untoward CVS effects. If treatment of arrhythmias is needed, amiodarone is recommended rather than lidocaine. Lipid infusion therapy has become a method of choice for treatment of local anesthetic-induced CVS toxicity [75]. The mechanism includes (1) lipid drawing the local anesthetic out of the myocytes into blood; (2) lipid increasing intracellular calcium, resulting in improved cardiac contraction; or (3) lipid overcoming the loss of cardiac energy due to the local anesthetic's inhibition of acylcarnitine transferase. Recommendation of lipid rescue is 1.5 mL/kg of 20% lipid emulsion as an initial dose, followed by a maintenance infusion at 0.25 mL/kg/min. The bolus dose may be repeated once or twice for continued CVS toxicity, and the infusion rate may be increased to 0.5 mL/kg/min. The practitioner should be aware of lipid-related metabolic abnormalities such as increased triglyceride or amylase, volume overload, fat embolism, and allergic reaction, which may occur.

High neuraxial blockade

High neuraxial blockade is caused by excessive spread of spinal/epidural medications or unintentional subdural administration of epidural dosage of anesthetic agents.

Table 19.6 Symptoms at various (increasing) concentrations of lidocaine

Plasma concentration (mcg/mL)	Symptoms
1–5	Analgesia
5–10	Light-headedness, dizziness, tinnitus, numbness around mouth/fingertips, agitation
10–15	Tonic–clonic seizures, unconsciousness
15–25	Coma, respiratory arrest
>25	Cardiovascular depression, cardiac arrest

It causes impairment of ventilation and phonation, hypotension, bradycardia, and unconsciousness. Immediate interventions include intubation, mechanical ventilation, and administration of vasopressors. Dyspnea and handgrip weakness are early signs of high neuraxial block. The anesthesiologist must carefully monitor patient's ventilation, hemodynamics, and the level of consciousness.

Traumatic neuropathy

Insertion of spinal or epidural needle and threading of an epidural catheter sometimes causes radiating pain and/or paresthesia. It is a sign of a needle or catheter touching the nerve roots or spinal cord. It is imperative not to go ahead with the procedure when the patient reports paresthesia. The needle or catheter should be withdrawn immediately. The second attempt at needle insertion or catheter placement should not take place until after paresthesia goes away.

The level of the tip of spinal cord is known to be the lower border of L1 vertebrae or L1/2 interspace, but there is a wide anatomical variation, and the spinal cord can extend to L2/3 or the upper part of L3 vertebrae [9]. In addition, interspace estimation by palpating the intercristal line is often higher than the anatomical level [28,39]. Therefore, it is emphasized one more time that L2/3 interspace should not be chosen for spinal needle insertion (to prevent spinal cord injury).

In the midline approach, keeping the spinal/epidural needle in the midline is crucial to avoid trauma of the nerve roots (Figure 19.11b). Damage to the nerve root may present with persistent paresthesia in the same dermatomal distribution. Symptoms involving more than one spinal segment suggest damage to the spinal cord.

Epidural hematoma

Epidural hematoma associated with regional anesthesia is a rare complication. It is mostly caused by trauma to epidural vessels, especially if the patient is coagulopathic due to anticoagulants or medical problems such as placenta abruptio or HELLP syndrome. The symptoms of an epidural hematoma include severe lower back pain with localized tenderness, radiculopathy, myelopathy, bilateral weakness/paralysis in the lower extremities, lack of block regression, and urinary/bowel dysfunction. Symptoms usually develop within 12 hours of the initial neuraxial procedure. Prompt imaging studies of the spine such as a magnetic resonance imaging (MRI) and/or computed tomography (CT) are essential for diagnosis. If external spinal cord compression is shown on the imaging studies, it strongly suggests epidural space occupying lesion (e.g., hematoma or abscess). A surgical decompression within 8 hours is mandatory to avoid irreversible nerve damage.

Epidural abscess

Epidural abscess associated with spinal, epidural, or CSE technique is an extremely rare complication. Transmission of bacterial flora to the epidural space may be via the hematogenous spread of infection or external contamination from the skin, urine, feces, amniotic fluid, oral flora from the practitioner's mouth, or contaminated equipment. Diabetic patients, patients on chronic steroid therapy, patients with a history of intravenous drug abuse, and/or a history of alcoholism are particularly at risk. When local infection is suspected, regional technique is contraindicated. Aseptic technique during all neuraxial blocks is mandatory. If catheter is left in situ for a prolonged duration, the risk of epidural abscess may increase. Therefore, the catheter should be left in situ no longer than 2–3 days (even if used for postoperative analgesia). There is no clear evidence that bacterial filters are effective in decreasing the incidence of epidural abscess [32].

The symptoms of an epidural abscess are similar to those of an epidural hematoma. The symptoms include severe lower backache with local tenderness, radiculopathy, fever with leukocytosis/increased C-reactive protein, headache, and neck stiffness, and weakness/paralysis in the lower extremities. Imaging of the spine such as a MRI is essential for diagnosis. Antibiotics may be the treatment of choice in cases without neurological deficits. However, laminectomy is generally accepted as the most effective therapy for the severe cases (with neurological deficits). Prompt diagnosis followed by appropriate treatment is crucial for good outcome.

Chemical neuropathy

Nerve roots inside the subarachnoid space are vulnerable to chemical injury because they are poorly demyelinated. *Cauda equina syndrome* after spinal anesthesia is caused by neurotoxicity of the injectate (Box 19.2). Patients usually present with pain or sensorimotor deficit in the lower back, legs, and buttocks, and urinary and rectal disturbances. There is no specific and effective treatment for this damage, and the symptoms often result in permanent impairment.

Symptoms of *transient neurologic syndrome* or *transient radicular irritation* are defined as pain or dysesthesia in the lower back, legs, and buttocks after spinal anesthesia. The symptoms usually resolve within a few days, in contrast to those of cauda equina syndrome. The cause of transient neurologic syndrome is controversial, however; one hypothesis is of chemical injury by noxious injectate into the subarachnoid space (with less neural damage than in cauda equina syndrome) [10].

Arachnoiditis

Arachnoiditis after spinal anesthesia is a rare, but devastating condition. It is a progressive inflammation of the

---

Box 19.2 Risk factors for chemical injury to the cauda equina

- Limited spread of a high-dose local anesthetic within the subarachnoid space
- Lidocaine, dibucaine, tetracaine
- Preservatives
- Unintentional administration of a large dose of anesthetic intended for epidural injection

arachnoid typically associated with an unintentional injection of noxious chemical substances, such as preservatives and antioxidants, contained in an epidural anesthetic. Patients usually present with bilateral lower limb weakness, and bladder and bowel dysfunction. The prognosis is poor.

POST-OP PAIN MANAGEMENT

Postoperative pain management should not be neglected after cesarean delivery. Good pain control promotes good quality of recovery and allows mothers to take care of their babies. Furthermore, it may prevent development of chronic pain, which may result from inadequate treatment of acute pain.

There are several options available for postoperative pain management after cesarean delivery. These include intravenous medications, neuraxial techniques, peripheral nerve blocks, and wound infiltration. Multimodal oral analgesia combined with the options listed above may be the best choice, although the safety of breastfeeding should be considered.

If spinal anesthesia is used for cesarean delivery, intrathecal morphine 100–200 mcg will provide superior pain relief for about 12–24 hours after surgery. If epidural anesthesia is used for the surgery, epidural morphine 2–4 mg is equipotent to intrathecal morphine dose of 100–200 mcg. Side effects include pruritus, nausea, and vomiting. However, the most important morphine-related adverse effect is respiratory depression. Therefore, arterial oxygen saturation should be monitored at least 24 hours after the drug administration. Fentanyl may be used instead of morphine. However, it should be used as a patient-controlled technique because of a shorter duration of action.

Local anesthetics (e.g., ropivacaine or levobupivacaine) can be used in transversus abdominis nerve block, ilioinguinal and iliohypogastric nerve blocks, and wound infiltration.

For intravenous analgesia, fentanyl or morphine may be used as a patient-controlled analgesia (PCA). Usually, initial PCA settings are bolus of fentanyl (25 mcg) or morphine (1 mg), with lockout time of 10 minutes, and no background infusion.

Concurrent nonsteroidal anti-inflammatory drugs and acetaminophen through various routes are often used. Oral oxycodone or tramadol can be used for stronger pain.

REFERENCES

1. Kuczkowski KM, Reisner LS, Benumof JL. Airway problems and new solutions for the obstetric patient. *J Clin Anesth* 2003;15:552–63.
2. Hawkins JL, Birnbach DJ. Maternal mortality in the United States: Where are we going and how will we get there? *Anesth Analg* 2001;93:1–3.
3. Kuczkowski KM. A review of obstetric anesthesia in the new millennium—Where are we and where is it heading? *Curr Opin Obstet Gynecol* 2010;22:482–6.
4. Hood DD, Curry R. Spinal versus epidural anesthesia for cesarean delivery in severely preeclamptic patients: A retrospective survey. *Anesthesiology* 1999;90:1276–82.
5. Visalyaputra S, Rodanant O, Somboonviboon W, Tantivitayatan K, Thienthong S, Saengchote W. Spinal versus epidural anesthesia for cesarean delivery in severe preeclampsia: A prospective randomized, multicenter study. *Anesth Analg* 2005;101:862–8, table of contents.
6. Kuczkowski KM. Labor pain and its management with the combined spinal-epidural analgesia: What does an obstetrician need to know? *Arch Gynecol Obstet* 2007;275:183–5.
7. Kuczkowski KM. Labor analgesia for the morbidly obese parturient: An old problem—New solution. *Arch Gynecol Obstet* 2005;271:302–3.
8. Kuczkowski KM, van Zundert A. Anesthesia for pregnant women with valvular heart disease: The state-of-the-art. *J Anesth* 2007;21:252–7.
9. Saifuddin A, Burnett SJ, White J. The variation of position of the conus medullaris in an adult population. A magnetic resonance imaging study. *Spine (Phila Pa 1976)* 1998;23:1452–6.
10. Drasner K. Local anesthetic neurotoxicity: Clinical injury and strategies that may minimize risk. *Reg Anesth Pain Med* 2002;27:576–80.
11. Zaric D, Pace NL. Transient neurologic symptoms (TNS) following spinal anaesthesia with lidocaine versus other local anaesthetics. *Cochrane Database Syst Rev* 2009;(2):CD003006.
12. Kato R, Shimamoto H, Terui K, Yokota K, Miyao H. Delayed respiratory depression associated with 0.15 mg intrathecal morphine for cesarean delivery: A review of 1915 cases. *J Anesth* 2008;22:112–6.
13. Hillyard SG, Bate TE, Corcoran TB, Paech MJ, O'Sullivan G. Extending epidural analgesia for emergency Caesarean section: A meta-analysis. *Br J Anaesth* 2011;107:668–78.
14. Kuczkowski KM. Ambulation with combined spinal-epidural labor analgesia: The technique. *Acta Anaesthesiol Belg* 2004;55:29–34.
15. Apfelbaum JL, Connis RT, Nickinovich DG et al. Practice advisory for preanesthesia evaluation: An updated report by the American Society of Anesthesiologists Task Force on Preanesthesia Evaluation. *Anesthesiology* 2012;116:522–38.
16. Kuczkowski KM. Labor analgesia for the parturient with lumbar tattoos: What does an obstetrician need to know? *Arch Gynecol Obstet* 2006;274:310–2.
17. Kuczkowski KM. Labor analgesia for the parturient with prior spinal surgery: What does an obstetrician need to know? *Arch Gynecol Obstet* 2006;274:373–5.
18. Moeller-Bertram T, Kuczkowski KM, Benumof JL. Uneventful epidural labor analgesia in a parturient with immune thrombocytopenic purpura and platelet count of 26,000/mm^3, which was unknown preoperatively. *J Clin Anesth* 2004;16:51–53.

19. Horlocker TT, Wedel DJ, Rowlinson JC et al. Regional anesthesia in the patient receiving antithrombotic or thrombolytic therapy: American Society of Regional Anesthesia and Pain Medicine Evidence-Based Guidelines (3rd ed.). *Reg Anesth Pain Med* 2010;35:64–101.
20. Regional anaesthesia and patients with abnormalities of coagulation: The Association of Anaesthetists of Great Britain and Ireland The Obstetric Anaesthetists' Association Regional Anaesthesia UK. *Anaesthesia* 2013;68:966–72.
21. Kuczkowski KM. Labor analgesia for pregnant women with spina bifida: What does an obstetrician need to know? *Arch Gynecol Obstet* 2007;275:53–56.
22. Practice guidelines for obstetric anesthesia: An updated report by the American Society of Anesthesiologists Task Force on Obstetric Anesthesia. *Anesthesiology* 2007;106:843–63.
23. Smith I, Kranke P, Murat I, Smith A, O'Sullivan G, Soreide E, Spies C, in't Veld B. Perioperative fasting in adults and children: Guidelines from the European Society of Anaesthesiology. *Eur J Anaesthesiol* 2011;28:556–69.
24. Law AC, Lam KK, Irwin MG. The effect of right versus left lateral decubitus positions on induction of spinal anesthesia for cesarean delivery. *Anesth Analg* 2003;97:1795–9.
25. Andrews PJ, Ackerman WE, 3rd, Juneja MM. Aortocaval compression in the sitting and lateral decubitus positions during extradural catheter placement in the parturient. *Can J Anaesth* 1993;40:320–4.
26. Armstrong S, Fernando R, Columb M, Jones T. Cardiac index in term pregnant women in the sitting, lateral, and supine positions: An observational, crossover study. *Anesth Analg* 2011;113:318–22.
27. Broadbent CR, Maxwell WB, Ferrie R, Wilson DJ, Gawne-Cain M, Russell R. Ability of anaesthetists to identify a marked lumbar interspace. *Anaesthesia* 2000;55:1122–6.
28. Lee AJ, Ranasinghe JS, Chehade JM, Arheart K, Saltzman BS, Penning DH, Birnbach DJ. Ultrasound assessment of the vertebral level of the intercristal line in pregnancy. *Anesth Analg* 2011;113:559–64.
29. Balki M. Locating the epidural space in obstetric patient—Ultrasound a useful tool: Continuing professional development. *Can J Anaesth* 2010;57:1111–26.
30. Boyce JM, Pittet D. Guideline for Hand Hygiene in Health-Care Settings. Recommendations of the Healthcare Infection Control Practices Advisory Committee and the HICPAC/SHEA/APIC/IDSA Hand Hygiene Task Force. Society for Healthcare Epidemiology of America/Association for Professionals in Infection Control/Infectious Diseases Society of America. *MMWR Recomm Rep* 2002;51:1–45.
31. Benhamou B, Mercier FJ, Dounas M. Hospital policy for prevention of infection after neuraxial blocks in obstetrics. *Int J Obstet Anesth* 2002;11:265–9.
32. Practice advisory for the prevention, diagnosis, and management of infectious complications associated with neuraxial techniques: A report by the American Society of Anesthesiologists Task Force on infectious complications associated with neuraxial techniques. *Anesthesiology* 2010;112:530–45.
33. Bacterial meningitis after intrapartum spinal anesthesia—New York and Ohio, 2008–2009. *MMWR Morb Mortal Wkly Rep* 2010;59:65–69.
34. Choi PT, Galinski SE, Takeuchi L, Lucas S, Tamayo C, Jadad AR. PDPH is a common complication of neuraxial blockade in parturients: A meta-analysis of obstetrical studies. *Can J Anaesth* 2003;50:460–9.
35. Kuczkowski KM. The management of accidental dural puncture in pregnant women: What does an obstetrician need to know? *Arch Gynecol Obstet* 2007;275:125–31.
36. Dickson MA, Moores C, McClure JH. Comparison of single, end-holed and multi-orifice extradural catheters when used for continuous infusion of local anaesthetic during labour. *Br J Anaesth* 1997;79:297–300.
37. Mhyre JM, Greenfield ML, Tsen LC, Polley LS. A systematic review of randomized controlled trials that evaluate strategies to avoid epidural vein cannulation during obstetric epidural catheter placement. *Anesth Analg* 2009;108:1232–42.
38. Spiegel JE, Vasudevan A, Li Y, Hess PE. A randomized prospective study comparing two flexible epidural catheters for labour analgesia. *Br J Anaesth* 2009;103:400–5.
39. Margarido CB, Mikhael R, Arzola C, Balki M, Carvalho JC. The intercristal line determined by palpation is not a reliable anatomical landmark for neuraxial anesthesia. *Can J Anaesth* 2011;58:262–6.
40. Kuczkowski KM, Benumof JL. Images in anesthesia: Headache caused by pneumocephalus following inadvertent dural puncture during epidural space identification: Is it time to abandon the loss of resistance to air technique? *Can J Anaesth* 2003;50:159–60.
41. Fettes PD, Jansson JR, Wildsmith JA. Failed spinal anaesthesia: Mechanisms, management, and prevention. *Br J Anaesth* 2009;102:739–48.
42. Mercier FJ. Cesarean delivery fluid management. *Curr Opin Anaesthesiol* 2012;25:286–91.
43. Lee A, Ngan Kee WD, Gin T. A quantitative, systematic review of randomized controlled trials of ephedrine versus phenylephrine for the management of hypotension during spinal anesthesia for cesarean delivery. *Anesth Analg* 2002;94:920–6, table of contents.
44. Van de Velde M, Schepers R, Berends N, Vandermeersch E, De Buck F. Ten years of experience with accidental dural puncture and post-dural puncture headache in a tertiary obstetric anaesthesia department. *Int J Obstet Anesth* 2008;17:329–35.
45. Miro M, Guasch E, Gilsanz F. Comparison of epidural analgesia with combined spinal-epidural

analgesia for labor: A retrospective study of 6497 cases. *Int J Obstet Anesth* 2008;17:15–19.
46. Hartopp R, Hamlyn L, Stocks G. Ten years of experience with accidental dural puncture and post-dural-puncture headache in a tertiary obstetric anaesthesia department. *Int J Obstet Anesth* 2010;19:118.
47. Zeidan A, Farhat O, Maaliki H, Baraka A. Does postdural puncture headache left untreated lead to subdural hematoma? Case report and review of the literature. *Int J Obstet Anesth* 2006;15:50–58.
48. Holst D, Mollmann M, Ebel C, Hausman R, Wendt M. In vitro investigation of cerebrospinal fluid leakage after dural puncture with various spinal needles. *Anesth Analg* 1998;87:1331–5.
49. Reina MA, de Leon-Casasola OA, Lopez A, De Andres J, Martin S, Mora M. An in vitro study of dural lesions produced by 25-gauge Quincke and Whitacre needles evaluated by scanning electron microscopy. *Reg Anesth Pain Med* 2000;25:393–402.
50. Richman JM, Joe EM, Cohen SR, Rowlingson AJ, Michaels RK, Jeffries MA, Wu CL. Bevel direction and postdural puncture headache: A meta-analysis. *Neurologist* 2006;12:224–8.
51. Schnabel A, Schuster F, Ermert T, Eberhart LH, Metterlein T, Kranke P. Ultrasound guidance for neuraxial analgesia and anesthesia in obstetrics: A quantitative systematic review. *Ultraschall Med* 2012;33:E132–7.
52. Liu SS, Ngeow JE, Yadeau JT. Ultrasound-guided regional anesthesia and analgesia: A qualitative systematic review. *Reg Anesth Pain Med* 2009;34:47–59.
53. Richardson MG, Wissler RN. The effects of needle bevel orientation during epidural catheter insertion in laboring parturients. *Anesth Analg* 1999;88: 352–6.
54. Norris MC, Leighton BL, DeSimone CA. Needle bevel direction and headache after inadvertent dural puncture. *Anesthesiology* 1989;70:729–31.
55. Hatfalvi BI. Postulated mechanisms for postdural puncture headache and review of laboratory models. Clinical experience. *Reg Anesth* 1995;20:329–36.
56. Ready LB, Cuplin S, Haschke RH, Nessly M. Spinal needle determinants of rate of transdural fluid leak. *Anesth Analg* 1989;69:457–60.
57. Apfel CC, Saxena A, Cakmakkaya OS, Gaiser R, George E, Radke O. Prevention of postdural puncture headache after accidental dural puncture: A quantitative systematic review. *Br J Anaesth* 2010;105:255–63.
58. Ayad S, Demian Y, Narouze SN, Tetzlaff JE. Subarachnoid catheter placement after wet tap for analgesia in labor: Influence on the risk of headache in obstetric patients. *Reg Anesth Pain Med* 2003;28:512–5.
59. Cohen S, Amar D, Pantuck EJ, Singer N, Divon M. Decreased incidence of headache after accidental dural puncture in caesarean delivery patients receiving continuous postoperative intrathecal analgesia. *Acta Anaesthesiol Scand* 1994;38:716–8.
60. Heesen M, Klohr S, Rossaint R, Walters M, Straube S, van de Velde M. Insertion of an intrathecal catheter following accidental dural puncture: A meta-analysis. *Int J Obstet Anesth* 2013;22:26–30.
61. Al-metwalli RR. Epidural morphine injections for prevention of post dural puncture headache. *Anaesthesia* 2008;63:847–50.
62. Dieterich M, Brandt T. Incidence of post-lumbar puncture headache is independent of daily fluid intake. *Eur Arch Psychiatry Neurol Sci* 1988;237:194–6.
63. Sudlow C, Warlow C. Posture and fluids for preventing post-dural puncture headache. *Cochrane Database Syst Rev* 2002;(2):CD001790.
64. Kuczkowski KM, Benumof JL. Decrease in the incidence of post-dural puncture headache: Maintaining CSF volume. *Acta Anaesthesiol Scand* 2003;47:98–100.
65. Basurto Ona X, Martinez Garcia L, Sola I, Bonfill Cosp X. Drug therapy for treating post-dural puncture headache. *Cochrane Database Syst* Rev 2011;(8):CD007887
66. Sudlow C, Warlow C. Epidural blood patching for preventing and treating post-dural puncture headache. *Cochrane Database Syst Rev* 2002;(2):CD001791.
67. Szeinfeld M, Ihmeidan IH, Moser MM, Machado R, Klose KJ, Serafini AN. Epidural blood patch: Evaluation of the volume and spread of blood injected into the epidural space. *Anesthesiology* 1986;64:820–2.
68. Beards SC, Jackson A, Griffiths AG, Horsman EL. Magnetic resonance imaging of extradural blood patches: Appearances from 30 min to 18 h. *Br J Anaesth* 1993;71:182–8.
69. Taivainen T, Pitkanen M, Tuominen M, Rosenberg PH. Efficacy of epidural blood patch for postdural puncture headache. *Acta Anaesthesiol Scand* 1993;37:702–5.
70. Chen LK, Huang CH, Jean WH, Lu CW, Lin CJ, Sun WZ, Wang MH. Effective epidural blood patch volumes for postdural puncture headache in Taiwanese women. *J Formos Med Assoc* 2007;106:134–40.
71. Paech MJ, Doherty DA, Christmas T, Wong CA. The volume of blood for epidural blood patch in obstetrics: A randomized, blinded clinical trial. *Anesth Analg* 2011;113:126–33.
72. Banks S, Paech M, Gurrin L. An audit of epidural blood patch after accidental dural puncture with a Tuohy needle in obstetric patients. *Int J Obstet Anesth* 2001;10:172–6.
73. Stride PC, Cooper GM. Dural taps revisited. A 20-year survey from Birmingham Maternity Hospital. *Anaesthesia* 1993;48:247–55.
74. Neal JM, Bernards CM, Butterworth JFt, Di Gregorio G, Drasner K, Hejtmanek MR, Mulroy MF, Rosenquist RW, Weinberg GL. ASRA practice advisory on local anesthetic systemic toxicity. *Reg Anesth Pain Med* 2010;35:152–61.
75. Bern S, Weinberg G. Local anesthetic toxicity and lipid resuscitation in pregnancy. *Curr Opin Anaesthesiol* 2011;24(3):262–7.

Characteristics of the postcesarean delivery uterine scar

ANTONIO MALVASI and GIAN CARLO DI RENZO

INTRODUCTION

The scar is the result of various chronologically related biological events that comprise two key moments: cell regeneration and connective tissue replacement. These two phases differ on the phylogenetically acquired capacity of each tissue to repair, and on the external events that may interfere with the scarring process.

It would therefore be wrong to imagine a simplistic process of "substitution" of connective tissue in the myometrial scarring area. What instead occurs is an active process of "regeneration" of the cellular and structural constituents. In fact, some pathologists prefer the more appropriate term "restitution" to the word "substitution." Mesodermal tissues, including the myometrium, which is formed by stem cells, have the ability to produce their normal component elements, which are not passively replaced with connective tissue and amorphous substance (Figure 20.1).

The repairing processes, including in the myometrium, are mediated by different cell growth factors and inhibitor factors. Therefore, quality of healing process and possible related endometrial, myometrial, and peritoneal complications are strictly dependent on the activity of growth and inhibitor factors [1–3].

The precise mechanism that involves these factors in the healing process is not completely known, and further studies are needed in order to determine whether exogenous or endogenous causes influence and handle the scarring process of hysteroraphy.

We can list other interfering factors, such as type of suture, suture material, possible peritoneal suture, cesarean delivery performed during labor or elective, endometriotic implantation on the suture, and blood extravasation occurred during the postnatal period in the area of suture. These factors can also influence the possibility of a vaginal birth after cesarean delivery (VBACS) [4].

The severity of complications related to the uterine scar during a vaginal delivery in women with a history of one or more previous cesarean deliveries, resulted in an increasing number of studies conducted with different diagnostic methods, in order to assess the existence of parameters for a safe vaginal delivery. In particular, the first diagnostic studies were performed with hysterosalpingography followed by ultrasound and other "imaging" methods (computed tomography [CT] and magnetic resonance imaging [MRI]).

Morphological studies have also been also conducted, although less numerous than clinical-instrumental ones, which have often been correlated with the observations deriving from other diagnostic techniques.

ASSESSMENT OF THE UTERINE SCAR WITH HYSTEROSALPINGOGRAPHY

The postcesarean delivery uterine scar was initially viewed by means of hysterosalpingography (Figure 20.2) [5–7]. The rationale for these studies was similar to that in studies currently being carried out with other imaging methods [8,9].

The most significant image that can be seen in hysterosalpingography x-rays is of a "plus area" located at the level of the anterior isthmus wall of the uterus in which the contrast agent penetrates. This is the postcesarean delivery scar area that can be more or less deep and which provides a "negative" image of myometrium thickness in that area.

The limit of a hysterosalpingography, in terms of assessing the cesarean delivery scar, is the inability to view the external wall of the scar area and therefore to only provide information on the inner wall and on the thickness of the uterus in that area.

In addition to this recurring image, deformations of the isthmus–cervical area resulting from a previous cesarean delivery or its complications can also be occasionally seen [1]. Therefore, in some cases, this plus area can in turn contain "minus areas" that correspond to rare exophytic formations that developed in the scar area, such as polyps, endometriotic implants, and neoplasia.

Hysterosalpingography after a cesarean delivery can also show other morphological abnormalities that may be related to the surgical procedure. Defects of the cervical canal can be observed, which are often associated with hypertrophic scarring or partial synechiae. A lengthening of the cervical canal can also be detected, but this could be prior to the cesarean delivery.

In some cases an "opening" of the isthmus can be detected, which is, however, less common than one might suspect. Last, tubal occlusions or filling defects of the uterine cavity, resulting from synechiae of the endometrial cavity, secondary to a postcesarean delivery infectious process, may also be detected.

The images of the uterine scar can be either below or above the internal uterine orifice, depending on the location of the uterine incision. Generally, if the cesarean delivery is performed during labor, the scar is located in the middle of the cervical canal. In case of an elective cesarean delivery the scar is located above the internal uterine orifice. The location of the scar is so tied to the

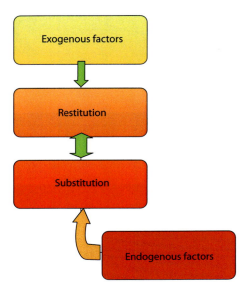

Figure 20.1 The two main healing factors: restitution and substitution in dynamic equilibrium with each other and influenced by exogenous and endogenous factors.

Table 20.1 Four classes of hysterography

Class	Condition
I	Hysterographies that are considered normal, no scar is noticed
II	Deformations with depth under 4 mm, or small alterations difficult to measure
III	Losses of substance that reach 45 mm and deformations that cannot be measured but whose morphology evokes defective scarring
IV	Depth abnormalities greater than 6 mm evoking poor scar quality

dilatation internal uterine orifice at the time of cesarean delivery. It is clear that in the presence of a dilatation the incision is made below the internal uterine orifice. On the contrary, in the case of an elective cesarean delivery, in which the uterine segment has not yet completed its morphological growth, the incision will be high and almost always between the uterine body and the uterine segment. Thus, over time a scar will remain above the internal uterine orifice. Finds of this type are becoming more frequent in the case of patients who undergo hysterosalpingography for secondary infertility due to the increase in cesarean deliveries.

The various morphological features described can be observed in anterior–posterior and sagittal or parasagittal x-rays. It is almost always possible to use x-rays to determine the depth in millimeters of the scar, in order to evaluate the thinning of the uterine wall at the level of the scar.

Four classes of hysterography (Table 20.1) have been identified based on scar depth:

This classification has currently been set aside in favor of less-invasive diagnostic techniques. However, VanVut [9] evaluating with hysterosalpingography 68 patients with previous cesarean delivery, considered this method useful in order to determine the thickness of the scar that, according to the author, was related to the gestational age, the surgical procedure that was performed, and the location of the incision.

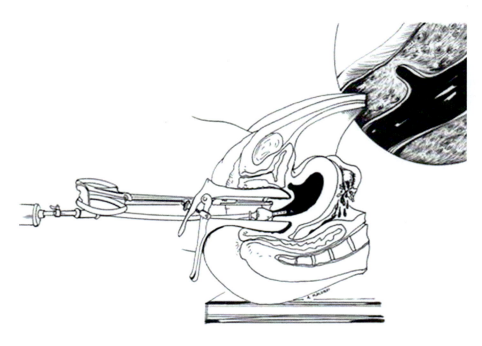

Figure 20.2 Hysterosalpingography performed on a uterus with uterine scar from cesarean delivery. At top right is the front uterine wall at the isthmus level which shows an area filled with the contrast medium, defined "plus area," corresponding to a thinning of the wall in the scar area.

In a study Barbot [5] claimed that in cases where hysteroscopy could not detect small abnormalities of the uterine scar and its contents, such as blood, hysterosalpingography could be an additional and valid method.

Negura et al. [10] have also used hysterosalpingographies in experimental animal studies on previously pregnant bitches, to verify the morphological characteristics of the uterine scar after traumatisms were induced for experimental purposes on the uterus.

In subsequent years the use of hysterosalpingography for the morphological study of the postcesarean scar in order to assess its suitability for VBACS has been abandoned in favor of other diagnostic techniques.

Currently the role of this method in evaluating the cesarean scar is mostly limited to the diagnosis performed by urologists of vesicouterine fistulae. Often these fistulae are the result of complicated cesarean deliveries.

Benchekroun et al. [11] diagnosed 30 vesicouterine fistulae, six of which were diagnosed with a hysterosalpingography, whereas Sefrioui et al. [12] reported three vesicouterine fistulae diagnosed by urography and hysterosalpingography.

ASSESSMENT OF THE UTERINE SCAR WITH ULTRASOUND

The majority of studies reported in literature on the evaluation of the uterine scar with imaging techniques concern ultrasound. Ultrasound is a noninvasive diagnostic tool that can be easily reproduced and implemented. The degree of specificity and sensitivity of ultrasound can be compared with diagnostic tools. Currently it is considered the "gold standard" for the evaluation of uterine scar in the postcesarean vaginal delivery.

In 1990 Brown et al. [13] published a study that asserted that transvaginal ultrasound was much more effective than transabdominal ultrasound in evaluating the lower uterine segment and the cervix, and was also not dependent on bladder filling. The study of the uterine scar involved radiologists who in some cases compared CT and MRI and ultrasound. For instance, Kawakami et al. [14] reported that unique uterine deformities displayed with MRI were significantly associated with transverse incisions from a cesarean delivery and could lead to a history of infertility found, with the help of CT scan, that a small population of women with a history of infertility had a unique uterine deformity, in which the cervix appeared elongated and fixed to the anterior abdominal wall, due to the incision in the lower uterine segment of a previous cesarean delivery, especially when this had been performed at late gestational age.

Still, Hebisch et al. [15], in comparing transvaginal ultrasound with MRI, concluded that transvaginal ultrasound was better in visualizing the uterine wall, in differentiating it from the vesical wall, and in measuring the thickness of the scar.

In conclusion, after it was established that ultrasound was the best diagnostic technique to use to study the uterine scar before and during pregnancy, the main purpose of further research aimed at determining the thickness of the uterine scar that could predict uterine rupture in patients who previously underwent cesarean deliveries.

Avrech et al. [16], described a case of a women with a history of a preceding cesarean delivery, who had, at 31 weeks' gestation, without uterine contractility, a corporeal uterine dehiscence of the previous scar, detected by ultrasound. This study showed how corporeal incision put the woman at higher risk for catastrophic events during further pregnancies, even without uterine activity during the third trimester. For this reason, when there is a history of corporeal incision, or the site of incision is not known, any abdominal pain should raise suspicion of uterine rupture, and ultrasound monitoring is required (Figure 20.3).

Still, Lebedev et al. [17], evaluated the morphological characteristics of the uterine scar of 86 patients with

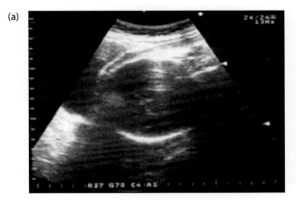

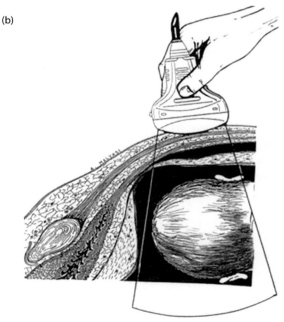

Figure 20.3 (a) Transabdominal ultrasound in the third trimester of pregnancy, (b) performed to evaluate the lower uterine segment in pregnant women with a previous cesarean delivery: the thin and extended lower uterine segment is visible.

previous cesarean delivery, including ultrasound, examination of the lower uterine segment during surgery, bimanual postnatal control, and the histological examination of the scar tissue. This study confirmed the high usefulness of ultrasound for the assessment of uterine scar and the risk of uterine rupture related to labor.

In a prospective study, Michaels et al. [18] evaluated "defects" of the lower uterine segment using ultrasound. They examined 70 pregnant women who would give birth by cesarean delivery, 58 of them at risk of rupture due to previous cesarean delivery and 12 nulliparous as control patients. Uterine defects were confirmed in 12 patients among the high-risk group (20.7%), while all patients belonging to the control group were normal.

Further, in a study by Fukuda [19], 84 pregnant women with a previous cesarean delivery were examined near term, in order to assess the risk of uterine rupture during labor. In 70 patients, ultrasound detected good thickness and good healing of the uterine scar, and 26 of them gave birth by vaginal delivery, whereas 46 women repeated cesarean delivery, for other obstetric complications. Among the 46 women, intraoperative findings in four women showed thinning of the uterine scar.

In 14 pregnant women, ultrasound demonstrated thinning and poor healing of the uterine scar and iterative cesarean delivery was performed, confirming during the surgical procedure thinning and loss of continuity of the lower uterine segment in all of them.

In another study Fukuda et al. [20] performed a series, starting from the 16th week, of transabdominal (longitudinal and transverse scans to assess the thickness of the uterine scar), transperineal, and transabdominal ultrasound scans, considering at risk of uterine rupture those scars with a thickness of less than 2 mm.

However, Alphen [21] reported another case of a woman with a history of two vaginal deliveries and two ectopic pregnancies with further left salpingectomy, who during her fifth pregnancy had cesarean delivery because of abdominal pain and left uterine cornual rupture at 29 weeks' gestation. Her sixth pregnancy was strictly monitored with ultrasound in order to evaluate any uterine wall changes at the cornual site, and the woman was told to refer any abdominal pain. At 28 weeks' gestation, abdominal pain appeared and ultrasound revealed fundal uterine rupture confirmed by laparotomy. In conclusion, women with risk factors for uterine rupture should be rigorously monitored, and any abdominal complaint could be a sign of this catastrophic event, even without uterine activity, anytime during the third trimester (Figure 20.4).

Tanik et al. [22] compared lower uterine segment wall thickness measured with ultrasound with uterine wall thickness assessed intraoperatively, confirming the accuracy and safety of sonography to detect women with a history of previous cesarean delivery, with high risk of uterine rupture during labor.

These authors reported a sensitivity of 100%, a specificity of 82%, with a positive predictive value of 87% and a negative predictive value of 100%.

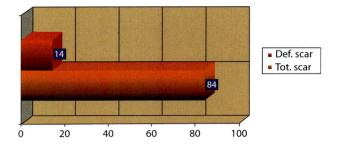

Figure 20.4 The results of the Fukuda study of the uterine scars detected with ultrasound (14) on the total sample (84), done by comparing the ultrasound report with the intraoperative report.

Cheung et al. [23] evaluated, with obstetric ultrasound performed between 36 and 38 weeks, in a prospective study of 53 women with a previous cesarean delivery, 40 nulliparas, and 40 multiparous with unscarred uterus. They concluded that the prenatal ultrasound examination of the lower uterine segment was related to delivery outcome and comparable with intraoperative findings as well as potentially capable of allowing diagnosis of an intrauterine defect and determination of the degree of thinning of the lower uterine segment in patients with previous cesarean delivery.

In another study, Cheung [24] examined 102 pregnant women between 36 and 38 weeks of gestation with one or more previous cesarean deliveries, to measure the thickness of the lower uterine segment. This thickness, evaluated as the distance between the outer wall of the bladder wall myometrium interface and the myometrium chorioamniotic membranes interface, was identified by obstetric ultrasound. If the ultrasound thickness of the lower uterine segment was less than 1.5 mm, the evaluation had a sensitivity of 88.9%, a specificity of 59.5%, a positive predictive value of 32%, and a negative predictive value of 92% in preventively determining dehiscence (in association with a 1.5-mm thickness of the lower uterine segment).

The author concluded that ultrasound could properly assess the thickness of the lower uterine segment in patients with a previous cesarean delivery, and, therefore, could potentially be used to predict the risk of uterine rupture during VBACS.

Ultrasound examination with different methods (transabdominal, transvaginal, and sonohysterography ultrasound) allowed a characterization and classification of morphology of the uterine scar. The morphology of the postcesarean delivery uterine scar can be divided into three groups (Table 20.2). The "axe-sign" expression represents an incision on the outer surface of the anterior wall at the isthmus level, which can be viewed with a transabdominal ultrasound, and which is generally accompanied by a lengthening of the cervical area and by ventrofixation [25] (Figure 20.5).

Monteagudo et al. [26] define "niche" as a triangular anechoic structure in the presumed site of the scar of the previous cesarean delivery. These authors used sonohysterography to study 44 patients with a history of

Table 20.2 Postcesarean delivery uterine scar morphologies

Type	Ultrasound condition
A	The axe-sign presents itself as a minus area, an incisure on the outer surface of the front wall of the uterus
B	"Niche," Anglo-Saxon term that indicates an incisure carved on the inner surface of the anterior wall, which appears as a minus area
C	Fluid ovoid areas in the thickness of the anterior uterine isthmus wall in the seat of the scar

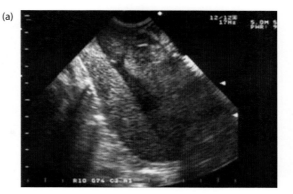

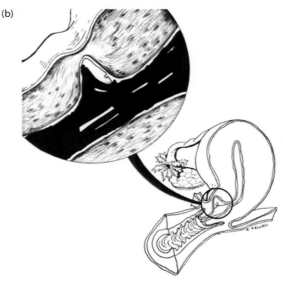

Figure 20.6 (a and b) The "niche" at the isthmus level in a uterus outside of pregnancy.

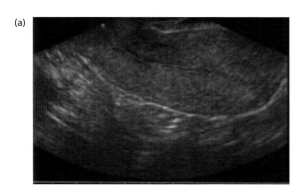

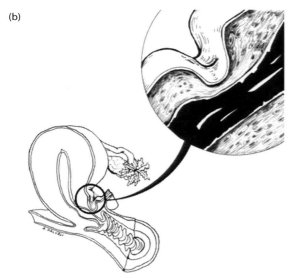

Figure 20.5 (a and b) The uterus outside of pregnancy, with previous cesarean delivery, which shows the "axe-sign" image at the isthmus level (more clearly visible in the enlargement).

previous cesarean deliveries and found a niche thickness of 6.17 ± 3.6 mm (standard deviation) (Figure 20.6).

Regnard et al. [27] defined "niche" as a triangular anechoic area in the previous incision site found with sonohysterography. They studied 33 patients with previous cesarean deliveries to find out the images that suggest the existence of dehiscence after a cesarean delivery in the site of uterine scar. These authors measured residual myometrium depth describing dehiscence when niche had a thickness of least 80% of the anterior myometrium. The conclusion of this study is that sonohysterography identified niche in 60% of patients, while prevalence of dehiscence was two out of 33 (6%), and risk of uterine rupture was 0.4% (Figure 20.7).

Sambaziotis et al. [28] examined the lower uterine segment of 24 patients during the second trimester of pregnancy with previous cesarean delivery, as well as 30 control patients with transvaginal ultrasound. In addition, these authors defined niche as a small triangular anechoic defect on the anterior wall of the uterus where the site of incision is supposed to be. The thickness of the uterine wall was measured where the bladder dome meets the lower uterine segment, and the measurement was obtained by placing the cursors between the outer surface of the bladder and the amniotic deciduous layer. The authors concluded that, as early as the second trimester of pregnancy, the lower uterine segment is significantly thinner in women with a previous cesarean delivery, and that identification is possible in most patients.

Sen et al. [29] assessed thickness of the lower uterine segment using transabdominal and transvaginal

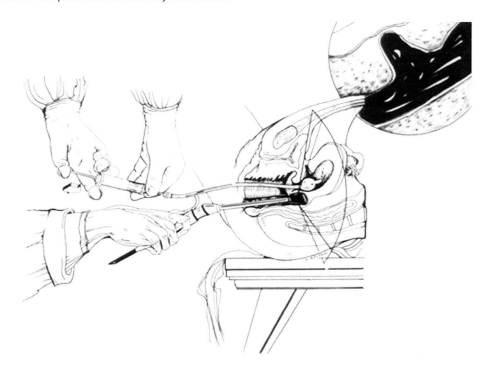

Figure 20.7 A sonohysterography carried out in a patient with previous cesarean delivery shows the area of the uterine scar and in particular the "niche" (enlargement). (Modified from Malvasi A, Di Renzo GC. *Semeiotica Ostetrica*, Rome, Italy: CIC Edizioni Internazionali; 2012.)

ultrasonography in 71 women with previous cesarean delivery and in 50 control patients in order to evaluate a reasonable cut-off over which vaginal delivery can be considered safe.

Results showed that a critical cut-off for a safe lower uterine segment was 2.5 mm, as revealed from curves obtained by various operators.

Other ultrasound findings that can be observed in the presumed site of the uterine scarring are fluid cystic areas. Armstrong et al. [30] used transvaginal ultrasound to study uterine scar, thickness, and defects comparing 38 patients with previous vaginal delivery and 32 with previous cesarean delivery, revealing a sensitivity of 100% and a specificity of 100% for this diagnostic test. They also detected defects represented by fluid collections within the site of incision, in 13 of 31 patients with a previous cesarean delivery, representing 42% of cases (Figure 20.8).

HYSTEROSCOPY AND EVALUATION OF UTERINE SCAR AFTER CESAREAN DELIVERY

In the last two decades the incidence of cesarean deliveries has increased considerably, reaching rates of over 40% in many obstetric departments.

The uterine scar can also be evaluated with hysteroscopy, which allows an internal and direct view of the scar. It can, therefore, detect any pathology developed after an abnormal wound healing process as a direct consequence of the scar itself (Figure 20.9).

Literature describes cases of localization of endometriosis over the site of uterine scars after a cesarean delivery, of polyps, as well as of localizations of endometrial carcinoma and ectopic pregnancies [31–55] (Figure 20.10).

Furthermore, previous cesarean delivery, especially when the incision is corporeal, represent a risk for rupture of the uterus (with abundant bleeding), often requiring emergency hysterectomy.

From 1978 to date, about 75 cases of ectopic pregnancy on cicatrix from previous cesarean delivery have been reported. The treatment, not yet standardized, included aspiration, curettage under ultrasound guidance, excision of the pregnancy, and even hysterectomy [37].

Successfully treated cases with correction of the uterine breach through laparoscopy or laparotomy have been reported, while other authors reported effective treatment with resectoscopy or uterine artery embolization, through endovascular procedure, laparotomy, or laparoscopy, in combination with methotrexate or solely with methotrexate-based chemotherapy treatment [34,39–41,49,53].

Nowadays hysteroscopy is increasingly required in cases of abnormal uterine bleeding.

During this examination we showed how spotting, which is mostly postmenstrual, can be sometimes related to the presence of a defect in the anterior uterine wall at the level of a uterine cicatrix of a previous cesarean delivery. This defect is highlighted during hysteroscopy as a "dimple" in the anterior wall, placed immediately after the internal uterine orifice. It can be more or less deep. It is usually not covered by endometrium (at most with a thin endometrium) and has a fibrous appearance.

By looking at the uterine "dimple," a loop of the vascular markings and a reduction of the endometrial thickness can be seen. This reduction can be correlated with formation of fibrotic tissue in varying degrees.

No other pathology, such as endometrial polyp, uterine myomas, and endometrial hyperplasias producing spotting, was observed in patients who underwent hysteroscopy. We also noted a collection of blood in the defect of the uterine wall, which was removed by the flow of saline solution during hysteroscopy. This diagnosis is correctly made when the hysteroscopy is performed in the immediate postmenstrual phase.

As we have seen, diagnosis of a hysterotomy scar defect of the uterine wall can also be performed with the help of transvaginal ultrasound. This diagnostic tool shows an anechoic triangular area at an inferior level on the anterior wall of the uterus, which can then be confirmed by hysteroscopy.

Fabres et al. [56] reported a case series of 24 patients with abnormal uterine bleeding, more specifically postmenstrual spotting, which were correctly diagnosed through hysteroscopy. These authors also confirmed our hypothesis that the presence of fibrotic tissue on the hysterotomy scar, which appears as a defect in the wall, can obstruct the flow of menstrual blood into the cervical canal, determining hematometra and delayed postmenstrual bleeding. The authors also believe that this anatomical defect, secondary to the process of cicatrization, can be corrected by hysteroscopic resection [56]. They treated 24 patients who underwent hysteroscopic resection of the fibrotic tissue at the level of the defect in the uterine wall. Spotting disappeared in a majority of patients (20/24) in a 24-month follow-up. The incidence and prevalence of

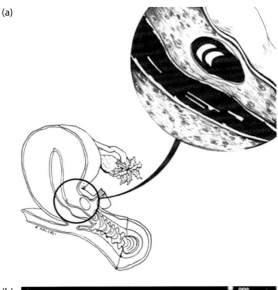
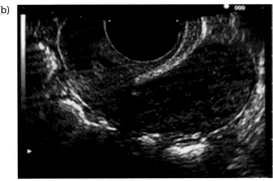

Figure 20.8 (a) The uterus outside of pregnancy in a patient with previous cesarean delivery; (b) anechoic fluid collection at the isthmus–cervical level.

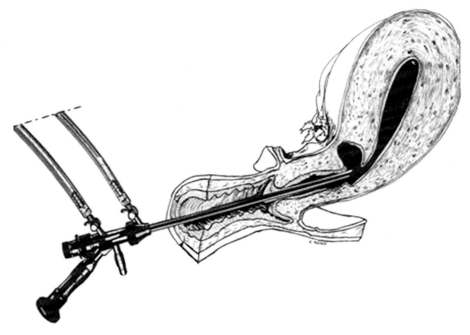

Figure 20.9 A hysteroscopy performed on a uterus with previous cesarean delivery, in which the scarring area shows a clear excavation with thinning of the myometrium at the isthmus–cervical level.

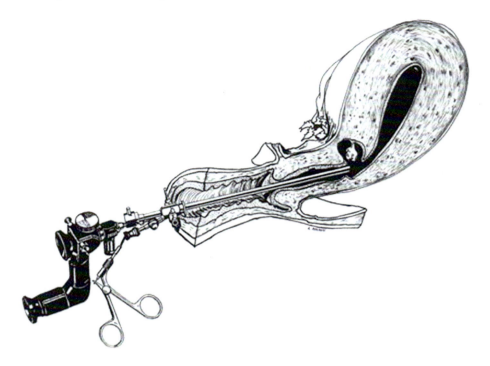

Figure 20.10 Hysteroscopy followed by resection of a polyp in the "niche" of the previous uterine scar from cesarean delivery. (Modified from Di Renzo GC. *Trattato di ostetricia e ginecologia*, Rome, Italy: Verduci Editore; 2009.)

this anatomical defect are unknown. As found, 82.6% of patients with this defect (76 patients out of 92) experience abnormal uterine bleeding [57].

A defect in the uterine wall after a cesarean delivery has also been suggested as a cause of infertility. This is because the accumulation of blood in the wall defect may produce alterations in the cervical mucus and in sperm transport [57].

Figure 20.11 shows a view of the internal uterine orifice and the defect of the anterior wall of the uterus corresponding to the scar from a previous cesarean delivery. These pictures show the prevalence of fibrous tissue with minimal glandular component and with a loop of the vascular markings.

MORPHOLOGICAL EVALUATION OF THE UTERINE SCAR
Macroscopic aspects

The macroscopic characteristics of the scar from a previous cesarean delivery are commonly observed during surgery but can also be seen in hysteroctomized uteruses in delivery of macrosomic fetuses. The macroscopic appearance of the uterine scar that can be seen during a repeated cesarean delivery presents some characteristics that are described here.

First, there can frequently be pathological adherences of neighboring tissues and, in particular of the posterior vesical wall and of the bladder dome, that must be detached and moved to the bottom so as to have access to the lower uterine segment. Therefore, the physiological cleavage plane, interposed between the bladder and the lower uterine segment, is frequently replaced by adherent connective

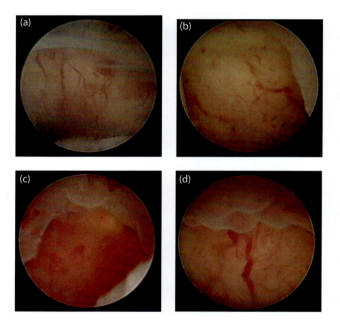

Figure 20.11 (a–d) Hysteroscopic view of the internal uterine orifice and the defect of the anterior wall of the uterus corresponding with the scar from a previous cesarean delivery.

scar tissue. It must be mobilized with instruments and very rarely are fingers able to lower it as during the first cesarean delivery.

Once the previous scar is freed from these adhesions, its shape varies depending on the time of the pregnancy, the number of previous cesarean deliveries, the quality of the previous scarring, and, in particular, the extension of the lower uterine segment and, therefore, whether there was labor. Indeed if the lower uterine segment is not thin, the presenting part can be felt through palpation, as it is still thinner than a nonscarred segment.

If the segment is stretched due to labor, the uterine scar site can be easily identified although varying degrees of thickness are present. When the scar is particularly thin, the presenting part (hair of the fetus in cephalic presentation), as well as amniotic fluid and flakes of vernix caseosa are visible.

In some cases there are small areas of less resistance from which the still intact membranes protrude. These "gaps" are defined by Anglo-Saxon authors as "windows," areas in which the myometrium or the fibrous connective tissue are absent. These correspond with a silent rupture of the uterus.

In particular, Fukuda et al. [19] in a 1988 study compared prenatal ultrasound findings with intraoperative findings classifying uterine scar thinness in three grades:

- Grade I: no thinning of the lower uterine segment
- Grade II: thinning and loss of continuity of the lower uterine segment but fetal hair not visible
- Grade III: thinning of the lower uterine segment and fetal hair visible

The thinness of scar tissue requires a delicate opening of the lower uterine segment in order to prevent instrumental iatrogenic injuries of fetus and an excessive lateral extension of edges of the hysterotomy which, due to the scar, can tear more easily.

In case of significant dehiscence, an imbibition of the hysterotomic edges can be observed; it is a type of tissue edema causing difficulty in recognizing the underlying surgical spaces, particularly for the bladder (so making difficult the bladder detachment from the uterus). After the fetus is extracted, the lower edge of the hysterotomy appears particularly thin compared with the considerable thickness of the upper edge, due to the extension of the lower uterine segment. Therefore, different depths between upper and lower edges, require a suture thread small enough to not tear the thin lower edge, but strong enough for the thickness of the upper edge.

In fact, the lower edge is often very thin and tears easily, when the suture thread passes through it or after the thread is tied. Therefore, sometimes a double suture is required to reinforce the hysterorrhaphy, often including the visceral peritoneum in favor of an increased thickness.

On the other hand, during a repeated cesarean delivery, some authors suggest an incision above the scar to prevent complications related to the different depths of lower and upper edges. The anatomopathological assessment of the uterine scar can show different alterations.

In a study of Morris, he evaluated 51 specimens of hysterectomy of women with history of one or more cesarean deliveries, revealing pathological findings in the area of the scar, responsible in part of those clinical symptoms that leaded to hysterectomy. His results showed distortion and widening of the lower uterine segment in 75% of cases, congestion of endometrium in 61% of cases, polyps located in the scar recess in 16% of cases, foci of adenomyosis, capillary dilation, and lymphocytic infiltration. Some of these findings, especially distortion of lower uterine segment, polyps, and congestion of endometrium, are the main causes of menorrhagia, dysmenorrhea, lower abdominal pain, and dyspareunia that lead to hysterectomy.

In another study, Monteagudo et al. [26] examined uterine scar areas of 44 patients who underwent cesarean delivery, using sonohysterography, founding that 36% of patients examined had myomas while 18% had associated polyps outside of the uterine scar.

Microscopic aspects

The microscopic aspects of the uterine scar after cesarean delivery were observed on both uteruses of pregnant and nonpregnant women.

The histological specimen obtained from the gravid uterus comes largely from biopsies performed on the lower uterine segment and, less often, from hysterectomies after complicated cesarean deliveries or complications that occurred during the puerperium. Histological findings of the uterine scar vary in relation to the quality of the healing process.

The most common characteristics found in scars of a cesarean delivery are the following: young collagen connective tissue, partially acellular in the subserosa, the cleavage plane with the myometrium is occupied by hemorrhagic extravasations and microhematomas are found between myometrium and the scar tissue. Collagen fiber bundles are mainly directed in the longitudinal direction and, therefore, are on axis with the uterus.

There is an abundance of intercellular substance which, due to the edema, in isolated cases results in pseudomyxomatous lesions. The architecture of some scars is instead significantly altered. In particular a rigid and inelastic structure is caused by the fusion of muscle fiber bundles and subsequent replacement with connective tissue which, at times, is young and rich in fibroblasts, while in other cases, is composed from acellular adult connective tissue.

In some cases these aspects are associated with a large reduction of scar thickness, so that one can observe the parietal decidua and the atrophic and very thin myometrium covered by edematous and highly vascularized visceral peritoneum. Some histopathological conditions show micronodular lesions within the superficial layers. These findings are single or multiple and are related to either granulomas, resulting from residual suture material (as foreign body) or surgical outcomes, such as, for example, homogeneous sclera-hyaline areas, chaotically intertwined, that are associated with a poor lymphohistiocytic inflammatory component with microcalcifications.

In the context of these images we also observe papillary proliferation in the visceral peritoneum, as a result of a reaction to the surgical trauma that originates "papillary mesothelial hyperplasia."

It is also possible to observe histopathological images on the lower uterine segment that can be attributed to changes induced by pregnancy; these conditions can be represented as images that show a striking abundance of intercellular matrix, local fibrinoid necrosis, with probable hypoxic pathogenesis, groups of myocytes, and of the wall of small vessels. We can also see in this context hyperplasia–hypertrophy of vascular endothelium simulating pseudoglandular images of adenomyosis. Furthermore, the last described finding is the Arias–Stella reaction, with ectopic location on cervical glands displaced higher in the thickness of the cervical isthmus musculature.

Morris reports, in a study of 54 cases of hysterectomy and previous cesarean deliveries [1], a moderate lymphocytic infiltration of the scar in 95% of cases, capillary dilatation in 65%, free red blood cells in the stoma scar (suggesting hemorrhage) in 59% of cases, fragmentation and detachment of the endometrium from the scar in 37%, and adenomyosis limited to the scar in 28%.

Morris reported that the pathologic changes developed as a result of the postcesarean delivery uterine scar, which are responsible, especially for endometrial hyperplasia, polyps, fibrous and inflammatory infiltration, and of several clinical symptoms such as menometrorrhagia, dysmenorrhoea, and dyspareunia, so much so that this author in another article talks about "Ceasarean scar syndrome" [58].

The scar of a cesarean delivery can be seen from a morphological point of view as the result of a healing process of reparative fibrosis. This type of scar affects the epithelial lining (mesothelium) as well as the mesenchymal tissue (smooth muscular tissue of the myometrium), and may own some morphological peculiarities that have been previously described and whose histological aspects are shown in Figures 20.12 through 20.17.

Unfortunately, even today, although there are indications for a "good" or "not good" postcesarean delivery scar, there are no clear parameters that can tell us when the scar is an indication for a safe VBACS.

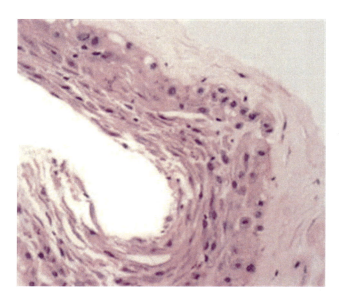

Figure 20.13 Hyperplasic mesothelium in uterine scar with visceral peritoneum closure.

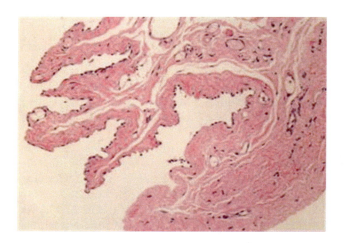

Figure 20.14 Peritoneum coated with normal mesothelium uterine scar without visceral peritoneum suture.

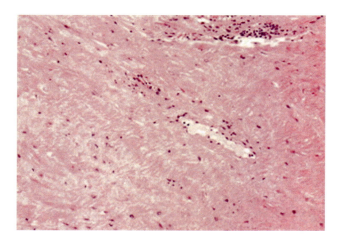

Figure 20.12 The scar is composed of hyaline hypocellular fibrous connective tissue.

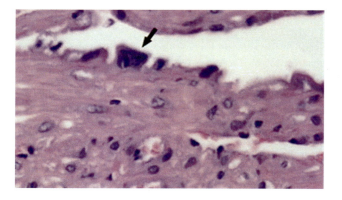

Figure 20.15 The mesothelium that covers the peritoneum shows reactive nuclear "atypias" (see arrow).

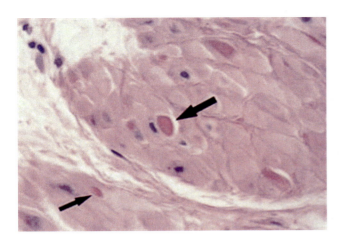

Figure 20.16 The smooth muscular tissue of the myometrium is hyperplastic and contains intracytoplasmic eosinophilic hyaline globules (see arrows); these images are reminiscent of the "inclusion body" reported in digital fibromatosis.

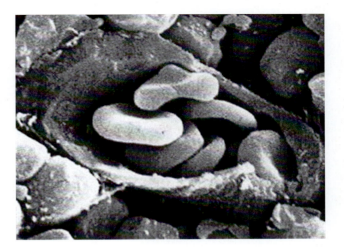

Figure 20.18 Electron microscope scanning shows a cross section of a normal capillary vessel in the lower uterine segment.

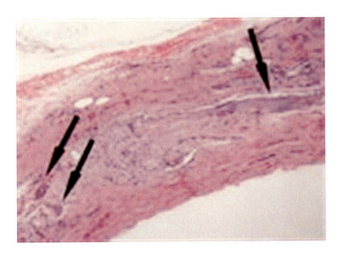

Figure 20.17 Presence of foreign body (arrows), presumably suture stitches surrounded by inflammation, in the context of the scar.

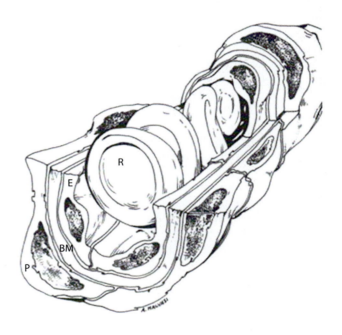

Figure 20.19 Image of a capillary vessel of a uterine scar from a cesarean delivery in the lower uterine segment. Many pericytes (P), thick basal membranes (BM), endothelial cells of increased thickness that restrict the capillary lumen (E), and red blood cells (R) are visible.

Interesting data come from electron microscopy studies (Figures 20.18 and 20.19) that identify the following elements as the main features of a postcesarean delivery scar tissue:

- Increase of vessel pericytes
- Increase in the thickness of the basal membranes of the vessels
- Increase of heavy proteoglycans, instead of light ones

These are not findings of a specific disease, but characterize aged tissue, of less strength, and clearly not suitable for a VBAC labor.

CONCLUSIONS

The increased rate of cesarean deliveries worldwide has increased scientific interest in the postcesarean delivery uterine scar and its related problems and complications.

Many studies have been conducted about the ultrasound assessment of puerperal uterine scar [59,60] as well as sometime after the cesarean delivery [61].

One aspect studied by several authors is the benefit of not suturing the visceral peritoneum, as a hematoma may form ("bladder flap hematoma") in the surgical pocket in the VUS (vesicouterine space) [62]. In the majority of cases these hematomas spontaneously disappear, but other times laparoscopic surgery [63,64] is required.

Malvasi et al. [65,66] demonstrated with optical and electron microscopy that the detachment of the vesicouterine fold and the suture of the visceral peritoneum determine an inflammatory process. This alters the healing process of the uterine scar and lowers the quality of the scar itself.

The same authors have shown that the detachment and suture of the visceral peritoneum, especially in cases of complete dilation, alters the local neurotransmitters, thereby modifying the physiology of the uterine scar tissue [67,68].

The unsutured visceral peritoneum has been determined to not cause more adhesions than the sutured one [69]. This has also been confirmed with experimental studies [70].

The postcesarean delivery scar can cause symptoms requiring hysteroscopic surgery [71].

There is a growing amount of literature describing ectopic pregnancies in the scar [72], in which the treatment is becoming increasingly conservative so as to preserve future fertility [73,74].

REFERENCES

1. Morris H. Surgical pathology of the lower uterine segment caesarean delivery scar. Is the scar a source of clinical symptoms? *Int J Gynaecol Pathol* 1995;14:16–20.
2. Ofir K, Sheiner E, Levy A, Katz M, Mazor M. Uterine rupture: Differences between a scarred and an unscarred uterus. *Am J Obstet Gynecol* 2004;191:425–9.
3. Tsenov D, Mainkhard K. Endometriosis in the surgical scar from caesarean delivery. *Akush Ginekol (Sofia)* 2000;39:50–1.
4. SOGC. Clinical practice guidelines. Guidelines for vaginal birth after previous caesarean birth. Number 155. *Int J Gynaecol Obstet* 2005;89:319–31.
5. Barbot J. Hysteroscopy and hysterography. *Obstet Gynecol Clin North Am* 1995;22:591–603.
6. Dellenbach P, Szwarcherg R, Walter JP, Alaoui T, Muller P, Main causes of repetitive abortion revealed by hysterography. *J Radiol Electrol Med Nucl* 1971; 52:522–3.
7. Gellpke W. Value of hysterography after cesarean delivery for the assessment of uterine scar. *Geburtshilfe Frauenheilkd* 1969;29:26–32.
8. Adeleye Ja, Ogunseyinde AO. Hysterography after lower-uterine-segment caesarean delivery. *Afr J Med Med Sci* 1984;13:155–60.
9. Van Vugt PJ. The protrusions from the cervical canal at the scar of a previous caesarean section. *Acta Obstet Gynecol Scand* 1979;58:327–34.
10. Negura A, Gavrilita L, Ardelanu D. The trauma of the hysterotomy incision. *Rev Fr Gynecol Obstet* 1988;8:161–4.
11. Benchekroun A, Lachkar A, Soumana A, Farih MH, Belahneech Z, Marzouk M, Faik M. Vescico-uterine fistulas. Report of 30 cases. *Ann Urol* 1999;33:75–79.
12. Sefrioui O, Benabbes Taarji H, Azyez M, Aboulfalah A, El Karroumi M, Matar N, El Mansouri A. Vesico-uterine fistula of obstetrical origin. Report of 3 cases. *Ann Urol* 2002;36:376–80.
13. Brown JE, Thieme GA, Shah DM, Fleischer AC, Boehm FH. Transabdominal and transvaginal endosonography: Evaluation of the cervix and lower uterine segment in pregnancy. *Gynecol Obstet* 1990;162:596–7.
14. Kawakami S, Togashi K, Sagoh T, Kimura I, Noguchi M, Takakura K, Mori T, Konishi J. Uterine deformity caused by surgery during pregnancy. *J Comput Assist Tomogr* 1994;18:272–4.
15. Hebisch G, Kirkinen P, Haldemann R, Paakkoo E, Huch A, Huch R. Comparative study of the lower uterine segment after Cesarean delivery using ultrasound and magnetic resonance tomography. *Ultraschall Med* 1994;15:112–6.
16. Avrech OM, Weinraub Z, Herman A, Ariely S, Tovbin Y, Bukowsky I, Capsi E. Ultrasonic antepartum assessment of a classical cesarean uterine scar and diagnosis of dehiscence. *Ultrasound Obstet Gynecol* 1999;4:151–3.
17. Lebedev VA, Strizhakov AN, Zhelenov BI. Echographic and morphological parallels in the evaluation of the condition of the uterine scar. *Akush Ginekol* 1991;(8):44–49.
18. Michaels Wh, Thompson Ho, Boutt A, Schreiber Fr, Mchaels Sl, Karo J Ultrasound diagnosis of defects in the scarred lower uterine segment during pregnancy. *Obstet Gynecol* 1988;71:112–20.
19. Fukuda M, Fukuda K, Mochizuki M. Examination of previous cesarean delivery scars by ultrasound. *Arch Gynecol Obstet* 1988;243:221–4.
20. Fukuda M, Shimizu T, Ihara Y, Fukuda K, Natsuyama E, Mochizuki M. Ultrasound caesarean of caesarean delivery scars during pregnancy. *Arch Gynecol Obstet* 1991;248:129–38.
21. Van Alphen M, Van Vugt JMG, Hummel P, Van Geijn HP. Recurrent uterine rupture diagnosed by ultrasound. *Ultrasound Obstet Gynecol* 1995;5: 419–21.
22. Tanik A, Ustun C, Cil E, Arslan A. Sonographic evaluation of the wall thickness of the lower uterine segment in patients with previous cesarean delivery. *J Clin Ultrasound* 1996;24(7):355–7.
23. Cheung VY, Constantinescu OC, Ahluwalia BS. Sonographic evaluation of the lower uterine segment in patients with previous caesarean delivery. *Ultrasound Med* 2004;23:1441–7.
24. Cheung VY. Sonographic measurement of the lower uterine segment thickness in women with previous caesarean delivery. *Obstet Gynaecol Can* 2005;27:674–81.
25. Giorlandino C, Gentili P, Russo N, Papparella P, Vizzone A. Il segno del colpo d'ascia come diagnosi ecografica di pregresso intervento cesareo. *Esper. Ultras. Ost. Ginec.*, 1983; Bios Ed., 349.
26. Monteagudo A, Carreno C, Timor-Tritsch IE. Saline infusion sonohysterography in nonpregnant women with previous cesarean delivery: The "niche" in the scar. *J Ultrasound Med* 2001;20:1105–15.

27. Regnard C, Nosbusch M, Fellemans C, Benali N, Van Rysselberghe M, Barlow P, Rozenberg S. Cesarean section scar evaluation by saline contrast sonohysterography. *Ultrasound Obstet Gynecol* 2004;23:289–92.
28. Sambaziotis H, Conway C, Figueroa R, Elimian A, Garry D. Second-trimester sonographic comparison of the lower uterine segment in pregnant women with and without a previous cesarean delivery. *J Ultrasound Med* 2004;23:913–4.
29. Sen S, Malik S, Salhan S. Ultrasonographic evaluation of lower uterine segment thickness in patients of previous caesarean delivery. *Int J Gynaecol Obstet* 2004;87:215–59.
30. Armstrong V, Hansen WF, Van Voorhis BJ, Syrop CH. Detection of cesarean scars by transvaginal ultrasound. *Obstet Gynecol* 2003;101:61–65.
31. Esquivel-Estrada V, Briones-Garduno JC, Mondragon-Ballesteros R. Endometriosis implant in cesarean delivery surgical scar. *Cir Cir* 2004;72:113–5.
32. Gaunt A, Heard G, McKain ES, Stephenson BM. Caesarean scar endometrioma. *Lancet* 2004;364:368.
33. Ishida GM, Motoyama T, Watanabe T, Emura I. Clear cell carcinoma arising in a caesarean delivery scar. Report of a case with fine needle aspiration cytology. *Acta Cytol* 2003;47:1095–8.
34. Sugawara J, Senoo M, Chisaka H, Yaegashi N, Okamura K. Successful conservative treatment of a caesarean scar pregnancy with uterine artery embolization. *Tohoku J Exp Med* 2005;206:261–5.
35. Passaro R, Battagliese A, Paolillo F. Ectopic pregnancy on previous caesarean delivery scar. Case report. *Minerva Ginecol* 2005;57:207–12.
36. Hwu YM, Hsu CY, Yang HY. Conservative treatment of caesarean scar pregnancy with transvaginal needle aspiration of the embryo. *BJOG* 2005;112:841–2.
37. Wang CJ, Yuen LT, Chao AS, Lee CL, Yen CF, Soong YK. Caesarean scar pregnancy successfully treated by operative hysteroscopy and suction curettage. *BJOG* 2005;112:839–40.
38. Wang YL, Su TH, Chen HS. Laparoscopic management of an ectopic pregnancy in a lower segment caesarean delivery scar: A review and case report. *J Minim Invasive Gynecol* 2005;12:73–9.
39. Arslan M, Pata O, Dilek TU, Aktas A, Aban M, Dilek S. Treatment of viable caesarean scar ectopic pregnancy with suction curettage. *Int J Gynaecol Obstet* 2005;89:163–6.
40. Noguchi S, Adachi M, Konishi H, Habara T, Nakatsuka M, Kudo T. Intramural pregnancy in a previous caesarean delivery scar: A case report on conservative surgery. *Acta Obstet Gynecol Scand* 2005;84:493–5.
41. Tan G, Chong YS, Biswas A. Caesarean scar pregnancy: A diagnosis to consider carefully in patients with risk factors. *Ann Acad Med Singapore* 2005;34:216–9.
42. Graesslin O, Dedecker F Jr, Quereux C, Gabriel R. Conservative treatment of ectopic pregnancy in a caesarean scar. *Obstet Gynecol* 2005;105:869–71.
43. Hasegawa J, Ichizuka K, Matsuoka R, Otsuki K, Sekizawa A, Okai T. Limitations of conservative treatment for repeat Cesarean scar pregnancy. *Ultrasound Obstet Gynecol* 2005;25:310–1.
44. Wang CJ, Yuen LT, Yen CF, Lee CL, Soong YK. Three-dimensional power Doppler ultrasound diagnosis and laparoscopic management of a caesarean in a previous caesarean scar. *J Laparoendosc Adv Surg Tech A* 2004;14:399–402.
45. Seow KM, Hwang JL, Tsai YL, Huang LW, Lin YH, Hsieh BC. Subsequent pregnancy outcome after conservative treatment of a previous caesarean scar pregnancy. *Acta Obstet Gynecol Scand* 2004;83:1167–72.
46. Maymon R, Halperin R, Mendlovic S, Schneider D, Herman A. Ectopic pregnancies in a Caesarean scar: Review of the medical approach to an iatrogenic complication. *Hum Reprod Update* 2004;10:515–23.
47. Yazicioglu HF, Turgut S, Madazli R, Aygun M, Cebi Z, Sonmez S. An unusual case of heterotopic twin pregnancy managed successfully with selective feticide. *Ultrasound Obstet Gynecol* 2004;23:626–7.
48. Doubilet PM, Benson CB, Frates MC, Ginsburg E. Sonographically guided minimally invasive treatment of unusual ectopic pregnancies. *J Ultrasound Med* 2004;23:359–70.
49. Chou MM, Hwang JI, Tseng JJ, Huang YF, Ho ES. Cesarean scar pregnancy: Quantitative assessment of uterine neovascularization with 3-dimensional color power Doppler imaging and successful treatment with uterine artery embolization. *Am J Obstet Gynecol* 2004;190:866–8.
50. Marchiole P, Gorlero F, de Caro G, Podesta M, Valenzano M. Intramural pregnancy embedded in a previous Cesarean delivery scar treated conservatively. *Ultrasound Obstet Gynecol* 2004;23:307–9.
51. Shih JC. Cesarean scar pregnancy: Diagnosis with three-dimensional (3D) ultrasound and 3D power Doppler. *Ultrasound Obstet Gynecol* 2004;23:306–7.
52. Seow KM, Huang LW, Lin YH, Lin MY, Tsai YL, Hwang JL. Cesarean scar pregnancy: Issues in management. *Ultrasound Obstet Gynecol* 2004;23:247–53.
53. Li SP, Wang W, Tang XL, Wang Y. Cesarean scar pregnancy: A case report. *Chin Med J* 2004;117:316–7.
54. Tsenov D, Mainkhard K. Endometriosis in the surgical scar from caesarean delivery. *Akush Ginekol* 2000;39:50–51.
55. Kafkasli A, Franklin RR, Sauls D. Endometriosis in the uterine wall cesarean delivery scar. *Gynecol Obstet Invest* 1996;42:211–3.
56. Fabres C, Arriagada P, Fernandez C, Mackenna A, Zegers F, Fernandez E. Surgical treatment and follow-up of women with intermenstrual bleeding due to caesarean delivery scar defect. *J Minim Invasive Gynecol* 2005;12:25–28.
57. Fabres C, Aviles G, De La Jara C, Escalona J, Munoz JF, Mackenna A, Fernandez C, Zegers-Hochschild F, Fernandez E. The cesarean delivery scar pouch:

57. Clinical implications and diagnostic correlation between transvaginal sonography and hysteroscopy. *J Ultrasound Med.* 2003;22:695–700.
58. Morris H. Caesarean scar syndrome. *S Afr Med J* 1996;86:1558.
59. Malvasi A, Tinelli A, Hudelist G, Vergara D, Martignago R, Tinelli R. Closure versus non-closure of the visceral peritoneum (VP) in patients with gestational hypertension—An observational analysis. *Hypertens Pregnancy* 2009;28:290–9.
60. Malvasi A, Tinelli A, Tinelli R, Rahimi S, Resta L, Tinelli FG. The post-cesarean delivery symptomatic bladder flap hematoma: A modern reappraisal. *J Matern Fetal Neonatal Med* 2007;20:709–14.
61. Rodgers SK, Kirby CL, Smith RJ, Horrow MM. Imaging after cesarean delivery: Acute and chronic complications. *Radiographics.* 2012;32(6):1693–712.
62. Malvasi A, Tinelli A, Guido M, Zizza A, Farine D, Stark M. Should the visceral peritoneum at the bladder flap closed at cesarean deliveries? A post-partum sonographic and clinical assessment. *J Matern Fetal Neonatal Med* 2010;23:662–9.
63. Tinelli A, Malvasi A, Vittori G. Laparoscopic treatment of post-cesarean delivery bladder flap hematoma: A feasible and safe approach. *Minim Invasive Ther Allied Technol* 2009;18:356–60.
64. Tinelli A, Malvasi A, Tinelli R, Cavallotti C, Tinelli FG. Conservative laparoscopic treatment of post-cesarean section bladder flap haematoma: Two case reports. *Gynecol Surg* 2007;4(1):53–56.
65. Malvasi A, Tinelli A, Guido M, Cavallotti C, Dell'Edera D, Zizza A, Di Renzo GC, Stark M, Bettocchi S. Effect of avoiding bladder flap formation in caesarean delivery on repeat caesarean delivery. *Eur J Obstet Gynecol Reprod Biol* 2011;159(2):300–4.
66. Malvasi A, Tinelli A, Farine D, Rahimi S, Cavallotti C, Vergara D, Martignago R, Stark M. Effects of visceral peritoneal closure on scar formation at cesarean delivery. *Int J Gynaecol Obstet* 2009;105: 131–5.
67. Malvasi A, Tinelli A, Cavallotti C, Bettocchi S, Di Renzo GC, Stark M, Substance P (SP) and vasoactive intestinal polypeptide (VIP) in the lower uterine segment in first and repeated cesarean deliveries. *Peptides* 2010;31:2052–9.
68. Malvasi A, Dell'Edera D, Cavallotti C, Creanza A, Pacella E, Di Renzo G C, Mynbaev O A, Tinelli A. Inflammation and neurotransmission of the vesicouterine space in caesarean sections. *Eur J Inflamm* 2013;11(1):247–6.
69. Malvasi A, Farine D, Stark M, Cavallotti C, Tinelli A. Adhesions and one layer suture in cesarean delivery. *J Matern Fetal Neonatal Med* 2010;23(Suppl 1):48.
70. Mynbaev OA, Eliseeva MY, Kalzhanov ZR, Lyutova L, Pismensky SV, Tinelli A, Malvasi A, Kosmas IP. Surgical trauma and CO_2-insufflation impact on adhesion formation in parietal and visceral peritoneal lesion. *Int J Clin Exp Med* 2013;6(3):153–65.
71. Wang CJ, Huang HJ, Chao A, Lin YP, Pan YJ, Horng SG. Challenges in the transvaginal management of abnormal uterine bleeding secondary to cesarean delivery scar defect. *Eur J Obstet Gynecol Reprod Biol* 2011;154(2):218–22.
72. Tinelli A, Tinelli R, Malvasi A. Laparoscopic management of cervical-isthmic pregnancy: A proposal method. *Fertil Steril* 2009;92(2):829.e3–6.
73. Tinelli A, Malvasi A, Vergara D, Casciaro S. Emergency surgical procedure for failed methotrexate treatment of cervical pregnancy: A case report. *Eur J Contracept Reprod Health Care* 2007;12(4):391–5.
74. Robinson JK, Dayal MB, Gindoff P, Frankfurter D. A novel surgical treatment for cesarean scar pregnancy: Laparoscopically assisted operative hysteroscopy. *Fertil Steril* 2009;92(4):1497.e13–16.

FURTHER READING

Fukuda M, Fukuda K, Shimizu T, Natsuyama E, Mochizuki M. Two types of translucent membrane of caesarean delivery scar tissue. *Lancet* 1992;(25)339:254–5.

Garanov M, Popovich D. Anatomical and clinical correlations in uterine cicatrix. *Akush Ginekol* 1978;17:119–25.

Garanov M, Popovich D. Histological study of the uterine cicatrix after caesarean delivery (I). *Akush Ginekol* 1978;17:14–20.

Iakutina MF. Vessels and nerves of the uterine scar following caesarean delivery (clinico-experimental study). *Vopr Okhr Materin Det* 1968;13:50–54.

Kiss D, Gyorik J, Kekesi G. Hysterographic examination of unilayer lointed wound margins following caesarean delivery. *Zentralbl Ginakol* 1978;100:303–8.

Klimenko ZS, Gitman GI. Histological structure of the scar of the uterus after caesarean delivery. *Pediat Akus Ginekol* 1969;31:45–47.

Lazarov L, Stratiev S. The morphological characteristics of the cicatrix in repeat caesarean delivery. *Akush Ginekol* 1993;32:12–14.

Ruiz-Velasco V, Rosas-Arceo J. Evaluation of the cesarean delivery cicatrix. *Rev Fr Gynecol Obstet* 1971;66:83–93.

Wanoriek A. Segmental transverse cicatrix. Study of nonpregnant uterine specimens. *J Gynecol Obstet Biol Reprod* 1972;1:457–67.

Wojodecki J, Grynsztajn A. Scar formation in the uterus after caesarean delivery. *Am J Obstet Gynecol* 1970;15:322–4.

Vaginal birth after cesarean delivery

ANTONIO MALVASI, GIAN CARLO DI RENZO, and LAURA DI FABRIZIO

INTRODUCTION

In 1916 Craigin expressed the following axiom in a work eloquently titled "Conservatism in Obstetrics": "once a cesarean, always a cesarean." This was a warning to his colleagues of the danger of abusing cesarean deliveries, as once the surgical approach was adopted, repeat cesarean deliveries would became a necessity in later pregnancies (risk of uterine rupture at the time was 5%) [1].

For this reason in the United States, before 1950, vaginal birth after cesarean was rare, although it was more commonly practiced in Europe.

In 1980 the National Institute of Child Health and Human Development conference attributed 25%–30% of increases in cesarean deliveries to repeat cesarean deliveries (about one-third of the total).

On a global level previous cesarean deliveries represent, respectively, approximately 6% of overall deliveries (Figure 21.1) and 30%–40% of indications to a cesarean delivery, and is the main indication for a repeat cesarean delivery (Figure 21.2) [2–4].

In order to reverse the current increase in cesarean deliveries, it would seem appropriate, first of all, to modify one's approach to a woman who had a previous cesarean delivery, because this subset of patients represents a significant portion.

The growing interest surrounding this debated topic has resulted in guidelines from major scientific organizations. These help the physician decide which therapies should be implemented. In 1985 the American College of Obstetricians and Gynecologists (ACOG) was the first scientific organization to publish guidelines that supported the "trial of labor" after cesarean, or vaginal birth after cesarean (VBAC), with the goal of reducing the overall rate of cesarean births.

WHY CHOOSE VAGINAL BIRTH AFTER CESAREAN (VBAC)?

Feasibility of the trial of labor derives from the observation of the high probability of success, which would significantly reduce the overall rate of cesarean deliveries.

VBAC has a 60%–80% probability of success [5–12]. It is essential to carefully evaluate the individual risks before opting for the trial of labor. It is also important that proper counseling be provided to each patient eligible for VBAC. Even though there seems to be less risk associated with VBAC compared to repeat cesarean delivery [7–14] randomized clinical trials support this.

It must, however, be noted that there are greater risks, in terms of maternal and fetal outcome (uterine rupture, hysterectomy, intraoperative complications), in case of failure of the trial of labor, at double the percentage than in elective cesarean deliveries [3,15].

It is also important to not underestimate the fact that a repeat cesarean birth affects the obstetric future of the patient, in that it subjects the patient to the risk of short- and long-term complications.

The comparison between vaginal birth and first cesarean shows significant advantages to the former. Similarly, the comparison between VBAC and repeat cesarean shows that VBAC is definitively advantageous, especially for the subset of patients who are able to successfully deliver. See Table 21.1.

CONDITIONS ASSOCIATED WITH A LOWER PROBABILITY OF VBAC SUCCESS

Two previous cesarean births on the lower uterine segment, previous infection in the postoperative course of the previous cesarean delivery, dystocia as an indication for the first cesarean delivery, suspected macrosomia, and polyhydramnios [6] are conditions associated with a lower probability of VBAC success.

CONDITIONS ASSOCIATED WITH A HIGHER PROBABILITY OF VBAC SUCCESS

Previous vaginal birth, young age of the patient, previous cesarean birth for nonrepetitive indication (nonreassuring cardiotocography [CTG]) (Figure 21.3), breech presentation, and a previous vaginal birth (Figure 21.4) are conditions associated with a higher probability of VBAC success.

"MANAGEMENT" OF THE PATIENT WITH PREVIOUS CESAREAN DELIVERY

Counseling

Informing the patient is an essential part of the treatment procedure and includes a thorough anamnesis of the previous obstetric procedures. It has been theorized, and in some respects demonstrated, that the percentage of success and of risks can be correlated to the patient's clinical history.

The patient with a previous cesarean delivery must be adequately informed on how to prepare for a trial of labor, on the risks and benefits of the procedure, and of repeat cesarean deliveries, as well as on the assistance and the monitoring that take place during labor.

It has been demonstrated that attending a birth preparation class contributes to increasing the percentage of success. Last, the decision must be made by the patient, together with the doctors treating the patient, while taking into account the individual risk factors.

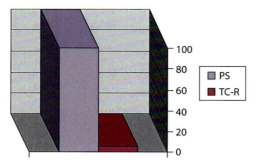

Figure 21.1 Percentage of repeat cesarean deliveries (R-CS) (6%) compared to the total amount of births.

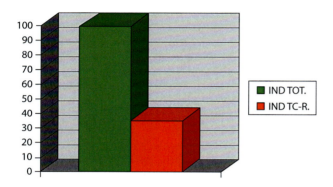

Figure 21.2 Percentage of total indications (TOT. IND.) compared to the percentage of repeat cesarean deliveries as an indication to cesarean delivery (R-CS IND.) which on average is 35%.

Table 21.1 Indications to VBAC

Indications	• Previous cesarean birth with low transverse incision
	• Presence of expert medical personnel and appropriate hospital facilities (level II or III center)
Absolute contraindications	• Presence of longitudinal/transfundal/T-shaped uterine incision
	• Previous dehiscence or uterine rupture
Relative contraindications	• Twin pregnancy
	• Two previous cesarean deliveries
	• Breech presentation

Maternal–fetal surveillance during labor

It is mandatory, during the active phase of labor, to continuously monitor (electronically) the basic fetal heart rate, even during the expulsive period as an alternative to intermittent auscultation between contractions. The goal of the continuous monitoring is to identify, early on, the

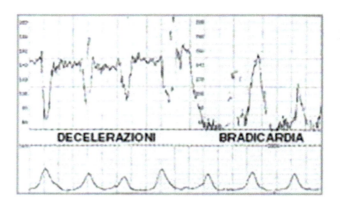

Figure 21.3 Previous cesarean delivery for nonreassuring CTG is an indication for VBACS—previous cesarean delivery for breech presentation.

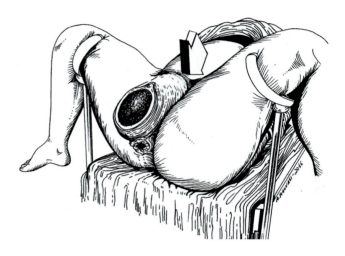

Figure 21.4 A previous spontaneous birth is a condition associated with higher probability of VBACS success. There should be no dystocia. (In the illustration the fetal head is being forced out in the occiput posterior position.)

clinical signs of uterine rupture, cardiotocograph anomalies, and the reduction and sudden halt of uterine contractions (Figure 21.5).

The clinical symptoms of uterine rupture that accompany cardiotocograph alterations are anomalous blood loss from the external genitalia or from the urinary tract, rising of the level of the presenting part, and state of shock. Pain localized in the surgical wound area is not pathognomonic to uterine rupture, whereas visceral uterine pain, located deeper than the surgical wound area, and which does not subside between contractions, is a cause for concern.

The Kristeller maneuver must always be prohibited, but the obstetric ventouse can be used to accelerate or facilitate the expulsive period (Figure 21.6).

Adequately trained staff that knows how to confront emergency situations and is readily available must be present. An emergency cesarean delivery needs to be completed in a very short amount of time—D-D (decision–delivery) time not over 30 minutes.

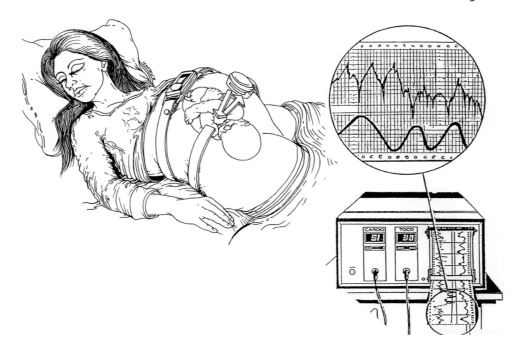

Figure 21.5 VBACS requires continuous cardiotocographic monitoring, even during the expulsive period of the second stage of labor in order to detect, from early on, rupture of the uterus. (The illustration shows variable fetal heart decelerations.)

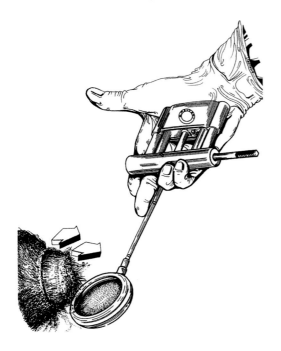

Figure 21.6 The obstetric ventouse can facilitate the expulsive period of the fetal head; the Kristeller maneuver is prohibited.

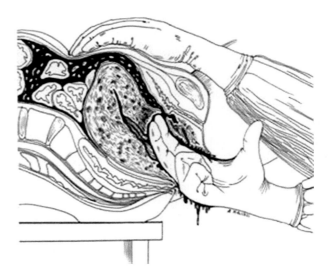

Figure 21.7 Digital intrauterine palpation of the previous scar is not recommended after VBACS, as there is the possibility of causing iatrogenic wounds or of worsening any present dehiscence.

Checking the structural integrity of the previous surgical scar after delivery, through digital examination, should not be performed. It has been proven, in fact, that it may cause a rupture or diastasis of any asymptomatic dehiscence present [16] (Figure 21.7).

In case of anomalous bleeding, or of signs of hypovolemia after delivery, pathologies of the placental stage or uterine rupture, for which the laparotomy is diagnostic, must be excluded.

ANALGESIA DURING LABOR

VBAC is not a contraindication to epidural anesthesia and may encourage patients to choose the trial of labor [17,18]. There do not appear to be differences in patients who undergo epidural analgesia compared to those patients who were not subjected to it. Analgesia does not seem to hide the clinical signs of rupture of the uterus [6,19] (Figure 21.8).

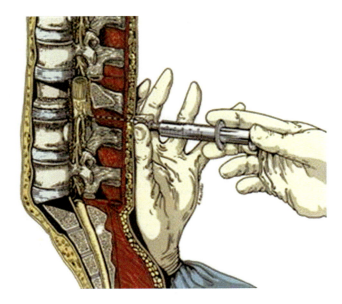

Figure 21.8 Analgesia during labor, if administered with a low dosage, is not a contraindication to VBACS—that is, it does not hide the pain of rupture of the uterus.

USE OF OXYTOCIN AND OF PROSTAGLANDINS

Administering oxytocin to induce or accelerate labor is a relatively safe option. There is no scientific evidence that supports an increased risk of maternal or fetal complications, even though its use is associated with a lower rate of vaginal birth success, especially when correlated with induction (68% versus 80%) (Figure 21.9).

Similarly, the use of prostaglandins seems to be associated with a lower probability of success, but the data in the literature are not sufficient (Figure 21.10).

Data from case-control and prospective studies, relative to the induction of labor in patients with a previous cesarean delivery, supported the efficacy and safety of prostaglandins up to 2001 [20–22], the year in which a retrospective study on 20,000 patients was published. The study showed a risk of uterine rupture five times greater in the group of patients who underwent induction with prostaglandins compared to the group of patients in which labor arose spontaneously (24/1000 versus 5/1000) [23].

This publication led major scientific organizations to review the management of women with a previous cesarean delivery during labor induction with prostaglandins. The ACOG in 2002, in an update of the VBAC procedure, advised against administering prostaglandins [24]. However, the limited amount of scientific data that back the dangers of induction with prostaglandins in trial of labor candidates, has led some scientific organizations, such as SIGO (Società Italiana di Ostetricia e Ginecologia) and the RCOG (Royal College of Obstetricians and Gynaecologists) to not completely ban this induction method. Instead, they recommend its use as an alternative to oxytocin (Figure 21.11) in favorable clinical situations and in informed and knowledgeable patients [25].

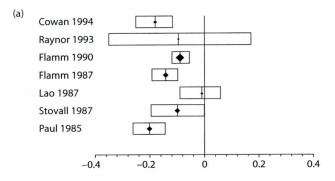

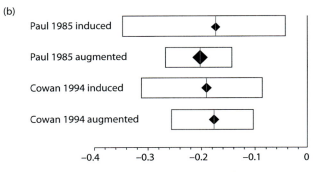

Figure 21.9 (a) Vaginal birth (VBAC): Comparison of prostaglandin E2 versus oxytocin; outcome of cesarean delivery. Difference with 95% CL. (b) Vaginal birth (VBAC): Comparison of prostaglandin E2 versus oxytocin; outcome of serious maternal morbidity or death. Difference with 95% CL. (Data derived from Jozwiak M. Dodd JM, *The Cochrane Library*, Issue 3, 1–22, 2013.)

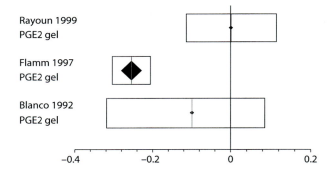

Figure 21.10 Vaginal birth (VBAC): comparison of prostaglandin E2 versus oxytocin; outcome of instrumental vaginal delivery. Difference with 95% CL. (Data derived from Jozwiak M, Dodd JM, *The Cochrane Library*, Issue 3, 1–22, 2013.)

RISKS AND COMPLICATIONS

The most dramatic consequence of failure of vaginal birth, after a previous cesarean delivery, is uterine rupture occurring during labor. The uterine rupture is defined as the opening of the previous hysterotomy scar, which leads to dramatic maternal and fetal consequences, if measures are not immediately taken (Figure 21.12).

It is a symptomatic event, separate from wound dehiscence that is asymptomatic and, usually, without negative

Risks and complications 359

consequences, which occurs during a repeat cesarean delivery performed due to other indications (Figures 21.13 through 21.15).

Existing studies in the literature do not allow an estimate of the frequency of the more serious maternal/fetal complications based on strong evidence. In fact, the data that have been used are not from randomized and controlled prospective studies, which are difficult to achieve given the relative scarcity of the more serious events (one every 1000/10,000 births), but instead from retrospective population studies or from cohort studies.

The difficulty in interpreting the data is also due to the different definitions and classifications used in describing obstetric interventions and maternal and fetal complications. Asymptomatic uterine rupture, also defined as dehiscence, is defined as the accidental finding of asymptomatic separation of the previous surgical scar (Figure 21.15).

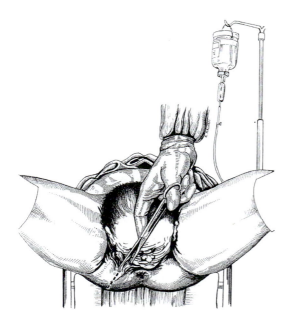

Figure 21.11 The induction of labor in VBACS with oxytocin can be performed in select cases. The use of prostaglandins is instead more problematic, as its effects on the uterine scar can lead to rupture of the uterus.

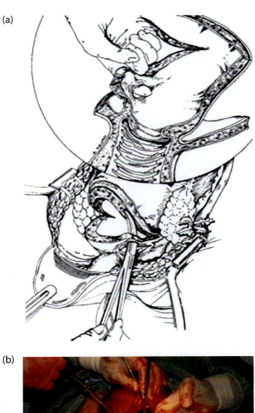

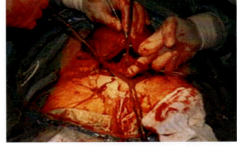

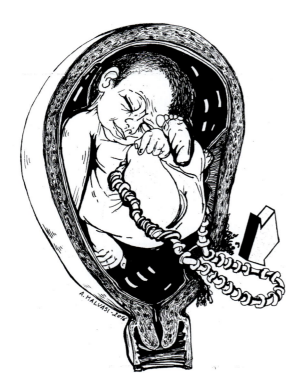

Figure 21.12 An anatomical model of rupture of the uterus at the 33rd week of amenorrhea, in a patient with three previous cesarean deliveries and placenta accreta, which caused hemorrhage during labor, death of the fetus, and cesarean delivery hysterectomy for the patient.

Figure 21.13 (a) Dehiscence of previous uterine scar during a repeat cesarean delivery, which silently ruptures after the removal of the membranes, due to the discontinuity of the uterine wall shown with the index fingers and a Moynihan forceps. (b) Photograph.

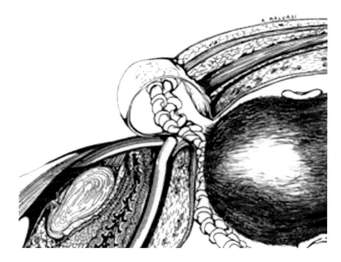

Figure 21.14 Uterine dehiscence at the level of the previous uterine scar from cesarean delivery, with only the amniochorial membranes and the prolapsed cord.

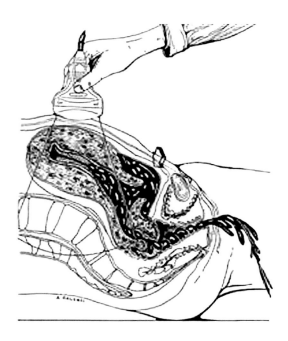

Figure 21.15 Ultrasound can reveal postpartum uterine rupture after VBACS with endoperitoneal effusion.

There is no significant difference in the rate of asymptomatic uterine rupture between the trial of labor and elective cesarean delivery (Figure 21.16). In terms of the rate of symptomatic uterine rupture during trial of labor in women with previous cesarean delivery, it varies from 0 to 7.8 per 1000 trials of labor (overall rate of 3.16/1000).

Comparing the outcomes of pregnant women subjected to the trial of labor with those of women with elective cesarean deliveries brings to light an additional risk of 2.7/1000 (Figure 21.17). Comparison studies of different labor induction methods with spontaneous labor in patients with previous cesarean deliveries shows a slight

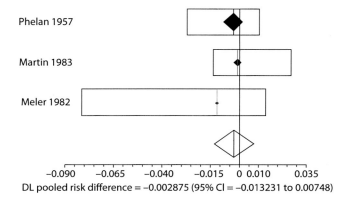

Figure 21.16 Asymptomatic uterine rupture: trial of labor versus elective repeat cesarean delivery.

nonsignificant increase in risk (Figure 21.18). The use of oxytocin does not seem to increase the risk of this complication (Figure 21.19). Although there are no highly accurate or precise studies on the use of prostaglandins, some retrospective studies suggest a concrete association with an increased risk of uterine rupture (Figure 21.20).

With regard to the rate of hysterectomies resulting from symptomatic uterine ruptures, an analysis of the literature shows that 3.4 out of 10,000 women who choose the trial of labor, will have a uterine rupture that will require a hysterectomy.

Perinatal mortality as a result of uterine rupture shows an additional rate of 1.4 out of 10,000 trials of labor. The results of the Scottish Morbidity Record and Stillbirth and Neonatal Death Enquiry show a perinatal mortality rate that is 10 times greater in women who choose the trial of labor, than in those women who underwent an elective cesarean delivery; though the absolute number of events remains acceptable (12.9 out of 10,000) and with serious reservations on the methods of collecting and analyzing the published data, which reduces the statistical significance.

PREDICTIVE FACTORS OF SUCCESS AND OF RISK IN VBAC

The primary goal of the obstetrician, faced with a patient with a previous cesarean delivery, is to identify the risk factors predictive of uterine rupture and of failure of the trial of labor, in order to minimize negative events and to correctly guide the patient to a safe and tranquil labor process. The predictive factors of uterine rupture identified in a more or less controversial and debated manner are the following: previous vertical surgical scar and high number of previous hysterotomies, period of time from the previous cesarean birth (according to some authors a period under 14–18 months is at greater risk), fever complication in the course of the previous cesarean birth, use of prostaglandins and of oxytocin, suspected fetal macrosomia, no previous vaginal birth, maternal age, gestational period [27–29], indication to previous cesarean birth (favorable for previous indication of breech presentation and nonreassuring CTG, unfavorable for previous indication of dystocia).

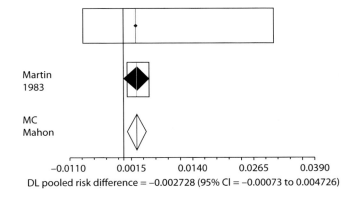

Figure 21.17 Symptomatic uterine rupture: trial of labor versus elective repeat cesarean delivery. Risk difference, 95% CL.

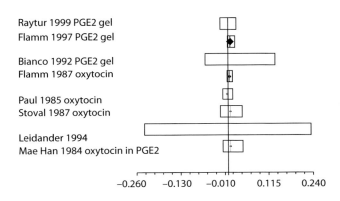

Figure 21.18 Induction and risk of uterine rupture. Risk difference, 95% CL.

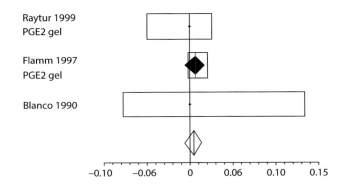

Figure 21.20 Uterine rupture: induction with prostaglandins versus spontaneous labor. Difference with 95% CL.

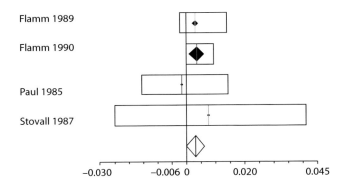

Figure 21.19 Use of oxytocin and risk of uterine rupture. Risk difference, 95% CL.

The use of various predictive factors, in the form of a score, has not yielded satisfactory results (see [5]).

The risks and benefits of VBAC compared with a repeat cesarean delivery are uncertain. The decision, therefore, on how to carry out a delivery after a previous cesarean delivery should consider the following:

- Maternal preferences and priorities
- A general evaluation of the risks and benefits of the cesarean delivery
- The risk of uterine rupture
- The risk of perinatal mortality and morbidity

Pregnant women with previous cesarean delivery who would like to give birth vaginally should be supported in their decision. They should be informed that

- Uterine rupture is a very rare complication; however, that is more likely in patients who undergo VBAC (35/10,000 women versus 12/10,000 women who undergo elective repeat cesarean delivery).
- The risk of perinatal mortality is low for women who undergo VBAC (circa 10/10,000) but is higher than in women who undergo elective repeat cesarean delivery (circa 1/10,000).
- The effect of VBAC or of elective repeat cesarean delivery on infantile cerebral palsy is uncertain.

Women with previous cesarean delivery should be guaranteed:

- That the fetus should be monitored during labor
- Assistance during labor from a center provided with blood transfusion; a center that can guarantee an immediate cesarean delivery

Women with a previous cesarean delivery can be provided with induction to labor, but both the patients as well as the medical staff must be aware that the likelihood of uterine rupture increases by

- 80 per 10,000 if labor is induced with nonprostaglandin drugs
- 240 per 10,000 if labor is induced with prostaglandin drugs

During labor induction, in women with a previous cesarean delivery, the fetus must be electronically monitored. There must be immediate access to the previous cesarean delivery in case of complications, as these women are at an increased risk of uterine rupture.

Women who have had a previous cesarean delivery as well as a vaginal birth should be informed that they have a better probability of success with vaginal birth than women with a previous cesarean delivery and no vaginal birth [29].

CONCLUSIONS

All the guidelines indicate that neither elective repeat cesarean delivery nor the trial of labor are without risks.

In particular, the benefits in case of success of the trial of labor, in terms of maternal and perinatal mortality and morbidity, are greater than for a cesarean delivery. In fact in this clinical circumstance, the outcomes of the two options can be compared.

A cesarean delivery is burdened with greater respiratory morbidity (RR 6.8) compared to vaginal birth, whereas vaginal birth has a greater risk of urinary incontinence and utero-vaginal prolapse (RR 0.6).

There are no significant statistical differences between the two methods of delivery in terms of fecal incontinence, back pain, postpartum depression syndrome, dyspareunia, neonatal mortality, intracranial hemorrhage, brachial plexus damage, and cerebral palsy.

In trying to determine the additional risks for those women who opt for the trial of labor instead of a repeat cesarean delivery, it can be deduced that elective surgery cannot completely eliminate the risk of uterine rupture or of maternal–fetal complications.

To prevent one symptomatic uterine rupture due to the trial of labor, 370 cesarean deliveries would need to be performed; 70,142 cesarean deliveries to prevent a perinatal death related to uterine rupture; 2941 cesarean deliveries to prevent a hysterectomy due to uterine rupture [30]; if, in theory, 7142 elective cesarean deliveries could be performed, there would be a maternal mortality of 0.8 out of 10,000 [31].

In order to avoid a single severe perinatal outcome (hypoxic–ischemic encephalopathy or perinatal death) due to the trial of labor, 588 cesarean deliveries would need to be carried out [32]. If all the data are analyzed it can be reasonably deduced that an elective cesarean birth would seem to be associated with only slightly better perinatal outcomes than with the trial of labor.

Note that the absolute numbers of risk cases are small, and this, therefore, leaves room for those who consider vaginal birth a valid option for women with a previous cesarean delivery. Vaginal birth after cesarean delivery is acceptable and comparable with elective surgical intervention in terms of complications.

The subset of patients that is most burdened with complications consists of patients who have unsuccessfully faced the trial of labor.

Generally, and not only in the medical profession, uncertainty in the outcome leads to decisions that follow rules that are not always easy to explain and that should belong to the realm of ethics and policy decision making. In certain circumstances, for example, individuals behave as though the risk threshold was unrealistically near zero. In other situations, patients are willing to accept the risks of elective surgical procedures with potentially catastrophic consequences, even though valid alternatives are available.

With regard to the decision-making process that leads the patient or the health-care professional to accept the risks of vaginal birth after cesarean delivery, or of a repeat cesarean delivery, it can be said, citing Michael F. Greene of the Massachusetts General Hospital in Boston, that "Risk, like beauty, is in the eye of the beholder" [32].

REFERENCES

1. Cragin EB. Conservatism in obstetrics. *NY Med J* 1916;104(1):1–3.
2. McMahon MJ, Luther ER, Bowes WA et al. Comparison of a trial of labor with an elective second cesarean delivery. *N Engl J Med* 1996;335(10):689–95.
3. Vaginal birth after cesarean delivery. *Obstet Gynecol Clin North Am* 1999;26(2):295–304. Review
4. Royal College of Obstetricians and Gynecologists (RCOG). The National Sentinel Caesarean Delivery Audit Report; October 2001.
5. American Congress of Obstetricians and Gynecologists (ACOG) practice bulletin. Vaginal birth after previous cesarean delivery. Number 115, August 2010 (replaces practice bulletin number 54, July 2004, and Committee Opinion Number 342, August 2006). Clinical management guidelines for obstetrician-gynecologists. American College of Obstetricians and Gynecologists. *Obstet Gynecol* 2010;116(2 Pt 1):450–63.
6. Cowan RK Kinch RA, Ellis B. Trial of labor following cesarean delivery. *Obstet Gynecol* 1994;83:933–6.
7. Flamm BL, Goings JR, Liu Y, Wolde-Tsadik G. Elective repeat cesarean delivery versus trial of labor: A prospective multicenter study. *Obstet Gynecol* 1994;83(6):927–32.
8. Nguyen TV, Dinh TV, Suresh MS, Kinch RA, Anderson GD. Vaginal birth after cesarean delivery at the University of Texas. *J Reprod Med* 1992;37(10):880–2.
9. Flamm BL, Newman LA, Thomas SJ, Fallon D, Yoshida MM. Vaginal birth after cesarean delivery: Results of a 5-year multicenter collaborative study. *Obstet Gynecol* 1990;76(5 Pt 1):750–4.

10. Rosen MG, Dickinson JC. Vaginal birth after cesarean: A meta-analysis of indicators for success. *Obstet Gynecol* 1990;76(5 Pt 1):865–9.
11. Stovall TG, Shaver DC, Solomon SK, Anderson GD. Trial of labor in previous cesarean delivery patients, excluding classical cesarean deliveries. *Obstet Gynecol* 1987;70(5):713–7.
12. Phelan JP, Clark SL, Diaz F, Paul RH. Vaginal birth after cesarean. *Am J Obstet Gynecol* 1987;157(6):1510–5.
13. Nielsen TF, Ljungblad U, Hagberg H. Rupture and dehiscence of cesarean delivery scar during pregnancy and delivery. *Am J Obstet Gynecol* 1989;160(3):569–73.
14. Hansell RS, McMurray KB, Huey GR. Vaginal birth after two or more cesarean deliveries: A five-year experience. *Birth* 1990;17(3):146–50; discussion 150–1.
15. Marconi AM, Natale N, Pardi G, Regalia AL, Scotto di Palombo V. Parto vaginale dopo taglioc esareo. *Proposta di Linee Guida Nazionali*. 2002;3:8–15.
16. Cheung VY, Constantinescu OC, Ahluwalia BS. Sonographic evaluation of the lower uterine segment in patients with previous cesarean delivery. *J Ultrasound Med* 2004;23(11):1441–7.
17. Flamm BL, Goings JR, Liu Y et al. Elective repeat cesarean delivery versus trial of labor: A prospective multicenter study. *Obstet Gynecol* 1994;83(6):927–32.
18. Sakala EP, Kaye S, Murray RD et al. Epidural analgesia. Effect on the likelihood of a successful trial of labor after cesarean delivery. *J Reprod Med* 1990;35:886–90.
19. Leung AS, Farmer RM, Leun EK et al. Risk factors associated with uterine rupture during trial of labor after cesarean delivery: A case-control study. *Am J Obstet Gynecol* 1993;168:1358–63.
20. Norman M, Ekman G. Preinductive cervical ripening with prostaglandin E2 in women with one previous cesarean. *Acta Obstet Gynecol Scand* 1992;71:351–5.
21. Rock SM. Variabiulity and consistency of rates of primary and repeat cesarean deliveries among hospitals in two states. *Public Health Rep* 1993;108:514–6.
22. Martin JN Jr, Morrison JC, Wiser WL. Vaginal birth after cesarean delivery: The demise of routine repeat abdominal delivery. *Obstet Gynecol Clin North Am* 1988;15(4):719–36.
23. Lydon-Rochelle M, Holt VL, Easterling TR, Martin DP. Risk of uterine rupture during labor among women with a prior cesarean delivery. *N Engl J Med* 2001;345(1):3–8.
24. ACOG Committee on Obstetric Practice. Committee opinion. Induction of labor for vaginal birth after cesarean delivery. *Obstet Gynecol* 2002;99(4):679–80.
25. Dodd JM, Crowther CA, Huertas E, Guise JM, Horey D. Planned elective repeat caesarean delivery versus planned vaginal birth for women with a previous caesarean birth. *Cochrane Database Syst Rev* 2004;(4):CD004224. Review.
26. Smith GCS, Pell JP, Cameron AD et al. Risk of perinatal death associated with labor after previous cesarean delivery in uncomplicated term pregnancies. *JAMA* 2002;287:2684–90.
27. Hammoud A, Hendler I, Gauthier RJ et al. The effect of gestational age on trial of labor after cesarean delivery. *J Matern Fetal Neonatal Med* 2004;15:202–6.
28. Loebel G, Zelop CM, Egan JF et al. Maternal and neonatal morbidity after elective repeat cesarean delivery versus a trial of labor after previous cesarean delivery in a community teaching hospital. *J Matern Fetal Neonatal Med* 2004;15:243–6.
29. Zelop CM, Shipp TD, Repke JT et al. Uterine rupture during induced or augmented labor in gravid women with one prior cesarean delivery. *Am J Obstet Gynecol* 1999;181:882–6. *Obstet* 2004;87(3):215–9.
30. Guise JM, McDonagh MS, Osterweil P et al. Systematic review of the incidence and consequences of uterine rupture in women with previous caesarean delivery. *BMJ* 2004;329(19):1–7.
31. National Institute for Health and Care Excellence (NICE). Caesarean delivery clinical guidelines. London, UK: NICE; April 2004.
32. Landon MB, Hauth JC, Leveno KJ et al. Maternal and perinatal outcomes associated with a trial of labor after prior cesarean delivery. *NEJM* 2004;351:2581–9.

FURTHER READING

Flamm B. Once a cesarean, always a controversy. *Obst Gynecol* 1997;90(2):312–5. Review.

Forensic aspects of cesarean delivery

22

ANTONIO MALVASI and GIAN CARLO DI RENZO

… After this first cut, see the body of the rectus muscle and cut that as well until reaching the peritoneum; once it is open you can see the matrix, which must also be cut, but slightly, so as to not harm the baby. The cut however must start at the top and must be pulled transversally to avoid cutting the testicles, the epididymis and the sperm vessels …

(*La Commare o Raccoglitrice*, Chapter XVIII, Second Book. Scipion Mercurii, 1601)

INTRODUCTION

The incidence of cesarean deliveries (CDs) has been steadily increasing in all countries around the world, including the least developed ones, with percentages much higher than the ideal 15% proposed by the WHO (World Health Organization).

Italy has gone from about 10% of CDs in the early 1980s, to 35.7% in 2002, with a decisive increase in estimates, making it one of the countries with the highest percentage of CDs in Europe and in the world: regional differences are significant with percentages ranging from a minimum of 21% in Friuli-Venezia Giulia, to 43% reported in Puglia, up to 56% in Campania [1].

The use of CD is, in general, directly proportional to the maternal age and to parity, with greater frequency in the primiparae.

The high frequency of CD is normally attributed to the increased number of complications related to advanced maternal age and to clinical indications such as repeat CD, multiple pregnancies, and pregnancies due to assisted reproductive techniques.

Other social, cultural, and economic factors have determined an increase in demand for CD from women, even beyond actual therapeutic needs, as well as a defensive attitude of the obstetrician, "threatened" by possible severe medical–legal implications, especially frequent in this profession.

It is not a coincidence that one of the main goals of the 2002–2004 national health plan is decreasing the frequency of CD, reducing the substantial regional differences that currently exist, and reaching within a three year period a national value of 20% in line with the average of other European countries.

In this same spirit of a declared "war on CD," some regions, such as Lazio, have even resorted to using economic incentives in order to promote the so-called natural childbirth.

In light of the excessive use of CDs facing such heavy condemnation from public opinion and media, we will now evaluate the main medical–legal implications associated with an issue that is so current and controversial.

CD AND "DEFENSIVE MEDICINE"

The term "defensive medicine" is the tendency of persons with medical liability to abuse the use of procedures or examinations in order to protect themselves from negligent behavior.

Obstetricians seem to be those most prone to this defensive attitude, most likely due to the large number of lawsuits in which they are involved.

The specter of legal disputes and court sentences severely influences traditional obstetric practices. In fact, every time a negative event occurs in a spontaneous or operative vaginal delivery, the failure to use CD as an unavoidable preventive measure is invoked.

These judiciary accusations continue to exist, though no correlation has been shown between an increased incidence of CD and a reduction in neonatal neurological disorders [2], or a reduction in the incidence of fetal trauma in case of macrosomia [3].

CD has played a significant role in defensive medicine for years and has, at times, been a defense against the risks of vaginal delivery, even if at the expense of the patient's health. The patient in fact undergoes surgery for situations in which there may have been no real need.

There is no doubt that physicians convicted for damages to pregnant women or to unborn children for failing to perform a CD which, if performed, would have solved "every situation," are numerous and constantly increasing [4].

One survey in Puglia on the role of defensive medicine in the choice of CD has shown there to be a greater predisposition of primary physicians with more years of experience, to accept the maternal choice of CD, with no apparent medical indications. In addition, a different degree of perception of the legal pressure by the physicians can be related to the increased number of CDs performed in each hospital [5].

CD AND COMPLICATIONS

The CD is the most frequent surgery in the obstetric field, and considerable efforts have been made to improve the surgical techniques, in order to reduce the duration of the intervention, possible complications, and related costs.

New procedures have in fact been proposed, such as the one in the Misgav Ladach General Hospital in Jerusalem, Israel, better known as the cesarean delivery "according to Stark." This reduces the surgical steps to those strictly necessary, with the indubitable advantage of rapid fetal extraction and of shortening the total duration of the intervention. The reduced surgical steps must always, however, be weighed against possible complications [6].

A greater risk of complications during a CD is associated with the following factors: high execution speed, operator inexperience, gestational period of less than 32 weeks, interventions performed in an emergency situation, premature rupture of the membranes, and very high (or very low) level of the presenting part [7].

There are different types of surgical difficulties during a CD, which are mainly tied to the opening of the peritoneal cavity in case of strong adhesions, to problems related to the limited exposure of the lower uterine segment, and associated with a stop in the progression of the presenting part, especially for abnormal presentations, and to premature rupture of the membranes.

Some phases of the surgical intervention are still controversial, such as the closure of the parietal and visceral peritoneum, the externalization of the uterus, manual or spontaneous afterbirth or with traction on the umbilical cord, the placing of the subfascial drainage, the suturing of the uterine breach in a single or double layer, and the suturing of the subcutaneous tissue [8].

We hope in this regard that there will be better answers at the conclusion of the randomized clinical trial "Caesarean Study" currently underway in Europe, coordinated at Oxford by the "National Perinatal Epidemiology" unit, with the participation in Italy of the University of Bari and Foggia. The trial is evaluating the three following surgical alternatives: single- or double-layer closure of the uterus, closure or nonclosure of the pelvic peritoneum, and restrictive or liberal use of subfascial drainage.

Another frequently discussed aspect in legal disputes is the amount of time between the decision to perform a CD and its implementation. The American Congress of Obstetricians and Gynecologists (ACOG) suggests, in this regard, a guideline based on 30 minutes; the expectant mother should be informed, in a clear and exhaustive manner, of the risks of surgery and of the possible obstetric and gynecological complications.

Accidental extension of the uterine breach

This occurs more frequently in case of repeat cesarean delivery due to the thinness of the lower uterine segment and when the fetus extraction maneuvers are excessively difficult (e.g., when the fetal presenting part is deeply engaged). In these cases, after the fetus has been extracted, there may be a tear in the central part of the lower edge of the uterine breach (below the bladder), the integrity of which should be carefully checked. After the edges of the tear have been precisely located, these must be sutured from the bottom up with a double layer, before closing the hysterotomy breach (Figure 22.1).

Compared to elective CD in which, generally, the lower uterine segment is thick, the uterine incision during CD in labor is performed on a thin and stretched lower

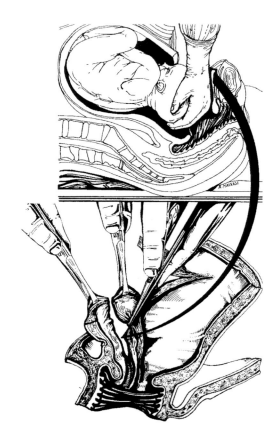

Figure 22.1 Tear of the lower uterine segment, downward to the cervix, during a cesarean delivery; the margins of the tear were extended with two Allis clamps before proceeding with the suture without involving adjacent structures. These tears are more frequent when the fetal extraction is performed at full dilatation with the head located at the pelvic cavity.

segment: the degree of these modifications obviously depends on the duration of labor and on the descent of the presenting part. The procedure is simpler technically, but requires the utmost attention when performing the incision to avoid sinking the scalpel in the underlying fetal tissues, especially with ruptured membranes. Due to the thinness of the lower edge and the frequent tears (which may also be caused by the needle), the suture of the hysterotomy must be performed with care and precision (Figure 22.2) [6].

Tear of the uterine vessels

The places in which a branch of the uterine artery may more commonly tear are the corners of the uterine breach, which may also have been enlarged by the fetus extraction maneuvers. In these cases one must pay special attention to hemostasis, taking care to start closing the uterine breach from a very lateral position so as to include the damaged vessels (Figures 22.3 and 22.4). If the tear affects a large vessel, the two severed branches must be ligated separately. This can be facilitated by the extraction of the uterus from the laparotomy breach, if this maneuver was not previously performed.

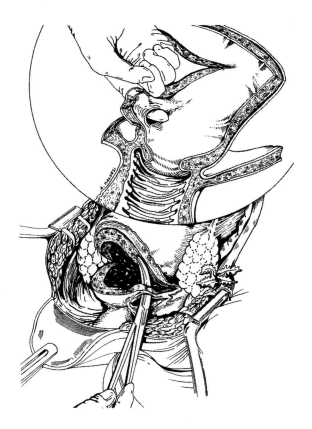

Figure 22.2 Dehiscence of a particularly thin hysterotomy scar; the disruption is highlighted with a Faure clamp (bottom) and digitally (top).

The failure to completely or partially ligate the torn vessel results in a hematoma of the broad ligament that may extend into the retro peritoneum up to the perirenal space. In such cases it may be necessary to ligate the ipsilateral hypogastric artery or, in extreme cases, to resort to a hysterectomy (Figure 22.5).

When the CD is performed before the 32nd week, it is often difficult to have sufficient space to perform a transverse cut at the level of the lower uterine segment. For this reason many authors recommend a low longitudinal incision or a traditional incision on the body, in order to avoid risks of lateral uterine tears and excessive trauma to the premature fetus (Figure 22.6) [6].

HEMORRHAGE

The average loss of blood during a CD is about 0.7–1.01 L and is generally underestimated, especially when there is a large amount. The risk factors associated with an increased blood loss are prolonged labor, emergency CD at stage II of labor, placenta previa, placenta accreta (Figure 22.7), chorioamnionitis, prepartum hemorrhage, previous postpartum hemorrhage, preterm CD, preeclampsia, uterine atony, general anesthesia, and obesity [9].

The recommended precautionary measures that should be taken in case of placenta previa are the presence in the operating room of an expert obstetrician and anesthetist and blood supply in the operating room (Figure 22.8).

In all these cases there is a particular need for an informed consent detailing the possible complications, as well as the risk of other interventions, such as a hysterectomy.

The most common cause of hemorrhage is uterine atony, which should be controlled in a systematic manner by following standardized protocols, such as oxytocic infusion, uterine massage, intramyometrial injection of prostaglandin F2α, thorough search for injuries to the uterine vessels, hemostatic suture of the placental bed, ligation of the internal iliac artery (Figure 22.9), and even, in extreme cases, hysterectomy. The problem of bleeding is, on the whole, easily contained, and only 1%–2% of CDs require transfusions; it must, however, be noted that most cases that require a blood transfusion are not a result of the surgical intervention per se, but of abnormal insertions of the placenta, of detachments of the placenta, and of various types of coagulation disorders [8,9].

POSTCESAREAN HYSTERECTOMY

In cases of severe postpartum hemorrhage, a hysterectomy may be necessary to save the life of the patient.

The most common causes of bleeding that bring about an indication to the intervention are uterine atony unresponsive to medical therapy, placental abnormalities including placenta previa and accreta, especially when associated with repeat CD, and hemorrhage secondary to the incision of the lower uterine segment, to laceration of prominent uterine vessels, to massive myomas, to severe cervical dysplasia, and to carcinoma in situ [10].

In addition, the complications associated with hysterectomy increase significantly when the operation is performed in emergency conditions. These complications include blood loss, duration of the intervention, as well as percentage of blood transfusions and infective problems.

Postpartum hysterectomy is performed in approximately 0.5%–0.8% of cases, with a relative risk that is greater in CD compared to vaginal delivery [11,12]. The intervention may be limited to a supracervical hysterectomy (subtotal) or extended to a total hysterectomy, which requires a greater mobilization of the bladder. Both techniques present the risks associated with increased uterine blood flow during pregnancy, but with the advantage that the tissue planes can be more easily detached.

The spectrum of indications for postcesarean hysterectomy has changed: in fact, atonies have been reduced thanks to the wide use of oxytocics and prostaglandins, while complications from placental anomalies have increased. During these emergency hysterectomies there is often considerable blood loss, resulting in blood transfusions and frequent damage to the bladder and urethras [11].

LESIONS OF THE BLADDER

Surgical damage to the urinary tract and to the gastrointestinal apparatus is rare in the course of a CD. In any case, early diagnosis and proper treatment are essential in preventing future morbidity (Figure 22.10).

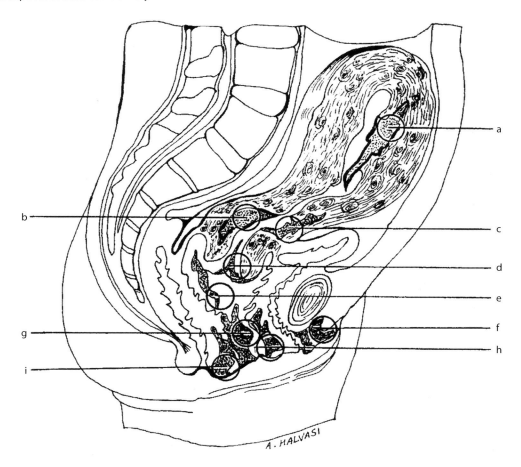

Figure 22.3 Parts of the puerperal genital tract that may be affected by tears that cause bleeding. (a) Tear of the anterior wall of the uterine body. (b) Tear of the posterior cervical wall. (c) Dehiscence of previous hysterotomy scar. (d) Tear of the esocervix. (e) Tear of the posterior vaginal wall. (f) Para urethral tear. (g) "Outbreak of the vagina." (h) Tear of the anterior wall. (i) Tear of the recto-vaginal septum.

The reported incidence of bladder injury (Figure 22.11) during CD varies from 0.0016% to 0.94% [13]. The risk of bladder injuries is greater in cases of CD performed in emergency conditions, repeat CD, previous abdominal surgery, prolonged labor, and in case of incisions according to Pfannenstiel (compared to longitudinal laparotomies).

However, bladder lesions may occur more frequently during the opening of the parietal peritoneum in the course of a laparotomy. This is especially true in case of dislocation at the top of the bladder due to adhesions resulting from previous cesarean deliveries, or other interventions, including, most frequently, previous myomectomies (Figure 22.12).

To prevent this complication it is appropriate to cut the peritoneum, when opening, as high as possible and then to detach the bladder lateromedially: for this reason transverse laparotomies, especially low ones, represent a predisposing condition if the abdominal wall is not detached at the top before entering the peritoneal cavity.

Another condition that can favor the onset of damage to the bladder is the scarring between the latter and the lower uterine segment, again, as a result of previous surgery. In these cases the bladder, generally, is damaged during the maneuvers required to isolate it from the lower uterine segment (prior to its incision), or during the extraction of the fetus, or during surgical detachment maneuvers of the bladder wall from the lower edge of the hysterotomy before suturing the breach [14].

In order to promptly recognize an injury to the bladder, it may be best to instill methylene blue into the bladder before the cesarean delivery. The site of the lesion is a factor that can affect the success of the suture. Disruptions in the bladder dome, in fact, can be easily repaired, while those of the base have a longer healing time due to insufficient vascularization of the area.

Sometimes it is also necessary to perform a ligation of the prevesical vessels in the course of a cesarean to avoid the formation of subfascial hematomas (Figure 22.13). It may also be necessary to perform, in the course of repeat cesarean or in prior laparotomies, a safety maneuver in which the lower wall of the Retzius space is cut in order to safeguard the bladder dome (Figure 22.14).

A simple cystotomy can be sutured in two layers with absorbable suture threads, size 2-0 or 3-0, in which the first layer includes the mucosa and the second layer the submucosa and muscle. After surgery, the catheterism should be maintained for 7–10 days to allow the healing of tissues and avoid overextension [6].

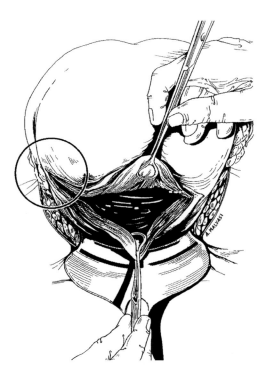

Figure 22.4 Extension of the hysterotomy toward the right corner during a cesarean delivery; the suturing of the uterine breach tear must be carried out after stretching the edge of the corner (the tear can be "undermined"), and by tying over the apex of the lesion.

URETHRAL LESION

Urethral lesions are rare, with an incidence that varies from 0.02% to 0.05% [15].

These lesions are generally linked to the maneuver that attempts to stop bleeding from the uterine incision corner, in direction of the broad ligament. According to some authors, the dextrorotation of the uterus and the relative anterior position of the left urethra, would expose it to more frequent surgical damage (Figure 22.15). Damage, when promptly repaired, is associated with a lower morbidity, thus avoiding the need for a second surgery. Lesions caused by ureter compression usually do not involve the devitalization of tissue and can be reversed. In these cases, however, urinary functionality should be checked and a urinary drainage should be left in the peritoneum.

An evaluation by the urologist may help indicate the position of a urethral catheter. More severe lesions with redelivery of the distal segment of the ureter may require a neocysto-ureterostomy intervention. Several urethral lesions, stenosis, bendings, and occlusions are diagnosed only after delivery.

Any complicated CD in which sutures have affected the parameters, might lead to urethral damage. A renal and pelvic ultrasound check should be performed prior to discharge, or if any sign of urinary obstruction is shown. It would be a good idea in all these cases to isolate the urethra, in the course of a CD, from the iliac bifurcation to the entry in the bladder (Figure 22.16) [15–18].

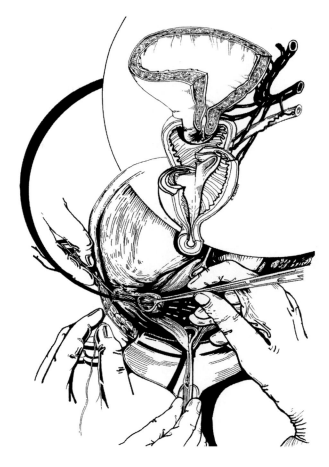

Figure 22.5 Ligation of the uterine vessels of the tubaric corner in case of tear of the breach; the hemostatic suture should be placed at the origin of the tubaric corner, and its effectiveness must be verified.

GASTROINTESTINAL LESIONS

The incidence of intestinal injury in the course of CD, in the large case studies reported by Nielson and Hokegard in 1984, is 0.08% [20].

The risk for inflammatory intestinal disease is higher in women with previous abdominal surgery. The intestine may adhere to the previous scar or to the uterus in the case of previous myomectomy, suture of a previous perforation of the uterus, and CD. An intestinal lesion generally occurs upon opening the abdominal cavity or during adhesiolysis between uterus and intestinal loops, or when extending the incision to the adherent intestine (Figure 22.17).

To avoid causing intestinal lesions, the peritoneal cavity should always be opened with utmost caution. Perform a vertical incision and a careful and meticulous adhesiolysis, especially in those women who have already undergone abdominal surgery [14].

When a lesion of the small intestine is detected before the extraction of the fetus, place a sign of recognition on the loop in question, which will then be covered with a damp cloth. The repair should be performed after closure of the uterine breach. Surgical management is based on

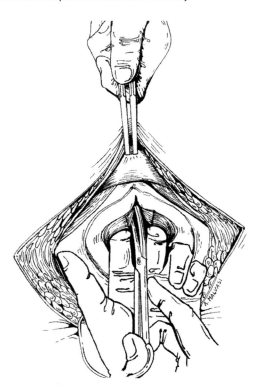

Figure 22.6 T incision of the lower uterine segment during a cesarean delivery on a preterm fetus of 32 weeks, in which the left hand of the surgeon protects the underlying fetal parts to avoid iatrogenic injuries.

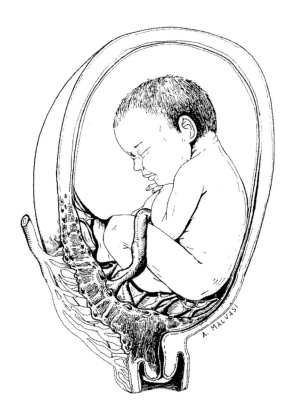

Figure 22.7 Frontal delivery of the uterus at 34 weeks of amenorrhea with the fetus in breech presentation and central placenta previa increta; in this case the pregnant woman must be transferred to a third-level center, as serious puerperal bleeding complications may arise.

the size, number, and location of the lesions and on the vascularization of the loop in question.

Small lesions of the serosa do not require repair, whereas larger defects are to be sutured using absorbable 2-0 sutures or nonabsorbable 3-0 sutures, in a direction perpendicular to the axis of the loop. If it is a full-thickness lesion, the suture can be performed in a single or double layer.

A single-layer closure with knots inside the intestinal lumen increases the blood flow and the width of the intestinal lumen and decreases phlogosis compared with a double-layer closure. If the injury affects more than half of the intestinal circumference, vascularization is compromised or, in case of multiple lesions, the concerned delivery must be redelivered and a termino-terminal anastomosis must be performed.

You should always rely on the collaboration of a general surgeon and remember to always make a careful count of the surgical pads employed in the abdomen, so as to not accidentally leave the pads inside (Figure 22.18).

Systemic antibiotics are usually not necessary. Early fluid intake is instead recommended.

It is essential to suture the lesions of the large intestine, regardless of fecal contamination; colostomy is no longer generally considered necessary [6,14,20,21].

NEUROLOGICAL LESIONS

The incidence of maternal neurological complications at childbirth is estimated to be, from the data in the literature, approximately 0.04%–0.03% [22,23]. It is difficult to distinguish peripheral neurologic abnormalities attributable to causes inherent in the birth itself from those due to surgery (or only to anesthesiology).

Birth is, in fact, accompanied by the risk of neurological complications that vary in type and severity. The fetal head, during its progression in the birth canal, can compress the nerve structures in the small pelvis (lumbosacral plexus) or the nourishing spinal arteries (spinal branch of the internal iliac artery), particularly in the case of maternal–fetal disproportion, prolonged labor, or when forceps are applied (Figure 22.19). This causes postpartum sensory–motor alterations in the lower limbs (Figure 22.20) and/or bladder disorders of varying duration.

A certain number of neuropathies are also caused by incorrect and prolonged positions of the parturient in the periparturient period (Figure 22.21), by nerve damage that arises from the use of retractors during CD or inadequate stretching of the abdominal wall (Figure 22.22), by dural or epidural hematomas under regional anesthesia, and by neurological pathologies, either known or unknown, and which are exacerbated by the pregnancy (multiple sclerosis, diabetes, spinal vascular malformations, etc.).

The progression of the fetus in the birth canal may, therefore, determine the compression of the lumbosacral

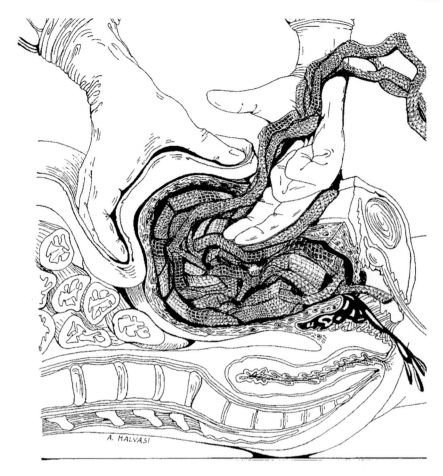

Figure 22.8 Intrauterine wadding pressed into the uterine atony during a cesarean delivery is one of the first instrumental means to cope with the loss of blood.

trunk, which descends in front of the sacroiliac joint. Although it is well protected by the promontory of the sacrum, it can be compressed in particular situations, such as fetal macrosomia or in the presence of a flat pelvis (platypelloid), and mainly involving the fibers originating from S1 (Figure 22.23).

This compression will clinically determine a skin and muscle deficit in the area of the external sciatic popliteal nerve (numbness of the external part of the leg and dorsiflexion deficit of the foot), lasting between 1 and 12 weeks.

The prolonged gynecological position of the legs on the brackets can cause a stretching of the femoral cutaneous nerve, in the point where it passes behind the inguinal ligament, with symptomatological repercussions in the form of paresthesia of the lateral wall of the thigh.

An incorrect lithotomic position with excessive external rotation of the hips can instead cause a sprain of the sciatic nerve, thus possibly resulting in paralysis of the muscles of the leg and of the posterior thigh compartment and hypoesthesia of the lateral half of the calf and foot [24]. In the lithotomic position, the excessive compression of the popliteal fossa by the metal brackets may damage the posterior tibiae nerve and result in a subsequent deficit in plantar flexion of the foot and anesthesia of the foot sole. The femoral and obturator nerves are, on the contrary, more easily damaged during a CD than during vaginal delivery [25,26].

It is good practice for the expectant mother to frequently change position during labor and to avoid maintaining the lithotomy position for long periods of time. This is especially true if the mother undergoes epidural anesthesia, due to the lower reactivity.

Obviously, in the case of CD during labor and neuropathy, it is difficult to clearly distinguish possible surgical causes from those relative to the preceding fetal engagement in the birth canal tied to an incorrect position (Figure 22.24).

Neuropathies associated with the use of epidural anesthesia generally involve a single spinal or peripheral nerve in the lumbar or sacral plexus, and occur with a frequency of 0.04%. These are generally caused by a trauma resulting from the epidural catheter or needle on the sensory nerve ending, with a frequency correlated to the type of catheter and the design of the needle tip. In 20%–40% of cases, transient paresthesias in the area of distribution of the affected nerve are present; in a small number of cases the paresthesias persist in the postpartum period for more than 24–72 hours.

Considering that delivery has an inherent risk of neurological complications of varying degree, and that

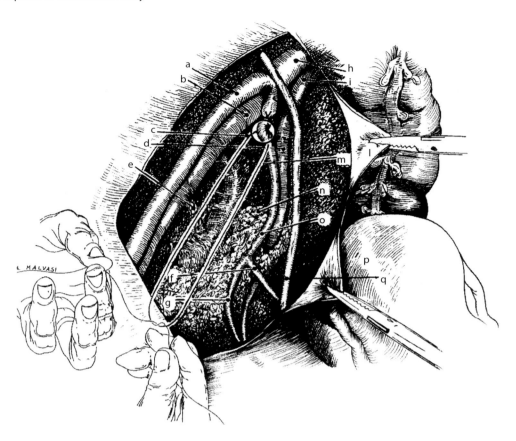

Figure 22.9 Ligation of the right hypogastric artery during postcesarean uterine atony in an attempt to avoid a postcesarean hysterectomy: (a) external iliac artery; (b) external iliac vein; (c) hypogastric artery, a suture thread is passed below (circumference) while another has already been affixed upstream; (d) hypogastric vein; (e) connective tissue; (h) common iliac artery; (i) common iliac vein; (l) medial edge of the incised pelvic peritoneum; (m) posterior branch of the hypogastric artery; (n) medium branch; (o) anterior branch; (p) uterus; (q) ureter.

epidural anesthesia carries an extrinsic risk of neurological sequelae, in order to distinguish obstetric causes from anesthesiological ones, it is extremely important to perform an early neurological evaluation in order to have a rapid diagnosis and therapeutic treatment.

It would, therefore, be useful to have a thorough medical history, physical examination, and imaging studies (computed tomography [CT], magnetic resonance imaging [MRI], etc.). In the case of peripheral neuropathy it is important to perform an electromyography of the lower limbs and paraspinal muscles, as it can determine whether the lesion lies within the spinal canal or is distal to the intervertebral foramina (Figure 22.25) [24–26].

HEMATOMAS

A postpartum complication, whether the delivery is carried out vaginally or by laparotomy, is the accumulation of blood with subsequent deposits. Hematomas, depending on when they are formed and deposited, may appear as simple fluid accumulations, corpuscular, or dense or complex, due to the presence of clots and septa.

More rarely, the deposits are intraperitoneal, in which case their differential diagnosis as physiological fluid layers, as in the case of intrapartum rupture of previously undiagnosed and voluminous ovarian cystomas, can be particularly laborious; the echogenicity and inhomogeneity of the deposit can help to define its hematic or purulent nature.

Extraperitoneal hematomas are the most frequent, following a CD, and can be localized in the subfascial, subcutaneous, pararectal, paravaginal, paravesical areas and at the Retzius level. A hematoma of the Retzius can be detected by transvaginal ultrasound and with semi-stretched bladder, whereas in a transabdominal ultrasound it is obscured by the pubis.

A uterine–bladder fold hematoma is significant only when it exceeds 2 cm, while the presence of hyperechoic spots indicates an infection. The hematoma can extend into the broad ligament laterally, grow posteriorly in the retroperitoneal space (Figure 22.26), and behave as a deep pelvic hematoma.

To diagnose these accumulations it is preferable to perform a transvaginal or transperitoneal ultrasound; the bladder should not be completely empty, so that the anatomical planes can be highlighted [27]. The suture material used for the uterine breach appears in an ultrasound as hyperechoic spots. The subfascial hematoma can instead best be seen with high-frequency transabdominal

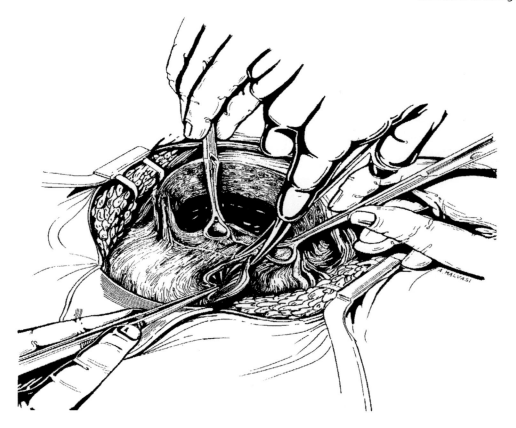

Figure 22.10 Accidental injury of the bladder dome with curved Mayo scissors, in the attempt to detach the bladder dome adherent to the uterine segment due to previous cesarean deliveries. One can see the significant difference between the thickness of the upper edge of the hysterotomy and the thinness of the lower edge that is "fused" with the bladder dome.

ultrasound (5–7.5 MHz); it can spread cranially over and under the rectus muscles or below in the retropubic or Retzius space.

Blood can sometimes reach the subcutis and emerge from the wound, as the transverse fascia is permeable, or it can spread into the abdominal cavity with ultrasound evidence of hemoperitoneum, especially when parietal peritonization has not been performed (Figure 22.27).

In the diagnosis of a subfascial hematoma the rectus muscle is a useful landmark for both the ultrasound and the CD [27]. The incidence of subfascial hematomas, as a complication of CD, varies in different studies from 1% to 3%. One survey, conducted in the obstetric clinics of the University of Bari, showed that this complication increases when CD is performed in hypertensive women, especially obese, and when the CD is performed in emergency conditions. On the contrary, the positioning of the drainage, the experience of the operator, and the type of incision do not constitute risk factors [28].

Last, subcutaneous hematomas occur more frequently in case of transverse laparotomies and intradermal or continuous sutures, which prevent spontaneous drainage of the wound.

RETENTION OF FOREIGN BODIES

Postoperative retention of surgical material ("gossypiboma") is among the less-frequent complications of a cesarean delivery and is especially significant in terms of its clinical and medicolegal consequences. Its actual incidence in obstetric surgery is not known, and in fact it is present in the literature only as case reports. Large case studies, however, report an incidence of about 0.5% in general abdominal surgery [29,30], with a risk nine times higher in emergency interventions. In approximately 70% of cases, the foreign body is gauze (Figure 22.18), while a surgical instrument, or part of it, is less frequent (30%) [29].

In addition, the nonspecific symptoms and the often unclear image diagnosis can make a correct diagnosis difficult to achieve [31]. Techniques such as ultrasound, radiography, MRI, or CT (including three-dimensional) may, at times, indicate the possible presence of a foreign body [32–34], especially in the absence of vascularization in the suspect formation and more or less recent abdominal surgery.

The clinical presentation of a retained "gossypiboma" can range from completely asymptomatic, with incidental diagnosis (x-ray, ultrasound), to an intense inflammatory reaction with intestinal obstruction or perforation [35]. Inflammatory reaction due to the presence of a foreign body (migration of polymorphonuclear cells and formation of a "gauzoma") or due to compression of blood vessels and/or hollow organs (intestine), can also lead to suprainfection.

The risk of fistulation increases with the persistence of the inflammatory process and the failure to restore initial

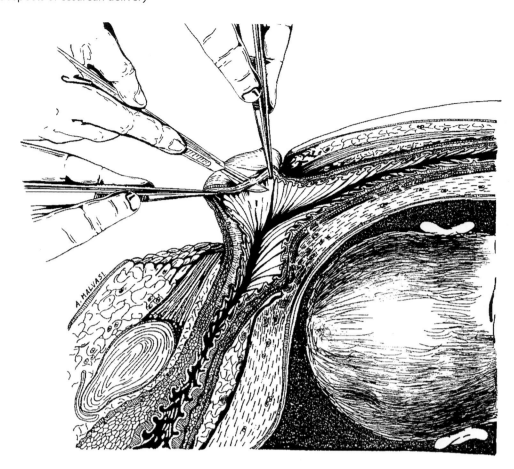

Figure 22.11 Accidental injury to the bladder dome with a scalpel blade during repeat cesarean delivery with Pfannenstiel laparotomy.

conditions [36]. About 70% of foreign bodies cause symptoms that require surgical removal of the foreign body by laparotomy or laparoscopy [37]. In rare cases, complications can even lead to the death of the patient [29].

The medicolegal outcome of this surgical incident is decidedly against the surgical team that performed the intervention, with severe consequences for the operators, even in the presence of extenuating circumstances (emergency and respect of protocols) [38,39].

MATERNAL MORTALITY

In the Western world maternal deaths related to CD have become rare, and are generally associated with serious systemic illnesses. The causes of maternal death by CD were, until a few years ago, related to anesthetic complications, hemorrhages, and infections.

These complications, with the improvement in anesthetic techniques, antibiotic prophylaxis, and the establishment of modern blood banks, have become less and less present and more easily resolved. On the other hand, thromboembolic diseases have taken a leading role and are now responsible for a quarter of maternal deaths from CD.

Maternal mortality occurs, generally, during emergency CD, while mortality in elective CD performed in epidural anesthesia, is below that of vaginal delivery. Currently, the overall incidence of maternal mortality, in women undergoing CD, is around 0.05/1000 interventions, of which 13% are attributable to anesthetic complications, 4%–6% to sequelae of infections, and 18% to thromboembolism; the remaining share can be attributed to preexisting diseases or complications of pregnancy and are independent from the CD event [6,8].

Maternal deaths due to anesthetic accidents have dramatically decreased due to the presence of anesthesiologists dedicated to obstetrics, to the widespread use of epidural anesthesia, and to the systematic preoperative administration of antacids for prophylaxis of the aspiration syndrome.

Pulmonary embolism is the most feared and least predictable complication. It is seven to nine times more frequent in CD compared to vaginal delivery. The expected deaths from pulmonary embolism are 1/100,000 after vaginal delivery and 5/100,000 after CD [40].

HEPARIN PROPHYLAXIS

Venous thromboembolism (VTE) is the leading cause of maternal morbidity and mortality, both during pregnancy and in the postpartum period. The highest incidence of fatal events occurs in the first 2 weeks after delivery, though a substantial proportion, approximately 40%,

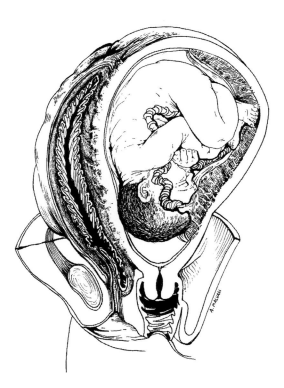

Figure 22.12 Abnormal postsurgical adhesion of the urinary bladder that covers almost the entire front wall of the uterus; this anatomic–surgical situation could be a result of previous myomectomies in which the suture was covered by the bladder. This situation favors bladder injuries in the course of a cesarean delivery, especially when performing a low transverse laparotomy.

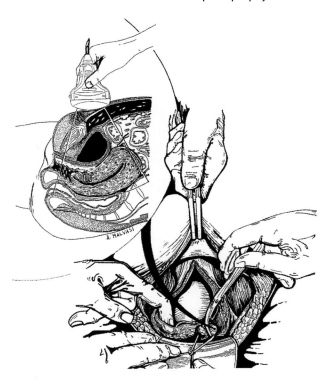

Figure 22.13 Ligation of prevesical vessels in the course of a cesarean delivery, needed to avoid the accidental formation of subfascial hematomas, which, when they are of a considerable size, require surgical draining (top left: subfascial hematoma viewed sonographically during puerperium).

occurs in the puerperium period, after hospital discharge, between the 15th and 42nd days.

The majority of postpartum deaths due to VTE take place after CD, with a risk three times higher than that associated with spontaneous delivery [41,42]. Even though pulmonary thromboembolism (PTE) continues to be the leading cause of maternal mortality, as shown in the latest report on maternal mortality conducted in the United Kingdom, it is clear that the percentage of postpartum deaths after cesarean delivery has decreased, suggesting that the adoption of antithrombotic guidelines has had a positive effect.

On the contrary, the effectiveness of prophylaxis on PTE in pregnancy (Figure 22.28) or after vaginal birth has not been clearly demonstrated [43]. Compared to non-pregnant women of the same age, the risk of thromboembolism increases about 10 times in pregnancy and 20 times in the puerperium.

It is known that several coagulation factors increase during pregnancy (V, VIII, fibrinogen, von Willebrand factors). There is also a reduction in protein S and an acquired resistance to activated protein C, in addition to an increase, of placental origin, in the PAI 1 and 2 factors [44]. The origin of the increase in clotting factors during pregnancy is mainly multifactorial and, in part, still unknown.

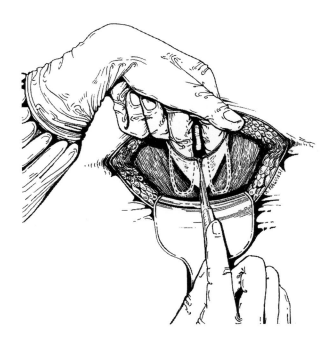

Figure 22.14 Safety maneuver that cuts the lower wall of the Retzius space and protects the bladder dome in the course of a repeat cesarean delivery, or in prior laparotomies, in which the space is adherent due to previous scarring.

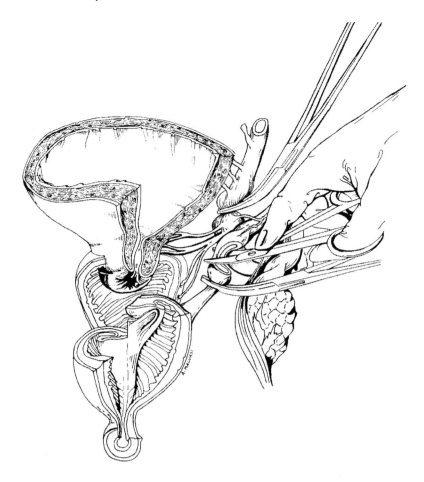

Figure 22.15 Accidental iatrogenic lesion with Mayo scissors of the left pelvic urethra following forcipressure with straight Foure tongs, in the course of a demolition cesarean delivery. These lesions, although rare, can occur more frequently when labor has resulted in complete dilation. In these circumstances, in fact, the pelvic ureter is fairly close to the uterine vessels, thereby causing accidental lesions.

Venous stasis occurs as early as the end of the first trimester and reaches a peak at the 36th week. About 90% of DVT during pregnancy involves the lower left limb and is of the iliofemoral type, corresponding to the course of ovarian arteries that cross the internal iliac vein to the left. In contrast, in 55% of cases referred to nonpregnant women, the femoropopliteal type is prevalently involved [40]. Some women are at a higher risk of thromboembolism during pregnancy due to additional individual risk factors; therefore, an appropriate estimate of the thromboembolism risk would be best, ideally, before pregnancy or during early pregnancy.

The Royal College of Obstetricians and Gynaecologists (RCOG) has defined categories of thromboembolism risk during pregnancy, with the goal of selecting women to subject to antithrombotic prophylaxis (Table 22.1).

In 2004, the same English body suggested specific guidelines for the clinical conduct of various risk categories of pregnant women [43], summarized as follows:

Women with previous VTE. It is recommended they should all be screened for congenital and acquired thrombophilia, ideally before pregnancy; the risk of VTE during pregnancy further increases for these women, in case of confirmed thrombophilia or atypical localizations of previous VTE.

Thromboprophylaxis in women with previous VTE that are negative to thrombophilia. Prophylaxis with low molecular weight heparin (LMWH) for 6 weeks after delivery is recommended; the usefulness of prenatal prophylaxis is still controversial, though it does not seem to be necessary when the previous episode of thromboembolism can be correlated to temporary causes, such as traumatic ones. However, in the case of estrogen-related risk (pregnancy or hormonal contraceptive therapy), or in the case of additional risk factors, such as obesity, prophylaxis seems to be beneficial.

In addition, women with previous and recurrent thromboembolic episodes, or with only one episode associated with a family history of VTE (first-degree relative), should be subjected to prophylaxis with LMWH during pregnancy and for 6 weeks after delivery.

Thromboprophylaxis in women with previous VTE and congenital thrombophilia. Prophylaxis with LMWH during pregnancy and for at least 6 weeks after childbirth is recommended; one must also consider that

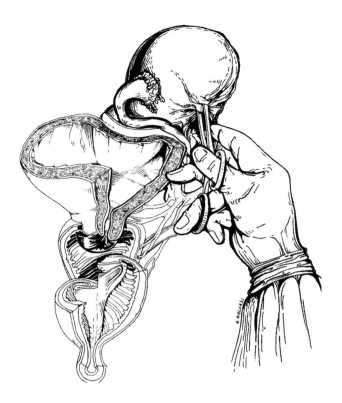

Figure 22.16 Accidental lesion of the left pelvic kidney with Collins forceps, in the course of a cesarean delivery, mistaken for a posterior subserosal uterine fibroma.

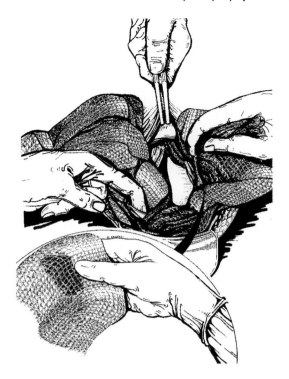

Figure 22.18 The use of laparotomy pads during a cesarean delivery requires careful verification before closing the abdomen, due to the possibility of accidentally leaving a piece of gauze in the abdomen.

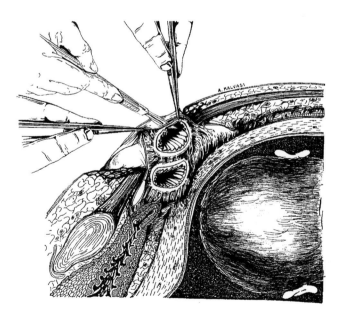

Figure 22.17 Accidental iatrogenic lesion, performed with scalpel blade, of an intestinal ileac loop adherent to the top of the lower uterine segment due to previous myomectomy.

the increased VTE risk varies in relation to the thrombophilic factor; for example, the Leiden factor V, the prothrombin factor, a deficiency in antithrombin, or a combination of the above, which would require different prophylactic doses.

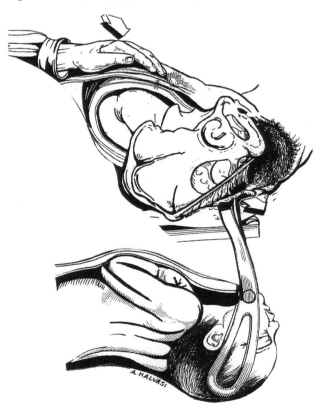

Figure 22.19 The application of forceps may induce alterations and vascular compression of the pelvic nerve branches with neurological sequelae.

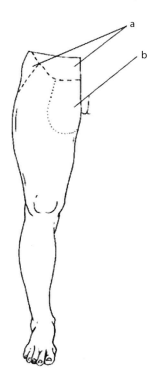

Figure 22.20 The areas of hyperesthesia and hypoesthesia of the iliac–hypogastric (a) and iliac–inguinal (b) nerve, after postcesarean transverse laparotomy.

Thromboprophylaxis in women with congenital thrombophilia and no prior VTE. In women with congenital or acquired thrombophilia, antenatal and postnatal thrombotic prophylaxis is useful, in relation to the specific thrombophilia and the presence of other risk factors. The risk of thrombosis in the absence of previous VTE is low, but varies with the type of thrombophilic factor involved, increasing significantly in the case of combined defects, homozygosis, or antithrombin deficiency.

Thromboprophylaxis in women with acquired thrombophilia (antiphospholipid antibody syndrome). Antiphospholipid antibody syndrome (APS) is defined as the presence of anticardiolipin antibodies or "lupus anticoagulant" at moderate/high titers, found on two occasions after a period of 8 weeks, in association with a previous history of venous or arterial thrombosis or an adverse outcome of pregnancy (three or more unexplained abortions before the 10th week of gestation, intrauterine fetal death after the 10th week of gestation, or preterm delivery (<35th week) due to severe preeclampsia or endouterine fetal growth restriction). The risk of recurrent thrombosis during pregnancy is very high in these women who, therefore, are in need of prenatal and postnatal prophylaxis with LMWH.

Low doses of aspirin appear to improve pregnancy outcomes in women with APS. In any case, the presence of antiphospholipid antibodies in the absence of previous negative obstetric or thrombotic outcomes, is not equivalent to APS, and does not necessarily require LMWH or aspirin at low doses.

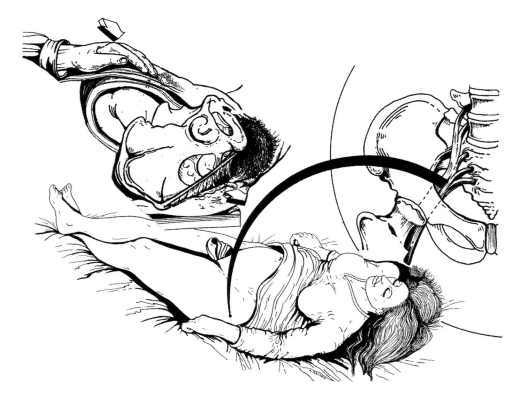

Figure 22.21 Compression of several roots of the lumbosacral plexus as a result of abnormal positions, during childbirth and/or the puerperium.

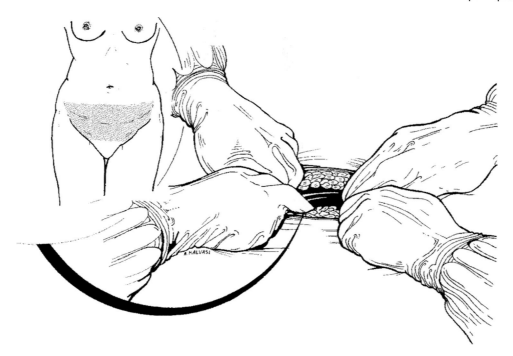

Figure 22.22 Areas of postcesarean hypo-/hyperesthesia, resulting from inadequate stretching of the abdominal wall and damage to the nerve branches of the iliac–hypogastric and iliac–inguinal nerves and the branches of the seventh intercostal nerve.

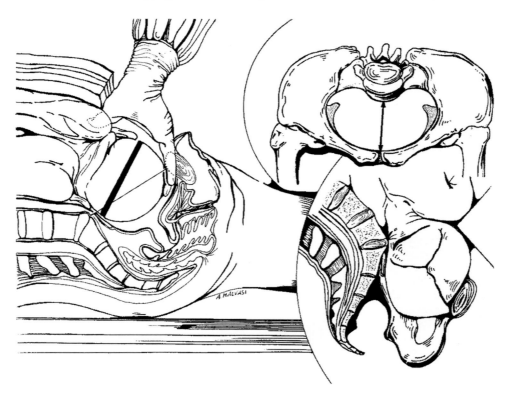

Figure 22.23 Compression of the fetal head during dystocic labor in a platypelloid pelvis (right top and bottom), due to anterior asynclitism in prolonged labor (right).

Thromboprophylaxis in women without previous VTE or thrombophilia. The indication for antithrombotic prophylaxis based on numerous individual risk factors (not including previous VTE or thrombophilia) is more controversial. In general, pregnant women with three or more persistent risk factors should be subjected to antenatal prophylaxis with LMWH and for at least 3–5 days after delivery.

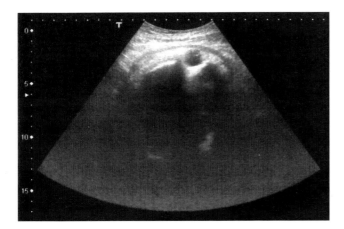

Figure 22.24 Intrapartum ultrasound: the occiput posterior position, in the second stage of labor, position is the most frequent cause of malposition and malrotation in the dystocic birth and may cause neuralgia and/or paresthesia from compression of the nerve branches of the iliac–hypogastric and iliac–inguinal nerves, even when the birth ends with a cesarean delivery.

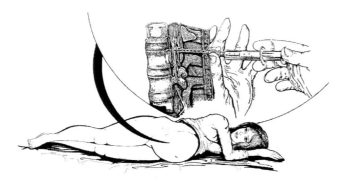

Figure 22.25 Maternal neurological lesions can result, albeit rarely, from the maneuvers for inducing locoregional anesthesia. Particularly dangerous is epidural hematoma, which can result from the accidental and unrecognized damage of a vessel in the epidural space.

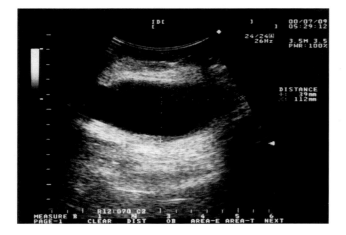

Figure 22.26 Subfascial hematoma with closed parietal peritoneum: transabdominal ultrasound image in sagittal delivery of the post-CD subfascial hematoma.

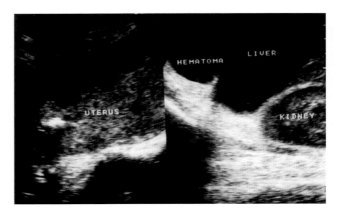

Figure 22.27 Subfascial hematoma with open parietal peritoneum; transabdominal ultrasound image of cross delivery of the hemoperitoneum: at left, parauterine blood collection and, at right, hemoperitoneum at the level of the hepatic and prerenal space.

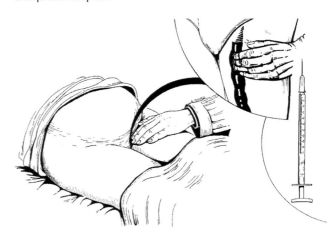

Figure 22.28 Prophylaxis with anticoagulants to reduce postcesarean puerperal thrombosis.

Table 22.1 Categories of thromboembolism risk

Low risk
- Age <35 years, negative family and personal history, elective cesarean delivery in uncomplicated pregnancy

Moderate risk
- Severe varicose veins, age >35 years, obesity, parity ≥4, concomitant infections, preeclampsia, preoperative immobility, concomitant pathology, emergency cesarean delivery

High risk
- Presence of three or more moderate risk factors, pelvic or major abdominal surgery, paralysis of the lower limbs, positive personal or family history for DVT, preeclampsia or thrombophilia, presence of antiphospholipid antibodies

Source: RCOG, from Hibbard, Handerson, Drife. *Report on confidential enquiries into maternal deaths in the UK. 1991–93.* London, UK: Her Majesty's Stationery Office; 1996. With permission.

In women over 35 a BMI (body mass index) over 30, or weight over 90 kg, are the most important and independent risk factors for postpartum VTE, even after a vaginal delivery.

Every time antenatal antithrombotic prophylaxis is performed, it should be started as early as possible and continued up to delivery, except when specific risk factors disappear.

Postpartum prophylaxis should be started after delivery as soon as possible, except in cases of postpartum bleeding or when regional analgesia has been performed, which requires an interval of at least 4 hours from the insertion or removal of the epidural catheter (6 hours when the removal or insertion is traumatic).

Generally, postpartum antithrombotic prophylaxis is continued in women at high risk for 6 weeks after giving birth. For low risk women 3–5 days are sufficient, though the data in this regard are more controversial. Oral contraceptive hormonal therapy should not be prescribed for women at risk during the first three postpartum months.

FETAL DAMAGE

Although cesarean deliveries are at times performed in cases of abnormal fetal presentation or suspected fetal macrosomia in order to avoid birth traumas, it should not be assumed that CD can consistently prevent such traumas.

Several studies report, in fact, cases of Erb's palsy (Figure 22.29), skull and other long bone fractures in infants delivered by CD. In other cases, inadequate maneuvers can result in temporary and limited damage to the fetus (e.g., sternocleidomastoid muscle hematoma) (Figure 22.30) [45,46]. In some cases operator inexperience, emergency conditions, the particular fetal presentation, or lack of proper care, can cause serious damage to the fetus (Figure 22.31).

Apropos brachial plexus palsy, reported in the course of CD, some are not iatrogenic, but originate during the intrauterine life. This is probably due to abnormalities of the uterine cavity and are, therefore, caused by prolonged

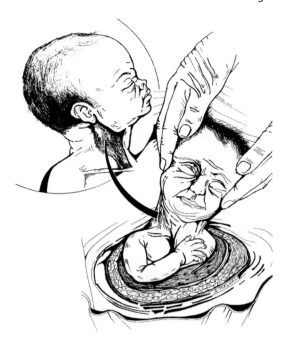

Figure 22.30 Hematoma of the sternocleidomastoid muscle of the fetus, resulting from inadequate fetal extraction during a cesarean delivery.

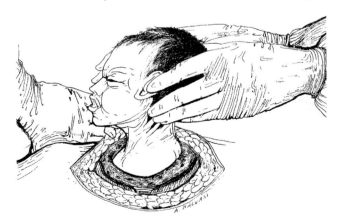

Figure 22.29 Erb's palsy following brachial plexus injury in the course of cesarean delivery in an obese patient with a macrosomal fetus from a low Pfannenstiel laparotomy.

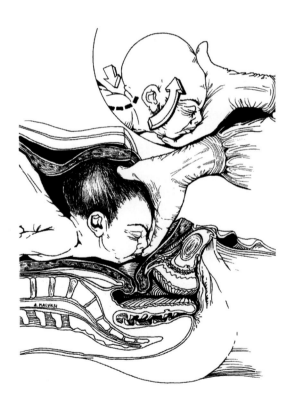

Figure 22.31 The extraction of a hyperflexed fetal head requires special attention by the operator, especially if the head is engaged in the pelvic cavity: in fact, an extraction maneuver that causes further hyperflexion can result, albeit rarely, in serious cervical vertebral and/or fetal bone marrow damage (image at top right).

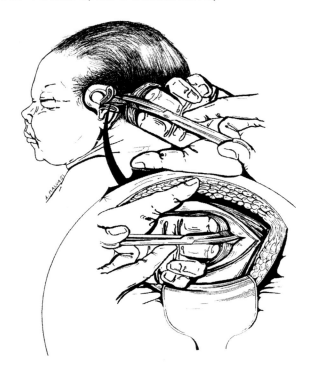

Figure 22.32 Accidental fetal lesion resulting from incongruous maneuvers of uterine breach extension with Mayo scissors.

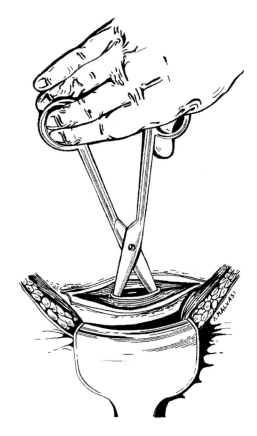

Figure 22.33 Divarication of the uterine breach with Mayo scissors is to be avoided; in fact the incision of the lower uterine segment performed "blindly," especially with surgical instruments, exposes the fetus to possible injury.

fetal malposition, or due to fetal decubitus of the second stage of labor, and have little tendency for postnatal regression [45].

During incision of the uterus, especially when the CD is carried out with the presenting part deeply engaged and with full dilation, it is possible that the surgical instruments may cause lesions, even severe ones, on the fetal presenting part (Figures 22.32 through 22.35). It is always therefore recommended to make use of the different nontraumatic maneuvers performed through blunt disdelivery, in order to open the lower uterine segment and ensure the integrity of the underlying fetal parts (Figure 22.36). Generally, surgeons prefer to access the fetal presenting part in the course of CD using fingers, which allows a tactile sensation of the underlying structures and is almost always nontraumatic.

In some cases, when the maneuvers and tractions are excessive, in addition to lesions on soft parts there may be injuries to fetal bones. In particular, these fractures can occur when the fetus is in a breech (Figure 22.37) or transverse presentation and therefore disengagement maneuvers of the "barred" limb become necessary (Figure 22.38).

Infants born from CD still show transient tachypnea in a percentage that is 4.5% higher compared to vaginal delivery. The incidence of intracranial hemorrhage is higher among babies delivered by vacuum extraction, forceps, and CD performed during labor, than in infants born from elective CD.

Various studies on CD and informed consent have shown that pregnant women are generally satisfied with both counseling and the decision-making process in case of elective CD, less so during an emergency situation or when the women are not involved in the choice [47–49]. Consent for the method of delivery is obviously more complex and different from consent in other medical areas, be it for the presence of the fetus, or for the psychological and emotional implications related to the birth event. In addition to consent on the method of delivery, risks involving anesthetic procedures in obstetrics, make it necessary to also mention the extremely important anesthesiological consent to epidural analgesia, in case painless childbirth is chosen, and the consent to locoregional anesthesia, in case operative delivery with CD is chosen (Figure 22.39).

In the selection of the delivery method two extreme and opposite situations are particularly controversial, that is to say, on the one hand, a refusal to CD due to fetal indications, and on the other, a request of CD in the absence of indications. Every pregnant woman weighs risks and benefits differently, and the choices are strongly influenced by family, ethical and religious factors, how long-term handicaps are considered, the rights of the fetus, and the female body and its integrity.

In light of the above, evidence-based medicine, bioethics, and the law should, rather than dictate individual

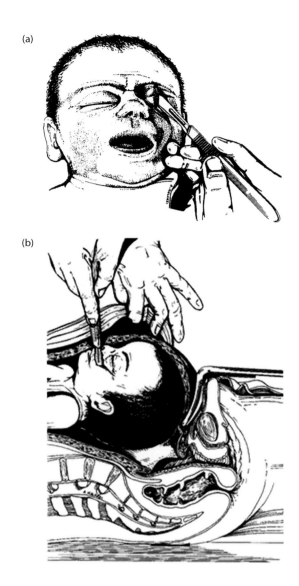

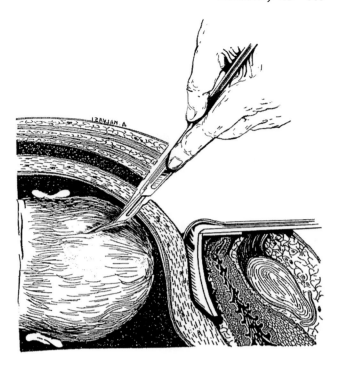

Figure 22.35 Accidental lesion of the fetal head in which the scalp of the fetal occiput is cut, can occur during an incision with scalpel blade of the lower uterine segment.

Figure 22.34 (a, b) Accidental fetal injuries from a scalpel, during the incision of the uterine segment, are much more serious from a medical–legal point of view when the lesions occur on the face, which causes a "scarring," i.e., a lesion on a visible part of the body. Such injuries can occur when the fetal head is in the occipital posterior position, the uterine segment is thin, the membranes are ruptured, and the surgery is performed in emergency conditions. For this reason, all nontraumatic maneuvers that allow the uterine segment to be opened to reach the presenting part are appropriate.

choices, set a range of acceptable decisions that are based on the choice of the patient as well as other factors.

"MANDATORY" CD

In the event of a situation that poses a danger to the health of the woman and/or the fetus the doctor is no longer free to choose between vaginal delivery and cesarean delivery, and the therapeutic option that saves the attended becomes mandatory. If the doctor were to opt for a certain mode of delivery, vaginal delivery rather than CD, and this were to determine a dangerous situation resulting in damage,

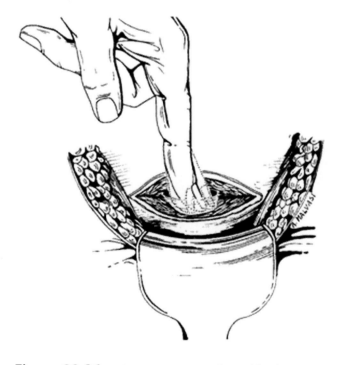

Figure 22.36 Safety maneuver performed by the operator with the index finger, after the lower uterine segment is incised to reach, in a nontraumatic way, the amniotic sac and the presenting part and to avoid accidental instrumental injury of the fetus.

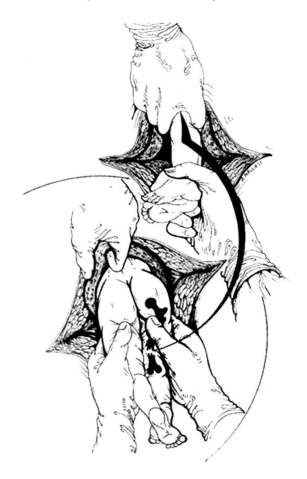

Figure 22.37 Accidental fracture of the right femur of the fetus, during fetal extraction in breech presentation (complete variant) in the course of a cesarean delivery.

culpability would be apparent from the initial choice with all its risks [4].

In these cases, professional negligence does not amount to having performed the procedure incorrectly, but in resorting to methods other than those considered more suitable for the treatment of the case and that could prevent dangerous situations.

This legal view, in which culpability originates from an erroneous initial choice that does not make use of more appropriate methods in order to avoid risk, as in the case of CD, has limited therapeutic possibilities and has certainly contributed to the increase in cases of professional liability of the obstetrician [4].

REFUSAL OF "MANDATORY" CD

In some cases, documented especially in the United States, women can refuse to undergo a CD due to fetal indication, with a number of ethical and legal consequences. An extensive American study shows that in cases where the choice of obstetric intervention has been sent back to the judge, following the refusal of a patient to undergo a CD, the indication for it was fetal distress in 47% of cases, previous CD in 20%, placenta previa in 13%, and in the remaining cases maternal–fetal isoimmunization and idiopathic thrombocytopenic purpura [50].

The possible moral and legal implications of clinicians involved in such cases are controversial:

- Can the fetal interest override the choice of the pregnant woman?
- Is it ethical to impose a choice?
- When does the moral obligation become a legal obligation?

Does the mother's right to privacy, integrity of the body, and self-determination come into conflict with the right of the fetus to be born alive and healthy? More than a mother–fetus conflict of rights, it comes down to a moral conflict of the doctor who is treating the fetus, as well as the mother, as a patient [51,52].

Chervenak and McCullough argue that when a pregnant woman refuses a CD the doctor can, on ethical grounds, supersede the refusal to therapy, and that it is right to appeal to a court if the intervention has a high likelihood of reducing fetal mortality–morbidity, the fetal risk associated with the intervention is low, or the risk of maternal mortality–morbidity is low [53,54]. Other authors, instead, believe that before the fetus is newborn, maternal autonomy should prevail in the "maternal–fetal conflict" [53,54].

In legal terms, CD in the United States is neither explicitly prohibited nor allowed on fetal indication, against the opinion of the pregnant woman. A juridical view referring to the law on abortion justifies the CD for fetal interest, arguing that, as in the decision to perform an abortion in the first and second trimester, once the pregnant woman decides to carry out the pregnancy, she has the obligation to protect the fetus and to undergo, when necessary, medical treatment, while the state must ensure these legal obligations [55–57].

According to another opinion, however, as there is no specific law that justifies the obligation to CD, the state cannot have unlimited authority to protect the fetus, albeit viable, and the woman cannot be legally forced to undergo a CD in order to increase the chances of fetal survival.

When maternal well-being comes into conflict with that of the fetus, the state must constitutionally ensure maternal interests over the fetus; there is no legal obligation for a person to undergo invasive or risky medical interventions on behalf of another person; therefore, a pregnant woman cannot be legally compelled to undergo a CD, even in the interest of the fetus [58].

As part of this controversial issue, let us now see the main guidelines proposed by the various international scientific bodies in regard to clinical management in similar cases of maternal refusal to CD. The general trend is to not accept the obligation for the pregnant woman to be subjected to CD against her own opinion [58].

In 1999 a Bioethics Commission of the American Congress of Obstetricians and Gynecologists (ACOG) [59] concluded that "it is justified to go to court to resolve cases of maternal–fetal conflict only in extraordinary circumstances," listed as the following:

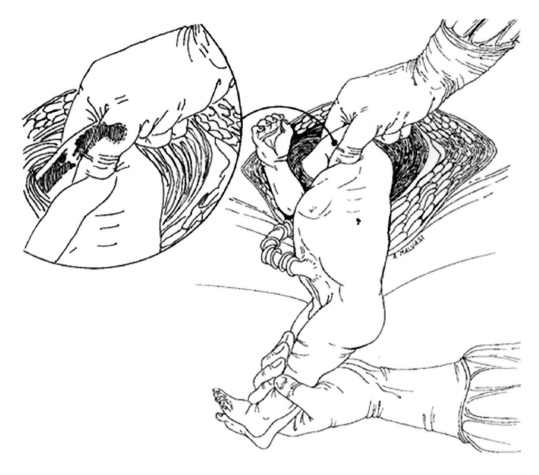

Figure 22.38 Accidental fracture of the right fetal humerus, during disengagement of the right shoulder in breech presentation in full-term baby in the course of a cesarean delivery.

- High probability of serious fetal harm
- High probability that the treatment will prevent or reduce the fetal risk
- The absence of less invasive and equally effective alternatives for preventing fetal damage
- High probability that the treatment is also beneficial to the mother or that the maternal risk is relatively low

It is also stated that, should the clinician make use of the courts to overcome the will of the mother, there is the risk of causing psychological and physical damage to the pregnant woman and of diminishing the faith in the national health system [60].

The American Medical Association (AMA, 1990) is even more in support of the autonomy of maternal decision making, further restricting the cases in which court intervention is justified, and only in those situations in which the medical intervention carries insignificant risks for the health of the pregnant woman, such as taking a drug orally [61].

Last, the ethics committee of the Royal College of Obstetricians and Gynaecologists (RCOG, 1994) establishes in its 1994 guidelines, in line with the AMA, that "it is inappropriate to resort to judiciary intervention to overcome the rejection of an informed and conscious woman to undergo a proposed medical treatment, even if the refusal is likely to endanger her health and that of the fetus at risk" [62].

CESAREAN DELIVERY "ON DEMAND"

The elective "on demand" CD, outside of maternal or fetal therapeutic indications, is one of the most sensitive and controversial issues. The expressed will of the pregnant woman to avoid labor of childbirth and the relative pain by performing an "on demand" CD raises many questions, such as

- Is this a legitimate practice?
- Does the doctor who performs a CD at the request of a woman incur criminal, civil, or disciplinary action?

While in many areas of medicine this same result is achieved by proposing different alternatives to patients, some of which are riskier, the same does not happen when deciding how to carry out a delivery [63]. A survey done in 1986 shows that 92%–95% of obstetricians would not perform a CD in the absence of recognized indications.

One wonders why women are not provided with choices in the method of delivery, by informing them of the potential benefits and risks of an elective CD.

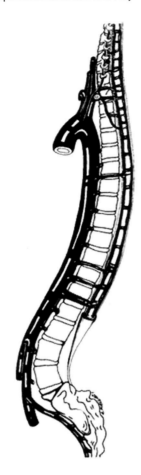

Figure 22.39 Anterior and posterior spinal arteries are subject to compression in the course of subdural hematoma, an anesthesiological complication than can occur during an anesthetic procedure of an obstetric intervention.

The percentage of CD on demand has been increasing in many countries. In the United Kingdom, CD on demand has taken on greater importance after the results of an anonymous questionnaire conducted in London were shown. The survey showed that 31% of female gynecologists prefer a CD for themselves in case of full-term pregnancy with fetus in cephalic presentation [64].

In 80% of cases the request for CD is motivated by fear of trauma to the perineal floor, with possible long-term consequences, such as prolapse and incontinence; in 58% of cases there is the fear of repercussions on sexual functions; in 38% of cases there is the fear of neonatal damage; and, last, in 27% of cases there is the simple desire for an elective birth.

The results from similar surveys conducted in Italy are more controversial: a first study on women lawyers, in fact, shows that only 4% would opt for CD on request [64], while another survey on the opinion of gynecologists revealed that a majority, especially older doctors, would be favorable to CD on demand [5].

This issue, actually, has been the subject of many debates, and to date there is no clinical or epidemiological evidence of the benefits of CD over vaginal birth. While there is a growing literature documenting the adverse effects of vaginal delivery on the pelvic floor, such as the increased risk over time of incontinence and pelvic organ prolapse, there are no randomized trials in which the long-term maternal and fetal outcomes of elective CD, of full-term fetuses in cephalic presentation, are compared with those relative to labor and vaginal delivery. Similarly, there are no cost–benefit analyses of the two methods of delivery.

In the absence of clinical evidence on the benefits and safety of elective CD, and following the ethical principle of not causing potential damage, it would seem to be questionable to meet the CD on demand request without precise medical indication. The main reasons *against CD on request* are listed below [10,65–69].

- It is a process of excessive medicalization when in the presence of a normal fear of labor, with an unnecessary increase of the relative risk of surgical procedures.
    - The data reported by the English are not representative of all women, for example, in the Netherlands only 1.4% of female obstetricians chose elective CD [65].
- The costs are greater.
    - Despite the relative safety of CD in developed countries, there is an increased maternal risk compared to vaginal delivery. Here 16.5% of maternal mortality from CD is attributable to elective CD. Possible complications involve the risk for future obstetric performance, such as an increased risk of placenta previa or accreta, the risk of uterine rupture in vaginal birth after CD, the surgical risk of bladder or bowel injury in the event of a repeat CD, decreased fertility, and increased abortions.
- There is a CD medical–legal problem of the responsibility of the clinician in the event of complications, following a CD, in the absence of a strict medical indication for intervention.
    - Increased risk of neonatal transient tachypnea and respiratory distress syndrome.

The main reasons *for CD on demand* are

- CD on demand now seems to part of the civil and reproductive rights of women, as with the right to vote, to contraception, to abortion. The active management of labor itself, the continuous monitoring of the fetal heart rate, and a series of diagnostic procedures make the woman feel as if she is losing control, which she would maintain with a responsible and independent choice of CD (and not submit passively to excessive medicalization of childbirth) [70,71].
- There is increased risk of perineal damage after vaginal delivery, with possible future genital prolapse and urinary incontinence problems.
- Many of the complications described in association with CD are not relative to elective primary cesarean but to old case studies that are not based on the most current anesthesiological, surgical, and antibiotic prophylaxis techniques.

- Costs cannot constitute a relevant factor.
- Women experience a less painful and safer childbirth.
- There is less risk, though not proven, of intrapartum hypoxia and birth trauma.
- There is less damage to the sexual sphere.
- There is improved planning of childbirth timing.

The problem of "on demand" CD is also tied to maternal and fetal complications, which unfortunately are much more frequent than in vaginal birth. Various studies have been carried out to evaluate the effects of CD on the health of the newborn [72–78]. These studies have shown that, compared to vaginal birth, there are more disadvantages than advantages.

A study performed by Morrison et al. over a period of 9 years on 33,289 pregnant patients, at approximately 37 weeks of gestation, showed that the incidence of respiratory morbidity was of 35.5 per 1000 live births from CD without labor, of 12.2 per 1000 live births from CD with labor, and of 5.3 for vaginal births [77].

Levine et al. have shown that the risk of post-CD pulmonary hypertension increases five times compared to vaginal birth. According to several pathophysiological hypotheses, this might occur because vaginal delivery favors the release of catecholamine and of prostaglandins, both of which favor the release of pulmonary surfactant. In addition, according to the same authors, vaginal delivery results in the lungs being pressed, due to compression of the fetal trunk during the passage through the birth canal, with releases (including from fetal epinephrine) of intrapulmonary fetal liquid, which facilitates postnatal adaptation [75].

Other risks that "on demand" CD would create for the baby include late neonatal neurological adaptation [78], possible harm to the fetus during the CD [72], and delayed breastfeeding [73]. One study [79], conducted in the United States over 4 years, from 1998 to 2001, on approximately 4 million births, focused its attention on CD "not motivated by medical causes." These interventions were performed without specific medical indications, but simply at the request of patients or by choice of the operators. The patients selected for the study did not show any notable diseases or disorders in their medical history, and the selected pregnancies presented no complications during labor or childbirth.

This study examined neonatal mortality by period of death in relation to the method of delivery (vaginal delivery or CD). The results of the study showed unexpected negative data. First, general infant mortality (within 1 year of life) was found to be surprisingly low in women defined as "low risk" (2.14 infant deaths per 1000 live births); post-CD infant mortality in primiparae was higher by 56% compared to vaginal delivery (2.85/1000 per CD versus 1.83/1000 per vaginal delivery) and for multiparae this ratio was double (4.51/1000 for CD versus 2.18/1000 for those born by vaginal delivery).

In general, the processed data showed an infant mortality rate for CD of 1.77 deaths per 1000 live births, compared to 0.62 per 1000 (in vaginal deliveries), with a death rate that is 2.9 times greater for CD; the majority of neonatal deaths (within the first 28 days of life) were caused by congenital malformations, deformations, and chromosomal abnormalities (in 54% of cases), while SIDS (sudden infant death syndrome) occurred in only 5% of total cases.

Besides this important data the debate over "on demand" CD must also include other disheartening scientific data: an increased risk, following a CD, of maternal postpartum death [80]. A study carried out to assess the potential risks of CD in terms of maternal mortality, has shown very interesting and incisive results, more than in all previous studies [19,81–90]. Obstetric data from the National French Registry were assessed over a period of 5 years (1996–2000). The registry provided important epidemiologic information on postpartum maternal deaths [91]: a group of researchers assessed all maternal deaths tied to CD and compared them with a control group (vaginal births).

After a thorough statistical analysis, the results showed that the risk of postpartum death for CD was 3.6 times higher than in vaginal delivery (odds ratio [OR] of 3.64, 95% confidence interval [CI] 2.15–6.19), while both prepartum CD and intrapartum CD were significantly associated with an increased risk of maternal death, due to anesthesiological complications, puerperal infections, and venous thromboembolism (the three most significant pre- and postoperative complications of major surgical interventions) [80].

The conclusions of the study were that CD was associated with an increased risk of death for the mother in the postpartum period, much greater than in vaginal delivery. The risk of death from postpartum hemorrhage, however, was the same between CD and vaginal delivery. (This is surprising data, in that it is not tied to the general amount of blood loss in the two types of delivery.) The most significant surgical complications were those related to the cause of death of the patient who underwent a CD.

Other studies on the complications of CD "on demand or *not motivated by medical causes*," have brought to light other very important aspects; it was found that there is an increase compared to vaginal delivery of endometritis in the postpartum period [92,93], as well as of rehospitalizations due to infections or thromboembolic events [94,95].

The degree of safety achieved by modern anesthetic techniques in the course of CD has greatly improved analgesia during and after CD. However, data from a French study [90] show an increased risk of maternal death from CD, due to complications of anesthesia with, in three cases out of four, patients dying from causes related to general anesthesia, while only one from spinal anesthesia.

As Marra holds, to better understand current jurisprudence in this regard in our country, it is best to start from an old and well-known judgment of the Court of Criminal Appeal (18/03/87 n.7415, known as the *Conciani sentence*), with which a gynecologist who practiced voluntary sterilization was acquitted of the imputation of deliberate injury because the fact did not constitute a crime [4]. Certain statements contained in the ruling can in fact be used as general principles for settling the legality problem of voluntary CD.

The Supreme Court stressed the difference between physical integrity and health (protected by article 32 of the Constitution much more than physical integrity) and concluded that the public interest in the protection of health is not harmed by interventions such as sterilization which, on the contrary, can benefit the mental stability of the individual who voluntarily submits to them.

The Court added that the trend in current law authorizes much more extensive interventions on physical integrity than those determined through voluntary sterilization, quoting as examples Law 164 of 1982 on transsexuals and Law 194/78 on abortion [4]. In regard to CD on demand, women seeking such an intervention do so to avoid pain, and therefore for alleviation purposes that cannot be refused by the law, which in fact already allows for a series of surgeries aimed at satisfying the needs of personal pleasure (cosmetic surgery, as an example).

In addition, CD on demand does not impact physical integrity as much as sterilization that blocks reproductive capacity, many times irreversibly, as it does not affect fertility or the ability to complete future pregnancies, which are, in the worst-case scenario, at risk of having to repeat the CD. In this perspective, CD is not contrary to the law, since no specific prohibition is expressed.

It is true, however, in light of the excessive number of CDs practiced in our health facilities, which so often worries public opinion, that the gynecologist should never lead the pregnant woman to choose a CD in the absence of medical indications, but should properly inform and explain all the possible maternal and fetal complications, including risks for future pregnancies.

If this does not occur, the behavior of the obstetrician would not follow deontological standards and would, therefore, be liable from a "disciplinary" point of view [4].

In conclusion, CD on demand involves a conflict between the moral obligation of the clinician to not routinely expose the patient to increased surgical risk and the obligation to respect the woman's decision-making autonomy.

CONCLUSIONS

The increase in medical–legal litigation in obstetrics that has taken place in the last few decades, prevalently in Western and developed countries, has resulted in an increase in the number of cesarean deliveries.

In Italy, and in particular in the south of the country, the increase in cesarean deliveries is in part motivated by a defensive reaction from many doctors.

On the other hand, a cesarean delivery is not without its risks, and can result in maternal and fetal complications.

Possible maternal complications include uterine lacerations; bleeding during and after a cesarean delivery [90]; iatrogenic urethral and bladder injuries [91–93]; intestinal lesions [94]; accidental lesions of abdominal organs next to the gravid uterus; foreign bodies and laparotomy patches "forgotten" in the abdominal cavity during surgery [95–97]; postsurgical infections [98–100]; uterovesical and abdominal wall hematomas [101,102]; surgical–anesthesiological neurological lesions; lesions of a thromboembolic nature, with the need for thromboembolic prophylaxis; anesthesiological complications in the course of general or locoregional anesthesia, such as, for example, the risk of subdural hematomas, neurological disorders, or technical complications associated with the introduction of the needle in the spinal and epidural spaces [103,104].

On the other hand, fetal lesions in the course of CD are much more serious from the medical–legal point of view. In the collective imagination it is in fact a contradiction that a cesarean delivery performed to protect the well-being of the fetus, can produce iatrogenic injuries to the same fetus [105]. Fetal lesions in the course of CD [106] include damage to the brachial plexus and to the sternocleidomastoid with paralysis [107,108], as well as damage to the cervical vertebrae after fetal extraction [109]. Moreover, clavicle, humerus, and femur fractures, as well as damage to other major organs [110], which can occur during particularly difficult fetal extractions or in abnormal presentations of the fetus, have also been reported.

Another particularly difficult medical aspect consists of cutting injuries on the fetal body during the incision, in particular those that occur on the face (scarring), which also constitute an aesthetic problem. It is, therefore, recommended to perform a series of safety maneuvers and to document them in case of medical–legal litigation [111]. These lesions occur more frequently during advanced labor, with rotation of the sacral occiput in a stretched and thinned uterine segment or, on the otherhand, in an unprepared uterine segment or, in the absence of amniotic fluid, following rupture of the membranes or oligoamnios [112,113].

Hypoxic fetal abnormalities have become increasingly important. Such abnormalities are a result of difficult intubation under general anesthesia in an emergency cesarean delivery, or of serious maternal hypotension affecting the fetus under general anesthesia.

Psychiatric alterations, depending on the type of anesthesia, have also been reported [114].

As a result of the progressive increase in BMI in developed countries, tied to an increase in CD, the current literature describes several cases of failed intubation in obese pregnant women [115–118]. In obese women there is the additional problem of cutting and suturing the excess adipose tissue and of using locoregional anesthesia [119–121].

In light of the aforementioned complications, it is essential to give the patient an appropriate indication of the obstetric situation and have them sign an informed consent form [122,123].

Consent is another factor that should be taken into account in case of iterative cesarean delivery, for the risks that are inherent with this intervention [124,125].

There are significant medical–legal differences between elective and emergency intervention CD: special attention is paid in emergency situations to "fetal distress" and to the CD execution time [126–128].

Cesarean deliveries indications, which in the last few years have steadily increased, include cesarean delivery on demand, which must, however, be appropriately discussed with the patient. In the discussion the cost–benefits of vaginal delivery versus cesarean delivery must be compared [129–131].

The progressive increase in the frequency of CD has resulted in the need for a specific qualification of both the medical and the obstetric staff, which has had to expand and increase its obstetrical and surgical skills. In fact there has been an increasing medical–legal involvement of the medical–obstetric team, thereby including the assisting obstetric staff [132].

Although cesarean deliveries have now become so common that they have been critically assessed and frequently opposed by a part of the media and public opinion, there is no doubt that the ability to extract the fetus by laparotomy, with a minimal risk for the mother, has been one of the most significant steps in the transition from traditional obstetrics to modern maternal–fetal medicine.

It is likely that the "birth" event, with its obvious sociocultural and health policy implications, should be better distinguished from the "delivery event," which instead remains an act of medical liability and, therefore, belongs exclusively to the medical realm.

REFERENCES

1. Scheda di Dimissione Ospedaliera, Ministero della Salute, Roma 2002.
2. Scheller JM, Nelson KB. Does cesarean delivery prevent cerebral palsy or other neurologic problems of childhood? *Obstet Gynecol* 1994;83(4):624–30.
3. Croughan-Minihane MS, Petitti DB, Gordis L. Morbidity among breech infants according to method of delivery. *Obstet Gynecol* 1990;75(5):821–5.
4. Marra A, *Il ginecologo e l'ostetrico.Diritti, doveri e responsabilità*. Rome, Italy: Passoni editore; 2003.
5. Vimercati A, Greco P, Kardashi A, Rossi C, Loizzi V, Scioscia M, Loverro G. Choice of caesarean section and perception of legal pressure. *J Perinat Med* 2000;28:111–7.
6. Rizzo N, Visentin A, Pilu G, De Jaco P, Bovicelli L. Il taglio cesareo: Tecniche e complicazioni. *J Prenat* 1997;1(3).
7. Dickason LA, Dinsmoore MJ. Red blood cell transfusion and caesarean delivery. *Am J Obstet Gynecol* 1992;167:327–32.
8. Hema KR, Johanson R. Techniques for performing caesarean delivery. *Best Pract Res Clin Obstet Gynaecol* 2001;15(1):17–47.
9. Ekeroma AJ, Ansari A, Stirrat GM. Blood transfusion in obstetrics and gynecology. *Br J Obstet Gynaecol* 1997;104:278–84.
10. Miller DA, Chollet JA, Goodwin TM. Clinical risk factors for placenta previa–placenta accreta. *Am J Obstet Gynaecol* 1997;177:210–4.
11. Baskett TF. Emergency obstetric hysterectomy. *J Obst Gynecol* 2003;23(4):353–5.
12. Forna F, Miles AM, Jamieson DJ. Emergency peripartum hysterectomy: A comparison of cesarean and postpartum hysterectomy. *Am J Obstet Gynecol* 2004;190(5):1440–4.
13. Magann EF, Dodson MK, Ray MA. Preoperative skin preparation and intraoperative pelvic irrigation: Impact on post-cesarean endometritis and wound infection. *Obstet Gynecol* 1993;81:922–5.
14. Davis JD. Management of injuries to the urinary and gastrointestinal tract during cesarean section. *Obstet Gynecol* 1999;26:469–80.
15. Briggs R, Chari RS, Mercer B, Sibai B. Postoperative incision complications after cesarean section in patients with antepartum syndrome of hemolysis, elevated liver enzymes, and low platelets (HELLP): Does delayed primary closure make a difference? *Am J Obstet Gynecol* 1996;175:893–6.
16. Department of Health. *Report on Confidential Enquiries into Maternal Deaths in the UK 1994–1996*. UK: The Stationary Office.
17. *Why Mothers Die*. London, UK: The Stationery Office; 1998:1–275.
18. Cox C, Grady K. *Managing Obstetric Emergencies*. Oxford, UK: Bios Scientific; 1999.
19. Lilford RJ, van Coeverden de Groot HA, Moore PJ, Bingham P. The relative risks of caesarean section (intrapartum and elective) and vaginal delivery: A detailed analysis to exclude the effects of medical disorders and other acute pre-existing physiological disturbances. *Br J Obstet Gynecol* 1997;97:883–92.
20. Nielson TF, Hokegard KH. Cesarean section and intraoperative surgical complications. *Acta Obstet Gynecol Scand* 1984;63:103–8.
21. Wheeless CR, Smith JJ. A comparison of the flow of iodine 125 through three different intestinal anastomoses: Standard, Gambee and stapler. *Obstet Gynecol* 1975;46:448–52.
22. Thornton FJ, Barbul A. Healing in the gastrointestinal tract. *Surg Clin North Am* 1997;77:549–73.
23. Holdcroft FB, Gibbert RL, Hargrove DF, Hawkins CI. Neurological complications associated with pregnancy. *Br J Anaesth* 1995;75:522–6.
24. Reynolds M. Maternal sequelae of childbirth. *Br J Anaesth* 1995;75:515–6.
25. Warner MA, Martin JT, Schroeder DR, Offord KP, Schute CG. Lower extremity motor neuropathy associated with surgery in a lithotomy position. *Anesthesiology* 1994;81:6–12.
26. Ong BY, Cohen MM, Esmail A. Paresthesias and motor dysfunction after labour and delivery. *Anesth Analg* 1987;66:18.
27. Lanza V, Pignataro A. Reazioni indesiderate e complicazioni dell'Anestesia Perdurale in ostetricia. *ESIA* 1999;1–11.
28. Arduini e Gruppo studio SIGO. *Trattato di ecografia ostetrica e ginecologica*. Poletto; 2002: 407–11.
29. Vicino M, Caradonna F, Vimercati A et al. Ematomi sottofasciali quale complicanza del TC in pazienti ipertese. *Medicina fetale*. Rome: CIC ed. Int. 1999:244–47.

30. Gawande AA, Studdert DM, Orav EJ, Brennan TA, Zinner MJ. Risk factors for retained instruments and sponges after surgery. *N Engl J Med* 2003;348:229–35.
31. Dux M, Ganten M, Lubienski A, Grenacher L. Retained surgical sponge with migration into the duodenum and persistent duodenal fistula. *Eur Radiol* 2002;12:74–77.
32. Prasad S, Krishnan A, Limdi J, Patankar T. Imaging features of gossypiboma: Report of two cases. *J Postgrad Med* 1999;45:18–19.
33. Vayre F, Richard P, Ollivier JP. Intrathoracic gossypiboma: Magnetic resonance features. *Int J Cardiol* 1999;70:199–200.
34. Kuwashima S, Yamato M, Fujioka M, Ishibashi M, Kogure H, Tajima Y. MR findings of surgically retained sponges and towels: Report of two cases. *Radiat Med* 1993;11:98–101.
35. Ariz C, Horton KM, Fishman EK. 3D CT evaluation of retained foreign bodies. *Emerg Radiol* 2004;10:212–23.
36. Dhillon JS, Park A. Transmural migration of a retained laparotomy sponge. *Am Surg* 2002;68(7):603–5.
37. Dux M, Ganten M, Lubienski A, Grenacher L. Retained surgical sponge with migration into the duodenum and persistent duodenal fistula. *Eur Radiol* 2002;12:74–77.
38. Olivier F, Devriendt D. Laparoscopic removal of a chronically retained gauze. *Acta Chir Belg* 2003;103(1):108–9.
39. Schmid C, Krempel S, Scheld HH. A forgotten gauze swab—Clinical and legal considerations. *Thorac Cardiovasc Surg* 2001;49(3):191–3.
40. Kaiser CW, Friedman S, Spurling KP, Slowick T, Kaiser HA. The retained surgical sponge. *Ann Surg* 1996;224(1):79–84.
41. Prisco G, ed., Linee guida SISET in Ostetricia e Ginecologia, *Haematologica* 2002;87(12): supplement.
42. Bonnar J. Can more be done in obstetric and gynecologic practice to reduce morbidity and mortality associated with venous thromboembolism? *Am J Obstet Gynecol* 1999;180:784–91.
43. Hibbard BM, Anderson MM, Drife JO. *Report on confidential enquiries into maternal deaths in the UK. 1991–93.* London, UK: Her Majesty's Stationery Office; 1996.
44. Royal College of Obstetricians and Gynaecologists (RCOG). *Thromboprophylaxis during pregnancy, labour, and after vaginal delivery. Guideline 37.* London, UK: RCOG; January 2004.
45. Toglia MR, Weg JG. Venous thromboembolism during pregnancy. *N Engl J Med* 1996;335:108–14.
46. Kaplan M, Dollberg M, Waintraub G, Itzchaki G. Fractured long bones in a term infant delivered by cesarean section. *Pediatr Radiol* 1987;17:256.
47. Depp R. Caesarean delivery. In Gabbe SG, Niebyl JR, Simpson JL. ed. *Obstetrics—Normal and Problem Pregnancies*, 3rd ed. New York, NY: Churchill Livingstone; 1996.
48. Graham WJ, Hundley V, McCheyne AL et al. An investigation of women's involvement in the decision to deliver by caesarean section. *Br J Obst Gynaecol* 1999;106:213–220.
49. Mould TAJ, Chong S, Spencer JAD, Gallivan S. Women's involvement with the decision preceding their caesarean section and their degree of satisfaction. *Br J Obstet Gynaecol* 1996;103:1074–7.
50. Wallace L. Psychological preparation as a method of reducing the stress of surgery. *J Human Stress* 1984;4:62–67.
51. Kolder VEB, Gallagher J, Parsons MT. Court-ordered obstetrical interventions. *N Engl J Med* 1987;316:1192–6.
52. *Jefferson v Griffin Spalding County Hospital Authority et al.* 247 Ga. 86, 274 S.E. 2d 457, 1981.
53. *In Re: Baby Boy Doe v. Mother Doe,* 632 NE2d 326 (III App I Dist 1994).
54. Chervenak FA, McCullough LB. Perinatal ethics: A practical method of analysis of obligations to mother and fetus. *Obstet Gynecol* 1985;66:442–6.
55. Chervenak FA, McCullough LB. Does obstetric ethics have any role in the obstetrician's response to the abortion controversy? *Am J Obstet Gynecol* 1990;163:1425–9.
56. Robertson JA. Procreative liberty and the control of conception, pregnancy and childbirth. *VA Law Rev* 1983;69:405–65.
57. Robertson JA. The right to procreate and in utero fetal therapy. *J Legal Med* 1982;3:333–66.
58. Schambelan B. *Roe v. Wade—The Complete Text of the Official U.S. Supreme Court Decision.* Philadelphia, PA: Philadelphia Press; 1992.
59. Nelson LJ, Milliken N. Compelled medical treatment of pregnant women. *JAMA* 1989;259:1060–66.
60. American College of Obstetricians and Gynaecologists (ACOG) Committee on Ethics. *Patient Choice and the Maternal Fetal Relationship.* Report 214. Washington, DC: ACOG; 1999.
61. Poland ML, Dombrowski MP, Ager JW, Socol RJ. Punishing pregnant drug users: Enhancing the flight from care. *Drug Alcohol Depend* 1993; 31:199–203.
62. American Medical Association Board of Trustees. Legal interventions during pregnancy. *JAMA* 1990;264:2663–70.
63. Royal College of Obstetricians and Gynaecologists (RCOG) Ethics Committee. *A Consideration of the Law and Ethics in Relation to Court-Authorised Obstetric Intervention.* London, UK: RCOG; 1994.
64. Johnson SR, Elkins TE, Strong C, Phelan JP. Obstetric decision-making: Responses to patients who request caesarean delivery. *Obstet Gynaecol* 1986;67:847–50.
65. Paterson-Brown S, Amu O, Rejendran B II. Should doctors perform an elective caesarean section on request? *Br Med J* 1998;317:462–5.
66. Editor's comment. What is the right number of caesarean deliveries? *Lancet* 1997;349:815.

67. Van Roosmalen J. Unnecessary caesarean deliveries should be avoided (letter). *Br Med J* 1999;318:121.
68. Idama TO, Lindow SW. Safest option is still to aim for vaginal delivery (letter). *Br Med J* 1999;318:121.
69. Sultan AH, Stanton SL. Preserving the pelvic floor and perineum during childbirth—Elective caesarean section? *Br J Obstet Gynaecol* 1996;103:731–4.
70. Hall MH, Campbell DM, Fraser C, Lemon J. Mode of delivery and future fertility. *Br J Obstet Gynaecol* 1989;96:1297–303.
71. Doherty EG, Eichenwald EC. Cesarean delivery: Emphasis on the neonate. *Clin Obstet Gynecol* 2004;47:332–41.
72. Jackson N, Paterson-Brown S. Physical sequelae of caesarean delivery. *Best Pract Res Clin Obstet Gynaecol* 2001;15:49–61.
73. McFarlin BL. Elective cesarean birth: Issues and ethics of an informed decision. *J Midw Womens Health* 2004;49:421–9.
74. Levine EM, Ghai V, Barton JJ, Strom CM. Mode of delivery and risk of respiratory diseases in newborns. *Obstet Gynecol* 2001;97:439–42.
75. Smith JF, Hernandez C, Wax JR. Fetal laceration injury at cesarean delivery. *Obstet Gynecol* 1997;90:344–6.
76. Morrison JJ, Rennie JM, Milton PJ. Neonatal respiratory morbidity and mode of delivery at term: Influence of timing of elective caesarean delivery. *Br J Obstet Gynaecol* 1995;102:101–6.
77. Otamiri G, Berg G, Ledin T et al. Delayed neurological adaptation in infants delivered by elective cesarean section and the relation to catecholamine levels. *Early Hum Dev* 1991;26:51–60.
78. MacDorman MF, Declercq E, Menacker F, Malloy MH. Infant and neonatal mortality for primary cesarean and vaginal births to women with "no indicated risk," United States, 1998–2001 birth cohorts. *Birth* 2006;33:175–82.
79. Deneux-Tharaux C, Carmona E, Bouvier-Colle MH, Breart G. Postpartum maternal mortality and cesarean delivery. *Obstet Gynecol* 2006;108(3):541–54.
80. Evrard JR, Gold EM. Cesarean section and maternal mortality in Rhode Island. Incidence and risk factors, 1965–1975. *Obstet Gynecol* 1977;50:594–7.
81. Frigoletto FD Jr, Ryan KJ, Phillippe M. Maternal mortality rate associated with cesarean delivery: An appraisal. *Am J Obstet Gynecol* 1980;136:969–70.
82. Harper MA, Byington RP, Espeland MA, Naughton M, Meyer R, Lane K. Pregnancy-related death and health care services. *Obstet Gynecol* 2003;102:273–8.
83. Lydon-Rochelle M, Holt VL, Easterling TR, Martin DP. Cesarean delivery and postpartum mortality among primiparas in Washington State, 1987–1996. *Obstet Gynecol* 2001;97:169–74.
84. Petitti DB, Cefalo RC, Shapiro S, Whalley P. In-hospital maternal mortality in the United States: Time trends and relation to method of delivery. *Obstet Gynecol* 1982;59:6–12.
85. Rubin GL, Peterson HB, Rochat RW, McCarthy BJ, Terry JS. Maternal death after cesarean section in Georgia. *Am J Obstet Gynecol* 1981;139:681–5.
86. Sachs BP, Yeh J, Acker D, Driscoll S, Brown DA, Jewett JF. Cesarean section-related maternal mortality in Massachusetts, 1954–1985. *Obstet Gynecol* 1988;71:385–8.
87. Schuitemaker N, van Roosmalen J, Dekker G, van Dongen P, van Geijn H, Gravenhorst JB. Maternal mortality after cesarean delivery in the Netherlands. *Acta Obstet Gynecol Scand* 1997;76:332–4.
88. Subtil D, Vaast P, Dufour P, Depret-Mosser S, Codaccioni X, Puech F. Maternal consequences of cesarean as related to vaginal delivery. *J Gynecol Obstet Biol Reprod (Paris)* 2000;29(Suppl):10–16.
89. Hall MH, Bewley S. Maternal mortality and mode of delivery. *Lancet* 1999;354:776.
90. Pollio F, Staibano S, De Falco M, Buonocore U, De Rosa G, Di Lieto A. Severe secondary postpartum hemorrhage 3 weeks after cesarean section: Alternative etiologies of uterine scar non-union. *J Obstet Gynaecol Res* 2007;33(3):360–2.
91. Phipps MG, Watabe B, Clemons JL, Weitzen S, Myers DL. Risk factors for bladder injury during cesarean delivery. *Obstet Gynecol* 2005;105(1):156–60.
92. Benchekroun A, Lachkar A, Soumana A, Farih MH, Belahnech Z, Marzouk M, Faik M. Vesico-uterine fistulas. Report of 30 cases. *Ann Urol (Paris)*. 1999;33(2):75–79.
93. Pelosi MA 2nd, Pelosi MA 3rd. Risk factors for bladder injury during cesarean delivery. *Obstet Gynecol* 2005;105(4):900.
94. Armentano G. Intestinal injury in cesarean delivery. *Clin Exp Obstet Gynecol* 1988;15(1–2):60–62.
95. Zantvoord Y, van der Weiden RM, van Hooff MH. Transmural migration of retained surgical sponges: A systematic review. *Obstet Gynecol Surv* 2008;63(7):465–71.
96. Salman M, Ahmed N, Mansoor MA. Gossypiboma in the early postoperative period: Computed tomography appearance. *J Coll Physicians Surg Pak* 2005;15(7):435–6.
97. Simpson KR. Surgical safety: Minimizing risk of retained foreign bodies during cesarean birth. *MCN Am J Matern Child Nurs* 2007;32(3):200.
98. Cho FN. Iatrogenic abscess at uterine incision site after cesarean section: Sonographic monitoring. *J Clin Ultrasound* 2008;36(6):381–3.
99. Mulic-Lutvica A, Axelsson O. Postpartum ultrasound in women with postpartum endometritis, after cesarean section and after manual evacuation of the placenta. *Acta Obstet Gynecol Scand* 2007;86(2):210–7.
100. Rivlin ME, Carroll CS, Morrison JC. Conservative surgery for uterine incisional necrosis complicating cesarean delivery. *Obstet Gynecol* 2004;103(5 Pt 2):1105–8.
101. Wagner MS, Bédard MJ. Postpartum uterine wound dehiscence: A case report. *J Obstet Gynaecol Can* 2006;28(8):713–5.

102. Yazicioglu F, Gökdogan A, Kelekci S, Aygün M, Savan K. Incomplete healing of the uterine incision after caesarean delivery: Is it preventable? *Eur J Obstet Gynecol Reprod Biol* 2006;124(1):32–6.
103. Hershan DB, Rosner HL. An unusual complication of epidural analgesia in a morbidly obese parturient. *Anesth Analg* 1996;82(1):217–8.
104. Yajima D, Motani H, Hayakawa M, Sato Y, Iwase H. A fatal case of hypovolemic shock after cesarean delivery. *Am J Forensic Med Pathol* 2007;28(3):212–5.
105. Alexander JM, Leveno KJ, Hauth J et al., National Institute of Child Health and Human Development Maternal-Fetal Medicine Units Network. Fetal injury associated with cesarean delivery. *Obstet Gynecol* 2006;108(4):885–90.
106. Dessole S, Cosmi E, Balata A, Uras L, Caserta D, Capobianco G, Ambrosini G. Accidental fetal lacerations during cesarean delivery: Experience in an Italian level III university hospital. *Am J Obstet Gynecol* 2004;191(5):1673–7.
107. Iffy L, Pantages P. Erb's palsy after delivery by Cesarean section. (A medico-legal key to a vexing problem.) *Med Law* 2005;24(4):655–61.
108. Noble A. Brachial plexus injuries and shoulder dystocia: Medico-legal commentary and implications. *J Obstet Gynaecol* 2005;25(2):105–7.
109. Okezie AO, Oyefara B, Chigbu CO. A 4-year analysis of caesarean delivery in a Nigerian teaching hospital: One-quarter of babies born surgically. *J Obstet Gynaecol* 2007;27(5):470–4.
110. Slobodian TV. A case of penetrating injury of the eye in a fetus during cesarean delivery [in Russian]. *Oftalmol Zh* 1988;(1):60–61.
111. Morini A, Cantonetti G, Spina V, Bonessio L. Fetal lesions due to the bistoury during cesarean delivery: A study of 58 cases. The 5-year case records of 3117 cesarean deliveries at the Institutes of Clinical Obstetrics and Gynecology of the University of Rome La Sapienza. *Minerva Ginecol* 1995;47(7–8):305–14.
112. Levy R, Chernomoretz T, Appelman Z, Levin D, Or Y, Hagay ZJ. Head pushing versus reverse breech extraction in cases of impacted fetal head during Cesarean section. *Eur J Obstet Gynecol Reprod Biol* 2005;121(1):24–26.
113. Blickstein I. Difficult delivery of the impacted fetal head during cesarean section: Intraoperative disengagement dystocia. *J Perinat Med* 2004;32(6):465–9.
114. Simon GR, Wilkins CJ, Smith I. Sevoflurane induction for emergency caesarean delivery: Two case reports in women with needle phobia. *Int J Obstet Anesth* 2002;11(4):296–300.
115. Patil S, Sinha P, Krishnan S. Successful delivery in a morbidly obese patient after failed intubation and regional technique. *Br J Anaesth* 2007 Dec;99(6):919–20.
116. Nicholson SC, Brown AD, MacPherson HM, Liston WA. "Classical" caesarean delivery at or near term in the morbidly obese obstetric patient. *J Obstet Gynaecol* 2002;22(6):691.
117. Porreco RP, Adelberg AM, Lindsay LG, Holdt DG. Cesarean birth in the morbidly obese woman: A report of 3 cases. *J Reprod Med* 2007;52(3):231–4.
118. Novoa L, Metge M, Estanyol N, Parramon F, Arxer A, March X. Difficult intradural puncture for urgent cesarean section in a morbidly obese patient. *Rev Esp Anestesiol Reanim* 2003;50(4):213–4.
119. Thornton YS. Caesarean delivery and celiotomy using panniculus retraction in the morbidly obese patient. *J Am Coll Surg* 2001;193(4):458–61.
120. Rajendra P, Popham P. Fracture of an epidural catheter inserted for labour analgesia. *Anaesth Intensive Care* 2008;36(2):245–8.
121. Abou-Shameh MA, Lyons G, Roa A, Mushtaque S. Broken needle complicating spinal anaesthesia. *Int J Obstet Anesth* 2006;15(2):178–9.
122. Mallardi V. The origin of informed consent. *Acta Otorhinolaryngol Ital* 2005;25(5):312–27.
123. Devendra K, Arulkumaran S. Should doctors perform an elective caesarean section on request? *Ann Acad Med Singapore* 2003;32(5):577–81.
124. Sobande A, Eskandar M. Multiple repeat caesarean deliveries: Complications and outcomes. *J Obstet Gynaecol Can* 2006;28(3):193–7.
125. Rozenberg P. The counselling of patient with prior C-delivery. *Gynecol Obstet Fertil* 2005; 33(12):1003–8.
126. Cohen WR, Schifrin BS. Medical negligence lawsuits relating to labor and delivery. *Clin Perinatol* 2007;34(2):345–60.
127. Onah HE, Ibeziako N, Umezulike AC, Effetie ER, Ogbuokiri CM. Decision—Delivery interval and perinatal outcome in emergency caesarean deliveries. *J Obstet Gynaecol* 2005;25(4):342–6.
128. Hillemanns P, Hasbargen U, Strauss A, Schulze A, Genzel-Boroviczeny O, Hepp H. Maternal and neonatal morbidity of emergency caesarean deliveries with a decision-to-delivery interval under 30 minutes: Evidence from 10 years. *Arch Gynecol Obstet* 2003;268(3):136–41.
129. Hankins GD, Clark SM, Munn MB. Cesarean section on request at 39 weeks: Impact on shoulder dystocia, fetal trauma, neonatal encephalopathy, and intrauterine fetal demise. *Semin Perinatol* 2006;30(5):276–87.
130. Ben-Meir A, Schenker JG, Ezra Y. Cesarean section upon request: Is it appropriate for everybody? *J Perinat Med* 2005;33(2):106–11.
131. Malvasi A, Tinelli A, Garzya V, Caprioli LC, Tinelli R, Pellegrino M, Colosimo E. Rischi di un taglio cesareo non motivato o "a richiesta." *Rivista di Ostetricia, Ginecologia pratica e Medicina Perinatale* 2008;23(1):16–22.
132. Moes CB, Thacher F. The midwife as first assistant for cesarean section. *J Midwifery Womens Health* 2001;46(5):305–12.

FURTHER READING

Vasa R, Kim MR. Fracture of the femur at caesarean section: Case report and review of literature. *Am J Perinatal* 1990;7:46–48.

Index

A

Abdominal aorta compression, 210
Abdominal birth, *see* Cesarean delivery
Abdominal muscle
    cutting rectus muscle, 11
    stretching of, 21
Abdominal palpation, 244
Abdominal towel usage, 164–165
Abdominal wall closure, 27, 31, 32
    Camper fascia closure, 33
    nonsutured peritoneum, 30–31
    parietal drain, 34
    peritoneal closure, 30
    rectus muscle closure, 32
    subcutaneous tissue healing, 35
    suture of visceral peritoneum, 32
    suturing subcutaneous tissue and skin, 33
Abdominal wall frontal section, 16
Abnormal placentation, *see* Placenta accrete; Placenta previa
    high-risk factor for, 209
Accidental fetal lesions, 45, 46, 47
ACOG, *see* American College of Obstetricians and Gynecologists (ACOG)
ACTH, *see* Adrenocorticotropin (ACTH)
Adrenocorticotropin (ACTH), 334
AFS, *see* American Fertility Society (AFS)
AGA, *see* Appropriate for gestational age (AGA)
Aintree intubation catheter, 315
AMA, *see* American Medical Association (AMA)
American College of Obstetricians and Gynecologists (ACOG), 88, 192, 222, 227, 316, 365
American Fertility Society (AFS), 180
American Medical Association (AMA), 385
American Society of Anesthesiologists (ASA), 307
Amnioreduction, 262; *see also* Twin pregnancy
Amniotic fluid effect, 139
Amniotic sac opening, 53
Anesthesia for obstetrics, 307; *see also* General anesthesia for CD
Anomalous presentation, 112; *see also* Breech presentation; Transverse presentation
Antenatal steroids, 283
Antibiotic therapy, 139, 140
    prophylaxis, 127
Antiphospholipid antibody syndrome (APS), 378
Appropriate for gestational age (AGA), 277
APS, *see* Antiphospholipid antibody syndrome (APS)
Arachnoiditis, 336–337; *see also* Local anesthesia for CD
Arteriovenous malformations (AVMs), 318
ARTs, *see* Assisted reproductive techniques (ARTs)
ASA, *see* American Society of Anesthesiologists (ASA)
Asian Global Survey data, 4
Aspiration pneumonitis (Mendelson syndrome), 318
Assisted reproductive techniques (ARTs), 257
Asymptomatic uterine rupture, 359, 360; *see also* Vaginal birth after cesarean (VBAC)
Asynclitism, 64, 69, 70, 220
    positions, 219
Atracurium, 311; *see also* Induction agents
AVMs, *see* Arteriovenous malformations (AVMs)
Axe-sign expression, 344; *see also* Postcesarean delivery uterine scar

B

Bakri balloon, 195, 196
Barnev cervicometer, 231–232
Bimanual stretching, 22
Bird concept, 104
BIS, *see* Bispectral Index (BIS)
Bispectral Index (BIS), 313
Bladder
    flap hematoma, 351
    injury, 212–213
Blocked limb, 95
B-Lynch ligature, 195
Body mass index (BMI) 11, 381
BPD, *see* Bronchopulmonary dysplasia (BPD)
Brain, impact of large, 237, 239
Breech presentation, 57, 76, 96; *see also* Anomalous presentation; Complete breech presentation; External cephalic version (ECV); Fetal extraction with instruments; Incomplete breech presentation
    blocked limb, 95
    contraindications of fetal adnexa, 89
    diagnosis, 76
    extraction maneuvers, 77
    funicle loop extraction, 85
    head extraction, 85–86
    hooking fetal inguinofemoral region, 77, 79, 80, 81, 82, 83
    locating fetal hand and foot, 83
    Mauriceau maneuver, 85, 86, 93, 94
    modified Piper maneuver, 82
    Pinard maneuver, 79, 85
    Piper maneuver, 90, 91
    rotation maneuvers, 82
    shoulder extraction, 85, 92, 93
    trunk extraction, 85
    version through external maneuvers, 86
    Wignard maneuver, 85, 86, 94
Bregma presentation, 62
Bronchopulmonary dysplasia (BPD), 284; *see also* Neonatal outcomes
    clinical presentation of new, 285
    incidence of, 285–286
    initial BPD in ELBW, 286
    pathogenesis of, 287
    prognosis, 286
    risk factors, 286
    severe, 286
Bumm pelvic fold, 11

C

Caesarean surgical technique, 11, 34; *see also* Abdominal wall closure; Joel-Cohen laparotomy; Pfannenstiel laparotomy; Misgav Ladach method
    abdominal wall frontal section, 16
    advantages of, 34
    advantages of transverse incision, 11, 12, 13
    aesthetic outcome, 34
    anterior fascia layer, 21
    bimanual stretching, 22
    caudocranial stretching of fascia to, 21
    Cherneyn laparotomy, 19
    cutaneous adhesion, 13
    cutaneous incisions, 11
    cutting fascia, 11, 12
    cutting peritoneum, 11, 22
    cutting rectus muscle, 11
    factor in fetus extraction, 13
    fascia preparation, 22
    hypertrophic skin removal, 19
    incision on parietal scarred peritoneum, 25
    intradermal suture, 31
    Kustner laparotomy, 21, 26
    laparotomy principle, 21
    linea alba, 21
    longitudinal incision, 17, 18, 24
    lower Pfannenstiel, 20
    Mackenrodt–Maylard technique, 13, 14, 16, 18
    paramedian incision, 21
    sagittal section of pregnant pelvis, 15
    space of Retzius, 11
    stretching, 20, 21
    surgical scar, 13
    suture of fascia, 31
    tissue healing, 35
    transverse laparotomies, 30
    uterine wall exposure, 25
    variant of Mackenrodt–Maylard technique, 15
    for wide surgical exposure, 16
California Perinatal Quality Care Collaborative (CPQCC), 292
Cannula cricothyroidotomy, 317
Caput succedaneum, 227
    in sagittal translabial section scan, 219
Cardiotocography (CTG), 89, 355
Cardiovascular system (CVS), 335
Cauda equina syndrome, 336; *see also* Local anesthesia for CD
CD, *see* Cesarean delivery(CD)
CDC, *see* Centers for Disease Control and Prevention (CDC)
Ceasarean scar syndrome, 350
CeDAP (Delivery assistance certificates), 279
CEMACH, *see* Confidential Enquiry into Maternal and Child Health (CEMACH)
Centers for Disease Control and Prevention (CDC), 307
Central incision of uterine breach, 46
Central nervous system (CNS), 287; *see also* Neonatal outcomes
    toxicity, 335
Central venous catheter (CVC), 195
Cephalic presentation, 57
Cervical dilation, 131, 134, 135, 227, 229
    curves, 230
Cervicometers, 230
    Barnev cervicometer, 231–232
    electrodes on fetal scalp and cervix, 231
    future applications, 232–233
    LaborPro, 232
Cesarean delivery(CD), 1, 123, 207, 297, 365; *see also* Cesarean delivery of twenty-first century; Childbirth
    according to Stark, 34
    allowed percentage, 1
    Asian Global Survey data, 4
    causes of, 225
    ceasarean scar syndrome, 350
    classification of, 226
    consequences of global inequalities, 2
    controversy in, 1
    elective, 297
    factors contributing to trends of, 6–7
    first, 161
    impact on mortality rate, 4
    and indications, 225
    and intrapartum death, 4, 5
    and maternal and perinatal outcomes, 3–6
    and maternal morbidity, 4, 5
    monitoring at local level, 7–8
    and neonatal admission to intensive care, 6
    postmortem, 242–243
    Robson 10-group classification system for, 7–8
    and sociological aspects, 225
    and subsequent delivery, 226
    trends worldwide, 1–2, 3
    variations in, 161

Cesarean delivery of twenty-first century, 161
  abdominal closure, 167–168
  abdominal incision, 162–165
  abdominal towels usage, 164–165
  anesthesia, 162
  classical music, 161
  clot removal, 168
  dangers of overused cesarean deliveries, 169–170
  delivery of baby, 165–166
  exteriorization of uterus, 166
  fascia closure, 168
  fascia opening, 162, 163, 164
  incision of fat tissue, 163
  lower segment incision, 165, 166
  modified Joel Cohen incision, 166
  optimal position for right-handed surgeon, 162
  pain at suture level, 168
  patient positioning, 161
  peritoneum non-closure, 167
  peritoneum opening, 164
  plica opening, 165
  recovery after surgery, 168–169
  repeated CD, 165
  scientific evaluation of, 169
  skin closure, 168
  transverse lower incision, 165
  uterine and adnexal examination, 167
  uterine single-layer suture, 167
  uterus closure, 166–167
Cesarean myomectomy, 175, 176, 178; see also Uterine fibroids
  blood tests, 187
  intracapsular, 180–183
  literature on 176–178
  pelvic irrigation, 182
  postoperative course, 182, 183
  removal by intracapsular, 181, 182, 183, 184
  sites of, 182
  suturing fibroid base, 182, 185, 186
  traditional technique of, 178–180
Chemical neuropathy, 336; see also Local anesthesia for CD
Chemo-antibiotic therapy, 39
Cherneyn laparotomy, 19
Childbirth; see also Cervical dilation; Cervicometers; Second stage of labor; Shoulder dystocia
  abdominal palpation, 244
  assisted, 237, 242
  disengagement maneuver of rear shoulder, 245
  dystocia, 240–241
  fetal head pushed back, 243
  finger exploration, 243
  front shoulder in anterior–posterior position, 245
  internal rotation, 237, 240
  impact of large brain, 237, 239
  latency, 240
  maternal-fetal childbirth stages, 240
  maternal mortality, 237
  oxytocic perfusion, 246
  pelvis in second stage of labor, 241
  postmortem childbirth, 242
  as private event, 237
  stations of fetal head in relation to pelvis, 242
Chorioamnionitis, 229
Chronic lung disease (CLD), 285
Clavicle fracture maneuver, 254
CLD, see Chronic lung disease (CLD)
CME, see Continuing medical education (CME)
CNS, see Central nervous system (CNS)
Coagulopathy, 326
Cobra-PLA, 316
Combined spinal epidural (CSE), 57, 323; see also Local anesthesia for CD; Obstetric anesthetic care issues
  anesthesia, 325, 331
  needles, 328–329
Complete breech presentation, 77; see also Breech presentation

  buttocks-only variant, 77, 78, 82
  feet variant, 84, 88, 89
Complications in low transverse incision extension technique, 48
Computed tomography (CT), 372
Conciani sentence, 387
Confidential Enquiry into Maternal and Child Health (CEMACH), 307
Congestion of uterine–ovarian venous plexuses, 137, 139
Contamination of suture threads, 145, 146
Continuing medical education (CME), 315
Continuous interlocking suture, 152, 154
Continuous Labor Monitoring (CLM)
Continuous positive pressure ventilation (CPAP), 297
Continuous suture, 151
Cord blood collection, 141
CPAP, see Continuous positive pressure ventilation (CPAP)
CPQCC, see California Perinatal Quality Care Collaborative (CPQCC)
Credé's maneuver, 123, 125
Critical point
  fifth, 246
  first, 238, 240–241
  fourth, 245–246
  second, 241–243, 244
  third, 243–245
CRL, see Crown–rump length (CRL)
Crown–rump length (CRL), 263
CSE, see Combined spinal epidural (CSE)
CT, see Computed tomography (CT)
CTG, see Cardiotocography (CTG)
Cutaneous
  adhesion, 13
  incisions, 11
CVC, see Central venous catheter (CVC)
CVS, see Cardiovascular system (CVS)

D
Dangers of overused cesarean deliveries, 169–170
D-D (Decision–delivery), 356
Decision–delivery, see D-D (Decision–delivery)
Defensive medicine, 365; see also Forensic aspects of CD
Dehiscence, see Asymptomatic uterine rupture
Delivery assistance certificates, see CeDAP (Delivery assistance certificates)
Dermatome, 332; see also Local anesthesia for CD
  landmark, 333
Difficult airway, 314; see also General anesthesia for CD
  aintree intubation catheter, 315
  airway equipment, 315
  cannula cricothyroidotomy, 317
  classification of airway devices, 315
  Cobra-PLA, 316
  EasyTube, 316
  Glidescope, 317
  I-Gel, 316
  laryngeal suction tube, 315
  Mallampati classes, 314
  management, 316–317
  obstetric airway assessment, 315
  predisposing factors, 314
  supraglottic devices, 315
  surgical cricothyroidotomy, 317
  Wilson sum score, 315
Digital examination, 216
Digital pull, 40, 42, 44, 45, 47, 48, 51
Disengagement
  of presenting part, 240
  of rear shoulder, 245
Double-layer suture, 147, 148, 149, 154
DRG classification system, 279; see also Preterm neonate
Dystocia, 65, 66, 215, 233; see also Cesarean delivery (CD); Intrapartum ultrasonography
  caput succedaneum, 227
  cause of, 215

  cervical dilation, 227, 229, 230
  chorioamnionitis, 229
  digital examination, 216
  engagement of fetal head, 226
  fetal abnormalities, 215
  fetal head position, 227, 228
  insufficient algorithms for management of labor, 229–230
  limitations in management of labor, 226
  vacuum extractor, 222
  vaginal bacteriological examination, 229

E
EasyTube, 316
ECV, see External cephalic version (ECV)
ELBW, see Extremely low birth weight (ELBW)
Elective CD, 297
Electrodes on fetal scalp and on cervix, 231
Emergency protocol for shoulder dystocia, 255
Endometritis, 127, 138, 203
Endotracheal intubation, 312; see also Induction agents
Engagement, 227
  beginning of second stage of labor, 240
  of fetal head, 226, 238
  of shoulder, 250
Epidural abscess, 336; see also Local anesthesia for CD
Epidural anesthesia, 324–325; see also Local anesthesia for CD
  procedures for, 331
Epidural hematoma, 336; see also Local anesthesia for CD
Epidural needles, 328; see also Obstetric anesthetic care issues
Episiotomy, 249, 255
Erb's palsy, 381
Etomidate, 311; see also Induction agents
Evolution in hysterotomy, 39
Exceptional situations after CD and PPH, 207; see also Placenta accrete; Placenta previa
  abdominal aorta compression, 210
  bladder injury, 212–213
  hysterectomy under hemorrhage, 210
  pelvisubperitoneal hematomas, 212
  placental invasions, 209
  retrovesical hematoma, 213
  secondary bleeding, 207, 209
  subperitoneal extension of hysterotomy, 210
  unexpected abnormal placentation, 207, 208, 209
  ureteral identification, 211
  ureteral injury, 213
External cephalic version (ECV), 88, 89, 90; see also Breech presentation
  contraindications, 89
  effectiveness, 88
  percentage of positive outcome, 96
  position, 89
  procedure, 95
  risks in, 95–96
Extraction from uterine breach, 60
Extraglottic devices, see Supraglottic devices
Extraperitoneal CD, 39
Extremely low birth weight (ELBW), 277

F
Face presentation, 60
Familial exudative vitreoretinopathy (FEVR), 291
Fascia
  anterior layer, 21
  Camper fascia closure, 33
  caudocranial stretching of, 21
  cutting, 11, 12
  opening, 162, 163, 164
  preparation, 22
  suture of, 31
FDA, see U.S. Food and Drug Administration (FDA)
Fentanyl, 324
Fetal abnormalities, 215
Fetal adnexa, absolute contraindications of, 89

Fetal extraction in CD, 57, 74; *see also* Fetal
position; Hand position in fetal
extraction; Head engagement; Head
extraction
- associated to upper left limb, 69
- head position, 57–58
- laparotomy retractors for, 73
- with left hand, 68
- risks of, 73
- strain on bladder, 66
- transverse presentation, 116–120

Fetal extraction with instruments, 98, 111–112
- Bird concept, 104
- forceps application, 98–102, 103, 104
- Kiwi OmniCup, 104, 107, 110
- occiput position, 110
- OmniCup-type Kiwi ventouse, 109
- ProCup, 104
- ProCup-type Kiwi ventouse, 108
- swelling of soft tissues, 108
- vacuum extractor, 102, 104, 105, 106, 110, 111

Fetal macrosomia, 68

Fetal position, 45–46
- head in occiput posterior position, 220, 221
- head in relation to pelvis, 242
- head position, 227, 228
- head pushed back, 243

Fetus extraction, factors in, 13

Fetus papyraceus, 261; *see also* Twin pregnancy

FEVR, *see* Familial exudative vitreoretinopathy
(FEVR)

Fibroids, *see* Uterine fibroids

Fibrosis, 165

FIGO, *see* International Federation of Gynecology
and Obstetrics (FIGO)

Finger exploration, 243

Flexion reduction, 60, 69

fMRI, *see* Functional magnetic resonance
imaging (fMRI)

Foot, holding blocked, 87

Forceps application, 98–102, 103, 104

Forcipressure and ligation of prevesical vessel, 42

Forensic aspects of CD, 365, 388–389
- areas of postcesarean hypo-/hyperesthesia, 379
- bladder dome injury, 373, 374
- bladder lesions, 367–368
- CD on demand, 385–388
- complications, 365
- defensive medicine, 365
- dehiscence of thin hysterotomy scar, 367
- divarication of uterine breach, 382
- effects of forceps, 377
- Erb's palsy, 381
- extension of hysterotomy, 369
- extension of uterine breach, 366
- extraction of hyperflexed fetal head, 381
- fetal damage, 381–383
- fetal head compression, 379
- fetal head lesion, 383
- fetal injuries, 382, 383
- frontal delivery of uterus, 370
- gastrointestinal lesions, 369–370
- hematomas, 372–373, 381
- hemorrhage, 367
- heparin prophylaxis, 374–381
- hyperesthesia and hypoesthesia of
iliac–hypogastric and iliac–
inguinal nerve, 378
- iatrogenic lesion, 376, 377
- intrauterine wadding pressed into uterine
atony, 371
- kidney lesion, 377
- ligation of prevesical vessels, 375
- ligation of right hypogastric artery, 372
- ligation of uterine vessels, 369
- lumbosacral plexus compression, 378
- malposition and malrotation in dystocic
birth, 380
- mandatory CD, 383–384
- maternal mortality, 374
- maternal neurological lesions, 380
- neurological lesions, 370–372
- postcesarean hysterectomy, 367
- postsurgical adhesion of urinary bladder, 375
- prophylaxis with anticoagulants, 380
- puerperal genital tract, 368
- refusal of mandatory CD, 384–385
- retention of foreign bodies, 373–374
- right fetal femur fracture, 384
- right fetal humerus fracture, 385
- risk categories of pregnant women, 376
- safety maneuver, 375, 383
- scarring, 383
- subfascial hematoma, 380
- tear of lower uterine segment, 367
- tear of uterine vessels, 366–367
- thromboembolism risk categories, 380
- T incision of lower uterine segment, 370
- urethral lesion, 369
- uterine atony, 367

FRC, *see* Functional residual capacity (FRC)

Frontal presentation, 60

Functional magnetic resonance imaging (fMRI), 289

Functional residual capacity (FRC), 314, 318

Fundal pressure, 60, 66, 68

Funicle loop extraction, 85

G

Gamete intrafallopian transfer (GIFT), 257

GDP, *see* Gross domestic product (GDP)

General anesthesia for CD, 307; *see also* Difficult
airway; Hypoxia; Induction agents
- aspiration prophylaxis, 308–309
- awareness during anesthesia, 313
- complications, 313
- denitrogenation/preoxygenation, 309–310
- effects on fetus and neonate, 312
- factors to intraoperative awareness, 313–314
- indications for, 307–308
- intravenous fluids, 309
- inverted traffic light difficult obstetric airway
management algorithm, 308
- maintenance of anesthesia, 312
- maternal monitoring, 309
- maternal mortality, 307
- pre-anesthetic evaluation, 308
- prevention of complications, 309
- prevention of fetal hypoxemia and acidosis, 313
- remifentanil, 319

Germinal matrix and intraventricular hemorrhage
(GMHIVH), 287–288; *see also* Neonatal
outcomes

GIFT, *see* Gamete intrafallopian transfer (GIFT)

Glidescope, 317

Global Positioning System (GPS), 231

Global Survey on Maternal and Perinatal Health, 4

Gloves effect, 127–128

GMHIVH, *see* Germinal matrix and intraventricular
hemorrhage (GMHIVH)

Gossypiboma, 373

Gottschalk–Portes CD technique, 132

GPS, *see* Global Positioning System (GPS)

Gross domestic product (GDP), 4

H

Halogenated agents, 312; *see also* Induction agents

Hand position in fetal extraction, 58, 65; *see also*
Head engagement; Head extraction
- asynclitism, 64, 69, 70
- bregma presentation, 62
- to change presentation, 60, 68, 69
- dystocia, 65, 66
- extraction from uterine breach, 60
- face presentation, 60
- fetal extraction, 68, 69
- fetal macrosomia, 68
- flexion reduction, 60, 69
- frontal presentation, 60
- fundal pressure, 60, 66, 68
- hyperextended head, 64
- locating fetal rima oris, 71, 72
- narrow laparotomy breach, 60
- operator's hand in occipital–pubic direction, 59
- progression toward uterine breach, 59
- raising presenting part, 58
- tilting movements to emerge shoulders, 72
- Zavanelli maneuver, 65–66

HDF, *see* Hospital discharge form (HDF)

HDI, *see* Human development index (HDI)

Head engagement, 64, 65, 70, 71; *see also* Hand
position in fetal extraction

Head extraction, 58, 85–86; *see also* Hand position
in fetal extraction
- with cup-like position, 69
- high head and narrow uterine breach, 66, 68
- high head position, 66
- with left hand by left-handed operator, 64
- in left occiput anterior position, 62
- in left occiput posterior position, 61
- in left occiput transverse position, 64
- in median occiput posterior position, 63
- in occiput median anterior position, 63
- in right occiput anterior position, 62
- in vaginal delivery, 60, 61, 62, 63, 64

HELLP syndrome, *see* Hemolysis, elevated liver
enzymes, and low platelet count
syndrome (HELLP syndrome)

Hemolysis, elevated liver enzymes, and low platelet
count syndrome (HELLP syndrome),
13, 308, 326

Hemorrhagic complications percentage, 155

Hemostatic sutures of lower uterine segment, 194

Herpes simplex virus (HSV), 300

HIE, *see* Hypoxic ischemic encephalopathy (HIE)

High head position, 66
- and narrow uterine breach, 66, 68

High neuraxial blockade, 335–336; *see also* Local
anesthesia for CD

HMG, *see* Human menopausal gonadotropin (HMG)

Hooking fetal inguinofemoral region, 77, 79, 80,
81, 82, 83

Hospital discharge form (HDF), 278

HSV, *see* Herpes simplex virus (HSV)

Human development index (HDI), 4

Human menopausal gonadotropin (HMG), 257

Hyperextended head, 64

Hypertrophic skin removal, 19

Hypotension, 333; *see also* Local anesthesia for CD

Hypoxia, 318; *see also* General anesthesia for CD
- aspiration pneumonitis, 318
- cerebrovascular stroke, 318
- chronic postcesarean pain, 319
- fetal and neonatal respiratory depression, 319
- and induction of general anesthesia, 318
- intracranial hemorrhagic stroke, 318–319
- intracranial ischemic stroke, 319

Hypoxic ischemic encephalopathy (HIE), 297

Hysterectomy under massive hemorrhage with
distorted anatomy, 210

Hysterosalpingography after CD, 341; *see also*
Postcesarean delivery uterine scar

Hysteroscopy, 347; *see also* Postcesarean delivery
uterine scar
- followed by resection of polyp in niche, 348
- four classes of, 342
- on uterus with previous CD, 347
- on uterus with uterine scar, 342

Hysterotomy incisions, 39, 48, 53
- accidental fetal lesions, 45, 46, 47
- amniotic sac opening, 53
- central incision of uterine breach, 46
- complications due to incision extension, 48, 52
- current techniques, 40
- digital pull, 40, 42, 44, 45, 47, 48, 51
- evolution in hysterotomy, 39
- fetal position, 45–46
- forcipressure and ligation of prevesical vessel, 42
- intraperitoneal adhesion, 42
- J incision, 47, 49, 50
- Kerr hysterotomy, 47
- laparotomy gauzes, 41
- locating placenta, 44, 45
- lower uterine segment, 45

Hysterotomy incisions (Continued)
  low vertical incision, 48, 49
  mass closuring technique, 42
  maternal morbidity percentage, 50
  myometrial delivery, 51
  myometrium, 45
  myometrium cut, 50
  safety maneuvers, 45
  transabdominal convex ultrasound probe, 45
  transverse incision of lower uterine segment, 47
  upside-down "T" uterine incision, 48
  uterine breach opening, 46, 47
  vesicouterine fold incision, 41–45
  vesicouterine plica, 42, 43, 44, 45
  visceral peritoneum incision, 44
  to widen breach, 50, 51, 52

I
Iatrogenic shoulder pseudo-dystocias, 245
ICD-9, see International Classification of Diseases, Ninth Revision (ICD-9)
ICM, see Intracapsular cesarean myomectomy (ICM)
ICU, see Intensive care unit (ICU)
I-Gel, 316
IGF-1, see Insulin-like growth factor (IGF-1)
IHDP, see Infant Health and Development Program (IHDP)
Incision
  cutaneous, 11
  extension and complications, 52
  longitudinal, 18
  paramedian, 21
  of uterus, 48
Incomplete breech presentation, 77; see also Breech presentation
  buttocks variant, 77, 78, 86
  feet variant, 79
  holding blocked foot, 87
  hooking maneuver in, 83, 84
  mixed, 78
Induction agents, 310; see also General anesthesia for CD
  atracurium, 311
  for cesarean delivery, 310
  endotracheal intubation, 312
  etomidate, 311
  inhaled anesthetic agents, 312
  ketamine, 310–311
  muscle relaxants, 311
  propofol, 310
  reversal agents, 311, 312
  rocuronium, 311
  succinylcholine, 311
  thiopental, 310
  vecuronium, 311
Infant Health and Development Program (IHDP), 290
Inhaled anesthetic agents, 312; see also Induction agents
Insulin-like growth factor (IGF-1), 291
Intensive care unit (ICU), 210
Intercristal line, 326
Intermediate vertex presentation, see Bregma presentation
Internal rotation, 219
  engagement at mid-strait, 240
  movement in birth canal, 237
International Classification of Diseases, Ninth Revision (ICD-9), 5
International Federation of Gynecology and Obstetrics (FIGO), 161
Intracapsular cesarean myomectomy (ICM), 187
Intracranial hemorrhage, 318–319
Intraparenchymal lesions (IPLs), 287
Intrapartum death, 4, 5
Intrapartum ultrasonography, 215, 216; see also Dystocia
  asynclitic positions, 219, 220
  caput succedaneum in, 219
  fetal head in occiput posterior position, 220, 221
  internal rotation, 219
  and medico-legal aspects, 223
  posterior fetal asynclitism, 220
  procedure, 215, 217
  role of, 222
  scientific role of, 217, 218, 219, 222
  in second stage of labor, 217
  timing of, 222
  transabdominal intrapartum, 217
  vaginal exploration, 219
  vertex presentation, 218, 221
Intraperitoneal adhesion, 42
Intrauterine
  balloon, 201, 202
  hemostasis, 203
  packing, 194
Intrauterine growth restriction (IUGR), 262, 263; see also Twin pregnancy
Intraventricular hemorrhage (IVH), 291
Inverted traffic light difficult obstetric airway management algorithm, 308
In vitro fertilization (IVF), 257
IPLs, see Intraparenchymal lesions (IPLs)
Italian National Institute of Heath–National System of Guidelines (SNLGISS), 191
IUGR, see Intrauterine growth restriction (IUGR)
IVF, see In vitro fertilization (IVF)
IVH, see Intraventricular hemorrhage (IVH)

J
Jacoby's line, see Intercristal line
Jacquemier's maneuver, 252, 255
J incision, 47, 49, 50
Joel-Cohen laparotomy, 16, 17, 20, 34; see also Modified Joel-Cohen laparotomy
  comparisons, 24
  less infection, 26
  less trauma, 26
  modified, 28, 29, 30

K
Kehrer incision, 39
Kerr hysterotomy, 47
Ketamine, 310–311; see also Induction agents
Kiwi OmniCup, 104, 107, 110
Kristeller maneuver, 251, 253, 254
Kustner laparotomy, 21, 26

L
LaborPro, 232
Laparotomy
  and CD, 11
  gauzes, 41
  retractors, 73
Large for gestational age (LGA), 277
Laryngeal suction tube, 315
LBW, see Low birth weight (LBW)
Leopold maneuver in transverse presentation, 113
LGA, see Large for gestational age (LGA)
Ligamentum flavum, 323
Linea alba, 21
Lipid infusion therapy, 335
Lipid related metabolic abnormalities, 335
LMA devices, 315
LMWH, see Low molecular weight heparin (LMWH)
Local anesthesia for CD, 323; see also Obstetric anesthetic care issues; Postdural puncture headache (PDPH)
  advantages and disadvantages, 324
  anesthetic agents and opioids, 325
  arachnoiditis, 336–337
  aspiration prophylaxis, 326
  chemical neuropathy, 336
  CNS toxicity, 335
  combined spinal–epidural technique, 323, 325, 331
  CVS toxicity, 335
  dermatome, 332
  epidural abscess, 336
  epidural anesthesia, 324–325, 331
  epidural hematoma, 336
  extension of epidural labor analgesia, 323
  high neuraxial blockade, 335–336
  hypotension, 333
  lipid infusion therapy, 335
  medications, 324
  monitoring, 326
  needle-through-needle CSE technique, 323
  physiological curvature of spine, 325
  postdural puncture headache, 333
  post-op pain management, 337
  pre-anesthetic evaluation, 326
  preparation for anesthesia, 325
  side effects and complications, 333
  single-shot spinal and de novo epidural technique, 323
  spinal anatomy, 323
  spinal anesthesia, 323, 324, 330
  symptoms at various lidocaine concentrations, 335
  systemic toxicity, 335
  traumatic neuropathy, 336
Locating
  fetal hand and foot, 83
  fetal rima oris, 71, 72
  placenta, 44, 45
  shoulder, 113, 115–116
Lochia discharge, 131
Longitudinal laparotomy, 24, 40
  advantages and disadvantages, 39
  and alba-line of fascia incision, 24
  apposition of abdominal muscles in, 32
  optimal exposure of uterine wall, 25
  vs. transverse, 34
LOR syringes, see Loss of resistance syringes (LOR syringes)
Loss of resistance syringes (LOR syringes), 329
Low birth weight (LBW), 277
Lower Pfannenstiel, 20
Lower segment incision, 165, 166
Low molecular weight heparin (LMWH), 376
Low transverse incision, 39
Low vertical incision, 48, 49

M
MAC, see Minimum alveolar concentration (MAC)
Mackenrodt–Maylard laparotomy, 13, 14, 16
  incision line, 18
  variant of, 15
Magnetic resonance imaging (MRI), 189, 372
Malgaigne triangle, 11
Maneuver
  clavicle fracture maneuver, 254
  Credé's maneuver, 123, 125
  disengagement of rear shoulder, 245
  extraction, 77, 116–120
  funicle loop extraction, 85
  head extraction, 85–86
  hooking in, 83, 84
  Jacquemier's, 252, 255
  Kristeller, 251, 253, 254
  Leopold, 113
  Mauriceau, 85, 86, 93, 94
  McRoberts' maneuver, 249, 250
  membrane extraction, 123, 130, 131, 132, 133
  modified Piper, 82
  Pinard, 79, 85
  Piper, 90, 91
  reverse Rubin maneuver, 254
  rotation, 82
  Rubin's II maneuver, 251, 252
  safety maneuver, 375, 383
  shoulder extraction, 85, 92, 93
  of suprapubic pressure, 250, 251
  therapeutic maneuvers, 248–249
  trunk extraction, 85
  twisting maneuver, 123, 126
  type I shoulder dystocia, 247, 248
  type II, 247, 248, 253
  version through external maneuvers, 86
  Wignard maneuver, 85, 86, 94
  Zavanelli maneuver, 65–66, 254, 255

Mass closure method (MCM), 42, 157
Massive placental invasions, 209
Maternal
 -fetal childbirth stages, 240
 -fetal dystocia, 241
 morbidity, 4, 5, 237
 and perinatal morbidity and mortality, 1
Mauriceau–Smellie–Veit maneuver, 85, 86, 93, 94
MCM, see Mass closure method (MCM)
McRoberts' maneuver, 249, 250
MDI, see Mental development index (MDI)
Membrane extraction, 123, 130, 131, 132, 133
Mendelson syndrome, see Aspiration pneumonitis (Mendelson syndrome)
Mental development index (MDI), 289
MFPR, see Multifetal pregnancy reduction (MFPR)
Minimum alveolar concentration (MAC), 313
Misgav Ladach method, 133
 modified, 26, 27
 principles in, 25–26
 surgery duration, 25, 26
Modified Joel-Cohen laparotomy, 22
Modified Piper maneuver, 82
MRI, see Magnetic resonance imaging (MRI)
Multifetal pregnancy reduction (MFPR), 263; see also Twin pregnancy
Multiple pregnancy, 257, 274; see also Twin pregnancy
 and embryonic reduction, 263
 uterine contractions, 264
Munro–Kerr technique, 133
Muscle relaxants, 311; see also Induction agents
Myomas, see Uterine fibroids
Myometrial delivery, 51
Myometrium cut, 50

N

Narrow laparotomy breach, 60
National Health and Medical Research Council (NHMRC), 277
National Institute of Child Health and Human Development (NICHD), 286, 289
NEC, see Necrotizing enterocolitis (NEC)
Necrotizing enterocolitis (NEC), 284, 291
Needle-through-needle CSE technique, 323
Neonatal intensive care units (NICUs), 6, 282, 297; see also Preterm neonate
Neonatal outcomes, 284; see also Bronchopulmonary dysplasia (BPD)
 assisted ventilation techniques, 284
 central nervous system, 287
 germinal matrix and intraventricular hemorrhage, 287–288
 periventricular leukomalacia, 288–290
 predisposing factors, 290–291
 prognosis, 291
 retinopathy of prematurity, 290, 291
Neonate, 278; see also Preterm neonate
Neonate from cesarean delivery, 297
 delivery at term, 297–298
 effect on other morbidities, 299
 fetal injury due to delivery mode, 300
 fetus at gestational term with giant sacrococcygeal teratoma, 303
 fetus with anterior cystic hygroma, 303
 fetus with hydrocephalus and macrocephaly, 302
 genitalis infection of herpes simplex virus, 300
 left facial palsy in baby, 301
 neonatal mortality, 298
 omphalocele with extracorporeal liver, 303
 outcome neonatal variables, 298
 in patient with HIV infection, 300
 planned vaginal vs. elective CD, 298–299
 in preterm, 300, 304
 rate of respiratory mortality, 299
 shoulder dystocia and brachial plexus injury, 302
 vacuum extraction failure, 301
Neuraxial opioids, 325
NHMRC, see National Health and Medical Research Council (NHMRC)
NICHD, see National Institute of Child Health and Human Development (NICHD)
Niche, 344, 345; see also Postcesarean delivery uterine scar
NICUs, see Neonatal intensive care units (NICUs)
NMR, see Nuclear magnetic resonance (NMR)
Nonsteroidal anti-inflammatory drugs (NSAIDs), 334
NSAIDs, see Nonsteroidal anti-inflammatory drugs (NSAIDs)
Nuclear magnetic resonance (NMR), 289

O

Obstetric anesthesia, 323, 307; see also Local anesthesia for CD
Obstetric anesthetic care issues, 326; see also Local anesthesia for CD
 catheters, 329
 confirming anesthetic block effects, 332
 CSE needles, 328–329
 epidural needles, 328
 hand washing by practitioner, 326
 inadequate spinal/epidural block, 332–333
 intercristal line, 327
 interspace estimation error in lateral position, 327
 locating needle insertion site, 326
 LOR syringes, 329
 masks, gowns, and gloves, 328
 needle placement, 329
 needles, syringes, catheters, 328
 patient positioning for neuraxial anesthesia procedures, 327
 positioning, 326
 pre-anesthetic antiseptic preparations, 326
 skin preparation at needle insertion site, 328
 spinal needles, 328
Obstetric malpractice, 140
Occiput position, 110
OmniCup-type Kiwi ventouse, 109
Opening abdominal wall, 11
Opening of uterine breach, 46, 47
Ovary inspection, 133, 138
Oxytocic perfusion, 246

P

Pain at suture level, 168
Paramedian incision, 21
Patient-controlled analgesia (PCA), 337
PCA, see Patient-controlled analgesia (PCA)
PDPH, see Postdural puncture headache (PDPH)
Pelosi retractor, 73, 74
Pelvis
 sagittal section, 15
 in second stage of labor, 241
Pelvisubperitoneal hematomas, 212
Percentage of maternal morbidity, 50
Perinatal epidemiology, 278; see also Preterm neonate
 DRG 391, 279
 ELBW at 26 weeks of gestational age, 282
 infant and neonatal mortality rate, 281
 infant mortality, 280–281
 mortality estimate of VLBW neonates, 282
 neonatal hospitalization, 279
 neonatal mortality and intensive care role, 281–282
 percentage of neonates with weight at birth, 280
 percentage of pathological neonates, 279
Peritoneum
 closure, 30
 cutting, 11
 incision on scarred, 25
 non-closure, 167
 opening, 164
 opening parietal, 22
Periventricular leukomalacia (PVL), 287, 288–290; see also Neonatal outcomes
Pfannenstiel laparotomy, incisions in, 11, 12, 20, 34
PHVD, see Posthemorrhagic ventricular dilatation (PHVD)
Pinard maneuver, 79, 85
Piper maneuver, 90, 91
Placenta accrete, 189, 192; see also Placenta previa
 Bakri balloon, 195, 196
 B-Lynch ligature, 195
 conservative management, 194
 diagnosis of, 192–193
 hemostatic sutures of lower uterine segment, 194
 intrauterine packing, 194
 MRI of, 193
 protocol to manage postpartum hemorrhage, 194–196
 surgical management, 193–194
Placenta examination, 129
Placental abnormalities, see Placenta accrete; Placenta previa
Placental removal, 123; see also Uterine exteriorization
 antibiotic prophylaxis, 127
 cervical canal dilation, 131, 134, 135
 cord blood collection, 141
 Credé's maneuver, 123, 125
 endometritis, 127, 138
 gloves effect, 127–128
 lochia discharge, 131
 manual removal, 123, 124, 126
 membrane extraction, 123, 130, 131, 132, 133
 placenta examination, 129
 postpartum hemorrhage, 125, 127
 risk of uterine inversion, 123
 umbilical cord detachment, 123, 124
 wiping, 128, 129, 130, 141
Placenta previa, 189; see also Placenta accrete
 diagnosis of, 189
 fetal head extraction, 192
 management of, 190
 mode of delivery, 191–192
 persistent bleeding in, 211–212
 to reduce blood loss, 192
 ultrasonographic section in uterus, 190
Platypelloid, 371
Porro method, 39
Postcesarean delivery uterine scar, 341, 351–352
 anechoic fluid collection, 347
 assessment with hysterosalpingography, 341–343
 capillary vessel of uterine scar, 351
 ceasarean scar syndrome, 350
 composed of hyaline hypocellular fibrous connective tissue, 350
 features of scar tissue, 351
 healing factors, 342
 hyperplasic mesothelium, 350
 hysteroscopy, 347
 hysteroscopy and evaluation, 346–348
 macroscopic aspects, 348–349
 microscopic aspects, 349–351
 morphology, 344–346, 348
 normal capillary vessel in lower uterine segment, 351
 peritoneum coated with normal mesothelium uterine scar, 350
 reactive nuclear atypias, 350
 repairing processes, 341
 smooth muscular tissue of myometrium, 351
 sonohysterography, 346
 ultrasound assessment, 343–346
 uterine dimple, 346, 347
 uterus outside of pregnancy, 345, 347
Postdural puncture headache (PDPH), 333; see also Local anesthesia for CD
 pharmacological therapy, 334
 prevention after accidental dural puncture, 334
 prevention in pregnant women, 334
 psychological support, 334
 therapeutic epidural blood patch, 334–335
Posthemorrhagic ventricular dilatation (PHVD), 288
Postmortem childbirth, 242
Postpartum hemorrhage (PPH), 125, 127, 202; see also Exceptional situations after CD and PPH; Uterine cavity balloon occlusion (UCBO)
 protocol to manage, 194–196
 reasons for CD hemorrhage complications, 199
 risk categories of, 376

PPH, *see* Postpartum hemorrhage (PPH)
PPROM, *see* Preterm prelabor rupture of the amniotic membranes (PPROM)
Prematurity, 277; *see also* Preterm neonate
Presenting, 112; *see also* Breech presentation
to change presentation, 60, 68, 69
Preterm fetus, 277; *see also* Preterm neonate
Preterm neonate, 277; *see also* Neonatal outcomes; Perinatal epidemiology; Preterm neonate survival rate improvement
classification, 277
communication and ELBW neonate, 292
communication before birth, 293
communication relative to potential neonatal outcomes, 292
criteria for gestational age and fetus weight determination, 278
incidence, 278
prematurity, 277
recommendations, 292–294
Preterm neonate survival rate improvement, 283; *see also* Preterm neonate
antenatal steroids, 283
cesarean delivery, 283–284
perinatal care regionalization, 284
surfactant therapy, 283
Preterm prelabor rupture of the amniotic membranes (PPROM), 283
Probe-Plug, 200
ProCup, 104
ProCup-type Kiwi ventouse, 108
Progression, 240
Propofol, 310; *see also* Induction agents
Protocol to manage postpartum hemorrhage, 194–196
PTE, *see* Pulmonary thromboembolism (PTE)
Puerperal
genital tract, 368
necropsies, 145
Pulmonary embolism, 139
Pulmonary thromboembolism (PTE), 375
PVL, *see* Periventricular leukomalacia (PVL)

R
RCOG, *see* Royal College of Obstetricians and Gynaecologists (RCOG)
RDS, *see* Respiratory distress syndrome (RDS)
Recovery after surgery, 168–169
Rectovaginal fistula, 237
Rectus muscle cut, 11
Reduction and engagement, 240
Regional anesthesia, 323; *see also* Local anesthesia for CD
Remifentanil, 319; *see also* General anesthesia for CD
Respiratory distress syndrome (RDS), 283
Restitution, 240
Retinopathy of prematurity (ROP), 290, 291; *see also* Neonatal outcomes
Retrovesical hematoma, 213
Retzius, space of, 11
Reversal agents, 311, 312; *see also* Induction agents
Reverse Rubin maneuver, 254
Robson 10-group classification system, 7–8
Rocuronium, 311; *see also* Induction agents
ROP, *see* Retinopathy of prematurity (ROP)
Rotation
maneuvers, 82
with shoulder engagement, 240
Royal College of Obstetricians and Gynaecologists (RCOG), 88, 189, 376
Rubin's II maneuver, 251, 252
reverse Rubin maneuver, 254

S
Safety maneuvers, 45
Sanger technique, 132
Scar, 341, 383; *see also* Postcesarean delivery uterine scar
Secondary bleeding by invaded tissues, 207, 209
Second stage of labor, 238; *see also* Childbirth
fifth critical point, 246
first critical point, 238, 240–241
fourth critical point, 245–246
second critical point, 241–243, 244
third critical point, 243–245
Sensorimotor deficits, 288
SGA, *see* Small for gestational age (SGA)
Short-acting opioids, 325
Shoulder dystocia, 237, 246, 255
clavicle fracture maneuver, 254
complications of, 246
emergency protocol for, 255
engagement of shoulder, 250
episiotomy, 249, 255
iatrogenic shoulder pseudo-dystocias, 245
Jacquemier's maneuver, 252, 255
Kristeller maneuver, 251, 253, 254
maneuver of suprapubic pressure, 250, 251
McRoberts' maneuver, 249, 250
prevalence of, 247
reverse Rubin maneuver, 254
risk factors for, 247
Rubin's II maneuver, 251, 252
therapeutic maneuvers, 248–249
therapy, 248
time for fetal body extraction, 248
type I shoulder dystocia, 247, 248
type II, 247, 248, 253
Zavanelli maneuvers, 254, 255
Shoulder extraction, 85, 92, 93
SIGO (Società Italiana di Ostetricia e Ginecologia), 358
SIMP, *see* Società Italiana di Medicina Perinatale (SIMP)
Simple continuous suture, 151, 152, 155, 156
Single-layer
closure, 154
suture, uterine, 167
Single-use vacuum extractor cup, 110, 111
Small for gestational age (SGA), 277
SNLGISS, *see* Italian National Institute of Heath–National System of Guidelines (SNLGISS)
Società Italiana di Medicina Perinatale (SIMP), 278
Società Italiana di Ostetricia e Ginecologia, *see* SIGO (Società Italiana di Ostetricia e Ginecologia)
SOD, *see* Superoxide dismutase (SOD)
Soft tissue swelling, 108
Sonohysterography, 346
Space of Retzius, 11
Spinal anesthesia, 323, 324, 325; *see also* Local anesthesia for CD
procedures for, 330
Spinal needles, 328; *see also* Obstetric anesthetic care issues
orifice position, 330
SS, *see* Subsymphysary space (SS)
Subcutaneous tissue
healing, 35
stretching, 20
Subperitoneal extension of hysterotomy, 210
Subsymphysary space (SS), 216
Succinylcholine, 311; *see also* Induction agents
Sufentanil, 324
Superoxide dismutase (SOD), 291
Supraglottic devices, 315
Surfactant therapy, 283
Surgery
cricothyroidotomy, 317
management, 369–370
scar, 13
wide exposure, 16
Suture thread contamination, 145, 146
Suturing uterine incisions, 145, 156, 157
complications observed, 145
contamination of suture, 145, 146, 152, 154
current techniques, 149
at different layers, 148
double-layer suture, 147, 148, 149, 154
excluding uterine mucosa, 152
fascia, 31
hemorrhagic complications percentage, 155
hemostasis, 154, 156
hemostatic function of, 148
intradermal, 31
margins of suture, 150
mass closure CD technique, 157
material used in, 148, 154, 155, 156
mortality rate in, 145
puerperal necropsies, 145
repositioning exteriorized uterus, 157
significance of, 147–148
silver thread, 145
simple continuous suture, 151, 152, 155, 156
single-layer closure, 154
transfixation of hysterotomy corner, 149, 150, 151
types of, 150, 151, 152, 153
uterine–parietal suture, 145
uterine rupture risk, 154, 155
utero-ovarian amputation, 145, 146, 147
visceral peritoneum inspection for hemostasis, 155
Suturing uterus, 136, 141

T
Tachypnea of the newborn (TTN), 297
Thiopental, 310; *see also* Induction agents
Third stage of labor, *see* Placental removal
Tilting movements to emerge shoulders, 72
Time for fetal body extraction, 248
T method, 309
Total expulsion of fetus, 240
Transabdominal convex ultrasound probe, 45
Transabdominal intrapartum ultrasound, 217
Transfixation of hysterotomy corner, 149, 150, 151
Transient neurologic syndrome, 336
Transient radicular irritation, *see* Transient neurologic syndrome
Transverse incision
advantages, 11, 12, 13
of lower uterine segment, 47
Transverse laparotomy, 30
longitudinal incision of fascia in, 17
Transverse lower incision, 165
Transverse presentation, 57, 113, 121; *see also* Breech presentation
extraction maneuvers, 116–120
Leopold maneuver in, 113
locating shoulder, 113, 115–116
ultrasound examination, 113, 114
Traumatic neuropathy, 336; *see also* Local anesthesia for CD
Trendelenburg position, 161
Trunk extraction, 85
TTN, *see* Tachypnea of the newborn (TTN)
TTS, *see* Twin transfusion syndrome (TTS)
Tuffier's line, *see* Intercristal line
Twin pregnancy, 257; *see also* Multiple pregnancy
amnionicity of, 259
amnioreduction, 262
with bilateral transverse lie, 266
biovular, dichorionic, diamniotic, 259
biovular, monochorionic, diamniotic, 259
blocked upper right limb, 272
cesarean birth in course of, 264–265
death of twin, 261–262
diagnostic problems of twins and anastomotic risk, 260–261
dichorionic diamniotic, 258
etiopathogenesis, 257
fetal lie and presentation in, 264, 265
fetuses in cephalic presentation, 266
fetus papyraceus at 37 weeks of gestation, 261
intrauterine growth delay in, 263
locking collision of twins in cephalic presentation, 271
locking of twins during vaginal extraction, 270
locking of twins in breech presentation, 271
locking of twins with second fetus in transverse lie, 272
lowering of blocked limb, 273
lowering of lower left limb, 273

maternal risk in course of CD, 263
monoamniotic, monochorionic, 267, 268, 269
monochorionic diamniotic, 258
monochorionic, monoamniotic twins, 261
monovular, monochorionic, diamniotic, 260
monovular, monochorionic, monoamniotic, 260
surgeon brings right foot toward uterine breech, 270
surgeon rotates by 90° fetus that is held by lower limb, 269
with transverse lie of single fetus, 266
ultrasound diagnosis of placenta in, 258–260
Twin transfusion syndrome (TTS), 262–263; see also Twin pregnancy
Twisting maneuver, 123, 126
Type I shoulder dystocia, 247, 248
Type II shoulder dystocia, 247, 248, 253

U

UCBO, see Uterine cavity balloon occlusion (UCBO)
U-D, see Uterine incision-to-delivery (U-D)
Ultrasound, 343; see also Postcesarean delivery uterine scar
    diagnosis of placenta in twin pregnancy, 258
    evaluation, see Intrapartum ultrasonography
    examination with different methods, 344
    postcesarean delivery uterine scar morphologies, 344–346
    results of Fukuda study of uterine scars detected with, 344
    transabdominal, 343
    in transverse presentation, 113, 114
Umbilical cord detachment, 123, 124
Unexpected abnormal placentation, 207, 208, 209
Upside-down "T" uterine incision, 48
Ureteral identification, 211
Ureteral injury, 213
U.S. Food and Drug Administration (FDA), 325
Uterine
    artery ligation, 203
    compressing sutures, 203
    dimple, 346, 347
    inversion risk, 123
    –parietal suture, 145
    sandwich, 203
Uterine cavity balloon occlusion (UCBO), 199
    abdominal insertion technique, 199
    device for, 199, 200
    efficiency of, 202, 204
    endometritis, 203
    indications for, 202
    intrauterine balloon, 201, 202
    occlusion, 201
    options for intrauterine hemostasis, 203
    placement of the balloon, 201
    Probe-Plug, 200
    vaginal balloon catheter, 201, 202
    vaginal catheter, 201
Uterine exteriorization, 132, 133, 136, 141; see also Placental removal
    amniotic fluid effect, 139
    antibiotic therapy, 139, 140
    congestion of venous plexuses, 137, 139
    failure to exteriorize, 138, 140
    inspecting ovaries, 133, 138
    inspection of uterine breach, 133, 137
    obstetric malpractice, 140
    positive aspect of, 137
    procedure, 133
    pulmonary embolism, 139
    studies on, 134, 137
    suturing uterus, 136, 141
Uterine fibroids, 173, 183; see also Cesarean myomectomy
    complications of, 173
    consequences in pregnancy, 173
    myometrial fibers overlying myoma, 179
    risk for CD due to, 173
    ultrasonographic scan of, 174, 180
    uterine-modified anatomy and physiology with, 173–174, 176
Uterine incision-to-delivery (U-D), 313
Uterine rupture, 358; see also Vaginal birth after cesarean (VBAC)
    risk, 154, 155
Utero-ovarian amputation, 145, 146, 147
Uterotonic therapy, 203

V

Vacuum extractor, 102, 104, 105, 106, 222
Vaginal bacteriological examination, 229
Vaginal balloon catheter, 201, 202
Vaginal birth after cesarean (VBAC), 5, 226, 341, 355, 362
    analgesia during labor, 357, 358
    anatomical model of rupture of uterus, 359
    asymptomatic uterine rupture, 359, 360
    cardiotocographic monitoring, 357
    comparison of prostaglandin E2 versus oxytocin, 358
    conditions associated with higher probability of success, 355
    counseling, 355
    digital intrauterine palpation of previous scar, 357
    indications to, 356
    induction and risk of uterine rupture, 361
    induction of labor, 359
    management of patient with previous CD, 355
    maternal–fetal surveillance during labor, 356–357
    for nonreassuring CTG, 356
    obstetric ventouse, 357
    percentage of repeat CD, 356
    postpartum uterine rupture, 360
    predictive factors in, 360–362
    previous spontaneous birth and success probability, 356
    risks and complications, 358–360
    success probability, 355
    symptomatic uterine rupture, 361
    use of oxytocin and of prostaglandins, 358
    use of oxytocin and risk of uterine rupture, 361
    uterine dehiscence at level of previous uterine scar, 360
    uterine rupture, 358, 361
Vaginal catheter, 201
Vaginal exploration, 219
Vanishing twin syndrome, 262; see also Twin pregnancy
VBAC, see Vaginal birth after cesarean (VBAC)
Vecuronium, 311; see also Induction agents
Venous thromboembolism (VTE), 374
Ventilation/perfusion ratio (V/Q), 287
Version through external maneuvers, 86
Vertex presentation, 218, 221
Very low birth weight (VLBW), 277
Vesicouterine fold incision, 41–45
Vesicouterine plica, 42, 43, 44, 45
Visceral peritoneum incision, 44
    for hemostasis, 155
Vision 2020 program, 290
VLBW, see Very low birth weight (VLBW)
V/Q, see Ventilation/perfusion ratio (V/Q)
VTE, see Venous thromboembolism (VTE)

W

WHO, see World Health Organization (WHO)
Wide surgical exposure, 16
Wigand–Martin variant, 85, 86
Wignard maneuver, 85, 86, 94
Wilson sum score, 315
Wiping, 128, 129, 130, 141
World Health Organization (WHO), 1, 277
Worldwide cesarean delivery trend, 1–2, 3

Z

Zavanelli maneuver, 65–66, 254, 255

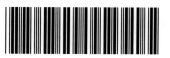